Introduction to
Veterinary Pathology

Introduction to Veterinary Pathology

NORMAN F. CHEVILLE

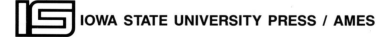 IOWA STATE UNIVERSITY PRESS / AMES

Norman F. Cheville, D.V.M., Ph.D, is Chief of the Pathology
Research Laboratory, National Animal Disease Center, Ames,
Iowa, and Professor of Veterinary Pathology, Iowa State Uni-
versity.

© 1988 Iowa State University Press, Ames, Iowa 50010
All rights reserved

Manufactured in the United States of America
⊗ This book is printed on acid-free paper.

First edition, 1988
Second printing, 1990

Library of Congress Cataloging-in-Publication Data

Cheville, Norman F., 1934–
    Introduction to veterinary pathology.

    Includes index.
    1. Veterinary pathology.   I. Title.
SF769.C473   1988   636.089′607   87-26152
ISBN 0-8138-0996-7

For Julie, Carol, John, and Anne

. . . who make it all worthwhile

CONTENTS

PREFACE

DURING the last two decades, teaching of veterinary pathology has made remarkable advances. There have been major improvements in textbooks, in color photography of gross specimens, and most important, in methods of teaching. Some instructors distribute entire lecture notes (although this to some degree preempts mental resynthesis during the lecture). As a result there seems to be no great demand for a didactic book that simply repeats lecture notes. In its stead, there is a need for a text that takes the student beyond the lecture, into the realm of how and why biologic things happen.

Introduction to Veterinary Pathology is constructed for the beginning student in veterinary pathology. The goal is to introduce new scientific information on mechanisms of general tissue injury into the basic language of pathology. Fundamental abnormalities are used repeatedly to explain the interaction of disease processes. Materials and illustrations are from nonhuman vertebrate animals, and most are from diseases in which the pathogenesis and etiology are relatively well known. The need to compare the biology of one species with another is a distinguishing character of the veterinarian; that character is an underlying principle in this book.

In conducting the necropsy, appropriate sampling is the important factor preceding the examination of tissue. Careless tissue collection and unscientific examination results in useless, and sometimes harmful, information. Veterinarians who use microscopy in this fashion run great risks in the legal and moral aspects of the profession. The clinician who, conditioned by familiarity with clinical signs, bypasses entirely the fundamental changes in tissue will ultimately be reprimanded.

Some students (and, I fear, some academicians) insist that an understanding of molecular biology and ultrastructure are not necessary for the practicing veterinarian. To refute that logic can be cited the difference between the scientific and the technical faces of veterinary medicine. Acceptance of the title "doctor" is acceptance of the responsibility for understanding disease, not merely knowing how to deal with it technically. One cannot condone those planners of curricula who, while insisting on rigorous preprofessional courses in mathematics and physics, willingly constrict the courses that provide the very foundation of medical knowledge.

Each element (the text, illustrations, vignettes, and references) of this book was prepared so that it can be studied independently. For example, as one progresses through illustrations, the legends provide a concise summary of general pathology.

One of the ways in which biology clearly differs from the physical sciences is in the need to deal conceptually with the variability of living organisms. A single stimulus does not produce the same reponse in different animals, because species and individuals differ in the capacity or magnitude of structural or functional responses. The study of pathology introduces students to the even more complex variations associated with disease.

As a student you will become aware of the special burden of the veterinarian—the lifelong need to keep one foot in science and one in clinical medicine. Avoid scientists who regard clinical work as "unscientific" and clinicians who disparage the basic sciences as "intellectual" or "academic." It is your responsibility to develop an intellect capable of distilling new science into clinical veterinary medicine well into the twenty-first century. This will not only enrich your professional life but will benefit your patients, as well as protect you legally.

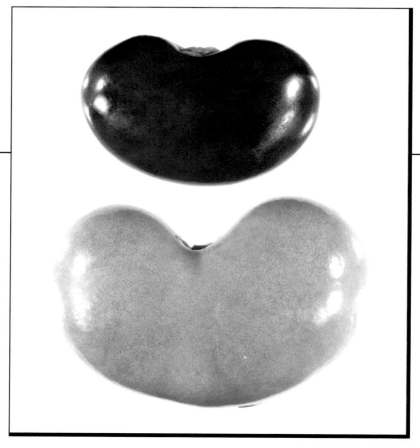

Normal kidney (*top*) and kidney with diffuse degeneration (acute cell swelling) and necrosis, tetracycline toxicity.

INTRODUCTION

1

PATHOLOGY, in the broadest sense, is abnormal biology. As a science it encompasses all abnormalities of structure and function. It involves the study of cells, tissues, organs, and body fluids and is the link between basic sciences and clinical studies. Pathology is essentially the search for and the study of *lesions,* the abnormal structural and functional changes that occur in the body.

The detection of lesions requires techniques of anatomy and physiology, and the discipline of pathology is divided into anatomic pathology and clinical pathology. Blood and urine from the animal bearing the swollen kidney on the facing page tells the clinical pathologist about the nature and extent of renal failure; tissue from a biopsy (or from a postmortem specimen) leads the anatomic pathologist to the same conclusion, though by far different methods.

The separation of pathologic structure and function is an artificial one. In some difficult cases, lesions are detectable only by microscopy and in others only by biochemical methods. For every chemical change in a cell, however, there is a corresponding structural change – the challenge to the anatomic pathologist lies in finding it.

Veterinary pathology requires knowledge of normal biologic variation, particularly differences due to age and species. *Ontogeny,* the normal development of an individual, involves specific controlled patterns of tissue growth and regression that must not be confused with pathologic changes. Disease produces great exaggerations in the spectrum of structural and functional responses considered normal. Disappearance of the thymus in young adults is a "normal" process, yet it involves degeneration and death of cells. Thymic regression is hastened by almost any severe disease, and this makes the interpretation of thymic change difficult. As animals age, limits of normality become increasingly vague; vascular lesions are present in aged animals, and although they are pathologic, they are part of the normal aging process.

Phylogeny, the evolution of a group of animals, is a basic concern of the veterinary student. It is impossible to develop a practical approach to pathology without an awareness of the differences (and similarities) among species. There is an intriguing tendency for closely related species to suffer similar metabolic, neoplastic, and infectious diseases. Specific pathogenic microorganisms generally also infect animals close, in the phylogenetic scheme, to the original host.

Here we deal with diseases of vertebrate animals. Occasionally disease processes in man or nonverterbrate species will be considered when they provide useful models for a basic process. Although the spontaneous diseases of these species are not mirrors of their counterparts in vertebrate animals, the biologic processes are similar and at the level of the cell may even be identical. One of the most exciting eras of pathology was begun by observations on the inflammatory response of the water flea.

1

Pathogenesis of Disease: The Host Response

1

PATHOGENESIS is the developmental process of a disease. To understand pathogenesis, both *causal agent* and *host response* must be identified. Determination of cause and tissue reaction must be followed by interpretation of their significance in the disease process. That is, are they primary causes and lesions or are they epiphenomena masking a subtler but more dangerous process that remains hidden? The goal of pathology is to understand the disease process sufficiently to provide a *diagnosis,* a conclusion regarding cause and pathogenesis, especially with a view to differentiating it from other diseases.

CAUSE OF DISEASE VERSUS HOST RESPONSE

Etiology

An understanding of pathogenesis is founded on *etiology,* the study of the causes of disease. An *etiologic diagnosis* provides the precise cause of a disease. A simple classification of *external* etiologic agents is a division into physical, chemical, and microbiologic types (Table 1.1). Some of these agents directly and consistently cause a pathologic reaction and a predictable series of consequences. Cyanide stops mitochondrial function and will kill an animal regardless of nutritional and immune status. Rabies virus, once established as an infection, replicates in neurons, invariably producing neuronal degeneration, inflammation of the brain, and death. The only determinants of disease for these dangerous agents are the total dose received by the host and the portal of entry.

It is rarely sufficient, however, to explain disease in terms of single causes and unremitting,

Table 1.1. Factors causing cell injury

EXTERNAL AGENTS	
Physical	
Mechanical trauma	Cutting objects, blows, compression
Electrical trauma	Lightning, high-frequency currents
Heat	Heatstroke, sunstroke, fever, burns
Cold	Local tissue freezing, cold shock
Radiant energy	Ultraviolet light, X-irradiation, cosmic radiation
Pressure	Increased, decreased
Chemical	
Biologic toxins	Bacterial and fungal toxins, arthropod and snake venoms
Pesticides	Organophosphates (parathion), organochlorine (DDT)
Herbicides	Chlorophenoxy compounds (2,4-D), paraquat, dinitrophenols
Environmental	Metals, nitrates, polychlorinated biphenyls
Nutritional	Excess vitamins A and D
Biologic	
Acellular agents	Viruses, prions
Prokaryotes	Bacteria, chlamydia, rickettsia, mycoplasma
Eukaryotes	Fungi, protozoa
Metazoan animals	Cestodes, nematodes, trematodes, insects
EXTERNAL DEFICIENCIES	
Nutritional	
Dietary deficiency	Protein, vitamins, calories
Environmental	
Water	Dehydration
Oxygen	Asphyxia
Sunlight	Vitamin D malfunction
INTERNAL DEFECTS	
Genetic	Spectrum, from single mutant gene to chromosome breaks

step-by-step progress. With most agents, production of disease is not uniform. The tubercle bacillus causes tuberculosis, yet only a small fraction of infected animals develop the disease.

Feline leukemia virus infects large numbers of kittens but induces lymphosarcoma or leukemia in only a few. In these diseases, pathogenesis involves a balance of agent viability and host defense.

The genetic, nutritional, immunologic, and environmental characters of the host animal determine, in large part, the development and extent of disease. Thus the pathologist must seek multiple factors as causes of disease, searching for patterns of lesions and groups of lesions that have combined to produce the clinical manifestations of disease.

Two or more agents are often involved in tissue injury.

Tissue evaluation is difficult in many diseases because of the need to search for more than one etiologic agent. In the liver, one drug may inhibit detoxifying enzymes that predispose to hepatotoxicity by another drug. For example, a single large dose of ethanol produces a markedly enhanced susceptibility to barbiturate anesthetics. A dose of barbiturate that is ordinarily anesthetizing may kill an animal already detoxifying ethanol.

Two or more infectious agents are commonly involved in tissue injury. Viruses may induce respiratory disease of little importance, yet in so doing predispose the lung to severe secondary bacterial infection, as when influenza is complicated by bacterial pneumonia. In the intestine, intracellular microbes (viruses, coccidia, treponemes) may destroy epithelium, permitting bacteria to colonize the gut wall. Bovine viral diarrhea virus replicates within intestinal epithelium to produce foci of destruction that support bacterial growth.

Viruses that suppress the host's immune system are especially dangerous because they lead to disseminated bacterial or fungal infections. Lymphoid tissue destruction produced in canine distemper permits growth of the protozoan *Toxoplasma gondii*. Bovine viral diarrhea virus also produces a smoldering chronic infection that destroys lymphoid tissues and permits widespread infection by several bacterial pathogens. When two or more of these processes are combined, they must be differentiated and the dominant causal factor of the lesion determined.

Antemortem disappearance of cause masks the relation between cause and effect.

Physical causes of disease such as heat and cold can be determined only by the pattern of tissue injury they produce. There is simply no direct evidence of the cause of tissue destruction. This is also true in many diseases in which the etiologic agent should be present but is not. Drugs may be catabolized after lesions arise in the liver but before death occurs. Microbial agents may be destroyed by host defenses between the times of infection and death. Microbial culture of the tissue may yield a bacterium that is involved only secondarily in the disease. Remember: *Isolation of a microorganism from a tissue does not necessarily mean that it has caused the lesion in question.*

Commonly, clinical treatment obliterates the cause. Bacteria can be killed by antibiotics, and thus cannot be cultured from even severe inflammatory foci in treated animals. In rare infections, antibiotic treatment may even promote death; in anthrax, treatment kills the circulating bacteria but the host may die from the ensuing massive liberation of bacterial toxins.

Host response

Gross and microscopic examination of lesions establishes the basic tissue response and provides clues to the etiologic diagnosis. In biopsy specimens, interpretation of lesions leads to a prognosis. A *pathologic diagnosis* tells the clinician about the severity, extent, and type of lesions. Encephalitis (inflammation of the brain) was the clinical diagnosis in the dog in Fig. 1.6. The pathological diagnosis was severe, diffuse, acute, purulent meningoencephalitis and ventriculitis, and the etiologic diagnosis was *Escherichia coli* with superinfection by *Corynebacterium* spp. Pathologic diagnoses are especially helpful to clinicians when etiologic diagnoses cannot be obtained.

Evidence of the host response changes as a disease progresses.

Host responses may vary markedly in different phases of the same disease. For example, circulating blood in the early stages of *septicemia* (septic bacteria in the bloodstream) has increased numbers of leukocytes; this *leukocytosis* is due chiefly to release of new cells from storage sites in spleen and bone marrow. As leukocytes are consumed in fighting bacteria, their numbers may return to normal (although the cells appear degenerate). In terminal stages of septicemia, there is a marked decrease in number of circulating leukocytes because these cells are trapped in the lung and viscera due to widespread capillary damage.

This pattern of "exhaustion reversal" occurs in many pathologic reactions, especially in secretory organs. Immediately after intense stimulation, the adrenal cortex undergoes an explosive response and its cells become vacuolated and degranulate. With slow, progressive stimulation, this tissue expands in response to the new work load and its cells become enlarged and granular. In contrast, during severe chronic stimulation, the adrenal cortex becomes exhausted and its cells are small and lack granule-forming organelles.

It is traditional to begin the study of pathology by examining basic categories of tissue response: cell degeneration and death, pathologic hemostasis, inflammation, disturbances of growth and development, and neoplasia. In examining abnormal tissue the first step is to answer the question, What is the basic process? To interpret an abnormal mass in tissue, all types of host responses must be considered. Did the lesion in question arise from a congenital growth defect or from an inflammatory process? Is it an abscess, a neoplasm, or a focus of necrosis?

DEGENERATION AND NECROSIS

Degeneration

Degeneration (L. *degeneratio*) literally means deterioration. It is a retrogressive change in tissues characterized by abnormal structural changes and decreased function. Historically, pathologists made the distinction between "true"

degeneration and *infiltration,* the deposition of abnormal matter in tissue. However, these processes overlap, and this distinction is not emphasized here.

Tissues with parenchymal cells diffusely affected by degeneration will reflect a particular type of injury. Organs undergoing acute degenerative changes tend to be larger and heavier than normal. The severity of enlargement reflects the diffuseness of the cellular injury. In the late stages of degeneration, large numbers of cells may have been killed and removed, so that the organ size does not always reflect the severity of injury.

Patterns of cellular degeneration used by the pathologist are grouped according to the dominant expression of injury: (1) *acute cell swelling,* due to water overload; (2) *metabolite overload,* degeneration involving overload of normal metabolic products such as fat, glycogen, or protein (hyalin, or proteinaceous) degeneration; and (3) *storage loading,* accumulation of complex nondegradable products such as pigments, minerals, and exogenous substances (Table 1.2).

Acute cell swelling causes organs to be enlarged, heavy, and pale (unless the tissue is also filled with blood). It is apt to be present in all types of injury but is most typical in severe toxic and febrile conditions in organs with intense rates of metabolism, such as liver, kidney, and brain; organs so affected bulge beneath their capsules and have rounded contours (Fig. 1.1). Acute cell swelling in epithelial surfaces is especially revealing because affected cells often bear other evidence of injury and may participate in the formation of characteristic blisters, ulcers, or other diagnostically useful lesions.

Necrosis

Necrosis is death of tissue in the living animal. It may be used to indicate dead tissue or the

Table 1.2.   Patterns of cell degeneration

Pattern	Cell Response	Mechanism
Water loading	Acute cell swelling Hydropic degeneration	Cell expansion due to loss of water intake control
Metabolite loading	Glycogen degeneration Fatty degeneration Hyalin degeneration	Degeneration with accumulation of normal metabolites
Storage loading	Lipidosis Mucopolysaccharidosis Mineralization Pigment loading	Accumulation of complex nondegradable products

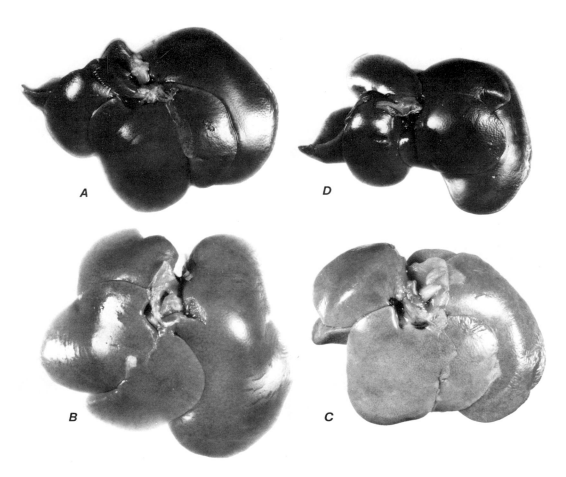

Fig. 1.1. Degeneration: diffuse degeneration, liver. A. Acute cell swelling, carbon tetrachloride toxicity. B. Glycogen degeneration, treatment with large dose of cortisol. C. Fatty degeneration, chronic carbon tetrachloride toxicity. D. Normal liver.

process of dying. Cell degeneration becomes necrosis when the point of irreversibility is reached in the degenerative process. Like the exact moment of death in the animal itself, however, that point is not precisely discernible.

Necrotic tissue may appear as a coagulated mass, as a creamy liquid, or as dry, crumbly material, and these differences are useful diagnostic clues. Toxins produced by bacteria, fungi, and venoms of poisonous insects and reptiles are common causes of necrosis. *Fusobacterium necrophorum* occurs in the rumen of normal cattle. When rumenal epithelium is injured, (for example, by bovine viral diarrhea virus), this large

bacterium can penetrate tissue to produce expanding foci of coagulation necrosis (Fig. 1.2). The architecture of the necrotic tissue can still be seen, but the varied detail and texture of the normal appearance are gone.

Foci of necrosis are often sharply delimited from surrounding normal tissue. In many cases, however, they are associated with inflammation, which tends to segregate necrotic from viable tissue. Liberation of peptides from dead cells can incite inflammation. Furthermore, most agents that kill cells simultaneously injure blood vessels, and when severe, inflammation and hemorrhage may mask the lesions of necrosis.

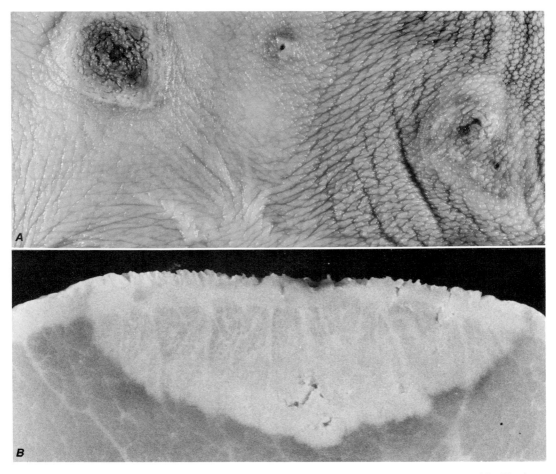

Fig. 1.2. Necrosis: *foci of necrosis* of rumen mucosa caused by *Fusobacterium necrophorum.* A. Preservation of tissue architecture in the necrotic mass typical of coagulation necrosis. B. Enlarged cross section of necrotic focus. Necrosis extends into muscle layers of the rumen wall. The causal bacteria are at the advancing edge of the necrotic lesion (see Fig. 3.2).

Necrobiosis

In *necrobiosis,* cell death is programmed, and the cytopathic changes evolve in orderly and reproducible sequences. Necrobiosis is required for the remodeling of tissue in organogenesis of the developing fetus. It occurs in adults as part of normal cell turnover, such as loss of cornified squamous cells of skin. Keratinocytes become filled with keratin, nuclei degenerate, and plasma membranes lose adhesiveness so that cells separate and desquamate from the skin surface. Necrobiosis occurs in erythrocytes, which die when hemoglobin molecules begin to precipitate and new hemoglobin cannot be syn-

thesized. In necrobiosis, cell death occurs without pathologic sequelae because cell function has been fulfilled.

BLOOD-VASCULAR DEFECTS
Hyperemia

Hyperemia is an increase in blood in tissue, which results in distension of blood vessels. It is referred to as *active hyperemia* when it is due to increased inflow of blood and as *passive hyperemia* when it results from decreased outflow when venous drainage is hindered. The unqualified term indicates active hyperemia, in which blood flows in to dilate and fill all capillaries of a tissue bed. *Venous congestion,* synonymous with passive hyperemia, is caused either by venous blockade or by cardiac failure. *Congestion* is an abnormal accumulation of fluid within vessels of an organ, usually blood but also applied to bile or mucus.

Ischemia

Ischemia, a local deficit of blood in tissue, is due to constriction of a blood vessel or obstruction of arterial inflow. Also called "local tissue anemia," it is commonly responsible for coagulative necrosis. If the blood supply to tissue is shut off, cells quickly die. For example, when the renal artery is experimentally clamped, renal tubules begin to degenerate within seconds. The lack of oxygen, in this case called *ischemic anoxia,* causes the mitochondria to swell and disintegrate. In the kidney this injury is reversible for about 60 minutes, but thereafter the tubule cells show signs of irreversible damage.

Infarction

An *infarct* is a local area of necrosis caused by ischemia due to obstruction in the arterial tree. Infarction may result from the local development of a clot or thrombus or by embolism (Fig. 1.3). Infarcts are classified on the basis of bacte-

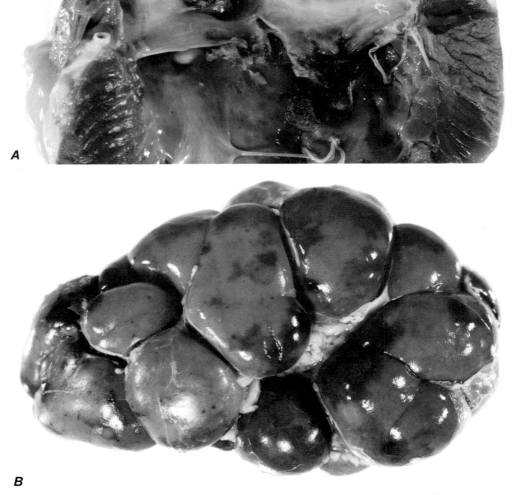

Fig. 1.3. Thrombosis: association of thrombosis, embolism, and infarction, cow with purulent metritis. A. *Vegetative valvular endocarditis* with thrombosis of heart valves. B. Acute pale *infarcts* in the lobulated kidney of the cow. These arise from thrombi lodged in the renal arcuate arteries.

rial contamination, either septic or bland, and color, either anemic (white) or hemorrhagic (red). Red infarcts are filled with blood. The amount of blood that escapes into the oxygen-deprived area is determined by age of the infarct, type of injury, and type of tissue. Infarcts of the kidney are usually white, those of the lung red. Most infarcts are transiently hemorrhagic but become pale in a very short period. Capillaries at the border of the infarct undergo dissolution, and blood may seep into the area of necrosis.

Rarely, infarction occurs due to blocks in veins. Venous infarcts are intensely hemorrhagic. Generally, peripheral venous drainage develops and prevents necrosis.

Embolism

Embolism is the sudden blockage of an artery or vein by an obstruction that has arrived in the bloodstream. Emboli can be thrombi, neoplastic cells, lipid globules, air bubbles, or foreign particles. *Thromboemboli,* which break away from some distant focus of thrombosis, are especially common causes of infarction and necrosis. Septic thromboemboli not only cause infarction but disseminate infection throughout the body of the animal. Emboli of neoplastic cells may dislodge from a primary tumor, circulate, and take up residence in the lung or other viscera to initiate secondary tumor growth.

Edema

Edema is the abnormal accumulation of fluid in interstitial spaces of body tissues. The tissues appear wet, and fluid seeps from a cut section. *Local edema* is usually due to lymphatic blockage, and evidence of lesions in efferent lymphatics should be sought. *Generalized edema,* on the other hand, results from either increased hydrostatic pressure of blood (as in the venous system of heart failure) or from decreased colloid osmotic pressure of plasma proteins. In heart failure, pressure in the veins rises and is transmitted to the capillary bed, where fluid exudes. Massive accumulation of edema fluid in the body tissues is referred to as *anasarca.*

Accumulation of edema fluid in the major body cavities is termed *hydroperitoneum, hydrothorax,* or *hydropericardium,* depending on the cavity involved. Hydroperitoneum (also called *ascites*) is the accumulation of fluid in the abdominal cavity. It is common in chronic heart failure, where it is caused by a rise in intrahepatic portal venous pressure. *Pulmonary edema,* seen as frothy, pale, massive lungs, leads to suspicion of either circulatory problems or sudden diffuse and direct damage to the capillary bed of the lungs. *Effusion* (L. *effusio,* a pouring out) is the escape of fluid into tissue. The term is used by some clinicians to distinguish fluid escaping from serous surfaces (e.g., pleural effusion).

Hemorrhage

Hemorrhage is commonly due to trauma. The blood vessel is torn and whole blood escapes. Hemorrhage may be external or internal and in either case may deprive the animal of blood (*exsanguination*). Accumulation of blood in the body cavities is called *hemothorax, hemopericardium,* or *hemoperitoneum,* depending on which cavity is involved.

When blood escapes into tissue (rather than through broken surfaces), it accumulates as a blood-filled space or *hematoma.* In dogs, hematomas are common on the concave surfaces of the pinna; they are a consequence of trauma, commonly due to violent head shaking and scratching from aural pain and usually develop in clefts formed by trauma in the ear cartilages.

Hemorrhage from surfaces may occur in abnormal tissue masses that protrude into lumens or onto surfaces in such a way that trauma easily causes already fragile blood vessels to rupture. Neoplasms of skin and intestine are prone to this kind of hemorrhage. Genital hemorrhage occurs in mares with varicose (enlarged and tortuous) veins of the vaginal wall; these varices probably arise during the physical impairment of venous return from the vagina during pressure from a gravid uterus.

Very tiny hemorrhages into the skin, mucous membranes, and serosal surfaces are designated *petechiae.* Their presence often indicates a severe generalized process. Petechiae are commonly seen in septicemia, where endothelium is destroyed by bacterial toxins, and in viral infections, in which the virus replicates in vascular endothelium. The viral diseases hog cholera, equine viral arteritis, Newcastle disease of birds, and epidemic hemorrhagic disease of deer are all characterized by multiple petechiation caused in part by necrosis of endothelial cells.

Hemorrhages slightly larger than petechiae, called *purpura,* are associated most commonly

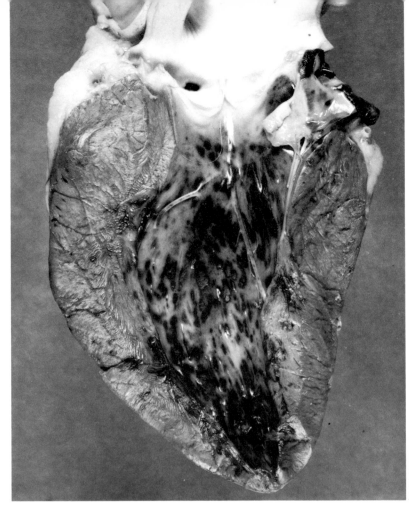

Fig. 1.4. *Ecchymotic hemorrhages,* endocardium, heart, horse given endotoxin of *Escherichia coli.*

with disturbances of the clotting mechanisms that allow more extensive escape of blood due to failure of blockage of the injured vessel. *Ecchymoses* are large hemorrhages (over 1 cm in diameter); large bruises are ecchymoses (Fig. 1.4).

Hemorrhages are rapidly resorbed. Bleeding into the skin produces a red ecchymotic blotch that gradually becomes darker and then purple, fading to brown-yellow and disappearing in 2–3 weeks. In the process of repair, erythrocytes are lysed or are phagocytized by macrophages (erythrophagocytosis). Hemoglobin is released and is degraded into bilirubin and hemosiderin, which impart their characteristic colors to the tissue. Bilirubin may form yellow crystals, called hematoidin.

The significance of lost blood depends on the acute or chronic nature of the hemorrhage and how much blood has been lost. The consequence of acute blood loss may be hypovolemic shock, that of chronic loss, anemia.

Thrombosis

Blood clots are the coagula formed when fibrinogen polymerizes into fibrin strands. The clot contains platelets, leukocytes, and erythrocytes trapped in the fibrin mesh. *Postmortem clots,* formed after death, are rubbery and homogeneous. Depending on whether the red cells have settled out after death, they are either solid red-blue (currant jelly clots) or clear yellow (chicken fat clots). Commonly, the upper part of the postmortem clot is clear yellow and the lower part into which erythrocytes have settled is red.

A *thrombus* is an antemortem clot formed by blood coagulation that remains at the point of its formation, usually attached to the blood vessel wall or to valves of the heart (Fig. 1.3). Thrombi are associated with damage to endothelium and contain many platelets and leukocytes. If platelets make up most of the clot, it is white; if erythrocytes dominate, it is red.

Thrombi are usually friable and conform to the shape of the vessel lumen. Alternating irregular strands of pale, gray-white fibrin and areas of massed, red-blue erythrocytes create a variegated tangled appearance. When thrombi are sectioned, the alternating layers of gray and red create a laminated effect. *Occlusive* thrombi are those that totally occlude vessels; they are most often found in small muscular veins and venous plexuses. *Mural* thrombi form plaquelike masses attached to walls and are seen in the heart and aneurysms of the larger arteries. Old clots appear as densely adherent masses of vascularized fibrous tissue, for they are gradually invaded by fibroblasts and new capillaries.

INFLAMMATION

The inflammatory response is a reaction to injury in which components of circulating blood are transferred across an abnormally permeable blood vessel wall. It is designed to destroy the cause of injury by dilution, immobilization, phagocytosis, and intracellular destruction. Inflammation begins when increased vascular dilation and permeability combine with activation of circulating leukocytes to promote passage of fluids and cells into tissue spaces. Redness and swelling of inflammatory lesions are manifestations of hyperemia and edema. In fact, the early phases of inflammation cannot be distinguished from hyperemia and edema until "inflammatory cells" and fibrin appear in the lesion.

Inflammatory exudates

Fluids, plasma proteins, and white blood cells that move into spaces and onto tissue surfaces constitute an *exudate.* An inflammatory lesion is characterized by the nature and amount of the exudate. Exudates are classified according to their dominant components.

Serous exudates contain chiefly exuded fluids and plasma proteins (the protein content is higher than that of plasma). For example, early stages of most upper respiratory infections begin as acute serous rhinitis. Blisters and vesicles of the skin contain serous exudates composed of water and albumin.

The shaggy mesh of a *fibrinous* exudate represents a more severe process in which fibrinogen has exuded and polymerized into fibrin (Fig. 1.5). Fibrinous exudates are characteristic of some acute bacterial infections, particularly in pasteurellosis. They are called "bread and butter" exudates because the rubbery fibrin adhering to surfaces resembles two slices of buttered bread when pulled apart (see Fig. 26.2).

Catarrhal exudates result from the outpouring of mucus onto surfaces and are seen only in mucus-secreting tissues of the nasopharynx, lung, and alimentary tract. Serous rhinitis and tracheobronchitis rapidly develop into catarrhal or seropurulent exudates in most cases of respiratory disease.

Purulent (or suppurative) exudates are thick, creamy, and some variant of white or yellow. The exudate, also called *pus,* is composed of large amounts of viable and necrotic neutrophilic leukocytes and necrotic tissue debris partially liquefied by proteolytic digestion. *Suppuration* (L. *sub,* under, plus *puris,* pus) is a gross diagnosis, and its use in microscopy requires clear histologic evidence of pus in the lesion. Certain bacteria are prone to pus formation: staphylococci, streptococci, and corynebacteria. For this reason they are commonly referred to as pyogenic (pus-producing) bacteria.

As neutrophils enter an otherwise serous exudate, the early transparent fluid becomes thickened, opaque, and whitish (Fig. 1.6). When most of the exudate is composed of neutrophils, it is termed *purulent.* Neutrophils distort interstitial tissues, distend tubules, and accumulate on epithelial surfaces. If the irritant cannot be overcome, large numbers of cells are destroyed. Fresh neutrophils from the blood continue to pour into the area, and there is extensive necrosis of the tissue and liquefaction of the exudate.

Granulomatous inflammatory lesions are composed of masses of macrophages (and their precursor monocytes), which do not form a fluid exudate but remain attached together and stabilized by newly formed vascularized connective tissue. On mucosal surfaces granulomatous lesions are shaggy, irregular masses (Fig. 1.7). Bacteria that notoriously produce granulomatous inflammation are those that replicate within cells: mycobacteria (tuberculosis), *Brucella* spp., and *Salmonella* spp.

Sequestration of exudates

An *abscess* is a pus-filled cavity formed by disintegration of tissue. As normal tissues die, large numbers of neutrophils invade the area and are rapidly walled off by fibrin networks and connective tissue (see Fig. 1.10). Abscesses

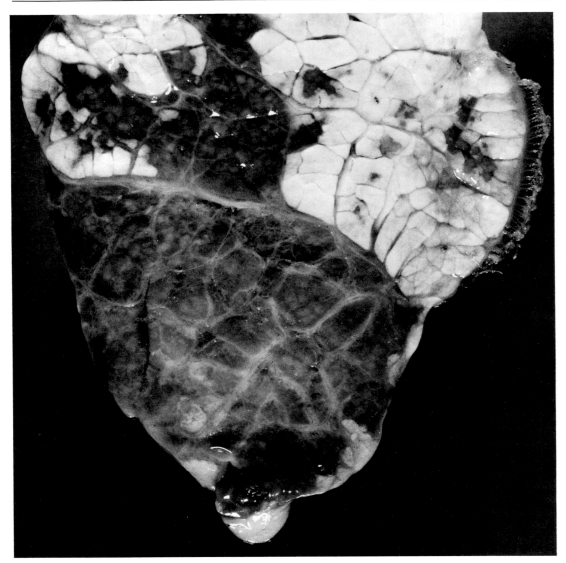

Fig. 1.5. Inflammation, lung, cow with *focal subacute serofibrinous pneumonia* caused by *Pasteurella multocida*. Septa contain large amounts of fibrin. Lesions at the lung periphery are older and are composed of macrophages and fibrous tissue. Lesions deeper in the lobe consist of hyperemia and alveoli filled with plasma proteins and large numbers of bacteria (see Fig. 18.4).

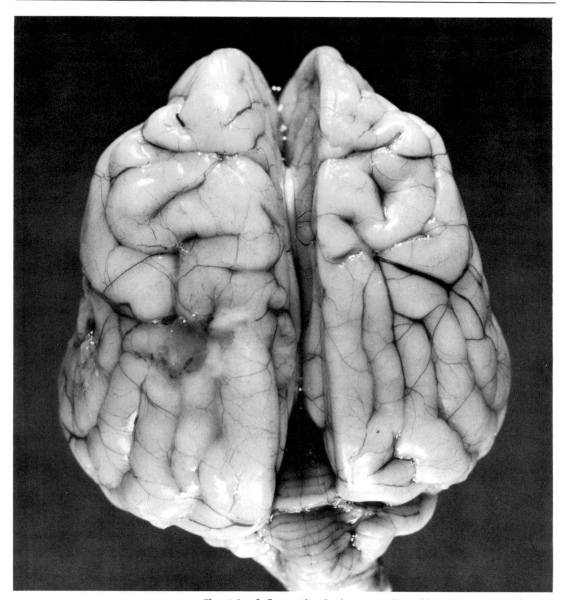

Fig. 1.6. *Inflammation,* brain, young dog with *severe acute purulent encephalitis.* Asymmetry is due to brain swelling; affected left side of brain is swollen (note the rounded gyri) compared with right side. Purulent exudate in the midcortex extends deep into the neuropil (see Fig. 18.6). *Escherichia coli* and *Corynebacterium* sp. were isolated from pus in the meninges.

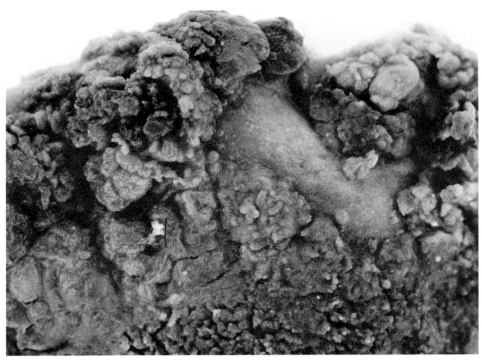

Fig. 1.7. Inflammation, peritoneum (over diaphragm surface), dog with *severe, diffuse chronic granulomatous peritonitis* (see Fig. 18.10) caused by *Actinobacillus* spp.

develop when invading bacteria are relatively low in virulence or when, for other reasons, they are contained by the inflammatory response of the infected animal.

Accumulations of large numbers of macrophages around a focus of infection is called a *granuloma,* a focal type of granulomatous inflammation. Granulomas commonly contain small numbers of lymphocytes and other leukocytes. If neutrophils make up a large part of the lesion, as they do in some fungal infections, the lesion is called a *pyogranuloma.*

Dissemination of exudates

When host defenses fail, inflammatory processes spread throughout the body. *Cellulitis* is the dissemination of pyogenic bacteria throughout the tissue. If untreated, cellulitis usually progresses to life-threatening disease and often causes death. Some bacteria (e.g., streptococci) contain hyaluronidase, which breaks down hyaluronic acid of the ground substances, allowing them to spread through tissue and lymphatics with appalling speed.

If the local inflammatory reaction and trapping by regional lymph nodes are insufficient, irritants are spilled into the blood, resulting in *bacteremia* (bacteria in the blood) or *toxemia* (toxins in the blood). Bacteria commonly gain access to the general circulation, but most are destroyed in the normal animal; that is, bacteremia occurs more often than disease because the highly responsive reticuloendothelial cells of liver, lungs, and spleen effectively process circulating bacteria.

Septicemia

Septicemia (septic bacteria in the blood) is the syndrome of septic bacteremia accompanied by fever, hemorrhages, and severe systemic illness. It is nearly always associated with some focus that provides a continuing supply of organisms (e.g., metritis, mastitis, or arthritis). Late stages of septicemia have a grave prognosis and are manifested by toxic signs, thrombocytopenia, disseminated intravascular coagulation, and shock.

Pyemia is pus in the blood.

Pyemia is a lethal variant of septicemia. Large numbers of neutrophils and bacteria circulate in the bloodstream. Emboli of bacteria lodge in tissues and initiate formation of secondary microabscesses in vascular organs such as kidney, lung, or liver. Bacteremia, septicemia, and pyremia are different pathogenetic processes, and they must be differentiated.

These severe diseases markedly affect leukocyte populations in the blood and storage sites of spleen and bone marrow. They induce increased granulocytopoiesis and massive release of neutrophils from splenic and marrow storage sites, both of which sustain high numbers of neutrophils in the blood (neutrophilic leukocytosis). If this increased supply of leukocytes is insufficient to combat disease, leukocytes are spewed out into the blood before they are mature. These immature neutrophils, called "band cells," indicate to the clinical pathologist that the systemic reaction is apt to be severe.

Healing

Late events of inflammation are concerned with healing, including repair and reconstruction by connective tissue and sequestration of debris by macrophages. Newly formed, highly vascularized connective tissue of inflammation is called *granulation tissue* because it appears to be composed of many tiny red granules. It is characteristic of skin wounds that fail to heal by primary closure. Granulation tissue is not the same as (and has no pathobiologic connection with) granulomatous inflammation.

Diagnosis of inflammatory lesions

The pathologist sums up the evaluation of an inflammatory lesion at the necropsy. Although an etiologic diagnosis may not be possible, the pathologic diagnosis transmits to the clinician the basic facts of abnormal anatomy. Lesions may be classified according to their extent, duration, distribution, type of exudate, and location. The proper pathologic diagnosis should therefore include this information (Table 1.3).

Adjectives such as *ulcerative, abscessing,* and *necrotic* are often used to characterize a lesion, but these are not proper adjectives for inflammation and should be used as separate listings (e.g., chronic granulomatous hepatitis with necrosis). *Hemorrhagic* is appropriate for some very severe exudates, such as the serohemorrhagic enteritis produced by *Clostridium perfringens.* Blood in an intestinal exudate may not be associated with the inflammatory process, and in this case the diagnosis should be serous enteritis with hemorrhage.

Like all things biologic, inflammatory lesions are seldom precisely classifiable. Most purulent lesions are also fibrinous, that is, fibrinopurulent. Description of lesion age is highly subjective, and the use of *acute* and *chronic* may be directed to the disease, to the gross lesions, or to the microscopic lesions, which are usually the same but not always since events may be seen by microscopy that are not visible grossly.

Chronic inflammation poses two special problems: (1) a chronic lesion that contains foci of acute inflammation (e.g., chronic dermatitis with foci of acute inflammation), which is properly diagnosed as chronic granulomatous dermatitis with foci of acute suppurative dermatitis, and (2) chronic inflammation that is actively laying down fibrous tissue (e.g., the connective tissue proliferation of an equine scar), which is best diagnosed as *chronic, progressive, fibrosing dermatitis.* Some pathologists call these lesions "chronic active dermatitis," but "active" implies that inactive inflammation exists, and that is wrong.

GROWTH DISTURBANCES

Abnormalities in growth and development of organs and tissues include both defective growth (e.g., hypoplasia and atrophy) and excessive growth (e.g., hyperplasia and hypertrophy). They may result from changes in the total number of cells or in the growth rates of individual cells (Table 1.4). Although cell size becomes ab-

Table 1.3. Classification of inflammation

Extent	Duration	Distribution	Character	Site
Slight	Peracute	Focal	Serous	Gastritis
Moderate	Acute	Multifocal	Catarrhal	Tracheitis
Severe	Subacute	Diffuse	Fibrinous	Pericarditis
	Chronic		Purulent	Epididymitis
			Proliferative	Cholangitis
			Granulomatous	Lymphadenitis

Table 1.4. Disturbances of growth

Type	Definition
Cell growth	
Hypertrophy	Increase in size of cells without increase in number
Hyperplasia	Quantitative increase in number of cells in a tissue
Metaplasia	Occurrence of normal cell type in tissue where not normally present; change to less-differentiated cell type
Cell regression	
Atrophy	Decrease in size of cells that have gained full development
Hypoplasia	Failure of organs or tissues to obtain full size
Aplasia	Complete failure of organ to develop

normal, growth is controlled and generally proceeds along patterns normal for the tissue involved. Because of its special nature, neoplasia is set apart from the above growth defects.

Growth disturbances are caused by many types of injury, the most prominent of which involve damage to the fetus, nutritional disorders, and endocrine dysfunctions. Usually the earlier growth is disturbed, the greater the deleterious effect. When development is altered in the embryo or early fetus, *agenesis* (the complete absence of a tissue anlage) may result.

Congenital diseases are abnormalities existing at or before birth. They may be hereditary or be caused by infectious, chemical, or physical agents. Congenital anomalies occur in young or newborn animals, do not show progressive expansion, have orderly tissue associations, and are usually associated with other defects.

Developmental changes sometimes cause organs to be *ectopic* (malpositioned). In dogs, ectopic thyroid tissue is frequently found in connective tissue of the mediastinum. Ectopic spleens are sometimes embedded in the pancreas. *Ectopia cordis* is displacement of the heart outside the thoracic cavity. *Ectopic testicles* are dislocated, usually outside the scrotum and retained within the abdominal cavity.

Neoplasia

A neoplasm (Gr. *neos,* new, plus *plasma,* formation) is literally a new and abnormal growth, specifically a new growth of tissue that is progressive and uncontrolled. *Neoplasia,* the formation of a neoplasm, involves progressive multiplication of cells. Growth is independent and competes for metabolic substrates with normal cells.

Neoplasms represent a pathologic overgrowth of tissue, occur as a spectrum of lesions varying from small solid masses to highly diffuse and infiltrative lesions (Fig. 1.8). The term *tumor,* used classically to describe any mass or swelling, is now used synonymously with *neoplasm. Cancer* is a noncommittal term that refers to all malignant tumors.

During the necropsy, pathologists must report all changes that indicate whether a tumor is *benign* or *malignant* (Table 1.5). This includes an examination of the extent of the mass or tissue infiltrate; of the regional arteries, veins, and lymphatics; of the draining lymph nodes; and of local tissue planes. Furthermore, evidence of *invasion* to adjacent tissue, of *implantation* along luminal or cavity surfaces, and of *metastasis* to lungs, liver, and other viscera must be sought.

Neoplastic cells show uncontrollable growth.

Factors controlling cell proliferation no longer limit mitotic activity in neoplastic cells. Cells grow into large masses visible as tumors. In host neoplasms, the pattern of growth clearly differentiates the tissue from hyperplasia and characterizes it as benign or malignant. In some, however, the borderline between hyperplasia and neoplasia is ill defined, and proper classification becomes lost in vague and imprecise definitions of the word neoplasm. The *differentiation* of neoplastic cells refers to the extent to which these cells resemble their normal ancestors. Tumors with poorly differentiated cells are

Table 1.5. Classification of neoplasms

Type	Designation	Examples
Benign	*-oma* added to cell type of origin	Fibroma, hemangioma, meningioma
	adenoma indicates gland origin	Thyroid adenoma, sebaceous gland adenoma, ovarian cyst-adenoma
Malignant	*carcinoma* indicates epithelial origin	Basal cell carcinoma, squamous cell carcinoma, pancreatic adenocarcinoma
	sarcoma indicates mesenchymal origin	Fibrosarcoma, osteosarcoma, liposarcoma, hemangiosarcoma
	Unspecified if origin uncertain	Malignant melanoma, malignant lymphoma

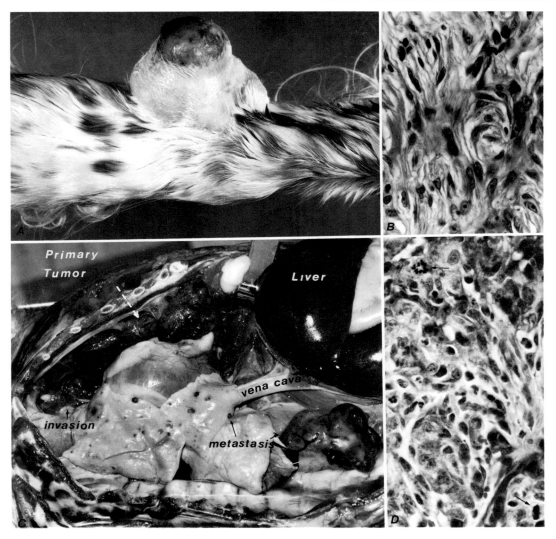

Fig. 1.8. *Neoplasia.* A and B. *Hemangiopericytoma:* benign vascular tumor originating from pericytes that surround capillaries, forelimb, dog. Neoplastic cells resemble and produce collagen like normal pericytes. C and D. *Hemangiosarcoma:* malignant vascular tumor of endothelial cells. Primary tumor has invaded the chest wall, producing intrathoracic secondary tumors. Metastatic tumors from hematogenous dissemination occur as dark spots on the lungs. Malignant cells are highly pleomorphic, contain mitotic figures (*arrow*), and lack any resemblance to normal cell types.

apt to be highly malignant. *Anaplasia* means lack of cell differentiation, and anaplastic tumors contain cells with marked pleomorphism (variations in size and shape).

VARIATIONS IN HOST RESPONSE

Characterizing the host response

Severity

Tissue responses may be slight (minimal), moderate, or severe (marked). Judgments of severity are often imprecise because there is no precise way to measure the rapidity with which an individual lesion has developed. Furthermore, there is often a discrepancy in the severity of the tissue lesion and the disease in the live animal. Nonetheless, information regarding the extent of lesions is critical to a good pathologic diagnosis.

Duration

The time involved in development of lesions is important in their structural appearance. *Acute* (sudden) processes may differ greatly from their *chronic* (slow, occurring over a long time) counterparts. For example, the cellular responses are markedly different in acute and in chronic inflammation. Inflammatory lesions may be especially confusing when acute and chronic processes are superimposed.

Acute processes tend to be less complicated than chronic ones. Acute necrosis of renal tubules may cause death, but the body lacks the widespread degenerative processes seen in animals dead from chronic kidney damage and uremia with its slowly progressive accumulation of toxic products.

Location

Similar pathologic processes in different organs may cause differences in clinical manifestations. Foci of acute and chronic inflammation confined within subcutis are often painful but, as space-occupying lesions, do not endanger the life of the animal. The same type of lesion in the brain is life threatening, for brain tissue cannot expand beyond the confining limits of the cranium.

In acute inflammation of the brain (encephalitis), fluids and cells of circulating blood seep into tissue, causing the brain to swell (Fig. 1.6).

Clinical signs of extreme pain, hyperesthesia, and paresis result more from brain swelling than from accumulation of inflammatory cells and fever.

Distribution

The extent and distribution of lesions are important characteristics of disease processes. *Focal* (localized) lesions are usually more controlled by the host than *diffuse* processes (those distributed throughout the tissue); the focal nature indicates that the pathologic process has been confined. Liver abscesses are less hazardous than diffuse hepatitis. A malignant neoplasm that is focal is less dangerous than one that is diffuse. In some diseases, a single focus of damage may spread to form several foci, or several foci may arise simultaneously. These distributions are called *multifocal.*

To prevent spread of processes such as necrosis, inflammation, and neoplasia, biological mechanisms have evolved to sequester causal agents in foci of initial contact. For example, as some parasites attach to gastrointestinal mucosa, they produce small foci of necrosis and ulceration (Fig. 1.9). These foci become underlined first by acute and then by chronic inflammatory tissue. Opportunistic bacteria attach to the site of epithelial damage, but this threat is largely neutralized by invasion of the tissue by plasmacytes that produce and release antibodies that initiate the process of bacterial uptake and killing.

Secondary foci of tissue damage via dissemination of microbes

Lesions often provide clues to secondary sites that may be affected. Local infectious processes and tumors may release cells into *lymphatic vessels,* so that lymph nodes draining the lesion should be examined for extension of the disease process. If bacteria escape from the parasite-induced gastric ulcer, foci of inflammation may be found in the gastric lymph node.

Dissemination commonly occurs *hematogenously* (via the bloodstream). Ulcers of the stomach and intestine are often associated with foci of necrosis in the liver. These areas of dead hepatocytes, which appear as round, pale, sharply delimited lesions throughout the liver parenchyma (Fig. 1.10), result from the seeding of pathogenic bacteria into the portal venous system. In cattle, rumen ulcers commonly arise from intraruminal acidosis. Bacteria, especially

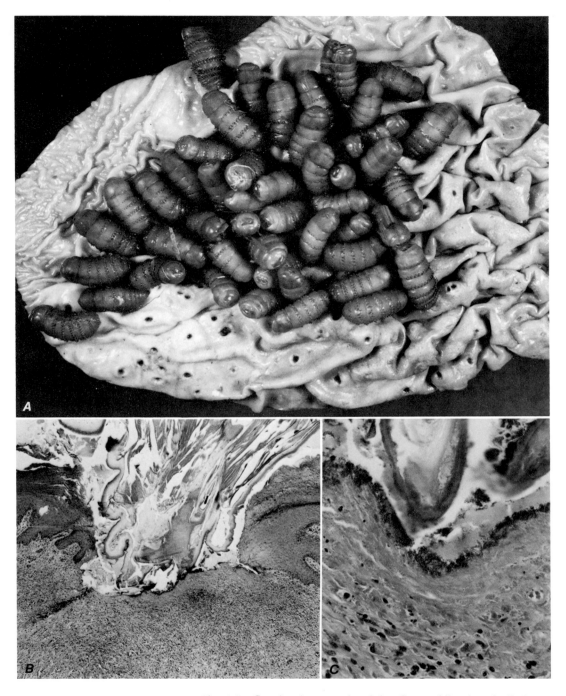

Fig. 1.9. Gastric ulcers produced by *Gasterophilus intestinalis* larvae ("bots") walled off by chronic inflammation. A. Detachment of larvae leaves ulcers on the gastric surface. B. Chitinous oral hooks of parasite produce erosions and ulcers surrounded by hyperplastic squamous epithelium and chronic focal fibrosing gastritis with many plasma cells. C. Surface of pit contains many aerobic and anaerobic bacteria.

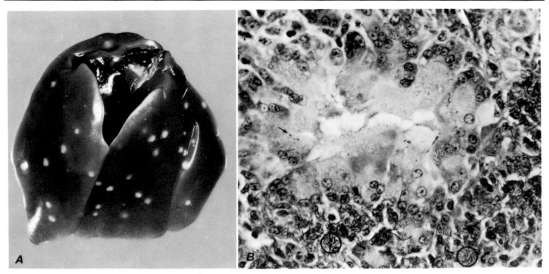

Fig. 1.10. Focal necrosis of liver resulting from dissemination of enteric bacteria through the portal vein. A. *Eubacterium* sp. turkey; bacteria originated in ulcers in the intestine, spread through the portal vein, and lodged in the liver. B. Histology: focus of necrosis in liver surrounded by zone of macrophages. *Eubacteria* sp. (*circles*) are associated with macrophages at the lesion periphery. Tiny cocci (*Staphylococcus aureus*) have superinfected the necrotic tissue (*arrow*). (Photographs: Larry Arp, *Vet. Pathol.* 20:80, 1983)

the opportunistic *Fusobacterium necrophorum,* enter the rumen wall, pass through the portal vein, and are trapped in the liver sinusoids where they initiate foci of liver cell degeneration and necrosis.

During the postmortem examination (necropsy), the pathologist must make associations among combinations of lesions. The findings of pus in the uterus, friable growths on heart valves, and wedge-shaped areas of tissue death in the kidney suggest a probable pathogenesis. A primary bacterial uterine infection has released bacteria into the bloodstream that localize on the heart valves. Infection of the valve causes thrombosis, and tiny pieces of thrombi are released from the heart, travel to the kidney, and obstruct the renal arterial tree, causing death of renal parenchyma.

FOCUS

Origins of veterinary pathology

Pathology is rooted in the anatomical theaters of the Italian Renaissance. In Padua, the chair of anatomy was occupied by a succession of great scientists: Vesalius, Malpighi, Valsalva, Fabricius, and Morgagni. Morgagni began the modern era of pathology with *Seats and Causes of Disease* in 1761, one year before the first veterinary school was founded in Lyon, France. The correlation of clinical signs with organic lesions was the turning point of ancient to modern medicine. Before Morgagni, physicians spoke of imbalanced mixtures of humors, and after him, of changes in organs that were constant for specific diseases. ▶

William Harvey studied in Padua and returned to London to discover the circulation of blood. The English legacy of experimental pathology extended into John Hunter's treatises on vascular pathology and William Osler's discovery of platelets in the 1800s. Hunter was on the founding board of the Royal Veterinary College in London. Osler was a staff member of the Montreal Veterinary College, where his contributions to veterinary pathology include important studies on verminous pneumonia in dogs.

Medical pathology ascended in the German-speaking world with a group around Johannes Muller in Berlin. Using the newly invented achromatic objective on the light microscope, Schwann, Henle, Ramak, Reichert, and Virchow established the cellular basis of tissue analysis. Rudolf Virchow introduced systematic analysis into the postmortem room. His book *Cellular Pathology,* published in 1848, opened new horizons and laid the foundations of medical and veterinary pathology. Involved in public health movements, Virchow was interested in infectious diseases of farm animals and advocated postmortem examinations as a form of meat inspection. By his presence on a Prussian commission for veterinary affairs, he was influential in the establishment of the first chair of veterinary pathology in Berlin in 1870. Because of a government regulation that all animals must be necropsied before compensation for disease loss was paid, Virchow's necropsy techniques spread through central Europe.

Virchow's pathologic concepts were carried to North America by several medical pathologists. A. W. Clement, a veterinary student of Osler in Montreal, spent time in Virchow's lab and returned to Canada. He wrote the first North American book on veterinary postmortem technique and was elected president of the American Veterinary Medical Association.

In the early 1900s, North American veterinary pathologists took advantage of the curiosity of staffs of large medical institutes such as the Rockefeller Institute, and Armed Forces Institute of Pathology, and the Mayo Clinic. From the latter came Dr. William Feldman, one of the outstanding veterinary pathologists and first president of the American College of Veterinary Pathologists. Founded in 1948, this organization has helped to guide the scientific development of veterinary pathology in the United States and Canada. The demands of its examination for certification influenced academic programs and endorsed the need for a lifelong goal of constant learning. It also emphasized the special burden of the pathologist: the need to keep one foot in the new technologies of science and the other in the observations of clinical medicine.

ADDITIONAL READING

Mouwen, J., and de Groot, E. *Atlas of Veterinary Pathology.* Utrecht: Weteschlappeliuke, 1982.

Saunders, L. Z. Some pioneers in comparative medicine. *Can. Vet. J.* 14:27, 1973.

Slauson, D. O., and Cooper, B. J. *Mechanisms of Disease.* Baltimore: Williams and Wilkins, 1982.

Trump, B. F., et al. *Cellular Pathobiology of Human Disease.* Stuttgart: Gustav Fischer Verlag, 1983.

Critical Defects in Homeostasis

2

SYSTEMIC changes such as fever, hypoglycemia, and increased heart rate commonly accompany local disease processes. Whatever causes these changes, they alter vital components of plasma and other body fluids. Many of these changes are important secondary contributors to disease. When superimposed on the primary or original cause of injury, they are often responsible for the death of the animal because of their effect on vital organ systems.

OXYGEN DEFICIT

Oxygen deficiency of tissue may be partial (hypoxia) or total (anoxia). When combined with increased body temperature, hypoxia becomes a potent cause of death. Oxygen deficit may be due to one cause or a combination of mechanisms that prevent oxygen from reaching its ultimate goal, the mitochondrion. The three types of mechanisms are *anoxic* (inadequate oxygen in the presence of adequate blood supply), *ischemic* (decrease of arterial flow and pressure with stagnation and decrease in oxygen consumption), and *cytotoxic* (interference with oxygen utilization by the cell) (Table 2.1).

The mechanisms involved in oxygen deficit may be generalized or precisely directed to specific cell organelles or enzyme systems. For example, cyanide quickly causes death of the animal by the precise and rapid inhibition of cytochrome oxidase in the mitochondria of brain cells. Cell anoxia develops because there is interference with the utilization of oxygen, which results in damage to neurons and white matter. Conversely, in death due to environmental oxygen deficiency from asphyxiation (suffocation), anoxia develops more slowly and tissue injury is much more widespread (Fig. 2.1).

Table 2.1. Mechanisms of anoxia in cell injury

Type	Mechanism	Examples
Anoxic	Circulatory failure	Shock, heart failure
	Venous stasis	Liver necrosis in heart failure
	Erythrocyte deficiency	Anemia, hemoglobin deficiency
	Lung disease	Pneumonia, edema, emphysema
	Blockade of upper respiratory tract	Foreign body obstruction, asphyxiation
Ischemic	Arterial blockade	Infarction due to emboli/thrombi
Cytotoxic	Mitochondrial lesion	Cyanide, fluoroacetate poisoning

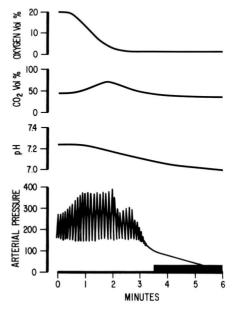

Fig. 2.1. Oxygen, carbon dioxide, and lactate in the blood of a drowning dog.

Cytopathology in oxygen deficiency

Cytopathology resulting from systemic anoxia varies according to severity and duration of the oxygen deficiency. The consequences are greater in visceral organs such as brain, heart, liver, and kidney, whose parenchymal cells are metabolizing to a high degree. These organs have elaborate vascular systems with shunts, anastomoses, and double blood supplies that protect them from lesser degrees of injury. They are vulnerable, however, when several mechanisms that produce anoxia are operable.

When anoxia occurs, cell ATP values approach zero within seconds due to absence of oxygen and substrates. As a result of loss of energy production, cell volume control is lost and pumping of sodium into extracellular spaces cannot occur. Crucial morphologic changes develop in mitochondria (the sites of ATP generation) and in the cytocavitary network (which accumulates water). Calcium homeostasis is especially important to degenerating cells, and as the level of calcium ions rises in the cytoplasm (because of the leaky cell membrane), widespread disintegration of cell membranes begins to occur (Table 2.2).

The brain is markedly sensitive to hypoxia.

Newborn primates may suffer brain damage with transient asphyxia in as little as 12 minutes during birth. The cerebellum, precentral gyrus of the cerebral cortex, and auditory colliculus are selectively injured (Fig. 2.2). Neurons become dense and shrink, and adjacent astrocytes appear watery and show evidence of dissolution of chromatin and Nissl substance. Similar cyto-

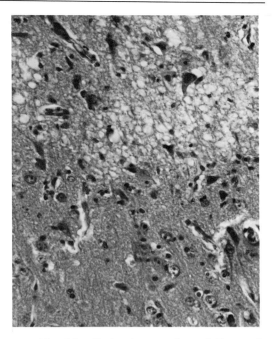

Fig. 2.2. Brain damage (vacuolation and laminar demyelination), dog with transient systemic anoxia.

pathic changes are produced by temporary clamping of the cat's middle cerebral artery, followed by reflow of blood for a time. Neuronal mitochondria undergo swelling and lysis of cristae, and rough endoplasmic reticulum dilates. Although capillary endothelium does not appear damaged, astrocyte foot processes that surround the vessels are markedly swollen.

Table 2.2. Cellular changes in anoxia

Event	Consequences
Mitochondrial shutdown	
Enzyme depletion	Loss of ATP, Ca^{++} flow altered
Ca^{++} pools altered	Loss of Ca^{++} from mitochondrial matrix to cytosol
Phospholipase activation within mitochondrial membranes	Arises from disturbed Ca^{++} homeostasis and leads to degradation of membrane phospholipids
β-oxidation of fatty acids inhibited	Long chain acyl-CoA esters accumulate and have detergent effect on membranes
Ion shifts in cytoplasm	
Entry of Na^+	
Gain of Ca^{++}	Microfilament depolymerization and uncoupling of gap junctions
Metabolic shifts	Increased glycolysis and inhibition of lipid metabolism
General membrane lysis	Occurs throughout cell, with loss of cytoplasmic protein, liberation of lysosomal enzymes, and necrosis

Centrolobular necrosis occurs in hypoxic liver.

Although the liver is supplied by both the portal vein and hepatic artery, it remains susceptible to hypoxic injury because of its intense rate of metabolism. Blockage of the hepatic artery (although this rarely happens clinically) will lead to hepatic necrosis. Experimental ligation of the hepatic artery in veins may be fatal in dogs within 2 days.

In most mammals, oxygen deficit hepatic necrosis is largely a result of four conditions: cardiac failure, severe anemia, shock with prolonged low flow rates, and hepatic ischemia due to obstruction of the portal vein. In old dogs, "cardiac necrosis" of the liver is a common finding in chronic heart failure (see Fig. 15.3). In young animals, anoxic liver damage is more apt to result from severe anemia, especially when coupled with agonal cardiac insufficiency and reduced hepatic blood flow (Fig. 2.3).

The renal medulla is sensitive to hypoxia.

In the kidney of an animal with hypoxia, lesions occur in the medulla and papillary areas. These areas are especially sensitive since blood pressure is lowest in the papillae. Furthermore, during hypoxia, prostaglandins (PGs) are synthesized, producing these events: PG release → local vasodilation → increased blood flow. Drugs that affect this path, especially in the sick animal with poor circulation or hypoxia, will exacerbate renal hypoxic damage.

Within the renal medulla, hypoxic injury is de-

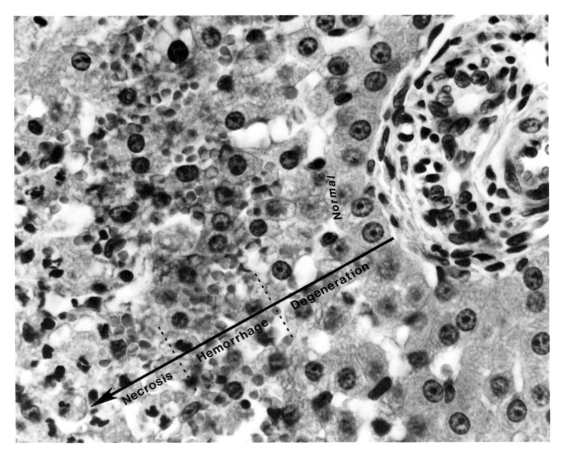

Fig. 2.3. Centrolobular liver necrosis, cat with severe anemia and heart failure. Stasis of blood in the hepatic vein causes degeneration to be progressively worse along the pathway of blood flow from the portal triad (*top right*) to the central vein (*arrow*). Zones of effect: normal liver cells, early degeneration, hemorrhage, and necrosis.

pendent on the rate of ion transport in the proximal convoluted tubules and Henle's loop; that is, the consequences of hypoxia are influenced by energy demand and oxygen utilization. In the renal medulla, the thick ascending limb of Henle's loop is selectively vulnerable to oxygen deficiency due to its high transport activity plus its meager oxygen supply.

Cardiac muscle extracts oxygen from blood efficiently.

Mammalian skeletal muscle uses about 40% of the oxygen in the blood that circulates through the muscle. In contrast, cardiac muscle uses nearly 100% of the oxygen in the blood circulating through the myocardial capillaries. This high oxygen demand makes myocardium susceptible to systemic hypoxia. Small random foci of necrosis of the ventricular muscle occur in shock and other diseases where blood pressure and blood circulation are compromised (Table 2.3).

The fetus is resistant to hypoxia.

The fetus has a remarkable resistance to hypoxia from midgestation to birth. Newborn animals have been known to tolerate 30 minutes of anoxia without permanent injury. Much of this is due to vascular mechanisms that redistribute blood during hypoxia. The lungs, liver, kidney, and intestine are not critical organs for survival of the fetus in utero because their functions are provided by the placenta. The ductus arteriosus and the ductus venosus shunt blood from the capillary beds of the lungs and liver respectively. In addition, thick muscular walls of the small arterioles and precapillaries of the lungs and intestine cause marked resistance to blood flow (postnatal development involves involution of the media with increased lumenal diameters). Anoxia increases the tone of these vessels. Resistance of fetal tissue to anoxia may be due in part to its capacity for rapid anaerobic glycolysis. There are large stores of glycogen in fetal tissues, which are largely absent from fetuses that have died with anoxia.

In those diseases in which cell degeneration is clearly due to exogenous agents, anoxia may still play an important secondary role in production of cell degeneration and necrosis. Anoxia is particularly important in embryos and fetuses that develop vascular damage of embryonic membranes. Abortion and defective embryogenesis may be the serious consequences.

ENERGY DEFICIT
Hypoglycemia

Any severe fall in concentration of glucose in plasma rapidly affects the central nervous system and results in progressive disorientation and prostration. Surprisingly, this is rarely a major clinical problem. Glucose levels are maintained within relatively normal ranges even in fasting and the early stages of starvation. Hypoglycemia may accompany the parasitemic phases of protozoal infections because of excessive glucose utilization within infected erythrocytes. Although precipitous drops in blood glucose occur in animals that die, this appears to play only a minor role in the process of death.

The mammalian nervous system consumes about two-thirds of the circulating glucose; most of the remainder goes to skeletal muscles and erythrocytes. Liver stores of glycogen can supply the brain's needs for only a few hours of fasting, and in the interval between night and morning feedings, amino acids from skeletal muscle protein breakdown provide material for hepatic glucose production. Free fatty acids derived from adipocyte triglyceride breakdown supply energy to tissues other than those of the nervous system.

Table 2.3. Lesions of systemic hypoxia in the dog

Organ	Lesion	Some Causes
Brain	Necrosis of neurons	Systemic anoxia
Liver	Centrolobular necrosis	Anemia Cardiac failure
Intestine	Necrosis at tips of villi	Opening of vascular shunts sends blood from central capillaries
Kidney	Necrosis of medulla	Hypoxia + natural low rate of blood flow in medulla + high metabolic rate
Myocardium	Shock	Hypoxia + high rate of metabolism + high utilization rate of oxygen

FOCUS

Pulmonary hypertrophic osteoarthropathy

This rare and curious disease involves new bone formation beneath the periosteum that progressively thickens and deforms long bones. Beginning at the distal ends of the limb bones, new bone grows outward in an interrupted manner, producing irregular and rough bony masses. The initial lesion is an overgrowth of subperiosteal vascular tissue that leads directly to osteoblast proliferation and bone formation. Treatment to correct this rapid increase in blood flow to the limb bones causes the lesion to regress. The case below was reported by Dr. Freddy Coignoul in *Ann. Med. Vet.* 128:545, 1984.

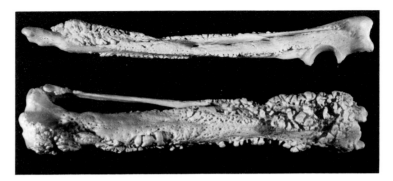

The prefix *pulmonary* indicates the unexplained association of bone lesions with lesions of the lungs. Thoracic neoplasms, pulmonary tuberculosis, granulomas of the esophagus, and lung abscesses have all been responsible. In a study of 60 canine cases, 58 dogs had intrathoracic lesions (36 secondary neoplasms, 18 primary neoplasms, 2 inflammatory lesions, and 1 case of dirofilariasis). Of the two dogs without thoracic lesions, one had bacterial endocarditis and one a sarcoma of the urinary bladder (see Brodey, *J. Am. Vet. Med. Assoc.* 159:1242, 1971).

When the thoracic lesion that underlies the periosteal change is removed surgically, the bone lesions of hypertrophic osteoarthropathy regress. Improvement correlates with the correction of increased blood flow to the bones. *Chronic anoxia* has been implicated as causal yet the magnitude of the pulmonary lesions is rarely of such extent that mechanical obstruction of the airways can explain the bone lesions. Vagotomy has been shown to suppress the bone lesions in both dog and man.

In rare cases, hypertrophic osteoarthropathy has developed without a thoracic lesion. The role of limb obstruction of these tumors has not been thoroughly investigated.

BODY TEMPERATURE

In all *homeothermic* (warm-blooded) vertebrates, body temperature is virtually independent of environmental temperatures. There is a selective advantage in having body temperature determined by the energy of metabolism and controllable by cellular mechanisms. Homeothermy is not without its price, for even under the least-demanding circumstances, birds and mammals devote over 90% of the heat produced by metabolism to maintenance of body temperature. The body temperature of *poikilothermic* (cold-blooded) animals varies directly with the environmental temperature. The rates of most chemical reactions double with each increase of 10°C. This is a particularly valuable influence on defense mechanisms such as phagocytosis. In most vertebrates the complex reactions of inflammation are plainly enhanced by the increases in body temperature known as fever.

In the cell, mitochondria are the major sites of heat production. Combustion within mitochondria, which is controlled by the ADP:ATP ratio, is dependent on adequate availability of substrates, oxygen, and calcium ions. Extracellular control is exerted by neuroendocrine systems, mainly catecholamines and thyroid hormones, which act directly on cells to modify thermogenesis. Catecholamines have a rapid effect that ceases when the hormone is removed, while thyroxin produces a slow, long-lasting action. Increased heat production in hyperthyroidism is due to the effect of thyroxin enhancing the operation of ion-pumping enzymes embedded in membrane on the mitochondria and on the cell surface.

Hyperthermia

Hyperthermia due to high environmental temperature is accompanied by increases in pH, hemoglobin, and erythrocytes in the bloodstream. All of these are consequences of water loss. In *heatstroke*, there may be degenerative changes in the myocardium, renal tubules, and brain due to the excessively high temperature in these rapidly metabolizing tissues. Heatstroke frequently occurs in small mammalian pets confined in a hot environment without water. Early signs of *hyperpnea* (abnormal increase in rate and depth of respiration), *tachycardia* (rapid heart action), and vomiting may be related to

brain injury. Several days after heatstroke there is often evidence of renal failure caused by degeneration and necrosis of renal tubules.

Mechanisms of heat loss and conservation

On a hot day a whippet can keep a rabbit running until the rabbit dies of heat exhaustion. Although running raises the temperature of both animals and both are cooled by airflow over oronasal mucosae, the dog's brain has a cooling system lacking in the rabbit. A network of blood vessels branching from the carotid artery, the carotid rete mirabile, to supply the brain passes through a venous sinus, drawing cooled blood directly from the nasal cavity, and the warm arterial blood loses heat to the cooler venous blood. These countercurrent heat-exchange networks occur in the brain of carnivores and artiodactyls (cattle and other even-numbered-hoofed mammals) but are lacking in horses, primates, rodents, and lagomorphs.

Hibernation, a precisely regulated lowering of the central thermostat in the hypothalamus is designed to conserve energy. Regulated by the effects of day-length cycles on the pineal gland, hibernation is mediated by a protein called thermogenen; stimulation of heat production in mitochondria-rich brown fat cells produces large amounts of heat because oxidative phosphorylation and respiration are uncoupled in brown fat mitochondria.

WATER DEFICIT
Water deprivation

A clinically significant decrease in body water is usually due to deficient intake. In mammals, clinical signs may appear after loss of 2% of body weight and become severe after loss of 10%. Some amphibians may lose water by evaporation equivalent to as much as 50% of body weight and survive if rehydrated. Mammals, in contrast, may die after losing 12%, especially if plasma sodium rises accordingly (camels, donkeys, and sheep tolerate up to a 25% loss).

The effects of water deprivation are enhanced by muscle work, fever, diarrhea, and high mineral intake. In large animals, cold winter temperatures often contribute. Gastrointestinal signs may appear before systemic effects of dehydration occur. For example, horses commonly suffer water deprivation in winter, partly be-

---

FOCUS

Hyperthermia and rhabdomyolysis in racing greyhounds

Focal *rhabdomyolysis* (lysis of skeletal muscle cells) and myoglobinuria can occur after severe, prolonged exercise, especially in hot climates. Potassium ions (K^+) are released from contracting skeletal muscle fibers and dilate arterioles. When K^+ release is subnormal, a relative ischemia may develop and tiny spots of coagulation necrosis begin to appear in the hardest-working muscle groups.

Focal rhabdomyolysis is a problem in racing greyhounds. Typically, a winning dog is returned to the kennel, fed, and watered. Over the next 48 hours the dog develops stiffness, anorexia, and excessive thirst. Urine is apt to be voided in excess and is often slightly pink. Mucous membranes are dry and rose or purple. The epaxial muscles are swollen, often more severely on the right side (because of the running pattern of the track). Such dogs are frequently destroyed because they rarely return to top racing form. At necropsy, foci of rhabdomyolysis are common and the lungs are congested. Blood taken during a period of severe signs show the following values:

Test	Hyperthermic Dog	Normal
Glucose	10.0	70–110 mg/dl
Blood urea nitrogen	83.0	5–28 mg/dl
Alkaline phosphatase	274.0	10–100 IU
ALAT[a]	101.0	0–40 mU/ml
ASAT[b]	194.0	4–66 mU/ml
LDH	4,234.0	100 mU/ml
CPK	14,028.0	8–60 mU/ml
Sodium	8.8	14–155 mEq/l
Potassium	5.9	3.6–5.6 mEq/l

[a]Aspartate aminotransferase (SGOT).
[b]Aminotransferase (SGPT).

---

cause of poor management but also because they tend to drink less in cold weather. Impaction of intestinal contents can cause signs of colic.

When animals do not drink, water is withdrawn from extracellular fluids to maintain blood volume. Extracellular fluids thus increase in osmoconcentration, and this in turn stimulates water-seeking behavior and renal mechanisms to decrease urine production. Water deficiency increases the osmotic pressure of plasma, which causes water to be retained and salts to be excreted. Despite an early increase in plasma osmotic pressure, plasma electrolytes remain within normal ranges in dehydration (because they are excreted in concentrated form in urine) until severe clinical signs occur. After long periods of dehydration, the animal is depleted of both water and electrolytes.

Hemoconcentration occurs in dehydration.

The number of erythrocytes per ml of blood increases as dehydration progresses, and any interpretation of hematocrit or packed cell volume of erythrocytes must consider the effects of dehydration on this clinical pathologic parameter.

Nervous signs occur in advanced dehydration.

In progressive dehydration, intracellular dehydration leads to enzyme defects that are reflected in mitochondrial degeneration. Certain areas of the brain are especially sensitive. Cellular water loss in these sites leads to unusually severe neurologic signs.

Water loss from skin occurs in hot weather.

Evaporation of water from skin is an important cooling mechanism and in host environments may be so active that it exceeds that amount of water taken in by drinking. Water loss from mammalian skin is impeded by lipid-rich substances in the stratum corneum (lipids are derived from expulsion of lamellar bodies from keratinocytes in the stratum granulosum). Deficiency of some dietarily essential fatty acids results in epidermal hyperplasia with impaired barrier function and increased water loss.

Excessive water loss

Dehydration can result from prolonged vomiting and diarrhea. Water and electrolytes are lost in both situations, and the clinical signs often are due more to electrolyte loss than to simple water deficiency. Dehydration also occurs in renal failure in which there is impairment of concentrating ability with excretion of large amounts of urine (e.g., the oliguric phase of acute renal failure).

Dehydration is important in fever.

The febrile animal requires greater amounts of water, yet if incapacitated is unable to drink. The skin is flushed in fever, and this causes increased water loss from skin. All these factors combined make maintenance of plasma fluid volume important in febrile infections.

Water loss or gain is controlled by the kidney.

Proximal convoluted tubules reabsorb more than 80% of the water of the glomerular filtrate. They shunt glucose and Na^+ across the luminal cell membrane by active transport (an energy-requiring process), diffusion of Cl^- accompanies Na^+, and the reabsorption of NaCl and glucose carries the water across the nephron passively, by osmotic diffusion (Fig. 2.4).

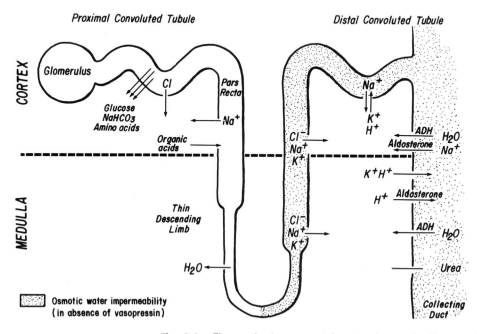

Fig. 2.4. Changes in glucose, protein, potassium, and sodium as glomerular filtrate passes through the nephron.

The hyperosmotic medulla withdraws water.

In mammals, many "long" nephrons are arranged to concentrate urine. The loop of Henle dips deeply down into the *vasa rectae* (the tips of the papillae accompanied by capillary loops). This peritubular capillary bed is a "low-pressure" bed (in contrast to the higher pressure of the glomerulus), and blood is sluggish in moving through it. By the retransport of Na^+ and Cl^- again and again from the lumen of the ascending to the descending loops of Henle (via the interstitium), water is removed in the highly permeable descending limb. This countercurrent osmotic multiplier mechanism functions in both the loops of Henle and the vasa rectae. The descending limb of the loop is highly permeable to water and to NaCl. The ascending limb has strong transport mechanisms to move these ions into the interstitium but is relatively impermeable to water. Tubule fluid in transit through the loops therefore passes through a hyperosmotic medulla. High urea and Na^+ in the interstitium allow water to be removed in the descending limb. In the ascending limb, the impermeability to water allows the tubular fluid to become progressively more dilute.

Antidiuretic hormone causes distal tubules to withdraw water.

In the distal tubules, reabsorption of water is controlled by the antidiuretic hormone ADH, or vasopressin, which originates in the posterior pituitary. ADH causes the otherwise impermeable tubules to become permeable to water (and, in the frog, increases permeability of the skin). Interstitial tissue must be hypertonic to provide osmotic gradients for water reabsorption. Exposure to the high osmolarity of the renal papilla causes water to be removed from the tubule. Increased permeability of the distal tubule epithelial cell is due to changes in the hormone-sensitive luminal surface of the collecting tubule epithelial cells. ADH appears to stimulate formation of cyclic AMP, which directly increases the permeability of the tubule membranes. ADH is packaged in secretory granules within nerve bodies in the hypothalamic supraoptic nucleus. Granules pass down the axon and into the posterior pituitary, where they are stored and eventually taken up by capillary endothelium. During dehydration and other hypovolemic conditions, depletion of granules in the hypothalamic neurons has been demonstrated.

Diabetes insipidus

In dogs this disease is characterized by excessive thirst, water intake, and urine formation (of low specific gravity). It is a result of either pituitary damage with deficiency of ADH or to failure of renal distal tubules to respond to ADH (nephrogenic diabetes insipidus). The most common cause is pressure atrophy of the pituitary from expanding tumors, which disturbs synthesis in hypothalamic nuclei and destroys neurosecretory pathways in the neurohypophysis. In 27 cases of canine pituitary neoplasms studied by Drs. Koestner and Capen at Ohio State University, 25 had evidence of diabetes insipidus. Diabetes insipidus can also be a consequence of cranial trauma when the pituitary and hypothalamus are damaged.

IMBALANCE OF INORGANIC IONS

The classic studies of Ringer utilizing the perfusion of isolated frog hearts clearly demonstrated the importance of sodium (Na^+), potassium (K^+), magnesium (Mg^{++}), and calcium (Ca^{++}) ions for normal function of the heart. Deficiencies of these cations can cause death due to myocardial failure. Early signs of ionic deficiency in the cardiovascular system include an irregular heartbeat, an abnormal electrocardiogram, and a drop in blood pressure.

Calcium
Ca^{++} in the cell

Ca^{++} is a critically important regulator of cell activity. Ca^{++} within the cell is controlled by mechanisms that regulate (1) passive influx into the cell cytosol from three compartments (extracellular space, mitochondrial matrix, and endoplasmic reticulum cisterna) and (2) active extrusion of Ca^{++} from the cytosol back into these zones by energy-requiring Ca^{++} pumps located within membranes of the cell surface, mitochondrion, and endoplasmic reticulum. Ca^{++} transport across the plasma membrane occurs by a Na^+-Ca^+ exchange transfer; transport across membranes of mitochondria and endoplasmic reticulum is chiefly achieved by energy-requiring Ca^{++} pumps. Even though intracellular and extracellular amounts of calcium may be similar, in ionic form the extracellular Ca^{++} is over 100 times the Ca^{++} in the cytosol.

Plasma Ca⁺⁺

Plasma Ca⁺⁺ is maintained by parathyroid hormone, which stimulates bone resorption and hypercalcemia, and by calcitonin, which inhibits resorption and leads to hypocalcemia. Calcium exists in plasma in ionic form (Ca⁺⁺) and bound to plasma proteins. When low levels of Ca⁺⁺ develop and persist, disturbances occur in skeletal and cardiac muscle contraction, blood coagulation, neural transmission, capillary endothelial junctions, and bone marrow. Ca⁺⁺ is also required for secretory activity in cells storing their secretory products in granules; thus inhibition of granule secretion will influence most endocrine cells.

Tetany

Tetany, a syndrome of convulsive seizures associated with twitching and spasm of skeletal muscle, occurs when there is a deficit of Ca⁺⁺ or Mg⁺⁺ in the circulating blood. The deficiency or imblance of these ions leads to irritability of the neuromuscular junction. In addition to their being required for muscle contractility, the inorganic cations also participate in maintenance of proper osmolarity of body fluids and proper acid-base balance.

Magnesium

Hypomagnesemia leads to muscular tetany and mineralization of soft tissues and arteries. It causes sudden death in horses and lactating cattle fed poor-quality winter rations and in calves on certain silages low in Mg⁺⁺. When tetany occurs in lactating cows grazing lush pasture, the hypomagnesemia is due to high dietary K⁺.

Hypomagnesemia is a major cause of disease in dairy and beef cattle. It often has a rapid course, and death occurs before clinical signs are observed. No specific lesions are present at necropsy.

Sodium

Sodium is the paramount cation in the extracellular fluid, a heritage from primitive unicellular organisms that evolved in seawater. Deficiencies occur as direct loss in severe vomiting and in diarrhea, which is most serious in newborn animals whose kidneys are less able to reabsorb Na⁺. Renal disease in adults may be accompanied by failure of Na⁺ resorption. In Na⁺ deficiency there may be excess intracellular

water because water passes into the cell by osmotic attraction.

Hyponatremia

Low blood Na⁺, acting via Na⁺-sensing mechanisms in the macula densa, increases renin synthesis and secretion by juxtaglomerular cells (see Fig. 15.5). This results in increased plasma angiotensin, which stimulates increased blood pressure (by peripheral vasoconstriction). Angiotensin also circulates in the blood to the adrenal cortex, where it stimulates aldosterone secretion by cells in the zona glomerulosa. Aldosterone, circulating back to the kidney, acts specifically on the ascending loop of Henle to increase the rate of Na⁺ reabsorption.

Small autonomic nerves ramify through the renal cortex, and adrenergic and cholinergic termini are associated with proximal and distal tubules to influence Na + reabsorption by central nervous mechanisms.

Hypernatremia

Elevation of plasma Na⁺ (hypernatremia) can be lethal. Degenerative lesions in the brains of piglets and human infants accidentally given excessive dietary salt illustrate the disastrous effects of Na⁺ on neurons. Sudden shifts from low plasma Na⁺ (hyponatremia) to normal levels may also mimic hypernatremia. When longstanding hyponatremia is rapidly corrected by administration of hypertonic saline, a syndrome of demyelination in the brain occurs. This syndrome can be reproduced experimentally in rats made hyponatremic with vasopressin (which causes renal loss of Na⁺). Subsequent treatment with a hypertonic Na⁺ solution leads to a sudden rise in plasma Na⁺ and death due to brain damage.

Potassium

Potassium is the chief cation of the animal's cells. Deficits affect the myocardium. Excesses that occur in renal disease may affect the cardiac conduction system. The kidney is designed to retain Na⁺ (by tubular resorption) and to excrete K⁺, contrasting mechanisms governed in part by aldosterone from the adrenal. Aldosterone promotes Na⁺ absorption at the expense of K⁺ loss.

Diarrhea causes loss of K⁺.

Diarrhea is the excretion of abnormally fluid

feces. It not only results from enteric disease (either enteritis or malabsorption diseases) but often accompanies gastric, pancreatic, and endocrine diseases. Mechanisms of enteric disease that commonly lead to diarrhea include (1) *inflammation* (enteritis), in which exudation of fluids occurs through a damaged intestinal wall; (2) *hypersecretion,* wherein enterocytes excrete massive amounts of fluids and electrolytes; and (3) *malabsorption,* leading to osmotic diarrhea.

The consequences of diarrhea are dehydration, acidosis, and electrolyte imbalance (Fig. 2.5). Dehydration causes hypovolemia, hemoconcentration, and inadequate tissue perfusion. As with shock, the terminal events of anaerobic

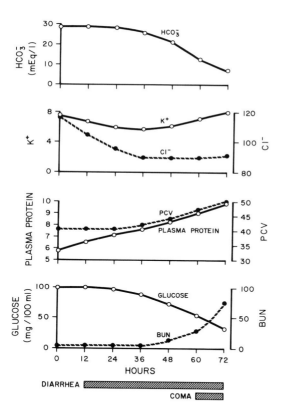

Fig. 2.5. Blood values during fatal enteric infection and diarrhea: acidosis, hyperpotassemia, hypochloridemia, hypoglycemia (due to shift to anaerobic glycolysis), and terminal renal failure. Increase in packed cell volume (PCV) and plasma proteins are related to loss of fluid from plasma. (Data from Tennant et al., *J. Am. Vet. Med. Assoc.* 161:993, 1972)

glycolysis, inhibition of gluconeogenesis, hypoglycemia, and ketoacidosis can lead to death.

Acidosis results from inadequate renal excretion of hydrogen ions (H^+) and absorption of bicarbonate (HCO_3^-). Direct massive losses of HCO_3^- in fecal fluids also contribute to acidosis. Intracellular acidosis occurs, and cells lose K^+, causing hyperkalemia. Extracellular K^+ excess interferes with neuromuscular activity and myocardial contraction, further adding to deficits in tissue perfusion and promoting the development of shock, often with hyperkalemia-induced cardiac malfunction as a major cause.

ACID-BASE IMBALANCE

In plasma and interstitial fluid, hydrogen ion (H^+) concentration must be maintained within narrow limits. The normal pH of body fluids in mammals is 7.4 (7.36–7.44). Death results below pH 7.0 and above pH 7.8. The H^+ constant of extracellular fluids results from a balance between acids and bases. Carbonic acid (H_2CO_3), formed from $CO_2 + H_2O$ is the most important acid in plasma. It is expired via the respiratory system as it is formed during metabolism of organic compounds. Bicarbonate (HCO_3^-) is the principal base. To combat disturbances of acid-base balance, the body uses three fundamental mechanisms: (1) chemical buffering, the major system being $HCO_3^- = H_2CO_3$; (2) release of blood CO_2 through the lungs; and (3) excretion of H^+ by the kidneys. Renal production of ammonia (NH_3) is one of the more important means of increasing H^+ excretion.

Cells are relatively tolerant to changes in pH. In terms of H^+, pH 7.8 is 40% and pH 7.0 is 250% of the H^+ at pH 7.4. Increase or decrease of H^+ causes cell degeneration by affecting the charge on enzymes and other reactive molecules. Cell pH thus influences rates of metabolic reactions, especially the important transport systems on membranes of the mitochondria and on the cell surface.

The state of acid-base balance between pH 7.35 and 7.45 may be disturbed in either direction. *Acidosis,* a drop in blood pH below 7.35, is usually characterized by disorientation, stupor, and coma. *Alkalosis,* an elevation in blood pH above 7.45, leads to excitement, tetany, and convulsions. Two general types of acidosis and alkalosis occur (Table 2.4); metabolic imbalances affect bicarbonate, while respiratory imbalances chiefly affect carbonic acid. Proper bal-

Table 2.4. Classification of acid-base imbalance

Type	Cause	Mechanism
Metabolic acidosis	Severe diarrhea	Bicarbonate loss in feces
	Renal failure	Retention of acid ions
	Ketosis: starvation, diabetes mellitus, severe infections	Ketone production
Metabolic alkalosis	Severe vomiting	Loss of H^+
	Hyperadrenocorticism	Loss of K^+
Respiratory acidosis	Impaired respiration: pneumonia, asphyxiation, respiratory paralysis	CO_2 retention
Respiratory alkalosis	Hyperventilation: fever, hysteria, respiratory center stimulation	Carbonic acid deficiency

ance thus depends largely on control of lung ventilation and cellular metabolism, particularly in the large skeletal muscle masses. During severe exercise, lactic acid builds up in muscle so that during postexercise rest the blood lactic acid is increased and the pH is temporarily lowered. In horses, blood pH may drop below pH 7.0 in venous blood up to 6 minutes after intense exercise. Even more drastic changes occur in greyhounds, which may suffer lethal effects after racing, due in part to large amounts of blood lactic acid and low blood pH.

Acidosis

Clinical signs of acid-base imbalance are usually vague. They include decreased neural transmission, depression of cardiac contraction, and relaxation of arterioles, which leads to decreased peripheral vascular resistance. Severe, acute *respiratory acidosis* may result in neurologic syndromes ("carbon dioxide narcosis") with fatigue, weakness, and tremors, and may end in coma. These signs arise from acidosis-induced increase in blood flow to the brain and are due to altered pH of cerebrospinal fluid (rather than of blood). Acute *metabolic acidosis* also results in neurologic dysfunction although signs are not as common as in the respiratory type.

In severe disease extracellular acidosis may have a protective effect on cells. Acidosis significantly retards the response of cells in culture to anoxic injury by partially stabilizing the plasma membrane, possibly as a result of interaction of H^+ with sulfhydryl groups.

The kidney regulates acid-base balance by controlling bicarbonate.

Secretion of (H^+) and acidification of urine, prime functions of the renal distal tubule, are immediate responses in defense of blood pH.

Renal acidification reclaims all filtered bicarbonate and excretes an amount of acid (H^+) equal to that produced endogenously. Both bicarbonate reabsorption and acid excretion are mediated by a single tubular operation: the exchange of H^+ (secreted) for Na^+ (reabsorbed).

In the proximal convoluted tubule lumen, the secreted H^+ spent in titrating HCO_3^- to H_2CO_3 is not excreted in urine as acid. The H_2CO_3 dissociates to H_2O and CO_2. Carbonic anhydrase located in the microvillous border of the proximal tubule cell reduces the concentration of luminal H_2CO_3 by catalyzing this dissociation. In the distal tubule, the H^+ secretory process further titrates the residual bicarbonate and the major urinary buffers: NH_3 and Na_2HPO_4 → NH_4^+ and NaH_2PO_4.

During metabolic acidosis, bicarbonate is titrated to extinction in the proximal nephron and excess acid is present in the filtrate. The distal secretion of H^+ adds to the increased net H^+ excretion. Urine pH decreases and net acid excretion increases: the classic indices of renal acidification.

END PRODUCTS OF PROTEIN METABOLISM

Plasma metabolites

Ammonia

High levels of ammonia are toxic to the citric acid cycle in mitochondria, especially in neurons. When ammonia arrives in the brain it shifts the reaction: NH_4^+ + β-ketoglutarate −(glutamate dehydrogenase)→ glutamate + additional NH_4^+ −(glutamine synthetase)→ glutamine. Depletion of β-ketoglutarate, a citric acid–cycle intermediate, leads to mitochondrial changes and ultimately to loss of ATP production.

Synthesis of urea in the liver is a major route of ammonia removal. Any step blocked in the urea cycle leads to elevated ammonia in blood (hyperammonemia), which, when prolonged, causes brain damage of a syndrome called *hepatic encephalopathy*. This syndrome progresses: liver destruction → hyperammonemia → accumulation of ammonia in brain → depletion of β-ketoglutarate → encephalopathy. It can be reproduced experimentally by surgically producing a portocaval shunt that diverts the blood coming to the liver in the portal vein away from the liver via the postcaval vein. Ammonia arising from the intestine is not detoxified in the liver and reaches the brain.

Urea and creatinine

Azotemia is the retention of nitrogenous wastes in the blood. It develops from the inability of the kidney to excrete these substances (or through their failure to reach the kidney, as in circulatory failure). The retention of nitrogenous wastes is reflected in elevations of blood urea nitrogen (BUN) and creatinine, and these laboratory tests are taken as indices of renal function. When azotemia becomes symptomatic, the condition is termed *uremia*.

Uremia

Uremia is the complex systemic disease brought about by decreased glomerular filtration and by failure of tubular reabsorption and secretion (Table 2.5). Alterations in uremia include (1) failure to conserve water, (2) electrolyte imbalance, (3) acid-base imbalance, and (4) failure in the excretion of urea and other nonprotein nitrogenous wastes. As renal tubules fail to resorb water, urine volumes may remain large until shortly before death. The ornithine-urea

cycle (Fig. 2.6) is shifted markedly, and failure of the kidney to secrete ammonia and to absorb Na^+ leads to progressive metabolic acidosis.

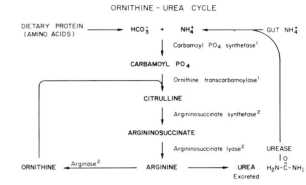

Fig. 2.6. Metabolic pathways of ornithine-urea cycle. Enzymes are located in mitochondria (*1*) or in the cytoplasm (*2*).

Vomiting, weakness, congestion of mucous membranes, and paleness and coolness of the skin are seen in animals with uremia. Neurologic signs range from drowsiness to coma. The abnormal electroencephalographic changes in dogs are related to increased Ca^{++} content in the brain. An ammonia odor of the breath is common. In dogs, ulceration and inflammation of the tongue, oral mucosa, and stomach are nearly always present in severe uremia.

Gastrointestinal lesions

Uremic gastropathy with edema and ulceration is common in dogs. There is striking diffuse arteriopathy with marked calcification of arte-

Table 2.5. Mechanisms of chronic uremia in the dog

Depression of		Leads to	Pathology
Glomerular filtration	PO_4 retention SO_4 retention H^+ retention Urea retention	→ Parathyroid hyperplasia → Bone resorption → OSTEOPOROSIS and hypocalcemia → Acidosis ══════════ → ACIDOSIS	
Tubular secretion and reabsorption	NH_4^+ retention	→ Hyperammonemia	
	K^+ retention	→ Hyperkalemia	→ CARDIAC DYSFUNCTION
	Na^+ loss	→ Hyponatremia	
Tubular detoxification	→ Toxin accumulation		→ ANEMIA and VASCULAR DAMAGE

FOCUS

Electrolyte imbalance and acidosis are life-threatening in uremia.

In most species, renal failure is associated with serum calcium concentrations that are either normal or moderately low. Metabolic acidosis or uremia tends to keep ionized calcium at normal levels and thus prevents tetany. The horse kidney is uniquely able to maintain serum calcium, and equine uremia may lead to hypercalcemia accompanying the hypophosphatemia.

The clinical pathologic findings below are from an 11-year-old male beagle with chronic dermatitis of 4 months over the rump. No ulcers were present in skin, but the haircoat contained fleas and large amounts of flea feces. For the previous 5 weeks the dog had been gradually losing weight. He refused food for the last 2 days yet continued to drink much water. The skin failed to return to normal contours when stretched (evidence of dehydration). The breath was foul, and the teeth had much tartar. The oral cavity had many ulcers, varying from a few mm to 3 cm in diameter, on the tongue, gingiva, and pharyngeal surfaces.

Clinical pathological findings:

Test	Uremic Dog	Normal
Blood urea nitrogen	228.0	30 mg/dl
Creatinine	2.1	1.5 mg/dl
Glucose	213.0	100 mg/dl
Calcium	7.2	9.9–12.0 mg/dl
Phosphorus	15.0	2.5–5.0 mg/dl
Potassium	6.0	3.6–5.6 mEq/l
Sodium	137.0	141–155 mEq/l
Chloride	91.0	96–122 mEq/l
Hematocrit	25.0	37–55%
Total leukocytes	21.3	6–17 thousand/cmm

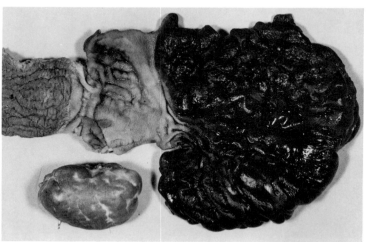

Diffuse edema, hemorrhage, and necrosis of gastric mucosa, corpus, and fundus (antrum spared), dog with uremia. Kidney (*bottom left*) with amyloid.

The clinical diagnosis on this dog was uremia, chronic nephritis, chronic dermatitis, and ulcerative stomatitis and glossitis. The pathologic diagnoses were chronic interstitial nephritis, gastric ulcers, and plasmacytic gastritis with glandular atrophy, plasmacytic cystitis with epithelial hyperplasia and cysts of the bladder epithelium, and uremia myopathy.

rial walls throughout the stomach; edema and hemorrhage correlate with the degree of vascular injury. Ulceration occurs via a mucosal energy deficiency due to vascular lesions superimposed over both local and systemic hypoxia (Fig. 2.7). These are compounded by bile reflux and back diffusion of H^+ from the gastric lumen. Gastric surface mucus, which acts as a diffusion barrier and inhibits the proteolytic action of pepsin, is diminished in uremia, and this contributes to ulcer formation. Mast cell histamine promotes gastrointestinal lesions via its functions in vascular permeability, calcification, and parietal cell chemostimulation.

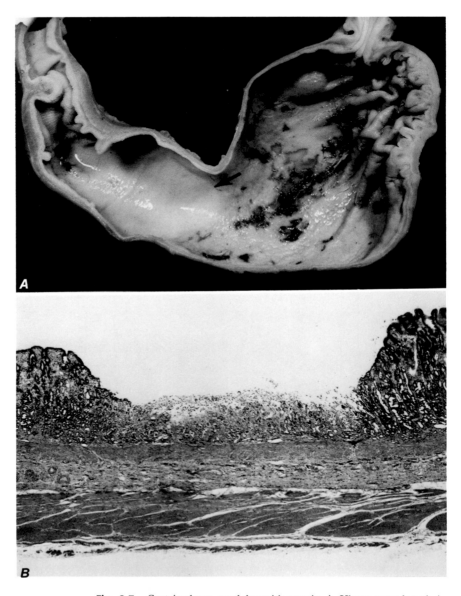

Fig. 2.7. Gastric ulcers, aged dog with uremia. A. Ulcers occur largely in fundus and body. B. Ulcer involves erosion of the mucosa and does not extend into deep layers of the gastric wall. Affected body and fundus are clearly demarcated from normal pylorus (*arrow*).

Lung

Pulmonary hyperemia and edema (and attendant dyspnea) are common manifestations of uremia. Acidosis depresses membrane transport mechanisms, which may explain injury to the alveolar wall. Lung function is also hyperactive in efforts to eliminate carbon dioxide. Diffuse calcium deposition in the alveolar wall may lead to solid, gritty, pale lungs ("pumice lung").

Muscle

Hyperkalemia and hypocalcemia are the most significant of the electrolyte imbalances in terminal uremia. They may influence myocardial contractility and be responsible for a twitching phenomenon of skeletal muscle. Progressive *myocardiopathy,* typical of final stages of uremia, results from the additive effects of plasma ionic changes, anemia, hypertension, and hypervolemia. Myocardiopathy produces and is further exaggerated by anoxia. Skeletal muscle is affected by the same degenerative changes, and because of its total mass, the products liberated from dying myocytes contribute to the clinical uremia syndrome.

Parathyroid

Progressive parathyroid hyperplasia and increases in serum parathyroid hormone during uremia are compensatory mechanisms that counter other factors suppressing serum calcium. Secondary hyperparathyroidism leads to increased osteoclastic bone resorption. It also suppresses dietary intake of phosphorus, which suggests that it is, in part, a consequence of adaptations to maintain phosphorus homeostasis in the face of nephron loss.

Bone

Osteoporosis ("renal osteodystrophy") occurs in uremia. Dr. Robert Norrdin, at Colorado State University, has clearly shown an increase in osteoid surfaces and increased osteoclastic resorption in uremic beagles. *Acidosis* in terminal uremia is a major contributor to osteoporosis; it suppresses bone matrix formation by osteocytes, and osteoclastic resorption leads to removal of mineral at a greater rate than its surrounding matrix. Affected bones, which become osteoporotic and soft, are responsible for the term "rubber jaw syndrome" in dogs.

Although *hypocalcemia* contributes to osteoclastic resorption, the changes in bone are independent of parathyroid hormone levels. The kidney is necessary for synthesis of the active metabolite of vitamin D. Failure of damaged tubular epithelial cells to produce this hormone prevents the intestinal epithelium from synthesizing the Ca^{++}-binding protein required for absorption. This contributes to the hypocalcemia-hyperparathyroidism-osteodystrophy pathway in uremia.

Renal lesions in diabetes suppress the enzymes needed to hydroxylate vitamin D, that is, $1,25(OH)_2D_3$ is not produced. Studies by Dr. Steven Weisbrode, at Ohio State University, indicate that target organs of vitamin D/parathyroid hormone may be resistant to hormone action; in uremic rats, increased osteoid covering of bony trabeculae in metaphyses produced resistance to the action of vitamin D (in stimulating osteoclastic removal of Ca^{++}).

Blood

Anemia is invariably present in uremia. It is caused both by the shortened life span of erythrocytes and by diminished erythropoiesis, which in turn is caused by low plasma levels of erythropoietin. The kidney, a potent source of erythropoietin, is damaged sufficiently to affect its synthesis. Destruction is not caused by an intrinsic property of the uremic erythrocyte. In man, transfusion of uremic erythrocytes into normal patients allows normal survival; normal erythrocytes transfused into uremic patients have shortened life spans.

Lymphoid system

Lymphoid tissue atrophy occurs in long-standing uremia. Immunoreactivity is depressed, allegedly due to a failure of interaction of antibody with antigen. Uremic animals have prolonged skin graft survival, diminished delayed hypersensitivity reactions, and decreased graft-versus-host activity—all associated with depression of cell-mediated reactivity. Cell proliferation is suppressed in all tissues in chronic uremia, and it is probable that this same effect is operating on macrophages and lymphocytes.

Pancreas

Acinar cell atrophy occurs in chronic uremia, possibly associated with cachexia. Focal and diffuse dilatation of acinar and centroacinar ductular lumens (pancreatic ectasia) is common. Dehydration and excess vagal stimulation have been suggested as contributory. In dogs, there may be an association between diabetes mellitus and *pancreatitis;* 40–50% of human uremic patients develop pancreatitis in association with acidosis and dehydration.

ADDITIONAL READING

Brobst, D. Pathophysiologic and adaptive changes in acid-base disorders. *J. Am. Vet. Med. Assoc.* 183:773, 1983.

Krum, S. H., and Osborne, C. A. Heatstroke in the dog: A polysystemic disorder. *J. Am. Vet. Med. Assoc.* 170:531, 1977.

Lage, A. L. Nephrogenic diabetes insipidis in a dog. *J. Am. Vet. Med. Assoc.* 163:251, 1973.

Lassen, E. D., et al. Effects of racing on hematologic and serum biochemical valves in greyhounds. *J. Am. Vet. Med. Assoc.* 188:1299, 1986.

Moore-Ede, M. C., et al. Circadian timekeeping in health and disease. *New Engl. J. Med.* 309:530, 1983.

Painter, E. E., et al. Exchange and distribution of fluid in dehydration in the dog. *Am. J. Physiol.* 152:66, 1948.

Sandals, W. C. D. Salt poisoning in cattle. *Can. Vet. J.* 19:136, 1978.

Strombeck, D. R., et al. Hyperammonemia and hepatic encephalopathy in the dog. *J. Am. Vet. Med. Assoc.* 166:1105, 1975.

Death and Dying

3

DEATH of an animal is based on irreversible cessation of activity in heart, lungs, or brain. Absence of function in any one of these organs will cause sudden collapse. After *somatic death* (death of the body), cells of an animal may live for several hours, although body fluids become so acidic and devoid of oxygen that the cells rapidly lose function.

Dying is the most complex process the pathologist must consider. When it is short, as in the action of cyanide on the cell enzyme cytochrome oxidase, the cell lesions produced are subtle and beyond the scope of routine pathologic methods. When dying extends over a long period of time, lesions are often so extensive, multiple, and interrelated that they are difficult to interpret. The excitement of discovering, studying, and integrating these pieces of evidence toward an acceptable thesis on the cause of death, however, is the reward of thorough pathologic examination.

The question, Why did the animal die? should not be carelessly dismissed. There is a tendency to prefer simplicity in determining causes of death for legal purposes. True, death can be initiated by specific agents that lead to processes such as inflammation, cardiovascular disease, or neoplasia. But the process of dying is much more complex. Kidney failure induced by mercury poisoning is responsible for death, yet determining the dying process is a demanding intellectual exercise, considering the effects of nitrogenous wastes, endogenous toxic peptides, and imbalances in electrolytes and acid-base equilibrium. The effects of these substances or events on brain centers for respiration and cardiovascular action—or directly on lungs, kidney, and heart—will answer the *why* in the question of dying.

PATTERNS OF TISSUE DEATH
Necrosis

Necrosis is death of tissue in the living animal. Foci of necrosis in tissue have characteristics that lead the pathologist in certain directions regarding etiology. Some of the distinct patterns of different etiologic agents are listed below.

Coagulation necrosis

In coagulation necrosis, affected tissue is pale and homogeneous and differs in texture from the surrounding normal tissue. Tissue architecture is preserved, and the outline of normal tissue components can be seen. Necrotic tissue often appears as granular irregular foci; for example, focal necrosis of the bovine placenta infected with *Brucella abortus* typically has dense granular white-tan areas that obscure the translucent membranes of the normal placenta (Fig. 3.1).

Focal necrotic areas are usually surrounded by zones of inflammation. While these lesions may be described according to their inflammatory component (focal purulent laryngitis), it is more precise to recognize the lesion as *focal necrosis* since that is the primary process. The pattern of focal necrosis in cattle is characteristic of infection of the bacterium *Fusobacterium necrophorum* (Fig. 3.2).

Necrotic lesions often contain hemorrhages. In focal necrosis, petechiae are at the periphery of the lesion. In diffuse necrosis, extravasted blood may color the entire organ red-black (see uremia, chapter 2). In severe uremic gastric necrosis, injury to the gastric vascular system leads to edema and hemorrhage that cause the necrotic gastric mucosa to be markedly thickened.

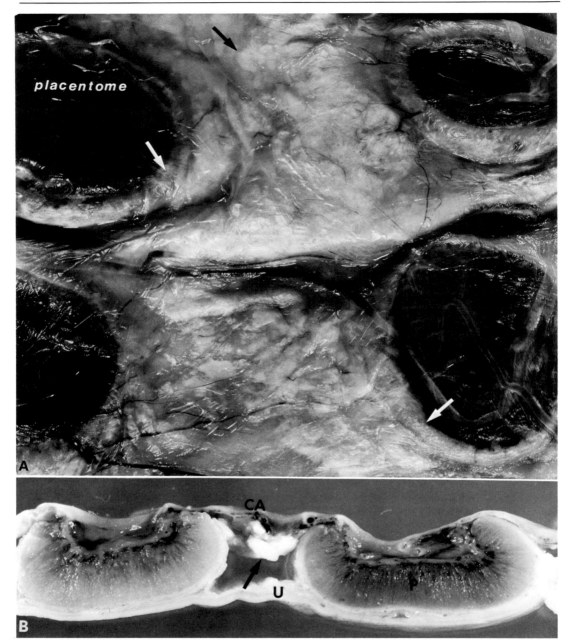

Fig. 3.1. Necrosis, placenta, cow infected with *Brucella abortus*. A. Necrotic tissue and exudate around placentomes (*white arrow*) and in interplacentomal spaces (*black arrow*). B. Cross section of placentome (*P*) appears normal, but there is necrotic tissue and exudate in interplacentomal spaces, between the uterine wall (*U*) and the chorioallantoic membrane (*CA*).

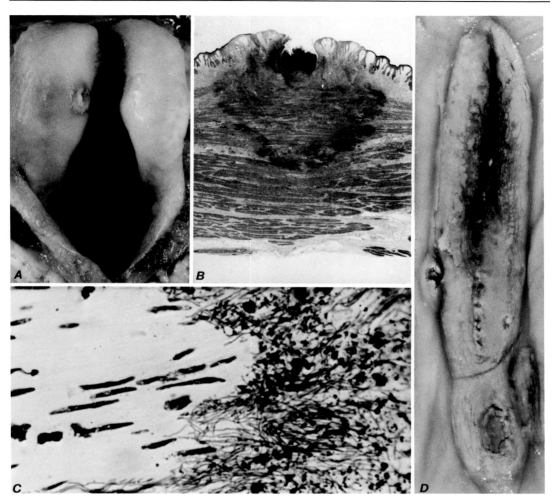

Fig. 3.2. Necrosis caused by *Fusobacterium necrophorum*, cow. A. Larynx. B. Histology: necrotic tissue deep in muscle layers. C. *F. necrophorum* located at margin of healthy and necrotic tissue. D. Linear foci of necrosis, esophagus.

Microscopically, necrotic cells are distorted, smudged, homogeneous, and opaque (because of coagulation of protein). The coagulated cell persists after cell detail has disappeared. Nuclei are contracted; they may be *pyknotic* (shrunken and dense with irregularities in the nuclear membrane), *karyorrhectic* (nuclear membrane rupture, with fragmentation and release of nuclear contents), or *karyolytic* (complete dissolution of the nucleus with loss of chromatin). If necrosis is recent, cells may stain deeply with eosin, but if *autolysis* (dissolution by their own enzymes) has occurred, cells take up little stain.

Some common causes of coagulation necrosis are bacterial toxins, foci of viral replication, and infarction. The appearance of necrotic cells depends not only on the type of degeneration but also on the time elapsing between injury and fixation for microscopic study. Sufficient time must elapse for pathologic changes to occur.

Caseation necrosis is a variant of coagulation necrosis in which dead tissue has a firm, dry, cheesy consistency. It occurs when dead cells are converted into a granular friable mass resembling cottage cheese. Caseation develops in diseases such as tuberculosis and tularemia.

The chronicity of the cellular reaction and the presence of special lipids prevents resolution or liquefaction.

Liquefactive necrosis

Rapid enzymatic dissolution of the cell that results in complete destruction is called liquefactive necrosis. It is seen in bacterial infections that lead to pus formation in which proteolytic enzymes are released from leukocytes; that is, pus is the evidence of liquefactive necrosis.

The brain responds to severe anoxic and toxic injuries with rapid enzymic digestion and foci of dissolution known as *malacia*. This too can progress to a form of liquefactive necrosis.

Enzymic necrosis of fat

In this pattern, lipases split the neutral fat in adipose cells, releasing the lipid and imparting a granular eosinophilic appearance to fat cells. This type of necrosis is seen in trauma of adipose tissue and commonly accompanies pancreatic injury. Unidentified enzymes released from damaged pancreatic acinar cells free the lipases in adipose cells, which cause autodigestion of triglycerides. Fat, free in connective tissues, incites inflammation and phagocytosis, which separate enzymic necrosis from autolysis. Cholesterol clefts, giant cells, and calcium are often present.

Gangrene

The superimposition of growth of saprophytic bacteria on necrosis results in a histologic pattern that is a mixture of coagulation and liquefactive necrosis. This *gangrenous necrosis* may occur because of bacterial invasion of an infarct or as a result of restriction of blood supply in an established bacterial infection, caused by collection of fluid and intravascular clotting.

Gangrene is also applied to necrosis of tissues in an extremity in which vascular occlusion has resulted in coagulation necrosis. When pus-producing bacterial infection does not occur, the tissue mummifies and the condition is referred to as *dry gangrene* (Fig. 3.3). Affected tissue is cool, dry, and discolored. There is a sharp demarcation of inflammatory tissue, preventing systemic infection. When pus-producing organisms invade, the combination of ischemia and infection produces putrefactive, foul-smelling tissues, a lesion called *moist gangrene.*

Necrobiosis

In *necrobiosis,* cell death is programmed, and the cytopathic changes evolve in orderly and reproducible sequences. Necrobiosis occurs in adult animals as part of normal cell turnover, such as the loss of cornified squamous cells of skin. Keratinocytes become filled with keratin, nuclei degenerate, cell surfaces no longer adhere, and cells desquamate from the skin surface. Necrobiosis is also seen in erythrocytes, which die when their hemoglobin molecules begin to precipitate and new hemoglobin cannot be resynthesized. The process actually begins immediately after maturation when erythocyte nuclei degenerate. The genome is no longer required for protein synthesis, and in mammals, nuclei are shed from the cell. Cell death occurs without sequelae because cell function has been fulfilled and the cells have been replaced with new erythrocytes.

Necrobiosis is a prominent feature of embryonic development. For example, tail breakdown during metamorphosis of tadpole amphibians has been used as a model for study. The tail regresses because of a thyroxin-dependent autolysis initiated in skeletal muscle cells. As myocytes disintegrate, their debris is removed by massive numbers of macrophages that infiltrate into the regressing tail. Similar changes occur in smooth muscle cells of the involuting uterus after pregnancy in mammals.

Postmortem degeneration

Interpretation of lesions is often clouded by degeneration that has taken place between the time of death and necropsy. Postmortem changes vary in the rapidity with which they occur, depending on environmental temperature and humidity (Table 3.1) and the condition of the animal (layers of fat, hair, or feathers act as insulators against heat loss after death).

Postmortem degeneration is due to total diffuse anoxia. Autolytic changes mimic early ischemic change and in fact have a hypoxic basis. Immediately after death, muscle cells show a massive uncontrolled burst of glycolysis. Uncoupled to oxidative phosphorylation, this energy is dissipated as heat. The body temperature (if measured in deep muscle masses) will be very high for several minutes after death (Fig. 3.4).

Cellular organelles degenerate according to their oxygen requirements, and the differences

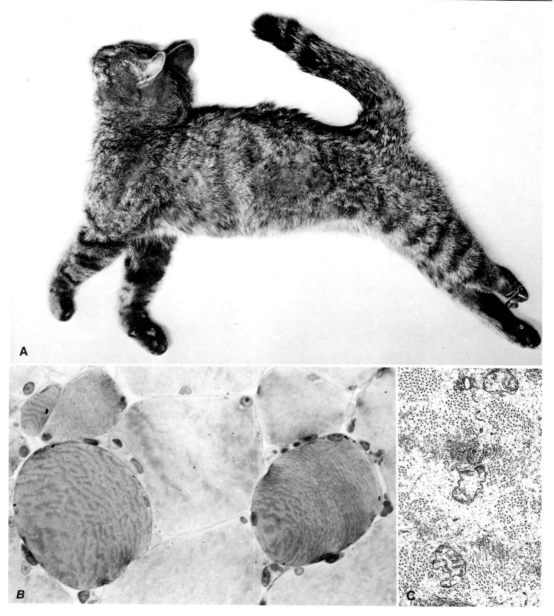

Fig. 3.3. Tetanus, cat. Gangrene of the hind leg (trap injury) provides the focus for growth of *Clostridium tetani*. A. Rigidity due to tetanic spasm (note tail and ear) caused by the neurotoxin *tetanospasmin*. B. Cell swelling and necrosis, skeletal muscle, produced by an uncharacterized myotoxin. C. Myofibrils disrupted by myotoxin.

Table 3.1.   Postmortem changes

Algor mortis (cooling)—aids in estimating time of death
Rigor mortis (rigidity)—begins 2–4 hours after death
Postmortem clotting (thrombi are antemortem)
Postmortem imbibition (hemolytic staining)
Hypostatic congestion (dependent lividity)—due to gravity
Pseudomelanosis—Fe + S = FeS, giving shades of green
    and black
Autolysis—invokes no inflammatory response
Putrefaction—rupture and displacement of organs
Emphysema (due to gas-producing bacteria)—may cause
    rupture of organs
Biliary imbibition

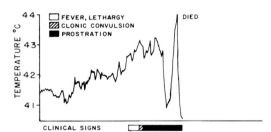

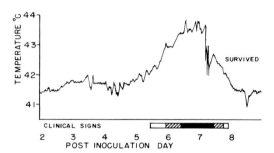

Fig. 3.4. Body temperature of two chickens with Newcastle disease (obtained by intraperitoneal implantation of radiotelemetric transmitter). The high terminal spike in the chicken that died occurred after death and is due to a burst of activity in muscle associated with anoxia.

in postmortem change are reflected in these requirements. The initial change occurs in mitochondria; in dog heart muscle it is due to accumulation of lactic acid and lower pH. Postmortem autolysis is characterized by relatively uniform destruction of the cell. Protein disintegrates into small granules and is distributed throughout the cells.

Rigor mortis

Rigor mortis, or stiffening of muscles, occurs 2–4 hours after death. Immediately after the circulation of blood ceases, there is a massive burst of metabolic activity as substrates are depleted. Much heat is produced in this period immediately after death, and there is a progressive decrease in the pH of muscle. Oxygen, adenosine triphosphate (ATP), and creatine phosphate are also decreased. Muscle fibers shorten as they pass into rigor. This movement resembles contraction in several ways: (1) it is initiated by an efflux of calcium from the sarcoplasmic reticulum into the cytosol of the myocyte, (2) it uses ATP as an energy source, and (3) the structural changes that occur resemble those of contraction.

Rigor begins earliest in cardiac muscle and expresses the blood from the left ventricle. Failure indicates antemortem degeneration. Of the skeletal muscles, the head and neck are first affected in most species, with progression to the extremities. Rigor disappears as putrefaction begins, a matter of 1–2 days, depending on external factors. Rigor mortis is enhanced by high metabolic activity and temperature before death and in diseases such as strychnine poisoning. It is delayed by starvation, cachexia, and cold.

Putrefaction occurs when dead tissue is invaded by anaerobic, saphrophytic organisms that digest proteins and form gas. Clostridia, which are normally present in feces, are common in putrefaction. Foul-smelling substances formed during putrefaction include ammonia, hydrogen sulfide, indole, skatol, putrescine, and cadaverine. Tissue turns green and brown from breakdown of hemoglobin and formation of hydrogen sulfide.

NECROPSY AND LABORATORY TECHNIQUES
The postmortem examination

The postmortem examination (*necropsy*) is often the most important factor in establishing a diagnosis. Evaluation of gross lesions tells the pathologist what type of disease process has occurred and to what extent it has damaged specific organ systems. The methodical examination of organs and tissues of the dead animal may be called either *necropsy* (Gr. *necros,* dead body, plus *opsis,* sight) or *autopsy* (Gr. *autopsia,* seen by oneself). Necropsy is preferred by veterinary pathologists; autopsy is used in medical pathology. *Biopsy* is the removal and examination of tissue from the living animal.

Lesions should be recorded in precise scientific language so that future reading does not require guesswork as to what a pathologist actually saw. Since pathology bridges the gap between science and clinical practice, its language is open to the misuse of "practicality." Words like sepsis, pneumonia, and nephrosis are often used differently by clinician and pathologist. It is imperative that scientific language be precise because blurring of language leads to blurring of our understanding of how biology works.

Although the language of pathology must be as accurate as possible, poorly characterized phenomena should not be defined with overzealous precision. In rare instances, lesions fall into a hazy borderland between two processes. If there is need to be deliberately vague the suffix -*pathy* (Gr. *pathos,* suffering or disease) is used. For example, when it is uncertain whether a lymph node lesion is neoplastic or inflammatory, lymphadenopathy is appropriate.

Gross pathology

The necropsy should begin with a careful inspection of the body surface, including orifices, hair, teeth, and eyes. Surface identification marks such as tattoos, ear tags, or ear notches should be noted and recorded, including notations of numbers that are faded or apt to be misread. Traumatic lesions should be specifically identified. Internally, organs should be examined systematically with attention to size, symmetry, color, and texture (Table 3.2). Organ surfaces or cross sections may be described as smooth, rough, granular, or pitted. An increase in size may indicate a controlled growth increase or a diffuse process of fluid exudation such as serous inflammation or edema. It may also suggest a deep-seated mass such as an abscess, cyst, hematoma, granuloma, or neoplasm.

The distribution of blood vessels, lymphatics, and nerves to a pathologic organ should be ex-

FOCUS

Statistics in pathology

Data derived from clinical pathology studies or from a series of necropsies, just as from an experiment, have practical value since it often provides a basis for decisions about patient care. Statistical analysis of the relative frequency with which kinds of lesions occur provides a standard way in which data are presented so that probability can be predicted with a reasonable degree of certainty.

In the early 1800s Gauss and de Laplace established curves of errors, the familiar symmetrical *bell-shaped curve,* believing that biologic phenomena could be described in these curves. Later, modified "wave-crest" curves were developed that were better suited to a particular situation. Much of how we use statistics in agriculture and medicine began in 1900 when Karl Pearson published his *chi-square test* of goodness of fit, a formula for measuring how well a hypothesis fits observations. In theory, dice will fall equally often on each of their six faces. When rolled 600 times, one number often comes up more frequently, for in practice there is chance and the ratios are almost always different. How well does the hypothesis that the die is fair fit the data? The chi-square test provided one measure of how well theory and data correspond. It is used for hypotheses and data where observations naturally fall into discrete categories. If, for example, you are testing whether a drug is toxic to the liver, animals must be divided among four groups: treated and liver lesions, treated and no lesions, untreated and lesions, and untreated and no lesions. If the treatment is not toxic, you expect no difference in recovery rate be-

▶

tween treated and untreated animals. But chance and uncontrollable variables in biologic activity dictate that there will almost always be some difference.

One of the most important judgments in using statistics is the initial decision as to whether the samples being used are independent or dependent. Repeated clinical measurements on a subject are usually *dependent* (i.e., the value of an early observation is related to the value of a later observation). The chi-square test, analysis of variance, the two-sample *t* test, and many statistical tests, however, require *independent* values. These values are more appropriate for analyzing lesions and other data from the necropsy.

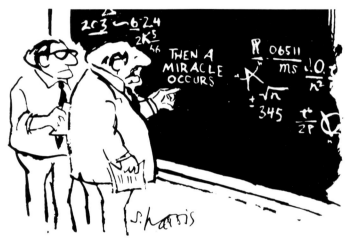

"I think you should be more explicit here in step two."

©1977 Sidney Harris, *American Scientist*

While of enormous value if used properly, statistics sometimes creates spurious impressions of objectivity, especially when scientists use soft data or inaccurate samples on which to base their mathematical manipulations. Critics suggest that this is a way of escaping the responsibility of admitting ignorance. Others point to the increasing use of complex models generated to "fit" reams of data in some statistical sense—models that can become a fantasyland without any connection to the real world. But no matter. Society today demands numbers to measure risk. Statistical inference provides a new style of reasoning, not by providing new facts but by changing the ways that we form our opinions.

Table 3.2. Necropsy protocol

The carcass is that of a (development, nourishment, color, sex, breed, species) of ___ years, measuring ___ cm in length. Temperature, rigor, lividity. *Skin* and *hair coat* in general. *Eye:* color, pupils, corneae, lens, sclerae. *Ears:* lesions, discharge. *Nose:* turbinates. *Oral cavity:* teeth, tongue, tonsils, salivary duct orifices. *Neck:* enlargements. *Lymph nodes:* general or local enlargement. *Thorax:* size, symmetry. *Mammary glands:* size, teats, masses. *Abdomen:* shape, scars (location, age). *Genitalia:* lesions (scars, discharge). *Limbs:* asymmetries, deformities, edema, paws/hooves. *Subcutaneous fat:* amount, color. *Peritoneal cavity:* fluid, surfaces, abnormal mesenteric relations. *Left pleural cavity:* fluid, surfaces, thoracic duct. *Right pleural cavity. Mediastinum.*

HEART
Weights ___ gm. *Epicardium:* surface, fat, chambers (size, content, clotting time if fluid). Congenital abnormalities. *Endocardium. Valves:* measurements and descriptions. *Myocardium:* thickness, color, consistency, lesions. *Coronary blood vessels:* caliber, lining, walls.

LUNGS
Left weighs ___ g; right, ___ g. *Left lung:* pleural surfaces, hilar blood vessels, bronchi, lymph nodes, cut surface (color, wetness, appearance of bronchi, vessels, general consistency). *Right lung:* "Similar to left lung with exception of ___."

SPLEEN
Weights ___ g. Surface. Consistency. Hilar vessels. Cut surface: color, trabeculae, white pulp.

GASTROINTESTINAL TRACT
Esophagus: dilatation. *Stomach:* mucosa (thickening of rugae, or edema), color. *Small intestine. Cecum. Colon.*

PANCREAS
Size, color, consistency. Lobulations, islets, ducts.

LIVER
Weighs ___ g. Surface and cut surface: lobule architecture, color, consistency. Local lesions.

GALLBLADDER
Bile amounts, color, consistency; mucosa, wall thickness. *Extrahepatic bile ducts:* caliber, wall thickness, abnormalities.

ADRENALS
Size, consistency. Cut section: color, width of zones. Lesions.

KIDNEYS
Left weighs ___ g; right ___ g (start with left, describe together if similar). Surface and cut surface: color, cortical thickness, striation, glomeruli. *Pelvis:* size, architecture, arcuate arteries. *Ureter:* size, color, thickness, lesions.

UROGENITAL SYSTEMS
Bladder: contents (volume, color, clarity), mucosa, wall and ureteral orifices. *Urethra. Prostate:* size, uniformity, location, appearance and consistency of abnormal areas. *Seminal vesicles. Testicles. Vagina. Uterus and cervix. Ovary and tubes.*

VASCULAR SYSTEM
Aorta: caliber, elasticity, intima, renal artery orifices, other branches. *Abdominal veins:* check anastomoses for portal hypertension (branch to vertebral veins, azygos vein). *Aberrant vessels.*

LYMPHATIC SYSTEM
General or local enlargement.

NECK ORGANS
Thyroid: size, color, consistency, nodularity. *Parathyroids. Thymus:* weight, color, consistency. *Larynx. Carotid bodies and carotid sinus* (visible?).

MUSCLE AND SKELETAL SYSTEMS
Important local or general abnormalities not covered under carcass description.

BONE MARROW
Color, consistency (mushy, cellular, firm, fibrous, gelatinous), quantity.

BRAIN
Weighs ___ g. *Skull. Meninges:* texture, fluid. *Convolutions. Sulci. Color. Consistency. Symmetry. Blood vessels.*

amined. Canals, ducts, major arteries, and intestines should be *patent* (open and unobstructed). They may show partial or total *stenosis* (narrowing or stricture) or *dilatation* (the condition of being dilated or stretched; *dilation* is the action of dilating) (Fig. 3.5). *Atresia* or imperforation indicates the absence or abnormal closure of an opening.

Torsion and intussusception

Organs suspended by ligaments of mesentery may be deprived of their blood supply by *torsion* (the twisting around of attachments). *Gastric torsion* occurs in large breeds of dogs and, because of pressure on the portal venous system, leads to ischemia of the stomach and intestine. *Torsion of the lung* occurs (rarely) in dogs and cats, usu-

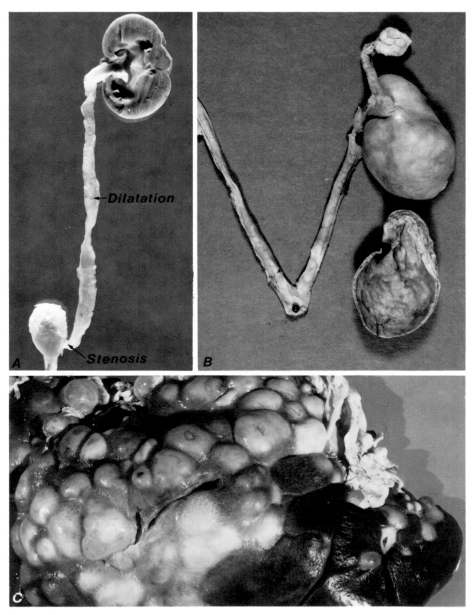

Fig. 3.5. A. Stenosis of ureter as it empties into bladder with hydroureter and hydronephrosis, cat. B. Cyst, uterine wall, dog. C. Parasite cysts caused by *Echinococcus granulosis,* liver, pig.

ally associated with pleural space disease, thoracic surgery, or trauma. Deep-chested breeds of dogs such as Afghan hounds are predisposed; the narrow right middle lung lobe, which is poorly fixed between the thoracic wall and mediastinum, is predisposed to rotation on its longitudinal axis.

In the intestinal tract, an *intussusception* is an invagination (infolding) of one segment of intestine into another. The character of the lesion is important because intussusception may occur as an *agonal* (occurring at the moment of or just before death) or even a postmortem event. Antemortem intussusceptions have marked inflammatory changes.

Color changes are important clues.

Aside from putrefactive changes, important color changes develop prior to death. Diffuse redness suggests *hyperemia* (congestion), an increased amount of blood in tissue. Conversely, pallor may indicate that the tissue is *ischemic* (bloodless). Hemorrhages also cause redness, but they usually are present as tiny foci of blood. Brown is caused by the pigments melanin and lipofuscin or, if combined with hues of yellow, by pigments released from degenerating erythrocytes. Green may be bile but can also be due to pigments produced by chromogenic fungi and bacteria that have invaded tissue or to large numbers of neutrophils that release greenish myeloperoxidase (e.g., the green tinge of bovine pus). Green discoloration of intestines can follow treatment with boluses of sulfonamides or antibiotics that contain green dyes.

Calculi

Calculi are abnormal masses (usually containing mineral salts) that develop in organs as a result of accretion or inspissation (thickening) of luminal contents. The combined effects of stasis, infection, and high mineral content of tissue fluids are usually associated with their presence. Classified by anatomic location, calculi may be biliary (gallstones), dental (plaque), intestinal (enteroliths), gastric (bezoars), renal (kidney stones), urinary bladder, or pancreatic duct. Varying shapes of calculi give rise to descriptive adjectives such as "hemp seed," "coral," and "staghorn." Renal calculi are especially important because they lodge in the ureter, producing hydroureter, hydronephrosis, and atrophy of the kidney (Fig. 3.6).

Cysts

A cyst (Gr. *kystis*, bladder) is a pathologic, fluid-filled sac bounded by a wall. Fluid is often secreted by epithelial cells lining the wall but it can arise by seepage into the space. Cysts are often derived from normal structures that become dilated. Renal cysts (Fig. 3.7) arise from dilation of the nephron and frequently occur in very old animals. Epidermal inclusion cysts filled with sebaceous and epidermal debris are found in skin. Cysts commonly arise in some neoplasms (e.g., the papillary cystadenoma of

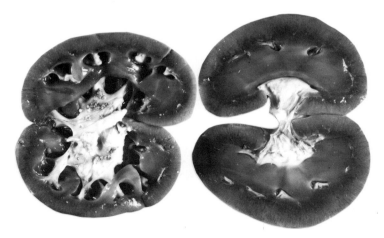

Fig. 3.6. Renal calculi, goat: normal kidney (*right*) and kidney with hydronephrosis due to calculi in the renal pelvis.

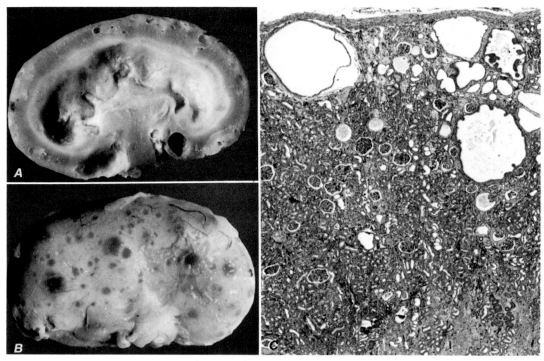

Fig. 3.7. A and B. Renal cysts in an aged dog associated with hydronephrosis. C. Histology.

the mammary gland). *Parasitic* cysts may form in viscera. The hydatid cyst in the liver, lungs, and other viscera is due to proliferation and growth of the larval form of the canine tapeworm *Echinococcus granulosus* (Fig. 3.5). The germinative layer secretes the "hydatid fluid."

Laboratory investigation

The observation of abnormal cells in vivo or in their living state after biopsy is tedious and time-consuming, and the results are not sufficiently reproducible for application to routine pathologic examination of sick animals. Limited use is made of cell cultures derived from pathologic tissues (particularly from tumors and viral infection), but the processes in vitro do not mimic cytopathology in vivo.

The evaluation of pathologic material therefore has been largely restricted to cells fixed by formaldehyde and other special solutions. Fixation of cells, followed by staining to accentuate special structures, allows the pathologist to evaluate degenerative changes in the basis of established and reproducible disease processes.

In examining pathologic tissue, it is essential to be aware of all abnormal conditions existing in the animal. Without this information, making a direct analogy between cellular change and its cause is likely to result in error.

Microscopic examination

For histologic examination, small tissue samples are collected and placed in 10% formalin (about 4% formaldehyde), which hardens and fixes proteins. Pieces should be less than 5 mm thick and the volume of fixative at least 10 times that of tissue. Formalin produces rapid penetration of tissue and is a reducing agent that forms bridging links between proteins. Other fixatives are used for special studies. Bouin's solution (picric acid, formalin, and acetic acid in a ratio of 15:5:1) induces brilliant staining and is excellent for photography. Glutaraldehyde is used for tissues that are to be processed for electron microscopy; tissues should collected within minutes of death and should not be larger than 1 mm^3.

After tissues have been properly fixed, they are washed in water for several minutes and processed by dehydration in ethanols and by infiltration with paraffin. In parasitic infestations, the fixative may need to be centrifuged and the sediment examined because nematodes can migrate out of brain and lung tissues into the solution during fixation.

Tissue sections are cut from the paraffin-embedded tissue blocks and stained, usually with hematoxylin and eosin. Special stains are used to detect specific substances in tissue. The periodic acid–Schiff, or PAS, technique stains carbohydrates including glycogen, glycoproteins, and glycolipids; it is especially useful for capsules on fungi and for the glycoproteins of basement membranes in the renal glomerulus. Gram stains are available for detecting bacteria in tissue.

Tissue selection determines accuracy of diagnoses.

Appropriate sampling is the important factor in analysis of biopsy and postmortem material. Fixation, staining, and microtomy are merely techniques to be mastered. Sampling, in contrast, differs in each necropsy, and demands a thorough knowledge of anatomy and cellular structure. Careless tissue sampling and unscientific examination result in useless and sometimes harmful information.

Surgical dissection for possible lymph node metastases of neoplasms requires careful search for nodes in the surgical biopsy. The tissue mass, if immersed in ethyl alcohol, can be radiographed to accentuate the location of lymph nodes.

Forensic pathology

During every necropsy the veterinary pathologists must be aware of potential legal consequences. The careless necropsy leads, at best, to a reputation of incompetence and, at worst, to legal responsibilities that may run to millions of dollars, especially when human health is involved. Situations can arise with consequences that are unpredictable at the time of the postmortem examination, as in the following three examples:

Case 1. A local veterinarian was asked to conduct a necropsy on a large reticulated python that had killed a small human infant. Months later, the parents of the infant were charged with homicide for permitting the large snake to have access to their child. The subsequent trial hinged on testimony by a veterinarian that a necropsy of the snake revealed atrophy of the liver, gastrointestinal tract, and musculature; this was evidence that the snake had been starved (so that it would more readily consume mice), which caused it attack the child.

Case 2. A valuable, highly insured thoroughbred stud was found dead in its stall. No cause of death was obvious, and the insurer considered that the horse might have been deliberately killed to collect insurance money. The veterinary pathologist was placed in a position of dealing scientifically with the horse and also with the press. Consideration of cause of death included agents such as succinylcholine, barbiturates, and insulin. In the end no definite cause of death was discovered. Small lesions were found in the heart, and the statement was made that they were "compatable with a cardiac death." In such cases the veterinary pathologist must release only information that is unequivocably documented and avoid statements that permit journalistic embroidery, that is, give no information that may later need to be retracted. In discussing areas of intense lay interest that have not yet been clarified, the pathologist should merely indicate that tests are under way.

Case 3. A veterinarian was asked to be present at the slaughter of a steer that allegedly had won a state fair competition and then been purchased at a high price by a meat company for publicity purposes. The company believed that a steer of lesser value had been substituted. In this case, muzzle print identification was used to establish that the steer in question was not the winning steer.

Lesions of trauma must be defined.

Traumatic causes of death often must be established for legal purposes. Flesh wounds may suggest deliberate injury but also occur during collapse of large animals due to natural causes. Wounds that occur at the time of death have sharp outlines and lack the detectable bruising, swelling, and inflammation that characterize wounds that occur antemortem. If body fluids are present in excess they should be examined for foreign matter. Fluid in the lungs should be centrifuged and examined for the algae and diatoms that are present when animals drown in river or lake water. These organisms can also enter the bloodstream from the lungs and may be found in the bone marrow.

Was the method for euthanasia responsible for tissue changes?

Barbiturates are a method of choice for the painless killing of small animals. These drugs may cause an enlargement of the spleen but produce little else that interferes with postmortem examination. For large animals, barbiturates are often considered too expensive and other means are used, including electrocution, succinylcholine, carbon dioxide, and stunning. Slaughter methods for animals often have involved stunning followed by exsanguination. Recent studies in England have shown that after cutting the common carotid arteries and jugular veins, unconsciousness (absent visually evoked cortical responses) was 17 seconds in cattle and 14 seconds in sheep. Other studies using electroencephalographic responses indicate ranges of 10–85 seconds before loss of consciousness.

Estimate of time of death

Time of death is often important in forensic pathology, but only crude assessments of muscle rigidity and postmortem autolysis are possible in most cases. Electrolyte concentrations in vitreous humor have been used to determine time of death. Drs. Wayne Crowell and Robert Duncan, at the University of Georgia, have studied potassium concentrations in vitreous humor of dogs' eyes at various postmortem intervals. Potassium was found to increase after death, but the technique was only reliable in dogs of 9 kg or more. Postmortem blood is unusable for measuring magnesium (Mg^{++}) because this ion increases rapidly after death due to leakage from cells. Use of postmortem vitreous humor has been suggested in suspected cases of hypomagnesemia since its Mg^{++} content remains stable for several hours.

Toxicologic analysis

Toxicologic analysis plays a large role in forensic pathology. Some of the samples that must be collected include (1) postmortem blood taken directly from the heart ventricles or atria (before the thorax is opened); (2) urine (since many drugs are excreted via the kidney); (3) stomach contents (to recover some drugs in nonmetabolized form), including a notation on odor (e.g., for solvents, alcohol, or insecticides); (4)

spleen (for drugs that bind to erythrocytes); (5) cerebrospinal fluid; and (6) vitreous humor from the eye, especially when putrefaction renders blood and cerebrospinal fluid unusable.

The species of animal can be identified by dried blood.

Reactions of aqueous solutions extracted from dried blood and specific antisera against animal proteins can identify animal species. Most forensic science labs keep a range of antisera against domestic and farm animals. Detection of a visible precipitation in liquid or gel media is a common method, but immunoelectrophoretic techniques are often more precise. Closely related animal species have a high degree of homology and are a problem for differentiation; that is, there is much cross-reactivity against sera of closely related species. Determination using isoelectric focusing patterns of erythrocyte enzymes or proteins can be used (e.g., sheep and goat and even closely related fish species can be differentiated on the basis of electrofocusing patterns of the erythrocyte enzyme superoxide dismutase).

In one recent report, an unidentified man was seen to shoot and batter to death a mute swan, a protected species. Police arrested a suspect whose clothes contained blood stains, which he insisted were from a mallard duck he had shot the previous day. Sent to a forensic laboratory, the stains were analyzed by immunoelectrophoresis and shown to be of avian origin. Hemoglobin and superoxide dismutase were then used as markers in the electrofocusing technique. Samples of blood from several swans and several ducks showed no polymorphism in a highly resolved banding pattern; the electrofocusing patterns of the two bird species were unequivocally different, and it was possible to compare them with that produced by the blood spot on the suspect's clothing–which was identified as swan's blood.

ADDITIONAL READING

Andrews, J. J. (ed). Necropsy techniques. *Vet. Clin. N. Am.* 2:1, 1986.

Blackmore, D. K. Energy requirement for the penetration of heads of domestic animals in the development of a multiple projectile. *Vet. Rec.* 116:36, 1985.

Crowell, W. A., and Duncan, J. R. Potassium concentration in the vitreous humor as an indicator of the postmortem interval in dogs. *Am. J. Vet. Res.* 35:301, 1974.

Divall, G. B. The application of electrophoretic techniques in the field of criminology. *Electrophoresis* 6:249, 1985.

Gregory, N. G., and Wotton, S. B. Time to loss of brain responsiveness following exsanguination. *Res. Vet. Sci.* 37:141, 1984.

Groote, A. D., et al. Radiographic imaging of lymph nodes in lymph node dissection specimens. *Lab. Invest.* 52:326, 1985.

Lincoln, S. D., and Lane, V. M. Postmortem magnesium concentration in bovine vitreous humor. *Am. J. Vet. Res.* 46:160, 1985.

van der Gaag, I., and Tibboel, D. Intestinal atresia and stenosis in animals. *Vet. Pathol.* 17:565, 1980.

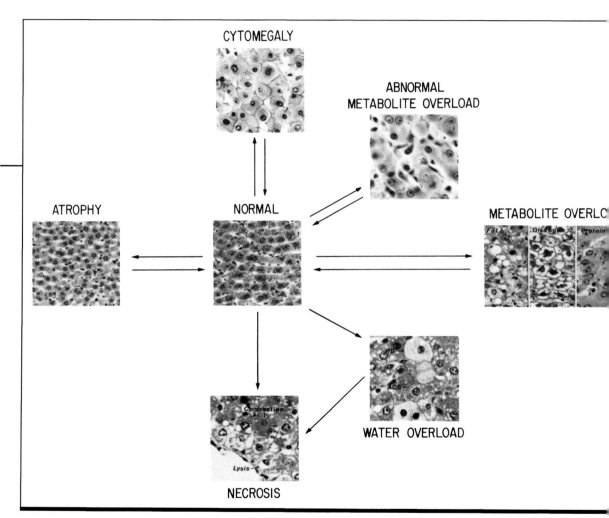

CYTOMEGALY

ABNORMAL
METABOLITE OVERLOAD

ATROPHY

NORMAL

METABOLITE OVERLC

WATER OVERLOAD

NECROSIS

Patterns of cell degener

DEGENERATION 2

CELLS respond to stimuli in one of two broad pathways: *cell regression,* and *cell growth*. Part II is concerned with regression, that is, with degenerative changes that are an aid in diagnosis. When tissue is injured its cells respond in ways that provide clues not only to the etiologic agent, but to the nature of the tissue reaction.

Degenerative changes occur in three basic cellular responses: defects in *water and electrolyte balance,* overload with *catabolic products* (glycogen, lipid, or protein), and defects in *cell processing and excretion,* in which complex nondegradable products accumulate in the cytoplasm. Each is an exaggeration of normal biological processes in the cell. Thus the greater the precision used to detect early subtle changes, the less clear the borderline between normal and pathologic changes.

Whatever the cause, the immediate cellular response to acute injury is a sudden, transient cell swelling. Metabolism is altered, electrolytes become imbalanced, and water is taken into the cell. This early process is so subtle that structural changes are not detectable by routine microscopy. That is, artifacts caused by biopsy, tissue fixation, and staining overshadow real pathologic alterations. As cellular degeneration progresses so that microscopic examination reveals meaningful structural changes, distinctive

patterns emerge that are the basis for differential pathologic diagnosis.

Cells that suffer *lethal injury* develop irreversible changes and collapse into shrunken, amorphous masses. Degeneration results both from direct damage to specific organelles and from secondary effects in cellular metabolism. In the classic sequence that follows lethal injury, the cell undergoes acute cell swelling, rapidly suffers irreversible injury, and collapses into a dark, eosinophilic mass called *coagulative necrosis.* If the cell survives for a longer time, water accumulates in the cytoplasm and the cell slowly expands and disintegrates by *lysis.*

As background information, one must remember that normal cells have varying appearances according to their rates of metabolism. The liver shows marked changes in size as food intake varies. Hepatocytes are large and plump during periods of good nutrition but shrink markedly during prolonged periods of food deprivation.

Cells vary in their response to injury. If in an active state of metabolism or a vulnerable position, they may be killed in a matter of seconds. In contrast, some cells, because of a protected location or an inactive metabolism, may suffer only slight damage from the same injury.

In *sublethal injury,* cells degenerate more slowly and changes involve accumulation of catabolic products and abnormal protein com-

55

plexes. The manifestations of injury are not severe swelling and lysis but more slowly developing shifts in metabolic pathways, which cause molecules of protein or lipid to accumulate and distort the cell.

In addition to changes in cells, there are clues in extracellular spaces. As cells are destroyed there are coincident changes in glycosaminoglycans of ground substance, deposition of fibrillar material, and reduplication of basement membranes. In *fibrosis* (or fibroplasia, the formation of fibrous tissue), collagen fibers are deposited, which stabilize tissue made friable by loss of parenchymal cells. The pathologist must distinguish various types of abnormal fibers, such as abnormal collagen, fibrin, amyloid, and various types of hyalin formed by inspissation of plasma proteins.

Cellular Degeneration

4

NEARLY all injurious substances cause damage at multiple sites in cells. In some cases, injury may be more specifically directed, that is, to cell surfaces, to mechanisms of nuclear control, to sites of energy formation in mitochondria, or to the protein-producing organelles of the cytoplasm. In the sections that follow, an artificial emphasis is placed on the early dominant sites of injury to explain mechanisms of cell responses. This must not obscure consideration of the complex interactions that occur in degeneration and recovery of damaged tissue.

After injury, degenerating cells suffer indirect injury because of the interdependency of cell structures and functions. Secondary factors that amplify the cascade of degeneration into death include *pressure* changes accompanying intracellular fluid and electrolyte imbalance, *lower pH* as lactate accumulates (acidosis), *increased metabolic rates* due to fever-induced temperature elevation, and *hypoxia,* which often results from decreased blood flow. When oxygen is lacking, there is a direct effect on oxidative phosphorylation and mitochondrial structure. Energy production is shunted to anaerobic glycolysis, and glycogen disappears from the cytoplasm. Whatever the complicating events, they ultimately lead to depletion of ATP, the common energy currency of the cell. In the end, all energy-requiring processes are halted, and degeneration becomes irreversible.

Pathologic changes that develop in response to injury depend on (1) duration of the injurious agent's effect and its concentration in tissue; (2) tissue vascular supply and blood flow to the cell, including oxygen availability, pH, and temperature; and (3) metabolic and structural characteristics of the cell. Metabolically active cells are, in general, most susceptible to injury, and that is why patterns of degeneration are so meaningful in liver, kidney, and muscle.

After sublethal injury, damaged cells recover and the pathologist must be able to detect even subtle evidence of tissue recovery. If the cell survives, the process of *autophagy* is stimulated; damaged bits of cytoplasm are sequestered in vacuoles and slowly digested by lysosomal enzymes and removed by expulsion from the cell. Cells that recover are apt to be larger than normal and have large nuclei and nucleoli. After severe, diffuse damage to the kidney tubules, renal epithelium may undergo necrosis but reduplication of adjacent tubular epithelial cells often permits survival. The presence of these large, hypertrophic cells in the nephron heralds the survival of the patient with nephrosis.

DEFECTS IN WATER AND ELECTROLYTE BALANCE
Acute cell swelling

Swelling is a universal manifestation of cell injury. It occurs in most types of acute injury as a prelude to more serious changes. Thus the term *acute cell swelling* is rarely helpful for diagnosis but is an aid to understanding how a lesion has progressed. For example, the blisters and ulcers induced by herpesviruses (e.g., bovine infectious rhinotracheitis) begin in small foci of kertinocyte swelling. These cells lyse and die to produce foci of necrosis in the germinal layer of epithelium. Plasma exudes into the necrotic area and a blister forms. The expanding process causes the blister to rupture and an ulcer to form over the epithelial defect. Even in these late stages of ulcer formation, when much of the lesion consists of necrotic tissue debris, swollen keratinocytes can still be identified at the expanding edges of the lesion (Fig. 4.1).

Acute cell swelling is expansion of cell volume due to loss of control of water intake.

Acute cell swelling is the fundamental expression of cell injury and is to the dying cell what electrolyte imbalance is to the dying animal, a basic killing mechanism over which are superimposed many other degenerative phenomena. Acute cell swelling includes a spectrum of changes that begins with water intake and ends with diffuse disintegration of soluble cellular proteins. With time, cells continue to swell uniformly or water may be sequestered in vacuoles formed by degenerating endoplasmic reticulum.

Microscopic changes include increased cell size and regression of organelles.

Water uptake dilutes the *cytoplasm* and gives cells a pale, transparent appearance. Tissue architecture is maintained, but the enlarged cells press on one another and normal tissue arrangement is distorted. With time, tiny granules of protein debris accumulate, and the cytoplasm becomes blurred and disorganized. Cells bulge from their normal limits and extend into lumens and cavities.

As *nuclei* degenerate, chromatin moves to the periphery of the cell and aggregates along the nuclear envelope. "Chromatin clumping" is a consequence of the decrease in cell pH that occurs as lactate builds up in the cell. As the cell dies, nuclear surfaces become irregular and invaginate. *Karyorrhexis* (rupture of nuclear mem-

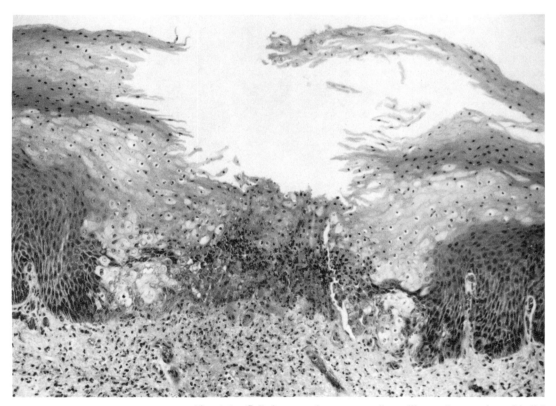

Fig. 4.1. Cell degeneration: acute cell swelling and necrosis, epithelial blister, cow with infectious bovine rhinotracheitis. A blister had formed due to accumulation of fluid (from exuded plasma with minor contributions from lysed epithelial cells) and ruptured during biopsy (note the defect in the stratum corneum).

branes and release of nuclear contents) and *kar-yoklasis* (total breakdown of the nucleus) are the important hallmarks of cell death.

Hydropic and vacuolar degeneration are variants of acute cell swelling.

Hydropic degeneration is applied to cells markedly swollen by water that is free in the cytoplasm. When severe, some pathologists refer to it as "ballooning degeneration." Central areas of the cell are cleared of protein, and nuclei are shrunken and lie along the cell margins. In epithelium, this pattern of degeneration is common to many injuries. For example, it is characteristic of blisters in epitheliotropic viral diseases. It also occurs in sunburn injury (e.g., the blistering of the exposed tongues that is often seen in dogs raised in temperate climates

and later moved to the tropics). The rumen epithelium of sheep and cattle that develop ruminal acidosis shows diffuse hydropic degeneration early in the disease. There is massive expansion of the epithelial cells and lysis of cellular proteins.

Vacuolar degeneration is very like hydropic degeneration except that the water is in large cytoplasmic vacuoles. It occurs in cells with large amounts of membranes that actively pump ions. As cell swelling progresses these membrane-bound pumps rapidly move ions and water out of the cytosol and into the cisternae of the endoplasmic reticulum. This organelle becomes fragmented, and water accumulates in large vacuoles, hence *vacuolar degeneration*. Both hydropic and vacuolar degeneration terminate by causing lysis of the cell (Fig. 4.2). These are often pera-

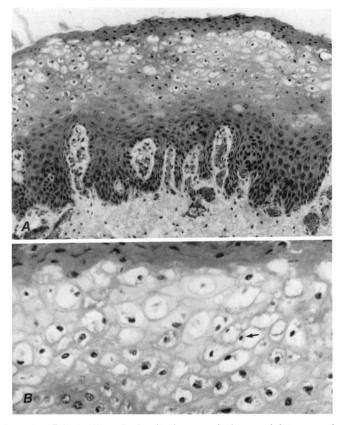

Fig. 4.2. Cell swelling (hydropic degeneration) caused by a poxvirus (bovine papular stomatitis), oral mucosa, cow. A. Swollen cells are in the upper squamous layers (in contrast to herpesviruses in the germinal layers (Fig. 4.1). B. Ballooning of cytoplasm is accompanied by pyknosis and eccentricity of nuclei (*arrow*).

cute changes, and in contrast to coagulation necrosis, in which in the architecture of the cell is preserved, the cell is deleted from the tissue.

Pathogenesis of acute cell swelling

The plasma membrane barrier is broken in acute cell swelling.

The basic event that underlies all forms of swelling occurs at the cell surface. The plasma membrane becomes leaky, sodium (Na^+) and calcium (Ca^{++}) enter the cell, potassium (K^+) is lost, and water enters the cell and dilutes the cytoplasm. To cause cell swelling, an injurious substance must have the capacity to damage the plasma membrane barrier that controls water and electrolyte transport at the cell surface. Injury may be direct, or it may be indirect, by inhibiting metabolic processes on which the membrane depends for its integrity.

Enzymes embedded in the plasma membrane maintain cell electrolytes.

Normally, water traverses the cell passively by diffusion equilibrium. Intracellular water is regulated by modifications of electrolyte composition, chiefly Na^+ and K^+, thereby regulating cell volume. The ionic concentration (in mEq) in the cell are Na^+ 12 and K^+ 155. In extracellular fluid the concentrations are Na^+ 145 and K^+ 4. This unequal distribution across the plasma membrane is maintained by the enzyme *Na-K-ATPase* (Na^+-K^+-dependent adenosine triphosphatase). Na-K-ATPase is an integral protein embedded in the lipid bilayer of the plasma membrane. As it interacts with ATP (its energy source), the configuration of the molecule changes to permit Na^+ to be pumped out of the cell; this again changes the molecule so that K^+ can flow into the cell in the same operation. Na-K-ATPase is called the "sodium-potassium pump" because the movement of ions is linked in actively pumping Na^+ out of and K^+ into the cell.

Damage to membrane ATPases leads to swelling.

Any process that depresses electrolyte-pumping ATPases results in acute cell swelling. A common cause involves *anoxia* (oxygen deficit) and depletion of ATP, the enzyme substrate. Some *drugs* and *toxins* may specifically react with cell surface ATPases to cause acute cell swelling (e.g., digitalis acts on membranes of the cardiac myocyte). In the brain, triethyl tin inhibits ATPases on astrocyte foot processes. Astrocytes swell, and because they do not pump fluids through the brain tissue, fluid accumulates and causes separation and unraveling of adjacent myelin lamellae, a process called *secondary demyelination*. In some of the rare *congenital diseases* of the brain, demyelination occurs because of an inherited deficiency of astrocyte ATPases.

Cells move more fluid by increasing membrane pumps.

In initial stages of swelling, cells increase ion transport by increasing the number of Na-K-ATPase pumps and by expanding pump-bearing membrane surfaces. In the colon of animals deprived of Na^+ or given excess K^+, epithelial cells show marked expansion of basolateral surfaces and increased ATPase activity. The new membrane surfaces are a response to move more Na^+ into the body from gut fluids or to rid the body of excess K^+ by the reverse process. *Thyroid hormone* causes increased amounts of ATPase pumps, and this mechanism underlies the increased cellular activity in hyperthyroidism. *Epinephrine* also suppresses cell swelling by regulating ATPase pumping on cell membranes.

Entry of Ca^{++} kills the cell.

When cell permeability is altered, Ca^{++} rushes in from higher amounts present in interstitial fluids, which is especially toxic to the cell. Ca^{++} regulates permeability of gap junctions between cells; in the presence of high Ca^{++}, rapid *uncoupling of gap junctions* occurs and isolates the injured cell from its neighbors, an attempt to prevent the spread of injury or infection. Increased amounts of Ca^{++} in the cytoplasm lead to *depolymerization of the cytoskeleton*; filaments and microtubules in the cell cortex disappear so they cannot function in cell movement, phagocytosis, and secretion as they normally do. Ca^{++} *activates endogenous phospholipases* present in cell membranes, which leads to a cascade of reactions that cause membrane breakdown.

Plasma proteins enter the cell during degeneration.

As severe cell swelling progresses to necrosis, large protein molecules from plasma and interstitial fluid enter the cells. When cardiac myocytes are killed by anoxia, for example, they can be shown to contain albumin and, in severe injury, even globulin and fibrinogen. Histochemical tests are used to quantitate the amount of albumin in the degenerate cardiac myocyte as a correlate of the severity of injury to the heart.

Enzymes leak from the injured cell into plasma.

Proteins and other large molecules normally present in the cell escape into the interstitium and circulating blood as cells degenerate. In injury to organs such as heart, skeletal muscle, and liver, certain enzymes in the bloodstream can be assayed to detect injury and to assess its extent. In *myocardial infarction,* for example, the rapid rise of serum creatine phosphokinase is useful in predicting the severity of tissue death. Massive damage to skeletal muscle leads to progressively increasing concentrations of muscle enzymes in plasma. In *exertional rhabdomyolysis* of racing greyhounds, soluble enzymes from myocytes appear in plasma early in the disease process (larger myoglobin molecules leak from the cell only after necrosis occurs).

Extensive skeletal muscle necrosis occurs in *clostridial myositis* ("blackleg") in sheep and cattle (Fig. 4.3). The clostridia secrete a powerful phospholipase that degrades cell surface membranes and causes massive necrosis. Clostridial phospholipases respect no component of tissue, and muscle, blood vessels, and erythrocytes are rapidly destroyed. Remarkably increased concentrations of aspartate aminotransferase and other intracellular enzymes appear in circulating blood as they are released from the dying cells.

METABOLIC OVERLOAD

Glycogen degeneration

Glycogen, a branched polymer of glucose molecules, accumulates when excessive amounts of glucose enter the cell. It is the storage form of glucose and a normal component in the cytoplasm of most cells. Major deposits occur in liver, muscle, and kidney, and glycogen degeneration is essentially limited to these organs.

Conditions where glycogen degeneration is prominent in the hepatocyte include (1) hyperglycemia of any cause (commonly that of early diabetes mellitus); (2) drug-induced metabolic disease with disturbed carbohydrate metabolism (e.g., liver cells of animals treated with corticosteroids); (3) enzymatic deficiencies associated with the hereditary glycogen storage disease; and (4) glycogen-storing tumor cells. Precise distinctions between overload and degeneration of glycogen are not practical. *Glycogen degeneration* is used for cells that are so distended with glycogen that degenerative phenomena occur in other organelles.

Probably the most common instance of glycogen degeneration occurs in the liver after the administration of massive doses of corticosteroids. The liver in treated animals becomes markedly enlarged and pale. Microscopically, all hepatocytes are affected and consist of massively enlarged cells with remnants of normal cytoplasm pushed to the periphery and large clear structureless areas (glycogen is leached out in aqueous fixatives).

Glycogen is detected in tissue sections with the periodic acid–Schiff (PAS) stain. Control slides digested with diastase (saliva will work) must be used to rule out glycoproteins that also accept this stain (diastase digests out the glycogen but not the more complex glycoproteins). In electron micrographs, glycogen occurs free in the cytoplasmic matrix as dense granules 10–30 nm in diameter.

Glycogen is sometimes seen in nuclei (e.g., in hepatocytes of aged ruminants and of dogs with diabetes mellitus). Intranuclear glycogen also occurs in some neoplastic cells where active glycogen synthetase has been found associated with nuclear chromatin.

Glycogenesis

Glycogen granules contain the enzymes that carry out glycogen synthesis (*glycogenesis*) and degradation (*glycogenolysis*). In glycogenesis, glycogen synthetase and a branching enzyme link glucose molecules into a large polymer. Glycogenolysis requires a different set of enzymes to destroy these branches and to break off molecules of glucose.

Glycogen breakdown in liver and skeletal muscle is markedly affected by two hormones: epinephrine and glucagon. Both hormones are transported to liver and muscle in the bloodstream. They attach to cell surfaces and activate the cell signal molecule *adenyl cyclase,* cytoplasmic cyclic AMP is increased, a protein kinase is activated that then phosphorylates an enzyme that in turn catalyzes glycogen breakdown, and the same enzyme also phosphorylates glycogen synthetase (which switches off this enzyme).

When blood glucose is high, glucose diffuses into insulin-independent hepatocytes and is

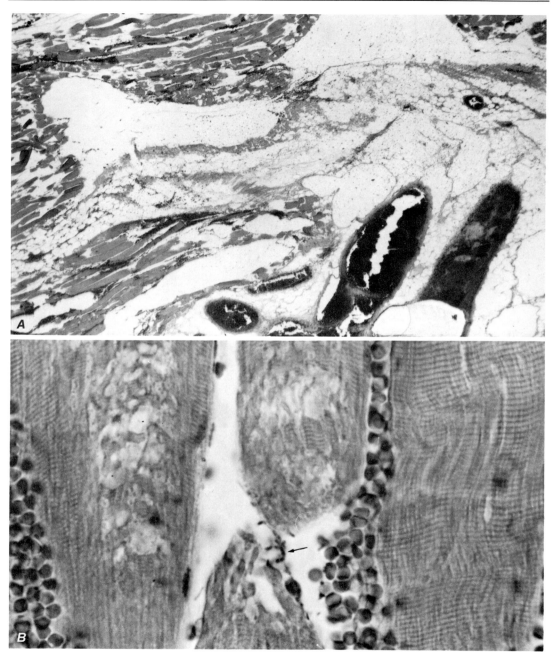

Fig. 4.3. Muscle necrosis caused by *Clostridium septicum,* lamb: severe edema, gas production, and hemorrhage. A. Dissection of gas and fluid throughout degenerate muscle fibers. B. High power: acute cell swelling with vacuolation of myocytes, extravasated erythrocytes (hemorrhage), and bacteria (*arrow*).

trapped in the cell by being forced into the glycolytic cycle. *Insulin* facilitates entrance of glucose into the metabolic pool by stimulating phosphorylation of glucose molecules to glucose-6-phosphate and prevents glucose synthesis by inhibiting the action of glucose-6-phosphatase.

Fatty degeneration

Fat is a normal product in most every cell. Fatty degeneration is an exaggeration of triglyceride production, and in theory, it can occur in any tissue. However, the swollen, yellow, greasy appearance of fatty degeneration is characteristic of liver and, less commonly, of kidney and heart. Nearly all tissues develop cytoplasmic lipids on injury, but few others develop them sufficiently to alter the gross appearance so strikingly.

Fatty degeneration is an important diagnostic clue.

Excess lipids in cells suggest (1) long-standing elevation of blood lipids, (2) chronic hypoxia in which lipid-metabolizing enzymes are inhibited, (3) acute sublethal toxic injury that suppresses lipid pathways, or (4) chronic progressive metabolic disease arising from defective cell enzymes. Liver and kidney are apt to be involved in acute injury or metabolic disease.

In hepatocytes with fatty degeneration, the distribution and size of lipid globules is a crude indication of the type of injury. Small-droplet degeneration is typical of acute metabolic disease and is always coincident with subtle acute cell swelling. Large-droplet fatty degeneration is characteristic of more slowly developing toxic or viral disease.

Special fat-soluble stains identify lipids.

Microscopically, lipid accumulation causes cells to be enlarged, pale, and lacy (Fig. 4.4). These foamy cells must be examined by special techniques to determine the type of lipid deposit, whether they are typical lipid triglyceride globules (neutral lipids) of fatty degeneration or the cholesterol, phospholipids, or glycolipids of the less common patterns of degeneration.

Solvents used in routine histologic techniques dissolve out fats, leaving clear spaces. To distinguish lipids from the clear spaces of hydropic or glycogen deposits, special techniques are used. Lipid globules of fatty degeneration are globules of triglycerides (neutral lipids) and must be stained in frozen sections with lipid-soluble dyes such as Sudan III and oil red O stains.

Triglycerides accumulate in fatty degeneration.

In normal hepatocytes, globules of triglycerides (also called "neutral fat") are formed as storage sites to await processing to more complex lipid structures synthesized in the liver (e.g., very low density lipoproteins). In fatty degeneration, triglyceride production exceeds the slower, more elaborate events involved in complex syntheses. When injury destroys any part of the lipid metabolic pathway, appropriate substrates (cholesterol, phospholipids, or fatty acids) accumulate. It is the massive backlog of triglycerides, however, that dominates the cytopathic changes of fatty degeneration.

Injuries that imbalance supply, utilization, synthesis, or release of lipids cause fatty degeneration.

Neutral fats accumulate from (1) oversupply of circulating fatty acids from blood lipids or nonlipid precursors such as alcohol; (2) interference with enzymes bound to membranes of smooth endoplasmic reticulum that transfer fatty acids to glycerol to form triglycerides; (3) blockade of protein synthesis in rough endoplasmic reticulum, of assembly of lipoproteins, or of release of lipoprotein granules at the cell surface; or (4) prevention of fatty acid activation by coenzyme A (CoA), with passage across the mitocondrial membrane to enter into mitochondrial matrix energy pathways in the citric acid cycle. Direct mitochondrial injury, for example, results in decreased fatty acid oxidation with increases in the fatty acid pool and accumulation of triglycerides.

Degeneration involving proteins

During the examination of pathologic tissues, protein inclusions are commonly encountered within abnormal cells. Pathologists are trained to recognize and differentiate these bodies in making an etiologic diagnosis (Fig. 4.5). Aggregates of protein or of proteins conjugated with carbohydrates (glycoproteins) or lipids (lipoproteins) are useful pieces of evidence for diagnosis. In some cases, the proteins represent an *excess accumulation of normal cellular proteins.* In many sublethal injuries, however, protein syn-

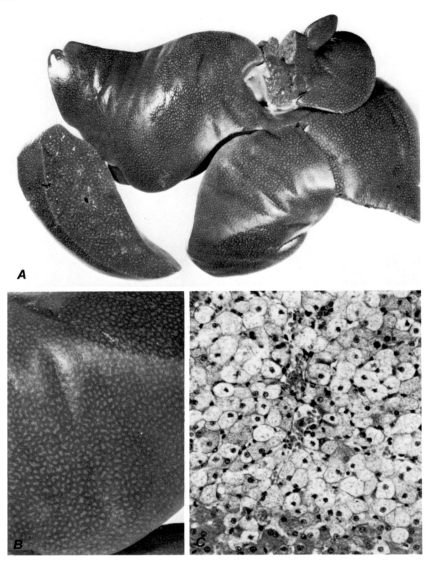

Fig. 4.4. Fatty degeneration, liver, dog with diabetes mellitus. A and B. Centrolobular distribution. C. Foamy, lipid-laden cells around the central vein.

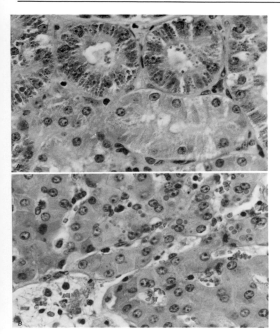

Fig. 4.5. Hyalin degeneration. A. Hyalin droplets in the proximal renal tubules, dog with chronic renal failure. The droplets represent inspissated protein acquired by the tubule cell from the glomerular filtrate. B. Hyalin droplets, hepatocytes, pig.

thesis proceeds but results in *abnormal peptide chains*. Masses of these defective proteins aggregate and appear as *inclusion bodies* in the cytoplasm or nucleus.

Inclusion bodies are evidence of defects in protein synthesis pathways.

When protein synthesis is disrupted, evidence of injury occurs in nucleoli, in ribosomes, and in the Golgi complex and its vesicles. Toxins can produce widespread cell injury by selectively damaging any of these structures. For example, agents such as aflatoxin that act on DNA or the polymerases that transcribe its genetic code tend to produce the most rapid and widespread changes throughout the pathways of protein synthesis. Destruction of the nucleolus is followed rapidly by that of ribosomes. The consequences of failure of ribosomes to produce enzymes and structural proteins required for normal cell maintenance extend the degenerative process into all organelles of the cell.

If abnormal protein fibrils are produced in

cells, they tend to polymerize and accumulate. This type of protein inclusion is common in neoplastic cells, toxic degeneration, and hypoxia. In aged dogs these proteins form enormous, crystalline lattice inclusions in the kidney and liver; although striking, these inclusions are not associated with known disease. The protein is laid down in repeating units, and the inclusions have a linear pattern as they are deposited.

Aging leads to defect protein assembly.

Protein filaments of aging form in cells of aged animals. Proteins polymerize into rigid, highly insoluble filaments in which specific amino acids are cross-linked by unusual covalent bonding of glutamyl-lysine side chains. It appears that the enzyme transglutaminase, which is activated by rising calcium concentrations in aging cells, promotes polymerization of otherwise normal peptide chains. Cataracts of the aging lens of the eye exhibit this reaction. The characteristic helical filaments in neurofibrillary tangles and plaques in brains of aged animals and man with senile atrophy are composed of glutamyl-lysine cross-linked proteins.

Hyalin inclusions

Hyalin degeneration refers to dense, amorphous globules of eosinophilic material in the cytoplasm. These heterogeneous changes have in common only the presence of a uniform, structureless material called *hyalin* (the term describes only physical appearance as seen by light microscopy and is not related to chemical composition or to a specific pattern of degeneration). Implicit in these materials is the lifeless nature of the substances involved; that is, there has been a physical change in cells or their products in which the cells have lost their identity and have fused to a structureless, homogeneous mass.

Hyalin droplets form in two ways.

Hyalin droplet degeneration develops because cells produce abnormal secretory granules. Hepatocytes that produce excessive amounts of proteins destined for plasma often contain hyalin droplets that are composed of albumin, fibrinogen, or components of complement.

Hyalin droplets also form when cells take up large amounts of proteins from surrounding fluids and sequester them within cytoplasmic granules (lysosomes). In renal disease, when plasma albumin passes into the glomerular filtrate and out in the urine (albuminuria), the proximal convoluted tubule cells resorb some of the protein. Massive accumulation of protein in some cells may fill and expand the cytoplasm into *hyalin lakes.*

Extracellular hyalin

The term *hyalin* is also applied to extracellular material. Hyalin substances in this connective tissue hyalin may be (1) collagen, in scars and tumors; (2) basement membrane, in arteriosclerosis, renal glomerulosclerosis, and many subepithelial lesions; and (3) plasma proteins, inspissated in albumin casts in renal tubules. Amyloid is often identified as hyalin but usually is sufficiently characteristic not to be confusing.

Viral inclusion bodies

The identification of inclusions is particularly helpful in viral diseases. Rabies is diagnosed, for example, by finding characteristic spherical, eosinophilic cytoplasmic inclusions in neurons of the brain. Viral proteins and virions aggregate in cells and have characteristic locations (cytoplasmic or nuclear), shapes (spherical or irregular), and staining affinities (eosinophilic or basophilic) (Fig. 4.6). By utilizing the Feulgen stain (for DNA) and the acridine orange stain (for single- versus double-stranded nucleic acids), viral inclusion bodies can be identified histochemically as containing DNA or RNA.

Viral inclusions can be specifically identified by immunocytochemistry.

Immunologic reagents such as fluorescent antibody techniques can be applied to tissue sections to identify *viral antigens.* The specificity of the test depends on the source of the antibody used in the test.

Monoclonal antibodies have been developed for some viruses and identify very precise binding sites on viral components. For example, a monoclonal antibody might be directed only to a specific glycoprotein molecule on the surface of a virus.

Electron microscopy will reveal the type of virion.

Ultrastructural studies show that most viral inclusions are remnants of viral protein "factories" composed of excess viral structural proteins and membranes with viral particles of varying maturity distributed around the mass

(see Fig. 28.3). Samples for this technique must be taken in early stages of infection (before necrosis masks the delicate cellular changes) and are best collected at the margins of the lesions, between viral and necrotic tissue.

ACCUMULATION OF COMPLEX NONDEGRADABLE PRODUCTS

These degenerative changes are not so much a response to acute injury as they are the end result of long-term abnormal metabolism. Instead of a rapidly developing cellular change that ends in necrosis, these changes lead to accumulation of amorphous, irregular aggregates in the cytoplasm. In most instances, these products arise from *excretory failure,* the inability of the cell to eliminate material accumulated in response to injury.

Lipofuscin

Lipofuscin is a golden brown lipid-pigment complex formed in cells undergoing excessive and prolonged auto-oxidation of unsaturated lipids. After peroxidation of double bonds on lipid molecules occurs, the oxidized forms are condensed into solid polymers that give the color and reactivity of lipofuscin. Deposits fluoresce brown in ultraviolet light and stain with fat-soluble dyes, acid-fast stains, and the PAS reaction.

Lipofuscins develop in rapidly metabolizing cells.

Lipofuscins occur most commonly in neurons, thyroid epithelium, and cardiac and skeletal muscle. They increase with advancing age and accrue as older cells must degrade more lipids and membranes at a time when their antioxidation mechanisms wane; hence they are called the "aging" or "wear-and-tear" pigment. The *brown bowel syndrome* occurs in dogs with chronic diarrhea, steatorrhea, and malabsorption. Large aggregates of lipofuscin granules develop in smooth muscle cells, giving the intestine a brown cast (see Fig. 7.1).

Phospholipid degeneration

In normal cells, all kinds of membranes are continually recycled. Tiny portions of membranes are sequestered by autophagosomes as part of normal cell reconstruction. This material

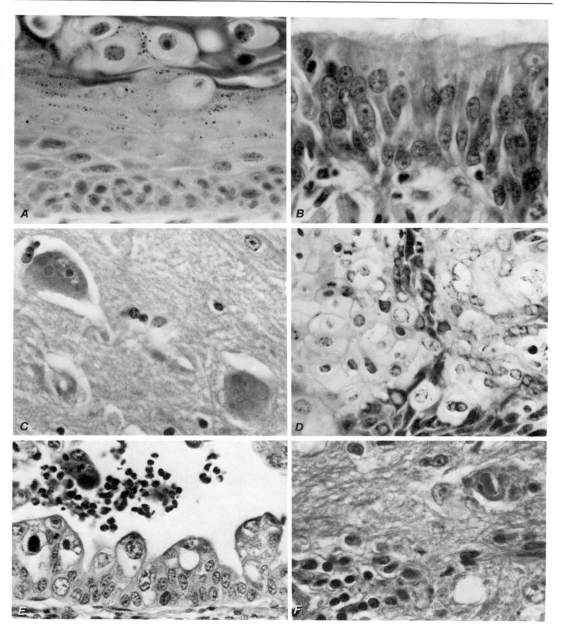

Fig. 4.6. Inclusion bodies are used in diagnosis: A. Pleomorphic, irregular, nuclear inclusions, oral epithelium, *canine oral papilloma*. B. Spherical, homogeneous (eosinophilic), cytoplasmic inclusions in respiratory epithelium, *canine distemper* (paramyxovirus). C. Large, irregular, cytoplasmic inclusions in neurons, bovine *rabies* (rhabdovirus). D. Diffuse, "ground-glass," nuclear inclusions, *infectious bovine rhinotracheitis*. E. Large, nuclear inclusions in markedly enlarged bronchiolar epithelial cells, *ovine adenovirus*. F. Large, nuclear inclusions in enlarged nuclei of neurons, chronic *canine distemper*.

is then shunted to enzyme-bearing lysosomes where they are degraded and either stored or released from the cell. Specific enzymes catalyse this normal breakdown of membrane phospholipids, glycolipids, and glycoproteins. When this membrane repair process is driven to excess, or when enzymes involved are missing or damaged, phospholipid fragments accumulate in lysosomes. Some tranquilizers and plant poisons produce phospholipid degeneration in neurons that leads to central nervous system signs.

Histologically, cells affected with phospholipid degeneration are called *foam cells* because they are massively enlarged and are packed with tiny vacuoles (which represent engorged autophagosomes). Individually they resemble cells with severe vacuolar degeneration or with small droplet fatty degeneration and must be identified with special stains. Phospholipid membranes usually stain with the PAS reaction (because of their high content of glycolipids and glycoproteins associated with the membranes), and the PAS-staining material is not removed with diastase. The vacuoles do not stain with oil red O or other fat-solvent stains.

Lipid storage diseases are caused by missing enzymes.

The familial, systemic lipid-storage diseases are due to the absence or diminution of enzymes that degrade glycolipidic cerebrosides and gangliosides. This deficiency is first seen in myelin, and lesions are characerized by accumulation of glia and macrophages filled with myelin membrane fragments and phospholipids. Degradation of myelin in the nervous system provides an extreme example of membrane breakdown and phospholipid degeneration. Schwann cells of peripheral nerves and oligodendrocytes of the central nervous system take up and process the disintegrating membranes of myelin.

Mucopolysaccharide inclusions

Glycosaminoglycans are polysaccharides containing amino sugars on their chains. Nearly all vertebrate glycosaminoglycans also contain

sugar groups with carboxylic acid units (e.g., glucuronic acid) and are referred to as *acidic mucopolysaccharides*. The strongly acid sulfate groups are bound to protein moieties and impart basophilia to cell structures. Their polyanionic nature is responsible for staining with alcian blue, which is used in identification.

Glycoproteins accumulate in mucopolysaccharide storage diseases.

The *mucopolysaccharidoses* are genetic storage diseases characterized by accumulations of incompletely degraded glycosaminoglycans in cells that normally degrade these mucosubstances. Storage results from diminished activity of specific hydrolases in lysosomes (see Chapter 6). Affected cells are massively enlarged, with pale, slightly basophilic foamy material.

Glycoprotein inclusions

Corpora amylacea are large, round bodies associated with secretory processes in brain, pineal, pituitary, and mammary gland. In bovine mammae, they occur within glandular acini. In the primate brain, corpora amylacea occur in the cytoplasm of astrocytes and other glia. They are derived by polymerization of acidic glycosaminoglycans of ground substance and appear to originate from degenerating neurons.

ADDITIONAL READING

Block, M. I. Myocardial myoglobin following coronary artery occlusion. *Am. J. Pathol.* 111:374, 1983.

Forman, H. J., et al. Roles of selenium and sulfur-containing amino acids in protection against oxygen toxicity. *Lab. Invest.* 49:148, 1983.

Kinoshita, J. H., et al. Aldose reductase in diabetic cataracts. *J. Am. Med. Assoc.* 246:257, 1981.

O'Brien, T. D., et al. Hepatic necrosis following halothane anesthesia in goats. *J. Am. Vet. Med. Assoc.* 189:1591, 1986.

5

Cytopathology: Structural Lesions in Cell Organelles

IN this chapter, the events of degeneration are described according to current knowledge of molecular biology and cell ultrastructure. For a professional person bearing the title *doctor of veterinary medicine,* it is no longer sufficient to interpret pathologic changes only at the level of the light microscope. To fully understand the biology of drug action, toxic injury, intracellular microbial infection, or any cellular injury, the basis of structure and function at the cellular level must be understood.

In eukaryotic cells the control of function and development resides chiefly in the nucleus; metabolic and synthetic processes occur in the cytoplasm. Cytoplasm is composed of a gel substance called the *cytosol,* a system of tiny filaments, and various organelles and inclusions. On the basis of tradition, *organelles* are considered the internal functioning organs. *Inclusions* are lifeless accumulations of metabolites (lipid globules, glycogen, protein crystals, and pigments) that are not required to maintain cell life.

The injured cell is considered as five distinct (but interrelated) operational systems: (1) the *cell surface* controls membrane barrier functions, receipt of chemical signals, and transport of molecules into and out of the cell, (2) *mitochondria* are sites of energy production, (3) the *nucleolus-ribosome–rough endoplasmic reticulum* systems are coding and production organelles for protein synthesis, (4) *lysosomes* carry out intracellular digestion, and (5) *smooth endoplasmic reticulum* is the detoxification system for the cell. Damage may be directed to any of these systems, and models will be used to illustrate how degeneration is initiated by *direct injury* to each system. Nearly all injurious substances cause damage at multiple sites in cells, and the emphasis on the early dominant sites of injury in this chapter must not obscure the complexity of advanced cell degeneration as it occurs in clinical disease.

PATHWAYS OF PROTEIN SYNTHESIS

Nucleus

The nucleus is the control center for the cell. From gene templates on its chromosomes the messenger molecules are formed that pass to the cytoplasm to control protein syntheses in ribosomes. Much of the gene activity occurs in the nucleolus, and when cell activities demand increased protein, the nucleolus enlarges.

Three sequential phases connect the reading of genes to the final release of protein chains into the cytocavitary network: (1) *Transcription* of DNA codes onto templates of messenger RNA (mRNA) occurs on chromosomes in the nucleus, (2) *translation* of the mRNA into the desired peptide chains occurs in ribosomes, and (3) the folding and conjugation of new peptides into the final protein product occurs in the rough endoplasmic reticulum and Golgi complex (Fig. 5.1).

Chromatin represents DNA-protein complexes.

Functional units of chromatin are the chromosomes, which become physically distinct only during mitosis. When chromatin fibers are experimentally stretched, they have the appearance of beads on a string. Called *nucleosomes,* the beads are protein cores of histones surrounded by several loops of DNA. Expression of genes is a consequence of selective unfolding of chromosomes. During inactivity, histones bind to DNA

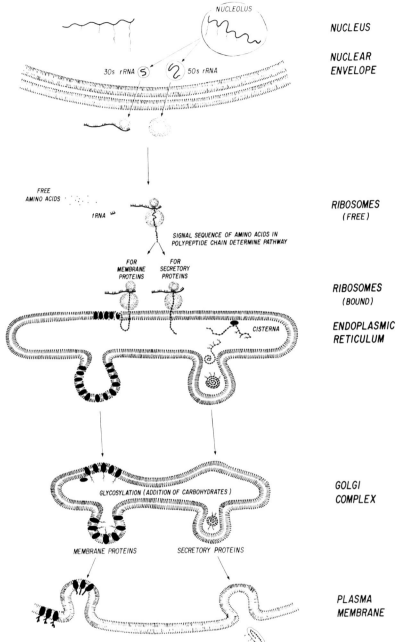

TRANSCRIPTION
FORMATION OF mRNA AND
rRNA FROM GENE CODES ON
DNA

TRANSLATION
ASSEMBLY OF AMINO ACIDS
INTO PEPTIDE CHAINS USING
CODES IN mRNA

CONJUGATION
GLYCOSYLATION OF PEPTIDE
CHAINS BY ADDITION OF
CARBOHYDRATE SPIKES

SECRETION
EXOCYTOSIS OF PROTEIN
MOLECULE

NUCLEUS

*NUCLEAR
ENVELOPE*

*RIBOSOMES
(FREE)*

*RIBOSOMES
(BOUND)*

*ENDOPLASMIC
RETICULUM*

*GOLGI
COMPLEX*

*PLASMA
MEMBRANE*

Fig. 5.1. Pathways of protein synthesis: transcription, translation, glycosylation, and secretion.

and by constraining it they physically prevent transcription.

Expression of genes is controlled.

The DNA in different cells of an individual contains the same genetic information but only a limited amount is expressed. The cells' genetic program not only can be switched on and off (as in mitosis) but also can be selectively expressed. Thus the neuron and the keratinocyte have the same genome but very different expressions of it.

RNA polymerase initiates gene reading.

A gene is transcribed when the massive enzyme *RNA polymerase* moves along the length of DNA, copying the sequence of nucleotide bases into their RNA equivalent. The first step in the process is the binding of the enzyme to the beginning or 5′ end of the gene, the *promoter region*. As the RNA transcript is completed, a *cap* is added to the 5′ end, and a string of 200 adenine molecules (the poly-A tail) is added to the back (3′) end. The RNA then associates with other proteins and exits from the nucleus through the nuclear pore.

Hormones can control gene action.

Steroid hormones cause cells with appropriate receptors to begin transcribing mRNA from their genes. They first diffuse into cells, and each is coupled to a specific receptor protein. The hormone-receptor complexes then are conveyed to the nucleus, where they bind to proteins of the chromosome. The two components of the receptor molecule separate, and one binds to the chromosomal DNA, causing translation to begin and new mRNA molecules to appear in the nucleus (Fig. 5.2). For example, estrogen diffuses into uterine epithelial cells to induce synthesis of new proteins.

DNA breaks occur during normal cell activity and must be repaired.

DNA molecules are not permanent but slowly undergo decay. This requires mechanisms of repair that, after toxic or irradiation injury to DNA, maintain normal cellular genomes. These elaborate procedures to protect the DNA molecule against mutagenesis include two major pathways: (1) the altered portion of the molecule may be repaired in situ (with or without enzymes), and (2) removal of the damaged seg-

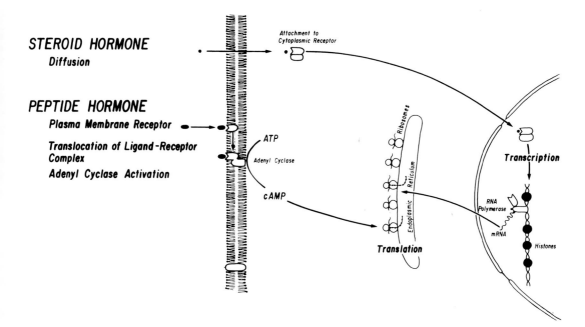

Fig. 5.2. Contrasting mechanisms of steroid and peptide hormone action. Steroids act by influencing the transcription of genes, and peptide hormones act on translation in ribosomes.

ment and replacement with newly synthesized DNA units may occur by complex enzymic processes called excision or "cut-and-patch" repair. This includes incision of damaged segments by an *endonuclease*, excision by an *exonuclease* with subsequent degradation, repair in which DNA replication is initiated by a *polymerase*, and rejoining of the new segment into the DNA molecule by a *ligase*.

The concept of DNA repair has enormous consequences in neoplasia. The genomes of cancer-causing viruses are passed from one cell generation to the next by becoming integrated into the host cell genome. DNA breakage facilitates integration of viral genomes into the host cell DNA, and the opportunity for insertion is extended when DNA repair is delayed.

Nucleolar degeneration is an early manifestation of injury.

Nucleoli are large bodies of nucleoproteins and chromatin in the nucleus that are sites of transcription and storage of new RNA transcripts. Composed of fibrillar and granular parts in association with chromatin (Fig. 5.3), they are largest in metabolically active cells and are prominent at sites where new cells are being formed and in neoplasms. In rapidly metabolizing cells, large, active nucleoli reside at the periphery of the nucleus, probably in order to facilitate nuclear cytoplasmic exchange.

When injured, nucleoli disintegrate in the following progression: (1) dissociation of the fibrillar zone, granular cortex, and intranucleolar chromatin, (2) segregation of fibrillar and granular components into distinct zones, and (3) disappearance of all structures. Nucleolar degeneration occurs when DNA or its polymerases are specifically injured and is prominent during infection by viruses that require a nuclear phase for replication. Some toxins (aflatoxin) and drugs (cyclophosphamide, actinomycin) produce specific DNA damage in which nucleolar injury is the first morphologic evidence of damage.

Ribosomes

When cells are appropriately stimulated, increased peptide synthetic activity is reflected in reduplication of ribosomes and rough endoplasmic reticulum. For example, when acidic digesta enter the gastric antrum and duodenum, the peptide hormones *secretin* and *pancreozymin* are discharged into the bloodstream where they stimulate pancreatic acinar cells to discharge zymogen granules and to increase synthesis of proteins by the ribosome. Acinar cells become basophilic, a manifestation of the increased mass of ribosomes.

Ribosomes detach from rough endoplasmic reticulum when injured.

Ribosomes disintegrate as a consequence of direct injury to their function of translating mRNA codes into peptide chains. This occurs after direct injury to ribosomal polymerases or indirectly after primary injury to nucleoli on which ribosomes depend for their formation. Ribosomes also disappear when the membranes of the rough endoplasmic reticulum (to which they are attached) are injured (Fig. 5.4).

Golgi Complex

The *Golgi complex* is the maturation site for newly synthesized proteins, glycoproteins, and glycolipids. Sacs of the Golgi complex act as condensation membranes for concentration into granules of products such as enzymes, hormones, bile, and yolk. On appropriate stimulation, product-bearing vesicles pinch off from the concave maturing face of the Golgi complex and are either stored in the cytoplasm or conveyed to the cell surface, where their contents are expelled.

Proteins acquire carbohydrate moieties as they pass through the flattened sacs of the Golgi complex, where membrane-bound glycosyl transferases catalyze transfer of sugar units to peptide chains (e.g., glucose is added to secretory glycoproteins of mucus). Just as they function as glycoprotein receptors on plasma membranes, these carbohydrate moieties function on membranes of lysosomes and other organelles to direct intracellular traffic. In effect these membrane-bound glycoproteins are address markers (comparable to postal zip codes) directing proteins to appropriate destinations in the cell—whether a particular protein goes to a lysosome or a secretory granule.

The Golgi complex degenerates when protein synthesis is inhibited.

Degeneration of the Golgi complex occurs secondary to any disruption of the protein synthetic pathway. This is most commonly seen when secretory cells become exhausted. For example, one of the early lesions in one type of diabetes

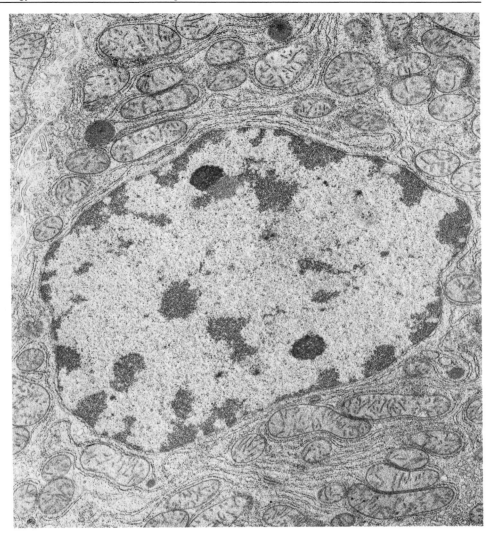

Fig. 5.3. Nuclear lesions. Liver, rat with actinomycin toxicity. Actinomycin intercalates into DNA molecules to cause (1) karyomegaly (enlargement of the nucleus), (2) destruction of nucleoli with segregation of nucleolar fibrous and granular components, (3) lysis of chromatin, (4) fragmentation of rough endoplasmic reticulum, and (5) swelling of mitochondria. (Photograph: Tim Bertram and Freddy Coignoul)

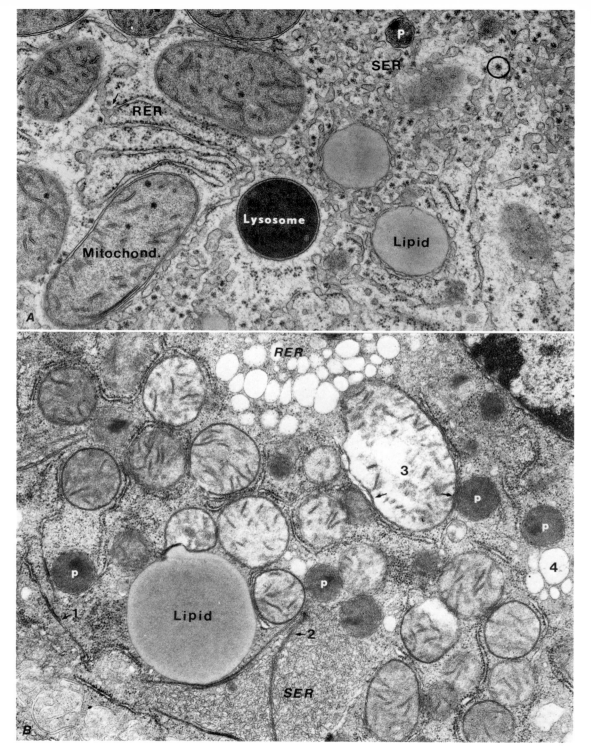

Fig. 5.4. Hepatocytes. A. Normal cell structure. Organelles include mitochondria, primary lysosomes, lipid globules, peroxisomes (*P*), glycogen
(*circle*), rough endoplasmic reticulum (*RER*), and smooth endoplasmic reticulum (*SER*). Note the connections of SER and RER (*arrow*). B. Acute
cell swelling, carbon tetrachloride toxicity. Cytoplasm shows degranulation
of rough endoplasmic reticulum (loss of ribosomes into surrounding cytoplasm) (*1*), replication and distortion of SER with formation of membrane
profiles (*2*), swelling of mitochondria with loss of cristae and inner membranes (*3, arrows*), vacuoles (*4*) form by accumulation of water in cisternae
of RER, and accumulations of peroxisomes (*p*) at sites of membrane injury
in mitochondria (*arrows*).

mellitus is vacuolation of the Golgi complex associated with extreme hyperplasia of the pancreatic islet beta cells. Only a few toxins directly affect the Golgi complex; the ionophore *monensin* is used experimentally to inhibit Golgi-associated activity.

THE SMOOTH ENDOPLASMIC RETICULUM AND DETOXIFICATION

Reduplication of the *smooth endoplasmic reticulum* (SER) is seen in early stages of poisoning, and chronic toxicity is often accompanied by massive development of this organelle (Fig. 5.3). Even cells in late stages of swelling and lysis show persistence of SER, which is evidence of a failed attempt to detoxify a lethal compound.

The catabolism of phenobarbital in liver cells is a widely studied model of detoxification. This barbiturate causes anesthesia by depressing synaptic transmission and neuronal metabolism. In brains of anesthetized animals there is a 50% decrease in oxygen utilization. Detoxification occurs in the liver. After intravenous injection there are parallel increases in SER and drug-metabolizing enzymes. Hepatocytes enlarge, and the greater cell volume is due to increased volume of SER. Cell recovery occurs after withdrawal of the drugs, and the SER returns to normal within 15 days (as seen by electron microscopy).

Biochemical events in detoxification can be correlated with structural changes by studying hepatocyte fragments of SER. When liver is ground, homogenized, and then centrifuged, SER breaks up and bits of membranes reseal to form tiny vesicles called microsomes. The microsomal fraction of the supernate is thus a convenient source of enzymes. *Mixed function oxidases* are an important detoxification enzyme complex in hepatocytes. They are nonspecific and require oxygen to function. The key enzyme of these oxidases is cytochrome P-450 (so named because in reduced form it binds carbon dioxide and then absorbs light most intensely at a wavelength of 450 nm; the amplitude of absorption is the basis of quantitative studies). This system detoxifies any poisons introduced from the environment, and the measure of cytochrome P-450 is a reliable index of detoxification reactions.

Species variability to poisons relates to differences in SER enzymes. A hexobarbital dose that makes mice sleep for 12 minutes puts rabbits to sleep for 49 minutes, rats for 90 minutes, and dogs for 315 minutes. When microsomes are isolated by differential centrifugation, the fastest oxidation reactions occur in mouse liver microsomes; rates of oxidation by microsomes of rabbit, rat, and dog are proportionally lower.

Some nonpoisons are converted to toxic intermediates in SER.

Many poisons are not directly toxic but are converted into toxic intermediate molecules within the SER and act directly on its membranes. Carbon tetrachloride is widely used as an industrial solvent, pickler, and coolant. Exposure occurs by inhalation and less often by skin contact and ingestion. Poisoning occurs when pets are left in airtight rooms after the toxin has been used to clean upholstery or clothing. When carbon tetrachloride is converted to toxic free radicals in the liver, smooth endoplasmic reticulum is one of the first organelles to degenerate (Fig. 5.4). The SER fragments into tiny vesicles, and ribosomes detach from the rough endoplasmic reticulum. A crucial effect also occurs on ribosomes where protein is synthesized. One of the earliest structural changes is the detachment of ribosomes from the rough endoplasmic reticulum.

Toxicologic enhancement

Single large doses of any of several drugs will suppress detoxification. Inhibition of detoxifying enzymes by one poison strikingly lowers the lethal dose of a second poison that acts directly on the cell. Heavy metals (e.g., lead and methyl mercury) inhibit the mixed-function oxidases and lead to increased susceptibility to other toxins. In acute alcohol (ethanol) toxicity, a single large dose inhibits drug-metabolizing enzymes and produces a markedly enhanced susceptibility to barbiturates. Ethanol, like many other toxins, has different effects on the SER at different doses and/or exposure times. Chronic alcoholics have increased liver concentrations of cytochrome P-450 and other alcohol-detoxifying enzymes that lead to stimulation of drug metabolism. For example, heavy drinkers may be less susceptible to phenobarbital.

MITOCHONDRIA

In nucleated living cells, energy coming from oxidation of carbohydrates and other organic compounds is invested in the manufacture of adenosine triphosphate (ATP). Molecules of ATP store energy in chemical form and serve as an energy currency that can be spent in powering cellular functions. Mitochondria provide the enzymes and structural framework for generating ATP by the citric acid cycle and by the coupled reactions of electron transport and oxidative phosphorylation. During phosphorylation, ATP is formed from adenosine diphosphate (ADP) at the surface of the inner membrane and is released into the mitochondrial matrix. It is then transferred to the cytoplasmic matrix and used to power most of the energy-requiring processes of the cell.

Mitochondria are located at sites of high energy utilization. Their outer membrane is porous and freely permeable to ions. The inner membrane, which contains the proton- and electron-carrier proteins, is extensively folded into ridges called cristae and has properties of highly reactive nonporous membranes. In most cells, there is a correlation between the number of cristae and the rate of mitochondrial respiration. Heart muscle cells have large numbers of mitochondria with long cristae. Tumor cells, which often depend more on glycolysis than on aerobic respiration for energy, usually have mitochondria that contain only a few stubby cristae (Fig. 5.5).

Mitochondrial pathology

Mitochondria are exquisitely sensitive to changes in factors controlling metabolic rates (e.g., oxygen tension, water and electrolyte balance, pH, temperature, and glycolytic products that feed into the mitochondrial pathways). Degeneration thus occurs secondary to almost every systemic insult to tissue and is widespread in conditions such as hypoxia, fever, acidosis, and toxemia.

Swelling and lysis

Mitochondria behave as osmometers, and the swelling that develops after injury reflects entry of solutes and water. In lethally injured mitochondria, there is swelling, shutdown of ATP production, cristolysis (breakup of cristae), and deposition of calcium-sequestering granules in

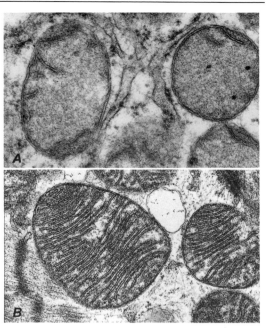

Fig. 5.5. Mitochondria. A. Mitochondria with short, stubby cristae, dog with hepatocellular carcinoma. Tumor cells obtain energy from glycolysis and do not produce large amounts of ATP in mitochondria. B. Enlarged mitochondria with increased numbers of cristae, myocardium, dog with cardiac hypertrophy.

the mitochondrial matrix. In severe swelling, excess water uptake transforms mitochondria into large, structureless vacuoles that give the cell the appearance of vacuolar degeneration.

Oxygen deficiency causes mitochondrial degeneration.

Mitochondrial swelling due to oxygen deficiency is a common lesion, especially in parenchymal cells of the heart, lung, brain, and other organs with high rates of metabolism. Oxygen is required at the end of the electron transport chain to accept electrons and to form water. Its absence suppresses oxidative phosphorylation, and these interruptions are rapidly translated as structural damage to mitochondrial cristae.

The effects of abolishing oxidative phosphorylation are magnified by its tight coupling with the citric acid cycle. NADH accumulates and exerts a powerful effect to inhibit dehydrogenases of the cycle; for example, pyruvate dehydrogenase no longer will catalyze the flux of pyruvate to coenzyme A (CoA). In acute anoxia, the damage to membranes of the mitochondria in electron micrographs suggests that shifts in ion balance are responsible for early damage in oxygen deficiency.

Metabolic poisons cause mitochondrial swelling.

Mitochondria are selectively poisoned by drugs and toxins that interrupt normal biochemical pathways, that is, pyruvate to acetyl CoA conversion, citric acid cycle reactions, and electron transport (Fig. 5.6). When these pathways are blocked, electrons are not passed to oxygen for formation of water and proton electrochemical energy is not generated to drive phosphorylation to produce ATP. Ultimately, the loss of ATP shuts down all cell processes.

ATP formation results from energy produced by proton flow at three sites along the electron transport chain. The reaction of phosphorylation, $ADP + P_i \rightarrow ATP$, actually occurs on specialized knobs that dot the surface of the matrix

side of the inner membrane of the mitochondrion. According to the prevailing chemiosmotic theory, the flow of electrons through the system of carrier molecules drives protons (H^+) across the inner membrane to create electrochemical gradients. The tight coupling of electron transport and oxidative phosphorylation occurs at the sites of proton flow. Specific poisons selectively affect these sites. If toxicity is systemic, the animal dies of cellular anoxia; the cell has oxygen but cannot use it.

Acetyl CoA formation is blocked by arsenic.

Arsenate is a classic mitochondrial uncoupling agent; that is, it uncouples the respiratory chain from oxidative phosphorylation. Arsenic poisoning from use of herbicides and insecticides is a common farm problem. In its inorganic form, trivalent arsenic combines with sulfhydryl groups of enzymes crucial to the citric acid cycle and to oxidative phosphorylation. Its dominant effect seems to be suppression of decarboxyla-

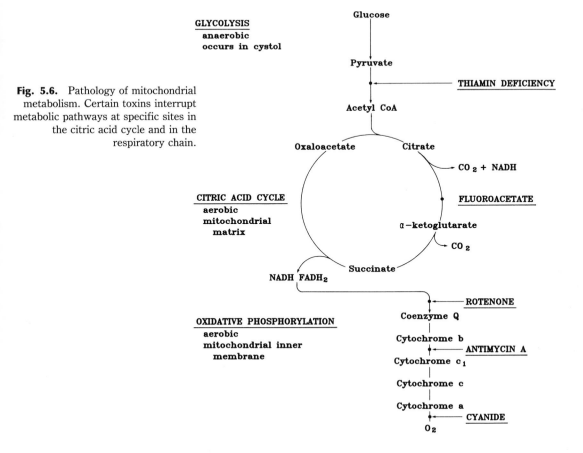

Fig. 5.6. Pathology of mitochondrial metabolism. Certain toxins interrupt metabolic pathways at specific sites in the citric acid cycle and in the respiratory chain.

tion of pyruvate, thus inhibiting formation of acetyl CoA and slowing the citric acid cycle. The hemorrhage and vascular lesions in gut, liver, and kidney are due to the rapid uptake of arsenic in these organs.

Citric acid cycles are blocked by fluoroacetate.

Sodium fluoroacetate is a rodenticide (sold commercially as compound 1080) limited in use to licensed pest control operators. It also occurs in leaves of some poisonous plants in Australia, South Africa, and South America. Accidental poisoning in mammals results in fatal ventricular fibrillation (although the dog tends to die with respiratory paralysis). Fluoroacetate is incorporated into the citric acid cycle (in place of normal acetate) as a fluoroacetyl CoA, which condenses with oxaloacetate to form the toxic fluorocitrate. Fluorocitrate inhibits the enzyme aconitrase and its conversion of citrate to isocitrate. Citrate accumulates, the cycle is blocked, and the animal dies with progressive cyanosis, cardiac irregularities, and convulsions. Ultrastructural examination of experimental animals poisoned by fluoroacetates clearly shows mitochondrial swelling and lysis.

Ammonia is toxic to the citric acid cycle.

Ammonia toxicity is manifest by its effects on citric acid cycles of brain cells. Synthesis of urea in the liver is the major route of ammonia removal; any steps blocked in the urea cycle lead to elevated ammonia in blood (hyperammonemia), which, when prolonged, is incompatible with life. When ammonia arrives in the brain it shifts the reaction: $NH_4^+ + \alpha$-ketoglutarate − (glutamate dehydrogenase)→ glutamate + additional NH_4^+ −(glutamate synthetase)→ glutamine. Depletion of α-ketoglutarate, a citric acid−cycle intermediate, leads to mitochondrial changes and ultimately to loss of ATP production.

Although hereditary urea cycle enzyme deficiencies have been reported in humans, *hepatic encephalopathy* is the most common disease resulting from diffuse liver injury. It progresses: liver destruction → hyperammonemia → accumulation of ammonia in brain → depletion of α-ketoglutarate → encephalopathy. Cerebral cortical astrocytes are most severely affected and show acute cell swelling. These lesions also result from portocaval shunts. Portal venous blood bypasses the liver to flow directly into the post-

caval vein. Ammonia arising from the intestine is not detoxified in the liver and reaches the brain.

Electron transport is blocked at three sites.

Rotenone (site 1), antimycin A (site 2), and cyanide, carbon monoxide, and azide (site 3) are drugs that block specific sites at which the electron transport chain is coupled to oxidative phosphorylation. *Rotenone,* an insecticide that acts as a respiratory depressant, specifically inhibits electron transfer from NADH dehydrogenase to coenzyme Q. Signs of toxicity, which are most often seen in pigs, include salivation, tremor, weakness, flaccidity, and coma without convulsions. Most deaths are due to respiratory failure, even though the toxicity involves mitochondrial damage in all organs.

Cyanide toxicity blocks site 3.

Cyanide is chiefly a problem when livestock graze plants with glycosides containing a cyanide moiety (e.g., arrowgrass, sorghums, and chokecherry). Like carbon monoxide, it inhibits the enzyme cytochrome oxidase by binding to its iron moiety (cyanide reacts with ferric iron, carbon monoxide with ferrous iron). Electron flow from cytochrome *a* to oxygen is blocked, and the affected animal develops dyspnea, salivation, trembling, and convulsions. Blood is well oxygenated and usually bright red; cyanosis occurs only in animals that survive for over 1 hour. Lesions of cyanide poisoning are seldom found, although laminar loss of neurons has been reported in the cerebral cortex and brain stem.

PATHOLOGY OF LYSOSOMES AND INTRACELLULAR DEGRADATION

Endocytosis is the uptake of material by invagination into the plasma membrane. Exogenous material contacts and dents into the cell surface. The pit so formed surrounds the material, separates from the cell surface, and moves deeply into the cytoplasm, carrying the material in a specialized vesicle called an *endosome. Phagocytosis* (the binding of large particles by triggering expansion of the cell surface to surround the particle) and *pinocytosis* (the nonspecific uptake of small amounts of fluids into tiny vesicles) are variants of endocytosis.

A very specific mechanism for acquiring material from the environment, termed *receptor-mediated endocytosis,* involves tight binding to substances outside the cell to specific receptor molecules on the cell surface. Specialized endosomes called *coated pits* form to envelop the material and carry it into the cytoplasm. The special coat of a protein called *clathrin,* like a postal zip code, helps to guide the new endosome to its proper destination in the cell. These endosomes lack digestive enzymes, and most are destined to combine immediately with lysosomes.

Lysosomes

Lysosomes are membrane-bound granules filled with digestive enzymes, structural proteins, and mucopolysaccharides. Because of their potent hydrolytic enzymes, they are essential for intracellular digestion. Lysosomal proteins (including their enzymes) are synthesized in ribosomes, transported into the rough endoplasmic reticulum, and put in proper order and packaged within the Golgi complex.

The *primary lysosome* is a small, dense granule with its enzymes in an inactive state. During intracellular digestion, primary lysosomes unite with phagosomes to form *phagolysosomes* (also called "secondary lysosomes"). Enzymatic degradation occurs in phagolysosomes, which either remain in the cell as "residual bodies" or excrete their digested debris from the cell by exocytosis (Figs. 5.7 and 5.8).

Lipid membranes are difficult to digest and usually accumulate in phagolysosomes (because appropriate lipases are not present); they appear as characteristic laminated bodies called *myelin figures.* Some intracellular lipids become oxidized to pigmented autofluorescent *lipofuscin* (aging pigment). Lipofuscin can be discharged from phagocytic cells or, as in the case of neurons and cardiac myocytes, remain within the residual body.

Autophagy is a general manifestation of injury.

Induction of lysosome formation as a mechanism of cellular repair occurs during all types of

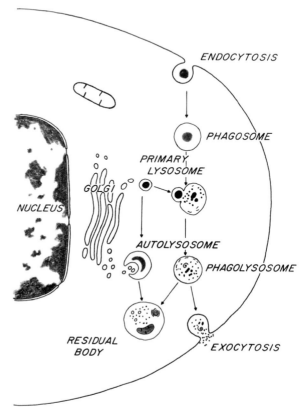

Fig. 5.7. Pathways of endocytosis, intracellular digestion, and exocytosis.

sublethal injury. The appearance of both primary and secondary lysosomes is paralleled by increased amounts of hydrolytic enzymes, which can be demonstrated either chemically in ground tissue homogenates or cytochemically by staining tissue section for enzymes such as acid phosphatase or α-glucuronidase. If injury is severe, the cell may not be able to process debris sufficiently because of overload or exhaustion of lysosomal enzyme stores. These cells are swollen and foamy due to masses of large phagolysosomes or autophagolysosomes filled with inspissated granular debris, membranes, and lipids.

Some drugs induce phospholipidosis.

Defects in phospholipid metabolism leads to production of abnormal membrane fragments, which accumulate as whorled masses of disconnected membranes within phagolysosomes. Most of these bodies result from foci of damaged or aberrant membranes of the rough endoplasmic reticulum.

Mechanisms involved in membrane injury

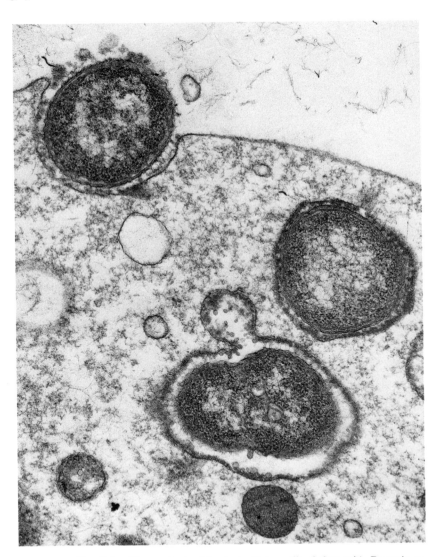

Fig. 5.8. Phagocytosis of bacteria (*Salmonella cholera-suis*). Bacteria occur at the surface of the cell, within a phagosome, and within a phagolysosome.

may be either stimulated uptake of phospholipids (which is rare) or inhibition of phospholipid degradation. The latter occurs by direct enzymatic inactivation (e.g., gentamicin) or by binding of drugs to lysosomal membrane phospholipids, rendering them resistant to degradation (e.g., chloroquine).

Drugs that commonly induce generalized lipidosis by complexing with polar lipids of lysosomal membranes are the depressants chloroquine, chlorpromazine, chlorphentermine, and iprindol. They are amphophilic compounds containing hydrophobic and hydrophilic moieties in close proximity. Chloroquine, used for treatment of malaria and some chronic immunologic diseases, induces side effects of degenerative myopathy and retinopathy. The basic lesions involve development of large lysosomes that appear histologically as foamy, granular, cytoplasmic inclusion bodies. They result from markedly increased autophagic activity with failure of enzymatic digestion and accumulation of membrane-bound aggregates of cell membranes.

Microbes and lysosomes

The sequence of bacterial killing by phagocytic cells includes attachment of the bacterium to the cell, phagocytosis with inclusion of the bacterium into a phagosome, fusion of phagosome and lysosome, and finally, intracellular degradation of the bacterium. The capacity of phagocytized pathogenic bacteria to prevent phagosome-lysosome fusion is a major factor of virulence; that is, it is a way in which the bacterium prevents the host cell from destroying it. For example, the virulence of tubercle bacilli correlates with the production (by the bacterium) of strongly acidic glycolipids containing sulfatide components, potent inhibitors of phagolysosome formation. These reactions paralyze macrophage function and sustain infection, and they operate most effectively for bacteria that replicate within cells.

Some protozoa survive intracellularly because of their capacity to resist digestion by lysosomal enzymes. In macrophages, the survival of different protozoa occurs by differing mechanisms: (1) *Trypanosoma cruzi* induces lysis of phagosomal membranes; (2) *Toxoplasma gondii* alters phagosomal membranes so that phagosome-lysosome fusion does not occur (the phagosomal membrane develops villous structures and is used for parasitic replication); and (3) *Leishma-*

nia spp. enter macrophages by being phagocytized, and when phagosomes fuse with lysosomes, mastigotes survive and replicate in the phagolysosome. The parasitophorous vacuoles of leishmaniae are a continuing part of the phagolysosome, open to extracellular menstruum from which exogenous substances can be brought in contact with the parasite via pinocytosis, rather than isolated at privileged sites as are *Toxoplasma* spp.

Hereditary lysosomal diseases involve defects in lysosomal enzymes.

These lysosomal diseases are caused by the absence or abnormality of specific enzymes and are manifest in one of two ways: (1) by the absence of a hydrolytic enzyme that causes the substrate of that enzyme to accumulate or (2) by defective enzymatic hydrolysis, wherein substrates are hydrolyzed to nondegradable products that accumulate in the cell.

Many lysosomal diseases are genetic defects, known as *lipid storage diseases,* that involve the brain or reticuloendothelial system. Affected cells are engorged with abnormal lipid complexes.

Lysosomes accumulate oligosaccharides in some plant poisonings.

Grazing animals develop striking cytoplasmic phospholipid granules in neurons and renal tubules after prolonged ingestion of certain species of locoweed (*Astragalus* and *Oxytropis* spp.) and the Darling pea (*Swainsona* spp.). Affected cells appear foamy and vacuolated because they accumulate large lysosomes filled with mannose-rich oligosaccharides. Locoweed, widely distributed in the western United States, produces a chronic neurologic disease known as locoism. Poisoned animals show lethargy, muscular incoordination, and a staggering gait, as well as the adverse effects of abortion and birth defects. Swainsonine, an indolizidine alkaloid in leaves of locoweed and Darling pea, is a potent inhibitor of lysosomal α-mannosidase. The intracellular accumulation of oligosaccharides resembles that of the hereditary mannosidosis.

Peroxisomes

These active, cell-protecting organelles are prominent around sites of membrane injury in the cytoplasm. They contain both oxidases and catalase (which converts hydrogen peroxide to water) and are especially important in oxidation and detoxification of alcohols. In vertebrates, peroxisomes are most prominent in hepatocytes, renal tubular cells, and steroid-synthesizing cells. The function of their enzymes is largely peroxidative, hence the name *peroxisomes.*

Two congenital peroxisomal diseases have been reported: acatalasemia in mice and an enzyme defect in human infants called the cerebrohepatorenal syndrome of Zellweger. Hepatic peroxisomes have dark central zones, which have been related to uricase storage. Dalmatian dogs, which have a hereditary uricase deficiency, have fewer of these dark centers than do other dogs.

Peroxisomes influence lipid metabolism.

An association between catalase-producing peroxisomes and serum lipids exists. Agents that inactivate catalase or block its synthesis produce *hyperlipemia* (catalase given intravenously has a hypercholesteremic effect). Reduplication of peroxisomes is induced by hypolipidemic drugs such as clofibrate, which is widely used for treatment of hyperlipidemia in man.

CELL SURFACE

The *plasma membrane,* its external glycocalyx, and the subsurface skeleton of filaments and tubules make up the cell surface. Large protein molecules embedded in the membrane actively regulate more specific functions (e.g., ion pumping and transmission of chemical signals to the cell). Sugar molecules attached to proteins project outward from the membrane to form a highly reactive feltlike layer over the surface that functions as a kind of immigration control; that is, their individual structures allow only a very selective attachment of specific hormones, toxins, or viruses to occur. These chemical instructions received at the cell surface are then translated into phenomena such as movement, secretion, and phagocytosis that are mediated through connections of the plasma membrane with microfilaments in the cortical regions of the cell. Cellular activities are thus *initiated* by surface glycoprotein receptor molecules and are *translated into action* by contraction of the subsurface cytoskeleton.

Plasma membrane
The membrane is a lipid bilayer, a double blanket of phospholipid molecules.

Membrane phospholipids have water-soluble polar heads and hydrophobic tails buried back to back in the interior of the membrane, a unique arrangement allowing the membrane surface to react with aqueous substances but making it impermeable to most water-soluble molecules because of the oily core (Fig. 5.9). Phospholipids are distributed asymmetrically between inner and outer layers of the membrane. In erythrocytes, choline phospholipids such as phosphatidylcholine are in the outer layer and amino phospholipids dominate the inner layer. Molecules are not static but move within the membrane. Individual phospholipids freely diffuse laterally and, when stimulated by certain signals, may flip-flop from inner to outer parts of the lipid bilayer.

Signal molecules attach to cells and induce phospholipid breakdown.

When hormones, cytokines, or other ligands bind to the cell surface, they initiate several important biochemical reactions in phospholipids. First, they *stimulate methyltransferases,* enzymes in the membrane that methylate the polar heads of phospholipids. This causes the newly methylated molecule to jump from inner to outer leaflet, reducing plasma membrane viscosity. Decreased viscosity, coupled with calcium influx, facilitates transmission of the appropriate chemical signal across the membrane. It permits ligand-receptor complexes to move more easily through the membrane to sites of enzymes, which then pass the appropriate signal into the cytoplasm.

Phospholipid degradation also leads to accumulation of *arachidonic acid,* a breakdown product of phospholipid tails. Arachidonic acid is the precursor for highly active molecules called *prostaglandins* that regulate many cellular activities. Arachidonic acid metabolites play major roles in regulation of all types of cells.

Ligand binding to surface receptors transmits signals inside the cell by a third and unique system, inducing turnover of *inositol phospholipids.* For example, the binding of a hormone causes breakdown of a key inositol phospholipid, phosphatidyl inositol biphosphate (PI-P$_2$):

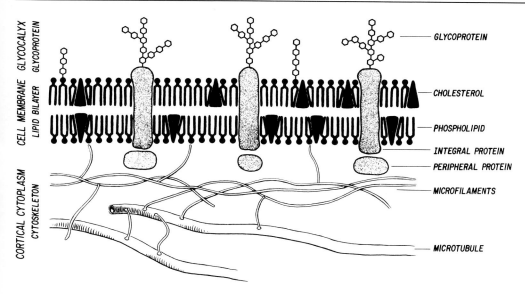

CELL MEMBRANE

GLYCOCALYX
GLYCOPROTEIN

LIPID BILAYER

CORTICAL CYTOPLASM

CYTOSKELETON

GLYCOPROTEIN

CHOLESTEROL

PHOSPHOLIPID

INTEGRAL PROTEIN
PERIPHERAL PROTEIN

MICROFILAMENTS

MICROTUBULE

Fig. 5.9. Plasma membrane. Polar lipid layers are interrupted by protein molecules and glycoproteins with reactive termini that function as receptor molecules. Complexing of hormones or other signal molecules with receptor glycoproteins causes changes in membrane fluidity and receptor molecule configuration that activate various cell processes (e.g., activation of microfilaments and microtubules leads to cell movement).

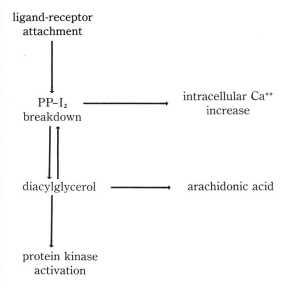

ligand-receptor
attachment

PP-I$_2$
breakdown

intracellular Ca^{++}
increase

diacylglycerol

arachidonic acid

protein kinase
activation

Cholesterol:phospholipid ratios determine membrane fluidity.

Cholesterol and other sterols are embedded in the lipid bilayer. They impose immobility on lipid molecules nearest the membrane surface but increase freedom of motion deeper within the hydrophobic core. Abnormal ratios of cholesterol-phospholipid or lecithin-sphingomyelin are responsible for abnormal plasma membrane rigidity and are especially important in erythrocytes, in which exchange diffusion of cholesterol between plasma and cell is common.

When large amounts of lithocholic acids are secreted into bile, the *cholesterol:phospholipid ratio* in plasma membranes of bile canaliculi is strikingly increased. Cholesterol molecules aggregate, which causes increased viscosity of the hydrophobic interior of the plasma membrane. Permeability to water and ions is reduced, and *cholestasis* (stoppage of bile flow) results. In icterus, where bile acids escape into circulating blood, erythrocytes may be affected by this same mechanism, that is, by increasing cholesterol in the plasma membrane of the erythrocyte.

Protein molecules are embedded in the membrane.

Most membranes contain about 50% protein, but nonreactive membranes such as myelin sheaths have less than 25% and membranes with high metabolic activities may have up to 75%. Most of these proteins are *integral;* that is, they traverse the bilayer to interact with both cell surface and submembrane cytoplasm. These integral proteins function as structural proteins, receptors, enzymes, and ion-transporting channels or pumps.

Structural proteins interconnect cells and maintain membrane stability. They form gap junctions, for example, which permit direct transfer of chemical messages between cells by allowing exchange of ions and small molecules. At gap junctions the intercellular space narrows and is filled with tiny cylindrical proteins, each with a narrow channel. In effect, the gap junction forms intercellular pipes that allow cells to coordinate activities and function as a tissue.

Charged molecules do not pass the lipid bilayer. As discussed earlier, critical ions such as Na^+, K^+, and Ca^{++} may pass directly through membrane proteins; these proteins alter their shape under certain stimuli to permit passage of ions. *Channel proteins* provide selective pathways through which specific ions diffuse. *Membrane pumps* are protein enzyme complexes that expend metabolic energy to move ions against concentration gradients. The enzyme Na^+-K^+-ATPase is an integral protein molecule embedded in the lipid bilayer of the plasma membrane. It is called the sodium-potassium pump because it pumps Na^+ out of and K^+ into the cell in a linked operation.

Receptor proteins recognize and cause specific molecules to attach to the cell surface. Their external surfaces provide binding sites with great specificity, and the protein stud exposed to the cytoplasm below the membrane provides communication for cellular events. Some large molecules move into cells by binding to receptor proteins, which then (through their connections with subsurface microfilaments) initiate endocytosis.

The glycocalyx is formed by sugars attached to membrane proteins.

Oligosaccharide chains project outward from the cell membrane. They are moieties attached to integral proteins (as glycoproteins) or more rarely to phospholipids (as glycolipids). Monosaccharide units of the oligosaccharide chains are arranged in specific sequences on different cell types. For example, on lymphocyte surfaces neuraminic acid is at the end of the chain, fol-

lowed by galactose and then mannose, which is linked to the integral proteins in the membrane. Neuraminic acid imparts a special reactivity to the lymphocytes; it is important for the attachment of certain viruses that bind to cell surfaces.

To determine which sugars are on cell surfaces, Dr. Joe Alroy, at Tufts University, has used special plant proteins called *lectins* that bind with high specificity to individual sugar units. Labeling of cells with these plant lectins provides a rough map of carbohydrate reactivity and which sugar units make up the cell surface.

Glycoproteins are receptors for most cell signals.

Glycoproteins are used as specific sites of contact by antibodies, hormones, and microorganisms. The carbohydrate moieties are well suited for this role because of their great structural diversity and extensive branching. In effect, the receptor plucks one type of molecule from the extracellular environment, even if it is present in very low concentration and mixed with large amounts of unrelated substances, and binds it tightly.

Substances that attach to glycoprotein receptor molecules on the cell surface by binding to oligosaccharide chains are called *ligands.* Ligand binding triggers remarkable changes in the viscosity of the plasma membrane, by causing phospholipid molecules to flip-flop in the membrane. As a result, phospholipids are pushed aside, and ligand-receptor complexes move to sites of further interaction with other membrane proteins.

At sites where ligand-receptor complexes cluster, *coated pits* are formed. Large molecules that have attached to specific receptors follow the pit and are brought into the cell by this *receptor-mediated endocytosis.* The material enters the cell in a vesicle or *endosome,* which is covered on the cytoplasmic side by a special protein called *clathrin.* Like a postal zip code, clathrin routes the new material to its proper destination.

The cortical cytoskeleton produces cell motion.

Microtubules and *microfilaments* (actin filaments) in the cell cortex (immediately below the plasma membrane) provide stability for the cell and also function in cell movement. The analogy has been made that they act as bone and muscle, respectively. They are involved in such diverse activities as cell migration, phagocytosis, granule secretion, lysosomal exocytosis, and membrane receptor movements.

The force that provides for movement of microfilaments is produced from the energy of ATP hydrolysis. ATP is used to power the sliding of filaments against one another. This ATP-driven motion is generated by two distinct groups of proteins: in microfilaments, by *actin* (and its coupling ATPase, myosin); and in microtubules, by *tubulin* (and its ATPase, dynein).

Microfilaments function in movement through connections with both plasma membrane and larger, more rigid microtubules. Actin is the major structural component of microfilaments in nonmuscle cells, just as it is in thin filaments of skeletal muscle fibers.

Long, rigid *microtubules* act in movement as stable guidelines, or tracks, along which particles are drawn by microfilaments or other contractile proteins. At cell surfaces microtubules operate in movement and changes of shape by cooperating with microfilaments. This interaction has been most studied in platelets and leukocytes, which change their shape by retracting and elongating their cytoplasm. Microtubules are responsible for orienting microfilament-induced movement along a particular axis.

Colchicine selectively poisons microtubules.

Colchicine, a toxic alkaloid from the meadow saffron (*Colchicum autumnale*), has been used since the 1800s by clinicians to treat human gout and by experimentalists to stop cells in mitosis. Specific binding sites for colchicine have been found on the tubulin dimer. The drug stops cell division in prometaphase by destroying the microtubules that make up the spindle apparatus. In poisoned tissue many mitototic figures are seen, not because mitosis has been stimulated but because there is an accumulation of cells blocked in midmitosis.

Intermediate filaments are used to identify cell origins.

Intermediate filaments are ubiquitous components of most cells. They are identified by their diameter (7–10 nm), which distinguishes them from the other two major filament systems, microfilaments (6 nm) and microtubules (23 nm). Intermediate filaments are a heterogeneous group composed of five major classes, each with distinct biochemical reactivity: (1) epithelial origin, *keratin*; (2) mesenchymal origin, *vimentin*; (3) muscle origin, *desmin*; (4) astrocyte origin, *glial fibrillary protein*; and (5) neuron origin, *neurofilament protein*. Using specific antibodies, these different proteins are useful in identification of unknown tissue specimens and are used to diagnose the correct classification of highly malignant tumors whose histologic source is not obvious on microscopic examination.

Pathology of the cell surface

Severe mechanical injury to the plasma membrane is lethal. In rupture wounds where the cytoplasm is not lost, however, the membrane can heal by reorientation. Molecules of the lipid bilayer move toward one another to seal the hole. The physicochemical nature of the membrane makes it self-sealing since a hole is energetically unfavorable. It is not necessarily a property of living cells, for the plasma membranes of erythrocytic "ghosts" are also self-sealing. With time, cells repair membrane defects by routing membranous vesicles to the cell surface. The vesicles fuse with and become patched into the plasma membrane at sites where injury has occurred.

Premature activation of autogenous enzymes leads to digestion of membranes.

Disastrous tissue lesions occur when potent enzymes of the digestive tract and its glands escape into the interstitium or are prematurely activated. Normally, these enzymes are segregated in secretory granules. Furthermore, the most dangerous proteases, such as trypsin, are synthesized as large, inactive molecules that must be activated, upon granule release, to be proteolytic.

During normal digestion of food, the gut releases two enzymes that enter the bloodstream and activate the pancreas: *secretin* stimulates secretion of fluid and electrolytes by centroacinar cells, and *pancreozymin* stimulates pancreatic acinar cells to release their potent enzymes (proteases, amylase, lipases, and nucleases). Proteases account for about 70% of the enzymes in pancreatic juice. One of these, trypsinogen, is normally activated to trypsin in the intestinal lumen by enterokinase, an enzyme secreted by the intestinal mucosa. Trypsin in turn can activate all other precursor proteolytic enzymes. When activated prematurely in the pancreatic ductules, it produces acute pancreatic necrosis.

Acute pancreatic necrosis is common in old dogs.

Excruciating abdominal pain, hyperlipidemia, and release of enzymes into circulating blood begin immediately after the premature activation of trypsinogen is triggered within the pancreatic canaliculi. Proteases and phospholipases injure the delicate ion- and water-pumping centroacinar cells located between acini and ductal epithelium. Rupture of canaliculi allows enzymes to leak into surrounding tissues and to destroy acinar cells and adipose tissue. The necrotizing process incites severe inflammation with edema, vasculitis, hemorrhage, and neutrophil infiltration (the condition is usually called *acute pancreatitis*). In severe cases, lesions are complicated by ischemia and by local intravascular coagulation and thrombosis, which promote shock and high mortality.

Toxic injury to membranes

Membrane structural damage due to direct destruction of phospholipid molecules in the lipid bilayers is produced by solvents and by several potent biologic toxins. All *snake venoms* contain a phospholipase A_2 (A_2 because of the specific bond it hydrolyzes in the phospholipid molecule) that destroys membrane phospholipids to release unsaturated fatty acids and lysophosphatides. These enzymes produce the same cell lesions at sites of envenomation that pancreatic acinar cell phospholipase A_2 produces in acute pancreatic necrosis.

Bacteria of *Clostridium* produce membrane toxins.

The highly lethal α-toxin produced by *Clostridium* spp. in gas gangrene, infectious necrotic hepatitis of sheep, and blackleg of cattle is a *lecithinase* that converts membrane lecithin moieties to phosphoryl choline and a diglyceride. Small holes and other defects in the plasma membrane associated with loss of selective permeability can be shown by vital dye staining.

Plasma membrane and immune reactions

Membrane injury can be produced when antibodies or lymphocytes are specifically directed to protein molecules (functioning as antigens) embedded in the membrane. In late stages of microbial disease, antibodies appear in the bloodstream and attack infected cells, which contain the specific microbial antigens on their surfaces. The reaction of antibody molecules with plasma membrane antigen leads to disruption of the membrane and lysis of the cell.

Complement causes cell injury.

To kill cells, antibodies act as recognition molecules; they attract a circulating group of proteins, known as *complement* (C), that actually produces the membrane injury that kills the cell. C is a self-assembling, extracellular system of serum enzymes that is present in most body fluids. The nine components of C (C1–C9) are attracted to the plasma membrane of cells in sequence by two related pathways: (1) the *classic* pathway, in which C activation is limited to sites where antibody is attached to cell membranes, and (2) the *alternate* pathway, which is initiated by direct interaction of particular material and a serum globulin. The later is antibody-independent and more primitive.

Both pathways generate an attack sequence of C, which actually forms holes in the plasma membrane (Fig. 5.10). The damaging effects of C activation are produced not only by cellular lysis but by release of C fragments into body fluids, which function as toxins and attractants on circulating leukocytes.

The classic C-activation scheme is a three-stage process: (1) reversible ionic interaction in which C1 components bind to antibody molecules that have attached to protein antigens in the plasma membrane; (2) enzymatic activation of the binding sites by serine esterases C2, C4, and C3; and (3) adsorption of the attach sequence complex of C5b–C6–C7–C8–C9. Cleavage of serum C5 to its derivative C5b, and attachment of this molecule to the target plasma membrane, initiates the terminal sequence of events that constitute the attack mechanism. After membrane attachment of C5b, serum C6, C7, C8, and C9 spontaneously complex to form a tightly membrane-associated, macromolecular C5b–C9 complex. The final complex forms a hollow tube in the membrane by dimerization of two C5b–C9 molecules. The hollow complexes are embedded in the glycocalyx with a thin rim extending through the membrane to create 100-nm-diameter pores that cause the cell to lyse.

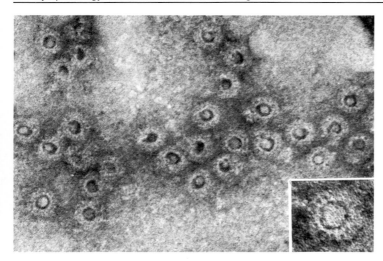

Fig. 5.10. Complement components in plasma assemble on surfaces of an erythrocyte. Holes formed by complement complexes are seen *en face* on lysed membrane, negative staining. Rings or annuli are outlined by the stain. Intermediate lines in some annuli appear as globular stain deposits in radiating patterns. (Photographs: J. Tranum-Jensen, *Scand. J. Immunol.* 7:45, 1978, used by permission)

ADDITIONAL READING

Baenziger, J. O. The role of glycosulation in protein recognition. *Am. J. Pathol.* 121:382, 1985.

Cheville, N. F. *Cell Pathology.* 2d ed. Ames: Iowa State University Press, 1983.

Freeman, B. A., and Crapo, J. D. Free radicals and tissue injury. *Lab Invest.* 47:412, 1982.

Martinez, J., and Barsigian, C. Carbohydrate abnormalities in N-linked glycoproteins in liver disease. *Lab. Invest.* 57:240, 1987.

Stanton, B. A. Regulation of ion transport in epithelia. *Lab. Invest.* 51:255, 1984.

Abnormal Metabolic Pathways

DEFECTS IN CARBOHYDRATE METABOLISM

Blood glucose

Blood glucose levels are maintained in normal animals by dietary sources of carbohydrate and by hepatic glycogenolysis, the conversion of stored glycogen to glucose. *Low blood glucose* is elevated by glucagon, epinephrine, and glucocorticoids, all of which cause glucose to flow out of the hepatocyte. In *high blood glucose,* glucose diffuses into and then is trapped in hepatocytes by being forced into the glycolytic pathway by insulin.

Insulin reduces blood glucose.

Insulin, a product of the pancreatic islet β cell, is the major anabolic hormone in mammals. It has two major functions: to stimulate carbohydrate and lipid metabolism by inducing cell enzymes (especially in hepatocytes) and to transport glucose across plasma membranes of insulin-sensitive cells (most significantly in fat cells and skeletal myocytes).

Hepatocytes, like neurons, erythrocytes, and lens epithelium, do not require insulin for glucose uptake. Glucose diffuses into the cell where insulin facilitates its entrance into the metabolic pool by stimulating phosphorylation of glucose molecules to glucose-6-phosphate (and prevents the overproduction of glucose by inhibiting the action of glucose-6-phosphatase). By being forced into the glycolytic pathway by insulin, glucose is trapped in the hepatocyte. Thus insulin depresses the critical blood level for the entry and exit of glucose molecules into and out of the hepatocyte; that is, it acts as a "glucostat," setting the blood level at which the liver is to control plasma glucose. When there are high levels of both insulin and glucose in plasma (as after feeding), glucose rapidly enters the liver. When blood glucose becomes low in the face of high insulin levels, glucose exits from the hepatocyte with equal ease to produce normoglycemia.

Insulin binds to surface receptors of insulin-sensitive cells.

In insulin-sensitive fat cells and skeletal muscle cells, insulin binds to glycoprotein receptors on the plasma membrane and markedly accelerates glucose transport into the cell. Insulin-receptor complexes are transferred to an effector molecule that transmits its message to the cell via adenyl cyclase and cyclic adenosine monophosphate (cyclic AMP). Once this process is initiated, insulin is rapidly degraded by insulinase. Insulin sensitivity is regulated by pituitary and adrenal hormones and by other factors.

Glucagon produces hyperglycemia and promotes gluconeogenesis.

Low insulin levels make the hepatocyte more sensitive to glucagon. Thus a declining insulin:glucagon ratio achieves two vital changes; it enhances gluconeogenesis and ketogenic capacity of hepatocytes, and it provides hepatocytes with precursors mobilized from muscle and fat that are needed for glucose production. Furthermore, there are other subtle interactions between liver and muscle. The increased use of glucose by skeletal muscle is matched by increased glucagon-mediated glucose production in the hepatocyte.

Adrenal glucocorticoids cause hepatocyte release of glucose by enhancing the sensitivity of *glucagon receptors.* They too are important in shock where they sustain the hyperglycemia initiated by epinephrine.

Blood glucose is erratic in the fetus and neonate.

In adult animals, a steady concentration of glucose is maintained in plasma. Regulatory factors control production and release in the liver and also the peripheral consumption by metabolizing cells. Normoglycemia is rapidly restored when glucose levels rise or fall to pathologic levels.

The newborn animal has lower and more erratic plasma glucose levels. Control mechanisms have not developed sufficiently to deal with rapid changes in demands for glucose. Newborns of some species may be particularly prone to *hypoglycemia* because of a low glycogen content in the liver after birth. In piglets, signs of hypoglycemia (e.g., weakness, convulsions, and coma) develop when colostrum is withheld too long. In contrast, newborn chicks, lambs, calves, and foals usually resist starvation for several days.

The mammalian fetus accumulates hepatic glycogen in the last few days of gestation. Glycogenolysis rapidly mobilizes glucose from these stores immediately after birth, probably due to the massive secretion of corticosteroids and epinephrine that accompany parturition. In cattle and sheep, the placental trophoblast converts glucose to fructose; that is, elevations in circulating glucose in the mother cause a rise in fructose in the fetal bloodstream.

Diabetes mellitus

Diabetes mellitus is *pathologic hyperglycemia* (the persistence of hyperglycemia during fasting). Excessive plasma glucose is eliminated by the kidney. The resulting *glycosuria* causes osmotic diuresis, polyuria, and polydipsia. Carbohydrate and lipid metabolism are abnormal, which leads to progressive emaciation and ketosis. In its total spectrum of pathologic metabolism, diabetes mellitus represents a set of complex syndromes of differing etiology, but with one common denominator—hyperglycemia.

Canine diabetes often follows acute pancreatitis.

Diabetes in dogs is commonly due to pancreatic islet β cell destruction and the resulting deficiency of insulin. In diabetic dogs, insulin is undetectable in plasma by most assays and does not increase after the stimulus of intravenous glucose infusion (Fig. 6.1). Glucose levels are high because glucose is not forced into the glycolytic pathway. In acute canine diabetes, β cells are vacuolated, devoid of granules, and filled with glycogen.

The pancreas is always affected in diabetes.

In rare cases, the islet β cells are normal and the diabetes results from suppression of insulin activity by some nonpancreatic factor. Whatever the case, the pancreas is always involved. If not affected primarily (when β cells are destroyed), the pancreas is affected secondarily by the elevated levels of blood glucose and shows elevated histologic evidence of β cell hyperplasia (with exhaustion in later stages).

Consequences of chronic hyperglycemia.

Acute elevations of blood glucose rarely lead to overt clinical disease. The excretion of massive amounts of glucose in urine tends to keep blood levels below life-threatening concentrations. In contrast, the chronic elevation of blood glucose leads to two serious changes. First, there is progressive thickening of capillary basement membranes throughout the body. The

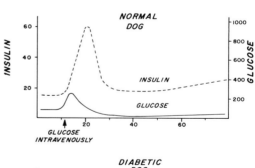

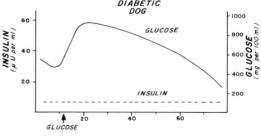

Fig. 6.1. Canine diabetes mellitus.

clinical significance relates to the renal glomeru-lus. Membranous glomerulopathy is often the killing factor in dogs that have survived for long periods on insulin therapy. Basement membrane thickening also affects the retina, but this is not the problem in dogs that it is in man.

A second consequence of hyperglycemia is the formation of sugar cataracts. Cataracts first appear as vacuoles and proceed to opacification of the lens nucleus. The earliest changes are acute cell swelling of lens fiber cells. The swollen fibers rupture and liquefaction of the fibers appears grossly as vacuoles. The osmotic change in lens fiber cells is due to accumulation of sugars by the polyol pathway: glucose −(aldose reductase)→ sorbitol −(sorbitol dehydrogenase)→ fructose.

Hemoglobin is also glycosulated excessively during hypoglycemia, although this is not associated with a known clinical consequence. The erythrocyte is an insulin-dependent cell, and intracellular glucose increases as plasma glucose rises.

Pancreatic β cell tumors cause hypoglycemia.

Neoplasms of the pancreatic islet β cells, called "insulinomas," create a situation that is the reverse of diabetes. Excess insulin is produced by the tumor cells, and this results in persistent *hypoglycemia*. The brain is very sensitive to diminished blood levels of glucose, so convulsions may occur. In tumor-bearing dogs, hypoglycemia is likely to occur in early morning prior to feeding. After eating, the production of hormones that promote elevations in blood glucose is stimulated.

Glycogen

Glycogen granules contain the enzymes that synthesize and degrade glycogen polymers. These enzymes originate in smooth endoplasmic reticulum, and glycogen is usually formed within this structure. The liver of starved animals loses its glycogen; on refeeding, there is rapid reduplication of new membranes of smooth endoplasmic reticulum and newly synthesized glycogen first appears in this labyrinth.

FOCUS

Diabetes mellitus

An 11-year-old intact male Chihuahua-terrier mongrel had been treated symptomatically for 1 year for cardiac failure. It was brought to a clinic because of a severe, seeping, ulcerating dermatitis, excessive thirst and urination, and abdominal pain. The dog had a serous nasal discharge and foul-smelling fluid feces.

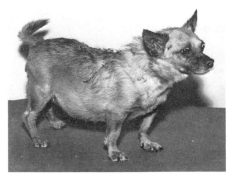

▶

Hematology		*Clinical Chemistry*	
Erythrocytes	$7.9 \times 10^6/\mu l$	Blood urea nitrogen	38
Hemoglobin	17.9 g	Glucose	371 mg/100 ml
PCV	44%	Cholesterol	300
WBCs total	42,200/μl	Van den Bergh	1.1
WBC diff.		total direct	0.1
neutrophils	76% (seg)	SGPT	28
neutrophils	10% (bands)	Amylase	2708
monocytes	4%	Lipase	4.6
lymphocytes	10%	Sodium/potassium	129/4.8
Platelets	543,500/μl	Phosphorus	5.1
Heartworms	neg.	Fibrinogen	500 mg/ml

The clinical pathology findings indicate that this dog had both pancreatitis and diabetes mellitus. The extensive pancreatic inflammatory lesions lead to diabetes. The long-term hyperglycemia is associated with several metabolic defects, one of which leads to increased staphylococcal infections of the dermis.

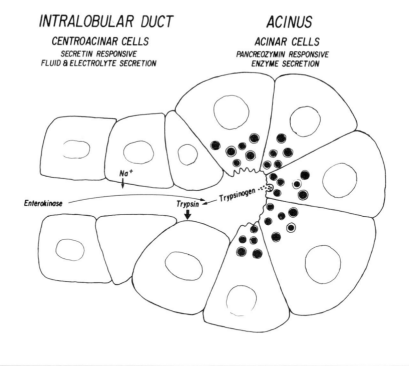

Glycogenesis: Synthesis of glycogen

Glucose molecules are joined into a chain by 1,4 glycosidic linkages, and branches are created by special 1,6 bonding to form the glycogen polymer (Fig. 6.2). The enzyme *glycogen synthase* catalyzes synthesis of 1,4 linkages. A *branching enzyme* is needed to induce the polymer-forming 1,6 linkages. Glycogen molecules are expanded as glucose units are added to terminal residues by uridine diphosphate–glucose (UDP-glucose). UDP-glucose, the donor, is the activated form of glucose, just as adenosine triphosphate (ATP) is the activated form of phosphate and acetyl coenzyme A (acetyl CoA) is the activated form of acetate.

Adrenal corticosteroids cause hepatic glycogen deposition.

Large doses of corticosteroids cause massive accumulation of glycogen in the liver (Fig. 6.3). Hepatocytes double in size, the nucleus moves to the periphery, and the cytoplasm becomes packed with glycogen particles. In dogs, corticoid hepatopathy is a serious complication of chronic steroid treatment.

Glycogenolysis: Breakdown of glycogen

The degradative pathway of glycogen to glucose begins with *glycogen phosphorylase,* which catalyzes cleavage of the linear glycogen chain (Fig. 6.4). Glucose units are sequentially removed from the end of the polymer by orthophosphate (P_i) to yield glucose-1-phosphate. Phosphorylase stops cleaving 1,4 linkages when it comes close to a branch. Branch points are degraded by the combined action of two other enzymes: a *tranferase* shifts blocks of glucose units from chain to chain, and the final breaking of the branch is accomplished by the debranching enzyme *1,6-glucosidase*. The transferase and debranching enzymes convert the branched structure into a linear one, which paves the way for final cleavage by phosphorylase.

Glycogenolysis is induced when ATP is depleted. ATP deficiency leads to increased cyclic AMP formation from breakdown products of ATP. Cyclic AMP activates a protein kinase that, in turn, phosphorylates both the synthetase (shutting it off) and the phosphorylase kinase (activating it).

Epinephrine causes glycogenolysis and hyperglycemia.

Epinephrine stimulates glycogenolysis in muscle, and to a lesser extent, in liver. In hepatocytes, it activates latent phosphorylases to begin breakdown of glycogen. Excitement, convulsions, and other stresses thereby tend to raise the blood glucose level. Chapter 13 discusses shock, in which a massive outpouring of epinephrine occurs in an effort to raise drastically falling blood pressure. Hyperglycemia invariably accompanies this phase of shock. Increased glucose is delivered to the underperfused brain to maintain life.

The liver is more responsive to *glucagon,* a polypeptide hormone secreted by the α cells of the pancreatic islets when blood sugar is low. Both epinephrine and glucagon are transported

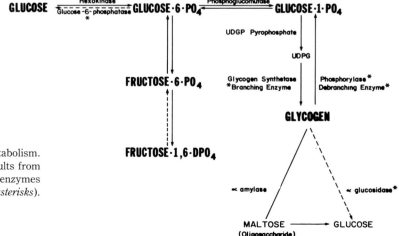

Fig. 6.2. Carbohydrate metabolism. Glycogen storage disease results from genetic deficiency of specific enzymes (*asterisks*).

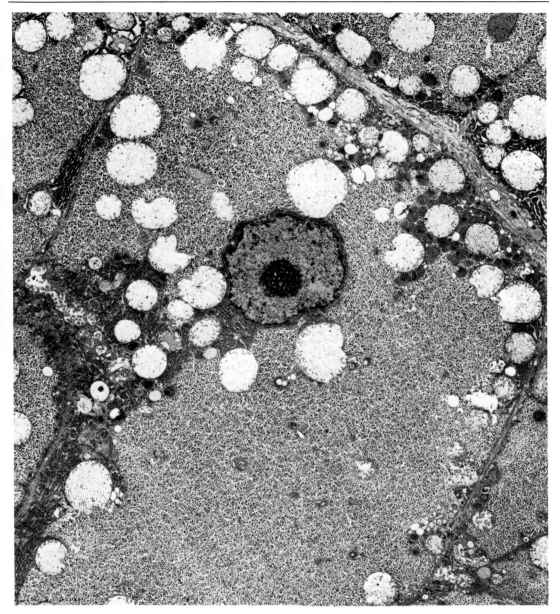

Fig. 6.3. Glycogen degeneration, hepatocyte, dog with cortisol treatment. Cell is enlarged by masses of glycogen. Mitochondria are swollen. Remnants of degenerate rough endoplasmic reticulum are around nuclear and plasma membranes.

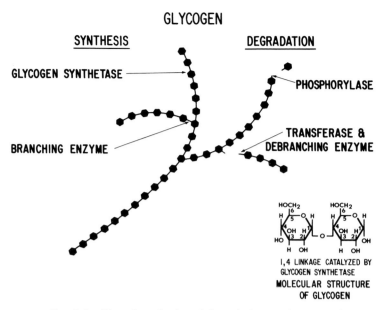

Fig. 6.4. Sites of synthesis and degradation on glycogen polymers.

in the bloodstream to muscle cells and hepatocytes. To initiate glycogenolysis, they attach to plasma membranes and activate adenyl cyclase, which increases cytoplasmic cyclic AMP.

Hereditary glycogenoses

Glycogen storage diseases are inherited syndromes caused by missing or defective enzymes of carbohydrate metabolism. Deposits of glycogen or other branched polysaccharides accumulate to produce massive amounts of foamy cytoplasm. Neurons, hepatocytes, renal cells, and leukocytes are especially affected, and their defectiveness is usually responsible for the clinical disease. At least 10 types of human glycogenoses have been described, and most types have a counterpart in animals (Table 6.1).

The first glycogen storage disease was elucidated in 1952 when it was shown that children with hypoglycemia and massive liver enlargement had a deficiency of *glucose-6-phosphatase.* Glucose was not formed properly from glucose-6-phosphate, and glycogen accumulated in the cytoplasm of hepatocytes and renal tubule cells. As a consequence of the block in glycogen degradation, lipids were mobilized and hyperlipidemia was common. Blood glucose levels did not rise after administration of epinephrine or glucagon. Convulsions occurred when hypoglycemia was severe (Fig. 6.2).

Type II glycogenosis is a lysosomal storage disease. The lysosomal enzyme *glucosidase* is missing and glycogen accumulates within large lysosomes called *glycogenosomes,* which give the cell a swollen, lacy appearance. In type III, the

Table 6.1. Glycogenosis: Hereditary storage disease of carbohydrate metabolism

Type	Deposit	Enzyme Defect	Animal
I	Glycogen	Glucose-6-phosphate	Dog,[a] mouse, man (von Gierke's disease)
II	Glycogen (lysosomal)	α-1,4-glucosidase	Cow, dog,[a] cat,[a] sheep,[a] man (Pompe's disease)
III	Glycogen (branched)	Amylo-1,6-glucosidase	Dog (German shepherd), man (Cori's disease)
IV	Glycogen (unbranched)	6-glycosyltransferase (branching enzyme)	Man (Andersen's disease)
V	Glycogen	Phosphorylase (muscle)	Man (McArdle's disease)
VI	Glycogen	Phosphorylase (liver)	Mouse, man (Hers's disease)
VII	Glycogen	Phosphofructokinase	Man
VIII	Glycogen (α-rosettes)	Phosphorylase (liver)	Man (α-particle glycogenosis)
	Oligosaccharide	α-mannosidase	Cow (Angus)

[a]Enzyme defect not clearly established.

lack of debrancher enzyme blocks degradation of glycogen beyond branching points and stored glycogen is abnormal in structure. Only the outermost branch of the glycogen polymer can be effectively utilized. German shepherds with this disease are dizzy, weak, and emaciated. Their debranching enzyme is only 0–7% of normal.

An oligosaccharide storage disease has been studied in Angus cattle with a deficiency of *mannosidase*. Dr. R. D. Jolly, then working at Massey University in New Zealand, demonstrated this to be an economically important disease and proposed testing programs to eliminate animals with this defect. Deficiency of mannosidase prevents cleavage of mannose from glycoprotein heterosaccharides. As a consequence, oligosaccharide-containing mannose accrues within secondary lysosomes and causes neurons and hepatocytes to become vacuolated.

Toxic glycogenolysis

Depletion of tissue glycogen and marked glycemia and glycosuria are characteristic of some intoxications. In clostridial enterotoxemia of lambs, extremely rapid hepatic glycogenolysis occurs. The mechanism involves rapid mobilization of glycogen due to a lysosomal response to anaerobiosis. The severe endothelial cell destruction caused by clostridial epsilon toxin is responsible for reduced transfer of substances between vascular lumen and hepatocyte, with a resultant stimulation of catabolic activity and breakdown of glycogen. Epinephrine and glucagon secretion play little role in toxic degradation of glycogen.

DEFECTS IN LIPID METABOLISM
Lipid mobilization

Fat cells (adipocytes) contain a single large locule of triglycerides that form from free fatty acids as they enter the cell. During lipolysis, triglycerides are again converted to fatty acids, which exit the cell. The continuous deposition and mobilization of adipose cell triglycerides provides an important storage and utilization system for energy. Plasma fatty acids are deposited in or removed from adipocytes under various influences, including blood lipid levels and genetic and endocrine factors (e.g., insulin stimulates triglyceride synthesis in addition to its effects on carbohydrate metabolism) (Fig. 6.5).

Lipolysis: Derivation of free fatty acids from adipocyte triglycerides

Lipolysis is promoted during starvation, short periods of fasting, and acute stress involving adrenal gland secretion. Epinephrine and other catecholamines initiate lipolysis by binding to plasma membrane receptors on adipocytes. Binding activates membrane adenyl cyclase, which catalyzes formation of cAMP from ATP at the cytoplasmic side of the plasma membrane; cAMP is the chemical messenger that initiates and regulates breakdown of stored triglycerides. As levels of cAMP rise in the adipoctye, a kinase is activated that in turn activates *triglyceride lipase*. The lipase then degrades the stored triglycerides into fatty acids. The adipose cell atrophies by the gradual segregation of the lipid locule into globules, even-

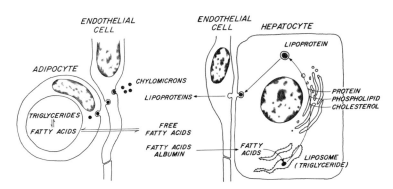

Fig. 6.5. Metabolic pathways of lipids. Triglycerides stored in adipose cells are constantly being mobilized and deposited.

tually returning to a more primitive mesenchymal type.

Epinephrine is a potent lipid mobilizer.

Injection of epinephrine is accompanied by an increase of free fatty acids in plasma. Lipolysis is also influenced by the sympathetic nervous system; when sympathetic activity increases (e.g., in stress, cold, emotional erousal, or trauma), plasma lipids increase. Alpha-adrenergic agents potentiate and β-adrenergic agents block lipolysis. The former is linked to vascular responses of adipose tissue; that is, vasodilation is induced by sympathetic nerve stimulation and facilitates diffusion of norepinephrine from nerve terminal to adipocyte.

Insulin is a potent inhibitor of fat breakdown, and its deficiency is accompanied by lipolysis. In dogs, acidosis suppresses lipolysis by inhibiting norepinephrine-induced fat mobilization.

Lipids in plasma

Two chemical classes of hydrophobic lipids are transported in the bloodstream: triglycerides (esters of long chain fatty acids + glycerol) and cholesterol esters (esters of cholesterol + long chain fatty acids). Triglycerides and cholesterol do not exist free during transport but are packaged into *lipoprotein* particles. Lipids form a hydrophobic core that is surrounded by a coat of apoproteins, phospholipids, and small amounts of free cholesterol. Apoproteins direct the lipoprotein particles to their proper destination for metabolism by binding to enzymes or receptor molecules on cell surfaces.

Triglycerides are delivered to adipocytes (for storage) and to muscle (for oxidation for energy). They are hydrolyzed at endothelial surfaces by the extracellular enzyme *lipoprotein lipase,* which liberates fatty acids. The lipase requires an activator peptide carried by the lipoprotein particle bearing the triglyceride.

Cholesterol esters go to many cells for use as membrane components, to glands for steroid hormone synthesis, and to liver for production of bile acids. They enter cells via receptor-mediated endocytosis. To deliver their cholesterol, circulating lipoproteins bind to specific receptor glycoprotein molecules embedded in coated pits on the surface of hepatocytes and other cells and are taken into the cell, where they are hydrolyzed within lysosomes by acid lipases.

Lipoprotein classes

Classes of lipoproteins transporting lipids in plasma are based on their size and composition (Table 6.2). They indicate the physical complex in which triglycerides and cholesterol esters circulate. Classes are based on electrophoretic migration and ultracentrifugation. For example, chylomicrons remain at the point of origin on paper or gel electrophoresis and float at a density of 0.95 in the ultracentrifuge. At the other extreme, high-density lipoproteins display greater α-electrophoretic migration and float at a density of 1.06–1.20.

Lipoprotein pathways

Transport paths can be divided into two systems, both of which begin with secretion of triglyceride-rich molecules: the *exogenous system* begins with secretion of chylomicrons from processing of dietary lipids by intestinal absorptive epithelium, and the *endogenous system* begins with secretion of very low density lipoproteins by hepatocytes. Each of these particles undergoes interconversion to other forms during circulation in plasma.

Chylomicron synthesis and degradation

In the intestinal lumen, dietary fats are cleaved by pancreatic lipase into fatty acids and monoglycerides. In the presence of bile acids, these form water-soluble micelles that attach to and enter intestinal absorptive cells by passive diffusion. Molecules composed of short chain (less than 12 carbon atoms long) fatty acids are released into the portal circulation. Long chain fatty acids are converted to triglycerides surrounded by a protein coat to form chylomicrons. Soon after a fatty meal, fats are resynthesized as triglycerides in the Golgi complex. As chylomicrons are formed they are secreted into lacteals of intestinal villi and enter the general circulation via the thoracic duct.

Chylomicronemia is common after a fatty meal. In cats and some other carnivores, transient *lipuria* may occur. In the laboratory, chylomicrons float during cooling of plasma to form a cream layer, a simple test for hyperchylomicronemia. Chylomicronemia is transient, however, because pathways of chylomicron metabolism are efficient and rapid. The half-time for clearance of chylomicrons and their remnants is only a few minutes in some species, and the

Table 6.2. Plasma lipoproteins

Type	Source	Composition	Catabolism
Chylomicrons (CM)	Intestinal epithelial cell	Triglyceride-rich Cholesterol-rich	Capillary endothelial surface: triglycerides hydrolyzed by lipoprotein lipase with conversion to CM remnants
CM remnants[a]	Capillary endothelial surface	Cholestrol-rich	Liver: cleared by receptor-mediated endocytosis
VLDL	Hepatocyte[b]: delivers endogenously synthesized triglycerides to adipose tissue	Triglyceride-rich Cholesterol-rich	Capillary endothelial surface via lipoprotein lipase
IDL[a]	Plasma: transformation of VLDL by action of lipoprotein lipase	Cholesterol-rich	Plasma
LDL[a]	Plasma: transformation of IDL by action of enzymes; delivers cholesterol to peripheral tissues	Pure cholesterol core with apoprotein coat	Taken up at cell surface by receptor-mediated endocytosis and catabolized in lysosomes
HDL	Hepatocyte[b]	Cholesterol-rich Protein-rich	Plasma interconversion with IDL

Note: Abbreviations: VLDL, very low density lipoprotein; IDL, intermediate-density lipoprotein; LDL, low-density lipoprotein; HDL, high-density lipoprotein.
[a]Atherogenic.
[b]Small amounts produced by intestine.

plasma level of cholesterol rises very little after feeding.

Too large to pass endothelial barriers (80–500 nm), chylomicrons are metabolized at endothelial surfaces. They bind to lipoprotein lipase molecules fixed on endothelial cells in capillaries of adipose tissue and muscle. A special apoprotein component activates lipoprotein lipase, which liberates free fatty acids and monoglycerides. Fatty acids then enter muscle for use in energy production or adipocytes for reesterification and storage.

Lipoprotein lipase activity on endothelial surfaces determines the uptake of fatty acids and varies with the animal's nutritional state. Normally lipase activity is high in adipose tissue capillaries but low in heart and skeletal muscle; thus free fatty acids tend to be taken up by adipocytes. During fasting, enzyme activity falls in adipose tissue but rises in muscle, so fats are diverted to muscle cells for energy.

Chylomicrons shrink as the triglyceride core is depleted. The remaining surface phospholipids and cholesterol are released from the endothelial surface, reentering the circulation as *chylomicron remnants.* Chylomicron remnants (30–80 nm) are carried to the liver, where they bind to receptors on hepatocyte surfaces. They are taken up by receptor-mediated endocytosis and degraded in hepatocyte lysosomes. Their cholesterol is liberated to be used by the hepatocyte to produce new lipoproteins, chiefly very low density lipoproteins. Thus the liver rapidly takes up dietary cholesterol in the form of chylomicron remnants. Much cholesterol is disposed of in bile and may be resorbed in the intestine and again delivered to the liver (enterohepatic circulation).

Very low density lipoprotein synthesis and degradation

Triglycerides produced in the liver are packaged into very low density lipoproteins (VLDLs) for transport to adipose tissue (Fig. 6.6). VLDL formation allows the liver to remove excess fatty acids from plasma and mobilize them for

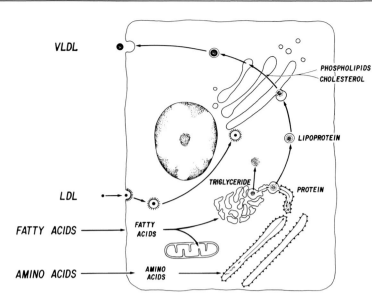

Fig. 6.6. Hepatocyte lipid metabolism. *Triglycerides* are formed from fatty acids and shunted from the site of their production in the smooth endoplasmic reticulum to storage sites in the cytoplasmic matrix (as lipid globules). *Low density lipoproteins* (LDLs), which carry cholesterol, contact hepatocytes. The LDL apoprotein interacts with LDL receptors on hepatocyte surfaces to initiate uptake by endocytosis via coated vesicles. LDLs are delivered to lysosomes where their proteins and cholesterol are hydrolyzed. Unesterified cholesterol thus liberated enters the cytosol where it is used in membrane synthesis (and suppresses further cholesterol synthesis). *Very low density lipoproteins* (VLDLs) are assembled by combination of triglycerides from smooth endoplasmic reticulum and apoprotein from rough endoplasmic reticulum.

storage in fat. In the bloodstream, VLDLs interact with endothelial lipoprotein lipase and release their triglycerides. VLDL-lipase interaction is less efficient than chylomicron-lipase interaction, so VLDLs persist in the circulation much longer.

As triglycerides are removed, VLDL particles diminish in size (and increase in density) and are converted to intermediate density lipoproteins (IDLs). Excess surface material, like that of chylomicrons, is transferred to high density lipoprotein (HDL) particles. IDL particles are released into the circulation. In hepatic sinusoids the remaining triglycerides are removed and most apoproteins are lost. The remaining particle of cholesterol ester and one specific apoprotein is called *low-density lipoprotein* (LDL). The cholesterol in the tiny LDL particle (22 nm) constitutes the bulk of plasma cholesterol in carnivores. LDLs thus deliver cholesterol to all cells. They

are removed from circulation only by cells containing specific receptor molecules on their surfaces. LDLs can also be removed from circulation and degraded by macrophages via a less efficient nonreceptor mechanism. This occurs when LDL levels are very high, as in familial hyperlipidemias, and the expanding macrophages appear as foam cells.

LDL receptors and species differences

LDL receptors and LDL metabolism are regulated by feedback mechanisms. When cholesterol is abundant inside the cell, new LDL receptors are not produced, cholesterol uptake does not occur, and enzymes that initiate cholesterol synthesis are suppressed. The reverse pathway occurs in cholesterol depletion. In dogs, as the demand for cholesterol rises, the number of receptors on the hepatocyte surface increases.

Hepatic LDL receptors are controlled by some hormones and drugs. Receptor fluctuations correlate with corresponding fluctuations in lipoprotein removal from plasma. Experimentally, drugs may increase the efficiency of hepatic LDL clearance and, in dogs, lead to a 75% drop in plasma LDL and cholesterol.

Hyperlipoproteinemia

Plasma lipids, both in amount and quality, are determined by varying and often cyclical contributions of (1) dietary lipids absorbed by the intestine, (2) lipoproteins produced by the liver, and (3) fatty acids released by lipolysis of triglycerides inside adipocytes. Although changes in diet and lipid caloric requirement alter blood lipid levels transiently, factors underlying serious and lasting pathologic hyperlipoproteinemia are more likely to involve endocrine imbalance, genetic mutation, or aging.

Primary hyperlipidemia results from endogenous defective lipoprotein metabolism. Although rare in most animal species, these defects are well characterized in man (Table 6.3).

Secondary hyperlipidemia results from defective lipid metabolism associated with diseases other than the genetically determined aberrations in lipoprotein metabolism. The lipolytic state associated with *food deprivation* and starvation causes free fatty acids and glycerol to be released into the bloodstream. This is followed by a rise in serum triglycerides as the liver takes up fatty acids and converts them to triglyceride-protein complexes.

Dogs with *diabetes mellitus* have increased serum cholesterol and triglycerides with a predominance of LDL. Diabetic hyperlipoproteinemia is caused by impaired removal of triglycerides secondary to lipoprotein lipase deficiency. Increased hepatic production of VLDL during elevations in plasma free fatty acids does not occur as it does in normal dog liver. Thus VLDL production does not contribute to hyperlipoproteinemia of diabetes. The role of diabetic hyperglucagonemia in canine diabetes mellitus is not known, although it may involve lipolysis (in the absence of insulin).

Hyperthyroidism is associated with hyperlipidemia, and thyroid hormones have widespread effects on lipid metabolism. They regulate the role of cholesterol synthesis and enhance hepatic degradation. Thyroxin is also required for lipoprotein lipase activation and for increased sensitivity to epinephrine, glucagon, and other hormones. Severely hypothyroid dogs usually have hyperlipoproteinemia, largely due to increased cholesterol, and have widespread deposits of cholesterol in arteries (see atherosclerosis, Chapter 15).

Turbid serum from hyperlipoproteinemia occurs in dogs with acute pancreatic necrosis and pancreatitis. Electrophoretic patterns reveal increased β-lipoproteins and altered migration of β_1-lipoproteins. Although pancreatic ductal enzyme reflux is thought to initiate pancreatitis, in some cases the hyperlipoproteinemia may precede the pancreatic lesion. Human pancreatitis is associated with the hyperlipoproteinemias of both chronic alcoholism and lipid metabolism defects.

Lipids in tissue: Fatty degeneration

In fatty degeneration, triglyceride production exceeds the slower, more elaborate events involved in VLDL production or in shunting of fatty acids into mitochondria for energy production. Normally, the amount of triglycerides awaiting processing is small and few lipid globules are in hepatocytes. When injury destroys any part of the lipid metabolic pathway, appropriate substrates accumulate (e.g., cholesterol,

Table 6.3. Mechanisms of primary hyperlipidemia

Defect	Substances Elevated in Serum	Pathogenesis[a]
Lipoprotein lipase defect	Triglycerides (TGs)	Missing enzymes for hydrolysis triglycerides carried on chylomicrons and VLDLs prior to entry into adipocytes
LDL receptors	LDL (cholesterol)	Failure to remove circulating LDL while hepatic cholesterol synthesis remains undiminished
Catabolism of LP remnants	LDL remnants	Apolipoproteins defective, LDL remnants not degraded
Apoprotein synthesis	Cholesterol and TGs *decreased*	Abnormal synthesis of apoprotein moieties, cholesterol esters deposit in tissues

[a]Most syndromes reported only in man.

phospholipids, or fatty acids). It is the massive backlog of *triglycerides,* however, that dominates the changes of fatty degeneration.

Injuries causing imbalance among supply, utilization, synthesis, or release of lipids may cause fat to accumulate. Thus in hepatocytes, fatty degeneration may result from (1) oversupply of circulating fatty acids from blood lipids; (2) interference with enzymes bound to membranes of smooth endoplasmic reticulum (triacylglycerolsynthetase complex) that transfer fatty acids to glycerol to form triglycerides; (3) block of protein synthesis in rough endoplasmic reticulum, assembly of lipoproteins, or release of lipoprotein granules at the cell surface; (4) prevention of fatty acid activation by CoA, or with passage across the mitochondrial membrane to enter into mitochondrial matrix energy pathways in the citric acid cycle.

Excess fatty acids: Starvation and diabetes

The abnormal carbohydrate metabolism that occurs in starvation and diabetes mellitus is accompanied by defects in lipid metabolism and fatty degeneration in the liver. Accumulation of fat begins around central veins, and the expanding lesion precisely outlining individual liver lobules is called *centrolobular fatty degeneration* (Fig. 6.7).

Insufficient sources of energy in the diet often lead to fatty degeneration, especially in lactating ruminants or in poultry during egg production. Fat accumulates in the liver of cows around the time of parturition, because of excessive mobilization of fatty acids from adipose tissue in response to the negative energy balance of early lactation. Lactating cows deprived of food for 1 week develop fat in the liver. The rapidly metabolizing hepatocyte has massive increases in cell volume caused by accumulation of lipid globules.

Carbohydrate stores in liver and muscle are depleted in starvation and diabetes mellitus (through continual loss of glucose via urine). In both diseases this leads to breakdown of fat and protein (gluconeogenesis, the formation of glucose and glycogen from noncarbohydrate sources). Lipolysis in adipose tissue accelerates,

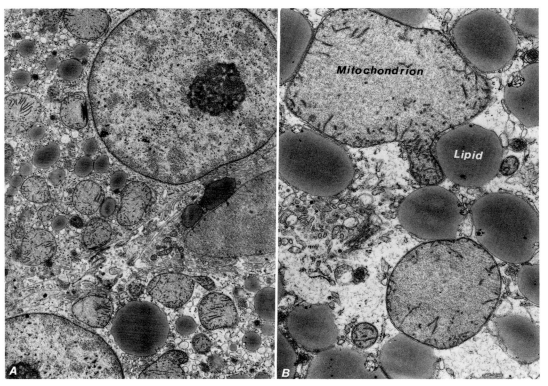

Fig. 6.7. Fatty degeneration, liver, dog with diabetes mellitus (see Fig. 4.4). A. Hepatocytes. B. High magnification of A.

and free fatty acids increase in the blood. In the liver, acetyl CoA fails to enter the citric acid cycle and is diverted to acetoacetate and hydroxybutyrate (ketone bodies), which diffuse out of the cell to circulate (see ketosis of starvation, Chapter 29).

Ketone bodies are normal fuels of mitochondrial respiration in organs other than liver. In fact, heart muscle and renal cortex use them in preference to glucose and brain adapts to their use. Liver, however, lacks the specific thiophorase required for utilization and can only supply ketone bodies in large amounts to the bloodstream.

Suppression of fatty acid oxidation: Hypoxia

Hypoxic cells, if not killed by acute cell swelling, attempt to accommodate to oxygen deficit. Mitochondria enlarge as precursor molecules that cannot enter the respiratory chain accumulate. A major defect in hypoxic cells is the inhibition of enzymes that catalyze fatty acid oxidation. This, plus other cell defects, promotes synthesis and accumulation of triglycerides.

The *hypoxic liver,* typified by venous hypertension and stasis of chronic congestive heart failure, develops fatty degeneration in the cells of centrolobular areas that are most susceptible to oxygen deficiency. In acute *myocardial infarction,* myocytes in the infarcted area are killed rapidly by lysis. Myocytes at the periphery survive and undergo fatty degeneration.

Suppressed protein synthesis

Sublethal doses of some toxins produce fatty degeneration in the liver by depressing protein synthesis. Toxins as diverse in mechanism as carbon tetrachloride (CCl_4) and aflatoxin ultimately affect ribosomes and their ability to produce peptide chains. If cells are not killed by acute cell swelling, they survive to develop massive triglyceride accumulation. Deprived of newly emerging peptide chains, the hepatocyte cannot conjugate triglycerides and is deprived of proteins that serve as enzymes in lipid metabolic pathways. Because apoproteins are not formed, lipoproteins cannot be synthesized; the continuing production of triglycerides results in a progressive accumulation of lipid globules in the cytoplasm.

Suppressed cell secretion

Any injury that interferes with intracellular transport and exocytosis will cause secretory granules to accumulate. In hepatocytes, membrane-bounded VLDL particles are moved out of the cell by exocytosis. When this is blocked, VLDL particles are packed into the cytoplasm. Ethanol toxicity produces defects in virtually all phases of lipid metabolism. In human chronic alcoholism, part of the liver damage is due to diminished hepatocyte excretion.

Hereditary lipidoses

The familial, systemic *lipid storage diseases* are due to defective or missing enzymes that degrade glycolipids, particularly cerebrosides and gangliosides that are components of cell membranes (Table 6.4). These complex lipids are degraded in lysosomes by the sequential removal of terminal sugar groups. Cells such as neurons that contain and catabolize large amounts of gly-

Table 6.4. Lipidosis: Hereditary storage disease of lipid metabolism

Deposit	Enzyme Defect	Animal
Glucocerebroside	β-glucosidase	Dog, man (Gaucher's disease)
Galactocerebroside	β-galactosidase	Dog, sheep, mouse (twitcher), man (Krabbe's disease)
Ceramide	Acid ceramidase	Man (Farber's disease, lysosomal sphingolipidosis)
Ceramide trihexoside	α-galactosidase	Man (Fabry's disease)
Ganglioside (GM_1)	β-galactosidase	Cat
Ganglioside (GM_2)	Hexosaminidase A Hexosaminidase A,B	Dog (German shorthair), pig, man (Tay-Sachs disease) Cat, cow, man (Sandhoff's disease)
Ganglioside (uncharacterized)	?	Cat, cow
Sphingomyelin	Sphingomyelinase	Cat, mouse, dog (poodle), man (Niemann-Pick disease)
Sulfatide	Sulfatidase	Mouse, man (metachromatic leukodystrophy)

colipids are first affected. *Cerebrosides* are present in large amounts in myelin, and deficiencies of cerebrosidases involve macrophages of the central nervous system. For example, globoid cell leukodystrophy is a hereditary central nervous system disease of dogs in which β-galactosidase is defective, leading to accumulation of galactocerebroside in macrophages of the brain.

Gangliosides are also present in large amounts in brain. Defects in degradation associated with deficiencies of appropriate enzymes are reflected in accumulation of the gangliosides GM_1 and GM_2 in nerve cell bodies.

These syndromes are defects of lipid *catabolism,* and mechanisms of synthesis of glycolipids are normal. Rare human lipid *anabolic* disorders have been described in which enzymes for formation of GM_2 and GM_3 are missing.

CALCIUM AND ITS ROLE IN METABOLIC DISEASE

Calcium in the cell

Calcium ions (Ca^{++}) are critical for many cell activities. The two major regulatory homeostatic mechanisms involve movement of Ca^{++} back and forth between cytosol and cytoplasmic organelles: (1) passive influx into the cytosol from three compartments (extracellular space, mitochondrial matrix, and endoplasmic reticulum cisternae) and (2) active extrusion of Ca^{++} from the cytosol back into these zones by calcium pumps in their membranes (Fig. 6.8).

Even though intracellular and extracellular amounts of calcium may be similar, in *ionic* form, extracellular Ca^{++} is over 100 times that in the cytosol. Ca^{++} transport across the plasma

membrane occurs by a Na^+–Ca^{++} exchange transfer. Transport across membranes of mitochondria and endoplasmic reticulum is chiefly due to energy-requiring calcium pumps.

Plasma calcium

Calcium exists in plasma in ionic form (Ca^{++}) and bound to plasma proteins. It is required for maintenance of skeletal and cardiac muscle contractility, blood coagulation, neural transmission, capillary endothelial junctions, and bone marrow activity. When very low levels of plasma calcium develop and persist, disturbances result in these systems (Table 6.5).

Plasma levels of Ca^{++} in mammals, birds, and reptiles are maintained directly by *parathyroid hormone* (PTH), which stimulates bone resorption and hypercalcemia, and by *calcitonin,* which inhibits resorption and leads to hypocalcemia. Other hormones elevate or depress high-affinity, Ca^{++}-binding proteins in plasma to indirectly influence Ca^{++} levels (e.g., plasma Ca^{++} in laying hens is 3 times that in male birds, a result of estrogenic stimulation of synthesis and release of circulating phosphoproteins with a high affinity for Ca^{++}).

Parathyroid hormone mobilizes Ca^{++} by bone resorption.

The parathyroids control the concentration of Ca^{++} in plasma. Parathyroid hormone mobilizes calcium from the skeleton; it also increases renal excretion of phosphorus and augments the rate of absorption and excretion of calcium from

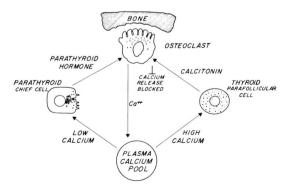

Fig. 6.8. Calcium pool.

Table 6.5. Calcium and phosphorus levels in blood expected in parathyroid disease

Disease	Serum Ca	Serum P
Primary hyperparathyroidism (neoplasm)	High[a]	Low
Renal secondary hyper-parathyroidism	Low[b] or low normal	High
Nutritional secondary hyper-parathyroidism		
Early	Low	High
Compensated	Normal	Normal
Low phosphorus osteomalacia		
Early	Low	Low
Compensated	Normal	Low

[a]Other causes of hypercalcemia: vitamin D toxicity, leukemic syndromes.

[b]Other causes of hypocalcemia: milk fever (cow), acute pancreatitis with fat necrosis, protein-losing gastroenteropathy.

the intestine. Parathyroid hormone is secreted in response to low levels of ionic calcium in plasma (hypocalcemia). The Ca^{++}-mobilizing activity is mediated through the activation of adenyl cyclase. In the kidney, parathyroid hormone also regulates the rate at which the renal tubule forms 1,25-dihydroxycholecalciferol, the active form of vitamin D.

In causing Ca^{++} to be removed from bone matrix, parathyroid hormone produces *osteolysis,* the absorption and destruction of bone; bone matrix is modified and bone calcium salts disappear. There is increased osteolysis by osteoclasts and osteocytes. Osteoclasts located on bone trabecular surfaces are stimulated to increase in numbers and activity. For example, when parathyroid hormone is given to cows, bone resorption is increased 5-fold by osteoclastic activity. Bone-absorbing osteoclasts have active and vigorous pinocytotic action on their cell surfaces, and these specialized areas of the plasma membrane cause active ion exchange.

Deep in bone, osteoblasts are also transformed into osteocytes, which may secrete proteases and collagenases that resorb bone. In osteocytic osteolysis the surrounding matrix of bone becomes less dense and is nearly devoid of mineral.

Parafollicular cells secrete calcitonin.

The parafollicular cells (C cells) of the mammalian thyroid gland secrete the hypocalcemic hormone *calcitonin.* Located between the thyroid follicles, they function independently of thyroid epithelium. The number and distribution of granules in C cells are responsive to the concentration of calcium in plasma. Experimental hypercalcemia in the dog results in rapid degranulation of C cells. C cells in cows made hypercalcemic by injections of vitamin D have reduced numbers of secretory granules. After long-term or chronic hypercalcemia, C cell hyperplasia will develop.

Calcium in plasma stimulates calcitonin secretion.

During hypercalcemia, C cells are induced to release *calcitonin.* A major action of this hormone is mainly on bone, where it acts to inhibit both matrix and mineral resorption. Osteocytes of animals given calcitonin experimentally become surrounded by star-shaped aggregates of calcium apatite crystals. The inhibition of bone matrix resorption by calcitonin is independent of, and in direct opposition to, the action of

parathyroid hormone. Complex interactions between these two hormones often lead to confusing tissue lesions. For example, during hypocalcemia-induced parathyroid hormone secretion, plasma calcium may be raised and secondary oversecretion of calcitonin occurs. This inhibits osteolysis (induced by parathyroid hormone), which in turn begins the cycle anew.

Calcitonin also acts on the lower nephron to cause calcium to be removed from the glomerular filtrate (Fig. 6.9).

Renal failure, secondary hyperparathyroidism, and osteodystrophy of dogs

In end-stage renal disease, the kidney fails to adequately excrete phosphorus from plasma to urine. The excess phosphorus in plasma depresses plasma calcium, and this in turn induces parathyroid hyperplasia and secretion of parathyroid hormone. Progressive hypocalcemia and hyperphosphatemia lead to increased destruction of cortical and trabecular bone and formation of new, poorly formed bone that is not functionally arranged. Affected dogs have bones that are soft and bowed.

High plasma phosphorus is caused both by failure of phosphorus to pass the damaged renal glomerulus and by failure of the altered renal tubule to respond to parathyroid hormone (which normally suppresses phosphate resorption and enhances calcium resorption). Thus, despite increased plasma PTH, phosphorus does not pass into the glomerular filtrate in sufficient amounts, and the phosphorus that does is resorbed. The calcium that manages to pass into the glomerular filtrate is not preferentially resorbed. To complicate the disease, hyperphosphatemia leads to excretion of a large amount of phosphorus into the gut where it combines with calcium to deprive the animal of its dietary source.

Calcium in tissue

When tissue encountered in postmortem dissection feels gritty and scrapes against the knife, it is probable that calcium deposits are present. They appear in histologic sections as granular or amorphous blue-black deposits. The von Kossa stain, which detects phosphates associated with calcium, is used to establish that the substance is calcium (Fig. 6.10).

Classically, students are taught that two forms of pathologic tissue calcification occur: *dys-*

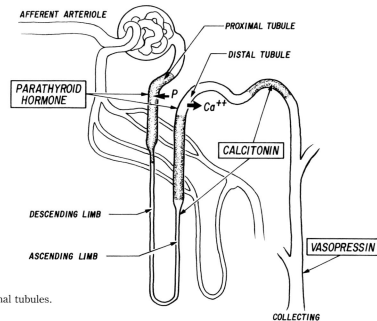

Fig. 6.9. Hormonal effects on renal tubules.

trophic calcification, in which calcium salts are deposited in degenerating cells, and *metastatic calcification,* in which they are deposited in normal tissues in the presence of hypercalcemia. This dichotomy is not entirely satisfactory, since hypercalcemia can rarely be directly correlated with tissue calcification. The role of cellular injury is difficult to assess, but it appears that nearly all forms of calcium deposition involve previous defects in cells.

Dystrophic calcification

Calcification is seen at sites of scarring, hemorrhage, and necrosis. Lesions of tuberculosis, trichinosis, histoplasmosis, and caseous lymphadenitis are frequently mineralized. Calcium salts develop within foci of damaged ground substance containing altered mucopolysaccharides, much as cartilage calcifies when certain glycosaminoglycans increase.

One of the most serious sites of dystrophic calcification is the degenerating smooth muscle layer of arteries. Calcium is deposited on the altered microfibrillar portions of elastic tissue, and calcification spreads to involve large portions of the artery.

Giant *laminated calcified bodies* called psammoma bodies or "sand bodies" are important

diagnostic features of some tumors and chronic inflammatory lesions. In tumors, they may form from calcification of thrombi or foci of dead tumor cells. They occur in normal thyroid, mammary gland, and avian embryonic yolk sacs and may be a source of calcium sequestration. In mammary glands they develop in late lactation but are not known to interfere with milk production.

Calcific metaplasia is a variant of dystrophic calcification in which tissues are converted into masses of calcium and in some cases into bone. These hard, circumscribed deposits are called tumorous calcinosis or calcinosis circumscripta.

Hypocalcemia and tissue calcification

Kidneys calcified by *hypervitaminosis D* have been used as models to study metastatic calcification. Vitamin D causes a progressive uncoupling of oxidative phosphorylation in mitochondria, which are the organelles first involved in the pathogenesis of this syndrome. Widespread soft tissue calcification occurs in a variety of diseases for which the mechanisms of calcification are not known.

Some plant toxins are calcinogenic.

Livestock grazing plants of the genera *So-*

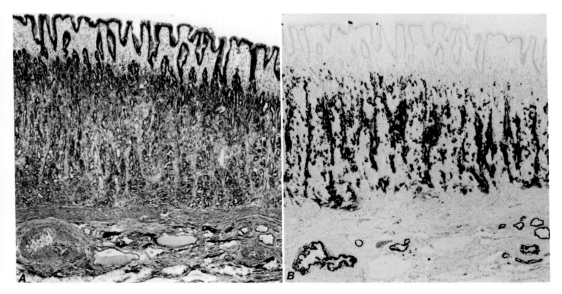

Fig. 6.10. Calcification in the stomach, dog with uremic gastropathy. A. Fundic mucosa: edema in foveolar (surface) regions, calcified pale areas in glandular regions, arterial lesions and dilated lymphatics in submucosa (see Fig. 3.2). B. Section adjacent to that in A stained by the von Kossa technique for calcium salts, which are deposited in mucosa and submucosal arteries.

lanum, Cestrum, and *Trisetum* develop hypercalcemia, hyperphosphatemia, and widespread tissue calcification. Soft tissue mineralization and progressive debilitation are due to the vitamin D–like action of toxins. Leaves contain a steroid-glycoside conjugate similar to 1,25 dihydrocholecalciferol (the active metabolite of vitamin D) that stimulates calcium-binding protein synthesis and enhances intestinal calcium absorption.

Bacteria can be calcinogenic.

Calcium-sequestering bacteria produce deposits of calcium salts in tissue, especially in late stages of inflammation. The extreme example of bacteria-induced calcification is the calcified microbial plaque on teeth. Dental calculi of dogs contain the calcite form of $CaCO_2$ mixed with small amounts of apatite ($CaPO_4$). Bacteria secrete peculiar acidic phospholipids that complex with soluble electrolytes in saliva to initiate precipitation of calcium carbonate and apatite in the calculus overlying the tooth surface. Some gram-negative rods produce extrabacterial debris and vesicles that become mineralized, and gram-positive rods sequester calcium within the bacterial cell.

Neoplasms can cause hypercalcemia.

Persistent hypercalcemia that accompanies disseminated neoplastic disease is often due to ectopic secretion of parathyroid hormone–like peptides by the tumor cells (see neoplasia, Chapter 10). Calcification is not common in these syndromes, and the hypercalcemia does not play a major role in mortality.

Pulmonary calcification

Diffuse pulmonary calcification, also called "pulmonary microlithiasis" or "pumice lung," is commonly seen in the dog. It occurs in young pups as a consequence of vitamin D toxicity and in aged dogs accompanying chronic renal insufficiency (uremia) and hyperparathyroidism. In rare cases, pulmonary calcification occurs as a component in adrenal cortical hyperplasia (Cushing's disease). Diffuse pulmonary calcification also is a sequel of viral pneumonitis and pneumonia in some species. Varicella pneumonia, a complication of severe chicken pox in man, is complicated by deposition of calcium in the lungs.

The lungs at necropsy are large, do not collapse, and have a granular gritty feeling. Micro-

scopically there are innumerable calcified con-
cretions (calcospheres) in the alveolar wall
throughout the lung. Despite this affection,
signs of respiratory disease are often surprisingly few. If unresolved, however, diffuse calcification induces a slowly progressive interstitial
fibrosis with increasing dyspnea.

In advanced pulmonary calcification, calcium
deposits are present throughout the alveolar
wall, which progressively thickens. Massive
nodular deposits project into the alveolus and
become large enough to be seen grossly. Granular pneumocyte hyperplasia accompanies deposition of calcium and adds to the thickness of the
wall. This process is an attempt at repair, and
the granular pneumocyte is rarely affected by
calcium deposits.

ADDITIONAL READING

Gilka, F., and Sugden, E. A. Ectopic mineraliza-
    tion and nutritional hyperparathyroidism in
    boars. *Can. J. Comp. Med.* 48:102, 1984.
Haskins, M. E., et al. Mucopolysaccharidoses in
a domestic short-haired cat. *J. Am. Vet. Med.
Assoc.* 175:384, 1979.
Howell, J. M., et al. Generalized glycogenosis
    type II. *Comp. Pathol. Bull.* 10:2, 1978.
Likar, I. N., and Robinson, R. W. Atherosclero-
    sis. Cattle as a model for study in man.
    Monogr. Atheroscler. 12:1, 1985.
Mattheeuws, D., et al. Diabetes mellitus in
    dogs. *Am. J. Vet. Res.* 45:98, 1984.
Rogers, W. A., et al. Lipids and lipoproteins in
    normal dogs and in dogs with secondary hy-
    perlipoproteinemia. *J. Am. Vet. Med. Assoc.*
    166:1092, 1975.
Schoen, F. J., et al. Onset and progression of
    experimental bioprosthetic heart valve calcifi-
    cation. *Lab. Invest.* 52:523, 1985.
Sheahan, B. J., and Donnelly, W. J. C. Enzyme
    histochemical and ultrastructural alterations
    in the brain of Friesian calves with GM_1
    gangliosidosis. *Acta Neuropathol.* 30:73, 1974.
Svenkerud, R., and Hauge, J. G. Glycogenosis
    type III. *Comp. Pathol. Bull.* 10:2, 1978.
Wood, P. A., and Smith, J. E. Glycosylated he-
    moglobin and canine diabetes mellitus. *J. Am.
    Vet. Med. Assoc.* 176:1267, 1980.
Woodard, J. C., et al. Calcium phosphate deposi-
    tion disease in Great Danes. *Vet. Pathol.*
    19:464, 1982.

Pigments and Crystals

7

IN many diseases, colored substances are deposited in tissue. Other than being pigments, they have little in common even though they are considered together here. The *endogenous pigments* are produced within the body. Of these, we will examine the melanins, lipochromes, and hemoglobin derivatives.

ENDOGENOUS PIGMENTS

In mammals, four major endogenous pigments accumulate in tissue: melanin, lipofuscin, hemosiderin, and bilirubin (Table 7.1). The last two pigments are derived from erythrocyte breakdown. In lower vertebrates chromatophores other than melanin are responsible for skin coloration and may be found in abnormal aggregates.

Melanin

Melanin is the brown pigment of skin, hair, leptomeninges, and choroid of the eye (Table 7.1). In lower vertebrates it is widespread, occurring in the interstitium of many organs. Melanin is a high-molecular-weight biochrome bound to protein. Formed in melanocytes, it resides in characteristic granules called *melanosomes*. In skin, melanin is also transferred from melanocytes to phagocytic storage cells called *melanophages*. In mammals, the only known function of melanin is protection against solar ultraviolet radiation. It is thought to capture injurious free radicals generated in the skin during injury. In lower animals, melanin has a protective effect in inflammation.

Melanocyte-stimulating hormone influences melanin production.

Melanocyte-stimulating hormone (MSH) is produced by the pituitary in two chains, αMSH and βMSH. It is formed as a precursor protein that contains sequences of ACTH (a corticotropinlike intermediate-lobe peptide), lipotropin, and several endorphins; selective proteolysis yields these smaller, individual peptides. MSH acts on the melanocyte to initiate melanin synthesis.

Melanin genes control production.

In most vertebrates, genes direct the production of black-brown insoluble *eumelanins*. Some avian and mammalian epidermal melanosomes (including those in human red hair) contain *phaeomelanin,* a light-colored, sulfur-bearing melanin.

The many different coat color mutations of animals are attributed to different genetic loci, which determine expression of genes for melanin synthesis. The *agouti* locus controls synthesis of eumelanin and phaeomelanin (in mice, a complex of 17 distinct alleles on chromosome

Table 7.1. Endogenous pigments

Pigments	Seen in
Melanin	Normal pigmentation
	Focal congenital pigmentary defects
	Tumors (melanomas)
Lipofuscin	Myocardium and neurons of aging animals
	Systemic metabolic disease (lipofuscinosis)
Bile pigments	Liver disease (congenital and acquired)
Malarial pigments (hematin-polypeptide complex)	Malarial infection

number 2 are active). Individual hairs of agouti animals are banded as a result of a switch from synthesis of yellow phaeomelanin to black or brown eumelanin, which occurs synchronously in every hair during the growth cycle.

The enzyme tyrosinase initiates melanin synthesis in melanocytes.

Tyrosinase, a copper-protein enzyme, facilitates oxidation of tyrosine to dioxyphenylalanine (dopa), and dopa to dopaquinone. Detection of tyrosinase (the "dopa reaction") is the basis of the histochemical identification of melanocytes and melanoblasts. In melanocytes, tyrosinase accumulates in small, membrane-bound Golgi vesicles called premelanosomes. During maturation of the melanosome, melanin develops into oriented protein strands and melanin polymers are deposited on the protein framework.

In the process of dermal pigmentation, melanosomes are transferred from the dendrites of melanocytes into keratinocytes. Increased transfer activity causes increased pigmentation. Tanning of human skin by ultraviolet radiation involves an increase in the length of dendrites and increases in melanosomes and tyrosinase activity but not in numbers of melanocytes.

Pathologic melanin

Abnormal melanin pigmentation can result from changes anywhere in the pathway of melanin production (Table 7.2). In chronic dermatitis, for example, the skin often shows pigmented defects caused by failure of transfer to hyperplastic keratinocytes. "Contact depigmentation" of skin is caused by some chemical, notably phenol.

Melanosis, the aberrant accumulation of melanin in foci, occurs in young animals of several species. In ruminants, melanosis of the brain is common (melanin arises from astrocytes), but these foci are not known to proliferate or cause disease. Melanotic lesions of the skin, in contrast, carry the potential for malignant transformation (see melanoma, Chapter 10).

Albino genes are mutations of melanin genes.

Albinism results from a structural gene mutation at the locus that codes for tyrosinase; that is, albino animals have a genetically determined failure of tyrosine synthesis. Animals that inherit an albino gene from both parents (are homozygous for albino) are unable to make melanin because the albino gene fails to direct synthesis of the enzyme tyrosinase. Albino cats are homozygous for a c-locus tyrosinase-negative allele. Heterozygotes have normal pigments but abnormal vision and can be identified with a tyrosinase enzyme assay.

Some albino animals have no tyrosinase, and others form tyrosine but no melanosomes (there are at least seven variants of human albinism). In *partial albinism,* there is a general reduction in skin pigmentation but no pigments are present in the eye. Epidermal melanocytes show retarded melanogenesis; their granules are immature fibrillar premelanosomes. It has been

Table 7.2.   Pathologic changes in melanization

Defect in	Occurs in	Pathologic Change
Melanoblast differentiation	Focal hypomelanosis (merle dogs, piebald mice, white spotting) Diffuse hypomelanosis (white tiger, gray collie syndrome)	Melanocytes absent due to inadequate differentiation or migration of melanoblasts from neural crest
	Vitiligo	Progressive loss of melanocytes throughout lifetime
Tyrosine synthesis	Albinism	Melanocytes do not synthesize tyrosine and melanin; any melanosomes present are normal and transferred normally to keratinocytes
Melanosome formation	Chediak-Higashi syndrome	Abnormal aggregation of melanin molecules with bizarre shapes
Transfer to keratinocyte	Chronic dermatitis	Melanocyte normal, but keratinocytes lack melanosomes; melanin not transferred to abnormal keratinocyte
Autoimmune destruction of melanosomes	DAM chickens	Lymphocytes destroy melanocytes

suggested that defective receptors for melanin-stimulating hormone are responsible for partial albinism.

The gene Himalayan, a variant of albino (and at the same locus on the chromosome), codes for an enzyme that can synthesize melanin at relatively low temperature only, so that affected mice, Himalayan rabbits, and Siamese cats (which have this gene) have pale or white bodies with darkened extremities.

Albino mammals have abnormal retino-geniculocortical pathways.

Siamese cats, white tigers, albino rats, and pearl mink all have genetic mutations characterized by reduced pigmentation and abnormal vision involving central visual pathways (some optic nerve fibers go to the wrong side of the brain). In all Siamese cats, the *lateral geniculate nucleus* (LGN), the main cerebral group that relays messages from the retina to the cerebral cortex, is abnormal. These cats often have crossed eyes, since it is in the LGN that inputs from the two eyes are matched and passed to the cortex (in mammals, correct alignment of the eyes requires a normal LGN).

Chromatophore pigments other than melanin

Chromatophores (contractile pigment cells) of cold-blooded vertebrates produce rapid color changes of skin by intracellular aggregation and dispersion of pigment granules. Dermal color changes are under hormonal control and are used for camouflage, sexual attraction, and protection.

In addition to melanophores, chromatophores of fish and amphibians include red *xanthophores* and refractile *iridophores*. Chromatophore movements are important in tissue responses to injury (they protect the subcutis from ultraviolet rays of sun, allowing it to recover), and in fish, massive aggregations of chromatophores are a characteristic of chronic inflammation.

Hemoglobin-derived pigments and iron

Hemoglobin, the oxygen-carrying pigment of erythrocytes, is a combination of globin and the pigment complex heme. During normal and pathologic breakdown, different types of pigment complexes are formed. Most of these are heterogeneous and, except for ferritin, are not chemically defined. Ferritin and hemosiderin are the principal *iron storage compounds* in animal tissue. Both contain trivalent iron in the form of hydrous ferric oxides $(FeOOH)_x$, and both are detected histochemically by the Prussian blue reaction.

Ferritin is a tiny (10–nm), iron-laden aggregate of the protein apoferritin. It is water soluble, and because it is distributed throughout the cytoplasmic gel, it is not easily demonstrable. Ferritin has a hydrous iron oxide core surrounded by several protein subunits.

In hemolytic disease, iron is sequestered by macrophages. Ferritin particles are formed as iron is added to apoferritin, and it accumulates in lattice arrays free in the cytoplasm. Intracellular transport may occur through the cytoplasmic matrix or in the cytocavitary network. These pathways converge in lysosomes, where ferritin is converted to hemosiderin. Cell iron overload may result either from massive accumulation of iron pigments or from a deficiency of lysosomal excretion of hemosiderin.

Hemosiderin (a brown, amorphous, granular, iron-containing pigment) forms when erythrocytes are lysed. It develops within macrophages anywhere in the reticuloendothelial system but is particularly common in spleen and liver and in any foci of hemorrhage. Hemosiderin consists of densely packed micelles of hydrous iron oxide derived from degenerating ferritin. Biochemical analysis is hampered because hemosiderin is always contaminated by other cell proteins.

Copper-containing pigments

Copper-bearing pigment granules (lysosomes) accumulate in hepatocytes in a genetic disease caused by inability to excrete copper into bile, the main route of disposal by mammals. Inherited copper toxicosis occurs in Bedlington terriers (and Wilson's disease of man). Affected dogs begin to accumulate copper as pups, and as hepatic copper exceeds 2,000 $\mu g/g$ dry liver, signs of liver failure appear. Copper localizes in centrolobular areas in the liver and also appears in kidney, cornea, and brain. Focal and periportal hepatitis develops, and finally cirrhosis appears.

Lipofuscin

Lipofuscin is a golden-brown pigment formed in lysosomes of cells undergoing progressive and prolonged autooxidation of unsaturated lipids (Fig. 7.1). After peroxidation of double bonds, oxidized forms are condensed into solid polymers that give the color and reactivity of lipofuscin. Deposits fluoresce brown in ultraviolet light and stain with fat-soluble dyes, acid-fast stains, and the periodic acid-Schiff (PAS) reaction. Ultrastructurally, lipofuscin appears as dense, amorphous autophagolysosomes packed with granules, vacuoles, and lipid globules.

Lipofuscins tend to develop in highly metabolizing cells such as neurons, thyroid epithelium, and all types of muscle. They increase with advancing age and are thought to accrue as older

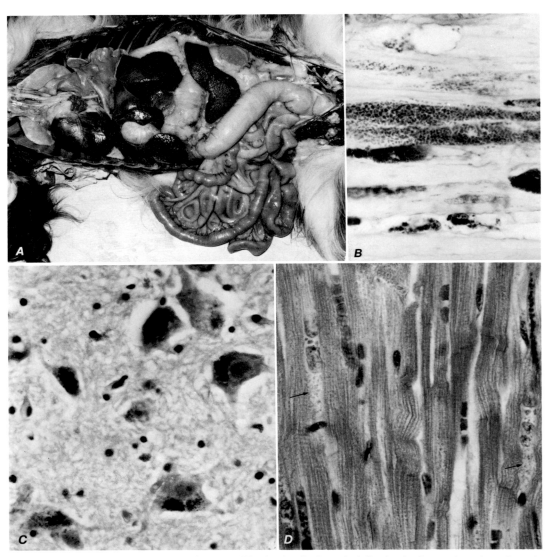

Fig. 7.1. Lipofuscin. A. Intestinal lipofuscin (brown bowel syndrome), aged dog with chronic relapsing pancreatitis (note the difference in color between the colon and jejunum). B. Histology: accumulation of granules in smooth muscle cells in the intestine. C. Neuronal lipofuscinosis, dog. D. Lipofuscin in cardiac myocytes, dog with dirofilariasis. Small granules around nuclei (*arrows*) are lipofuscin. Larvae of *Dirofilaria immitis* (*top right* and *bottom left*).

cells must degrade more lipids and membranes at a time when their antioxidation mechanisms wane (hence the terms "aging" and "wear-and-tear" pigment).

Lipofuscins are actually a group of complex lipopigments with variants, (e.g., ceroid, hemofuscin, and cytolipochrome). As oxidation proceeds in lipofuscin-bearing lysosomes, histochemical reactivity of the pigments changes. Early forms with many lipid globules and strong acid fastness (called *ceroid*) give way to dominance of membranogranular debris and weak acid-fast staining. Although lipofuscin is negative for iron, some lipofuscins stain weakly with the Prussian blue reaction, since iron may be incorporated into the lysosome during the initial autophagocytic process.

Ceroid, an early form of lipofuscin, consists of partially oxidized and polymerized unsaturated fatty acids. It develops in macrophages, hepatocytes, and other cells and is associated with vitamin E deficiency in several species. Hepatic ceroidosis is common in salmonids and catfish fed rancid diets. Livers are large, pale, and brown-orange with autofluorescent, acid-fast pigments distorting the hepatocytes. This fish disease can be reproduced by feeding large amounts of polyunsaturated fatty acids.

The *brown bowel syndrome* occurs in dogs in some chronic cases of diarrheal disease, steatorrhea, pancreatic acinar deficiency, and malabsorption. Large aggregates of lipofuscin granules develop in the smooth muscle cells, giving the intestine a brown cast (Fig. 7.1). Peculiar deposits of lipofuscin in specific organs (for which the cause is unknown) occur in various species of animals (e.g., "black kidneys" of cattle).

Neuronal ceroid lipofuscinosis

This disease is an autosomal recessive syndrome in English setter dogs characterized by intracellular accumulation of lipopigments (predominantly in neurons) and associated with progressive loss of cells and cerebral function. Autofluorescent pigments are about 50% acidic lipid polymers. The precise mechanism is a disturbance in detoxification of peroxides, based on markedly decreased tissue levels of *p*-phenyldiamine-linked peroxidase. Neuronal ceroid lipofuscinosis has also been reported in beefmaster cattle, cats, and South Hampshire sheep (Table 7.3).

Table 7.3. Neuronal ceroid lipofuscinosis

Species	Type
Sheep	South Hampshire
Cat	Domestic shorthair
Cow	Beefmaster breed
Dog	English setter, dachshund, chihuahua
Man	Infantile type, juvenile type, adult (Kufs' disease)

Bilirubin

This yellow-brown or brown-green pigment develops from breakdown of hemoglobin as macrophages process senescent erythrocytes. Porphyrin, the heme pigment, is cleaved, iron is released, and bilirubin is produced after a series of oxidation-reduction reactions within lysosomes. Although the hemoglobin-bilirubin conversions can occur in any reticuloendothelial cell, the principal organ of production is the spleen. Bilirubin enters the bloodstream, is bound to albumin, and is transported to the liver. Being insoluble in water, it is not passed through the renal glomerulus and is either processed in the liver or, if the liver is abnormal, accumulates in the bloodstream.

Bilirubin is conjugated in the liver and excreted into bile.

The albumin-bilirubin complex dissociates at the plasma membrane of the hepatocyte, and bilirubin enters this cell to be conjugated, largely to glucuronide. Conjugated bilirubin, which is water soluble, is secreted into biliary canaliculi (it can also be excreted in urine). As bile reaches the duodenum, the diglucuronide is cleaved and bilirubin is converted by bacteria to urobilinogen. Most urobilinogen is resorbed in the distal small intestine and transported to the liver (the *enterohepatic circulation*). Some is excreted by the kidneys. The nonabsorbed urobilinogen is transformed in the gut to urobilin and excreted in the feces.

Hyperbilirubinemia can be due to conjugated or unconjugated bilirubin.

The two major forms of hyperbilirubinemia, conjugated and unconjugated, have important diagnostic and prognostic implications. They can be distinguished by a specific test of serum. The *van den Bergh* test shows a *direct* reaction with conjugated bilirubin and an *indirect* reaction with unconjugated bilirubin.

In *conjugated hyperbilirubinemia,* bilirubin is present in urine. The disorder that causes this form involves some derangement in excretion of conjugated bilirubin into the gut, and urinary urobilinogen is decreased. In *unconjugated hyperbilirubinemia,* there is no bilirubin in urine; as the liver conjugates and secretes the increased amounts of bilirubin delivered to it, more urobilinogen is formed in the gut, which leads to increased urinary urobilinogen.

Bilirubin stains tissue yellow.

Bilirubin accumulates because of excessive production or failure of removal by normal amounts of bilirubin by damaged hepatocytes. Bilirubin appears in cells only when there is some derangement in its secretion by the liver or by obstruction of the biliary tract. When deposited in peripheral tissues it is responsible for the yellow color of the animal in *icterus* (also called *jaundice*) (Table 7.4).

Histologically, bilirubin appears in cells as brown-to-black, amorphous, globular cytoplasmic deposits. Commonly limited to hepatocytes (Fig. 7.2), it also develops in renal tubules and other tissues when icterus is severe.

Table 7.4.   Mechanisms of hyperbilirubinemia

Excess production of bilirubin — hemolytic disorders

Impaired uptake of bilirubin by the liver

Impaired conjugation of bilirubin

Impaired excretion of conjugated bilirubin (cholestasis)

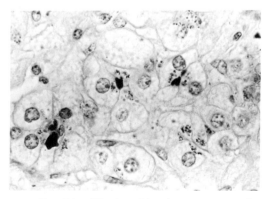

Fig. 7.2.   Bile thrombi and secretory granules bearing bilirubin, liver, aflatoxicosis.

EXOGENOUS PIGMENTS

Exogenous pigments enter via the skin, lung, and intestinal tract. They are most common and most serious in the lung, where the diseases are known collectively as *pneumoconioses.* Some of these diseases, such as *anthracosis* (caused by coal dust pigment), cause little tissue reaction. Others, including *silicosis* (silicon dioxide), may produce severe inflammation with extensive fibrosis. In dogs, accumulation of carbon dust in lungs is an indication of environmental contamination. Carbon pigments in macrophages of alveoli and lining the lymphatic vessels of alveolar septae blacken the lungs; pigments are also trapped in draining lymph nodes in the hilar region of the lungs.

Asbestosis is of particular concern to human populations not only because of chronic inflammatory lesions but because it is clearly associated with a lethal neoplasm called mesothelioma.

Silicosis

Desert atmospheres are rich in silicate dusts, and animals that roam these areas commonly have crystal-laden macrophages in peribronchiolar tissues in their lungs. The deposits are complex silicates and aluminum-potassium silicate. These lesions are especially common in animals that root about in the ground. In clinical disease resulting from silicates, animals usually have multiple granulomas in the lungs, composed of large foamy macrophages. The granulomas often have necrotic centers, some with multinucleate giant cells.

Histologically, macrophages contain refractile, crystalline particles, usually smaller than 1 μm, both free in the cytoplasm and within lysosomes. Dr. Les Schwartz, then at California, used a backscattered electron detection system on a scanning electron microscope to show that these crytals were silicon dioxide and aluminum silicate; other silicates also present contained iron and other metals.

Silica exists in dust in amorphous and crystalline forms. The latter is particularly important in induction of fibrosing alveolitis in the lung. Following phagocytosis by alveolar macrophages, necrosis occurs due to damage by crystals of 0.5 μm or less to lysosomal membranes. Hydrolytic enzymes leak into the interstitium of alveolar septa and produce lysis. Cycling of the silica that cannot be broken down results in prolonged destruction of macrophages. Silica and necrotic debris are finally walled off by a granulomatous reaction. Collagen production is stimulated, and there may be diffuse pulmonary fibrosis.

Exogenous pigments in other tissues are less important.

Pigments entering the *intestine* are generally of less import to health than are those in lungs. Metallic poisons such as lead (which causes plumbism) and silver (which causes argyria) may cause pigmentation following ingestion and absorption. Poisoning by these metals can produce a lethal disease in which intestinal pigmentation plays little role.

Tetracyclines, used widely as broad spectrum antibiotics in antimicrobial therapy, are known to be incorporated into *bone* where they form a fluorescent compound and stain the tissue yellow in visible light. This characteristic, which is unrelated to antibacterial effects, is used by experimental pathologists as a tool and specific label for calcifying tissues.

Only a few pigments enter through the *skin.* The best examples are Prussian blue, India ink, and mercuric sulfide (vermillion), which are used in tattooing and reside both in macrophages and free in the dermis.

Parasite pigments

Several parasites excrete pigmented compounds into tissue. *Pneumonysis simicola,* the lung mite of monkeys, is surrounded by dense deposits of excreta (Fig. 7.3). Brownish *malarial pigment* is formed by excretion of catabolized hemoglobin from certain species of plasmodia. In infected animals, massive deposits develop in reticuloendothelial cells of spleen and liver. Malarial pigment arises from degradation of hemoglobin, usually within lysosomes.

CRYSTALS
Oxalosis

Crystals of calcium oxalate are deposited in tissue in toxic diseases, causing increased oxalic acid in blood (oxalemia) and urine (hyperoxaluria). Causal agents are most often poisons of plants that contain large amounts of oxalic acid (e.g., halogeton, rhubarb, greasewood) or the

antifreeze component ethylene glycol (Table 7.5).

Sheep are commonly poisoned by ingestion of oxalate-containing plants, dogs and cats by drinking ethylene glycol. In the latter case, oxalate is derived thus: ethylene glycol $CH_2OH-CH_2OH \rightarrow$ oxalic acid CO_2H-CO_2H. Cattle are resistant to oxalate poisoning because of oxalate-utilizing bacteria in the rumen and oxalate-metabolizing enzymes in the liver.

Dietary ingestion of oxalates causes three patterns of disease.

Different patterns of disease depend on the species of animal and the amount of oxalate ingested. *Peracute toxicity,* due to corrosive action of oxalate on gastrointestinal mucosa, is associated with gastroenteritis, hemorrhage, and ulceration. This syndrome occurs in horses, which are resistant to oxalate nephropathy. *Acute toxicity* is due to hypocalcemia, the initial systemic effect of oxalates. Hypocalcemia and metabolic acidosis caused by formation of acidic products of oxalate metabolism combine to produce ataxia, convulsions, tetany, and abnormalities of cardiopulmonary function. If animals survive the above episodes, they are prone to develop a third manifestation, *oxalate nephropathy.*

Renal oxalate deposits cause tubular necrosis.

Deposits of doubly refractile, translucent, yellowish oxalate crystals occur in tubular lumens, interstitium, and tubular epithelium (Fig. 7.4). Tubular necrosis is particularly prominent, but cortical necrosis may also occur, caused by a secondary ischemic phenomenon. Anuria results from obstruction of tubule lumens by crystals, and uremia kills the animal.

Sulfonamide crystals

Nephrosis and uremia may result from ingestion of large doses of sulfonamides, particularly if associated with deficient fluid intake. It is apt to occur in calves that are febrile and dehydrated. Sulfonamide crystals are often visible grossly in the pelvis and as pale, yellowish, radial lines in the medulla. Tubular degeneration and plugging of the nephron, especially of the collecting ducts, cause anuria. Sulfonamides also produce renal disease by an allergic mechanism (see immunopathology, Chapter 23).

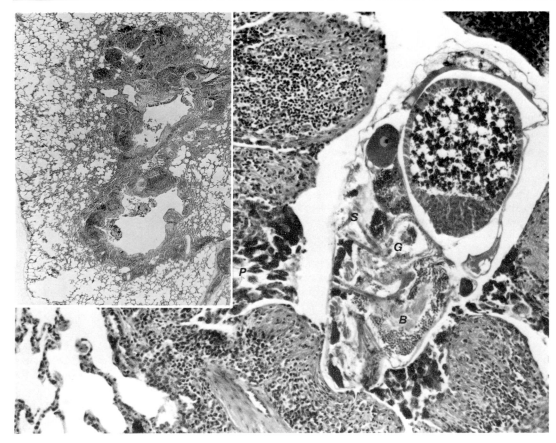

Fig. 7.3. Parasite pigments, pulmonary acariasis, rhesus monkey with *Pneumonyssus simicola*, longitudinal section. The mite is in a dilated bronchiole that is surrounded by histiolymphocytic inflammatory tissue and masses of excretory pigment (*P*). Midgut (*G*), brain (*B*), and striated muscle (*S*) of parasite. Inset: peribronchiolar lymphocyte aggregates.

Table 7.5. Classification of oxalosis

Type	Mechanism	Examples

Primary	Metabolic defect in oxalate metabolism	Inborn metabolic error
		  Primary hyperoxaluria[a]
		Vitamin deficiency
		  Thiamine deficiency[a]

Secondary	Ingestion of substances high in oxalates	Poisons
		  Ethylene glycol
		  Diethylene glycol
		  Methoxyflurane
		Plants
		  Halogeton
		  Setaria sp.
		  Bassia sp.
		Fungi synthesizing oxalic
		  acid
		  Aspergillus sp.

[a]Demonstrated only in man.

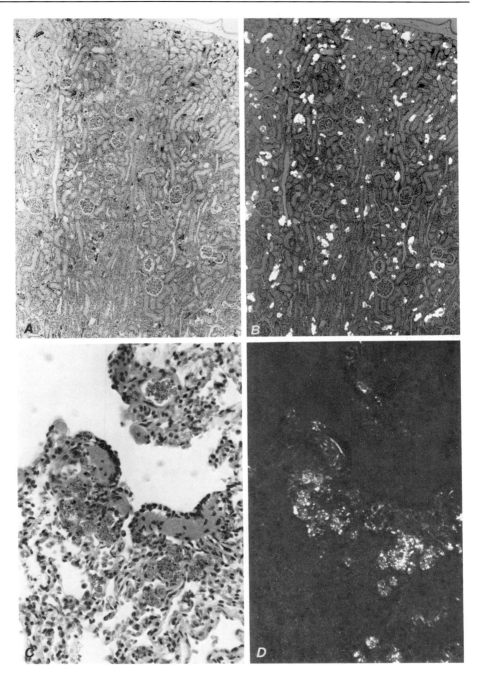

Fig. 7.4. Crystals in tissue. A. Oxalate nephropathy, cat with ethylene toxicity, routine H & E section (crystals not apparent). B. Same section using polarizing optics (crystals show clearly). C. Peribronchiolar crystals. D. Same section in polarized light.

Urates and uric acid

Deposits of uric acid crystals and urates characterize *gout,* a disease of purine metabolism. Seen most commonly in birds, snakes, and humans, it is due to excessive production or insufficient excretion of uric acid. Chalky white masses of uric acid (referred to as "tophi") develop in tissue and cause local inflammatory reactions.

Avian gout

Birds normally excrete much uric acid, which predisposes them to gout. Avian gout occurs in two forms. *Visceral gout* is common; plasma uric acid is increased, and urates are deposited in kidney, liver, joints, and pericardium. It is a common sequela to dehydration. *Articular gout* is limited to synoviae and tendon sheaths of joints, especially of the foot and hock. The diagnosis can be established by identification of urate crystals by polarizing microscopy of synovial fluid or renal tissues.

Both forms of avian gout are initiated by renal failure in uric acid secretion and are promoted by dehydration and diets high in protein. Occurrence depends on hereditary variations; strains susceptible to gout have defective renal uric acid secretion. Experimentally, avian gout can be produced by administration of nephrotoxic agents and diets deficient in vitamin A and high in calcium.

Gout in other species

Urate nephrolithiasis has been reported in mink and is probably due to an inherited defect in uric acid metabolism. In snakes, the nephrotoxic antibiotic gentamicin is associated with a high incidence of gout. In the dog, uric acid is converted to allantoin in the liver by uricase (Dalmatian dogs differ in that hepatic metabolism lacks this conversion and dogs excrete uric acid in urine).

Human primary gout is caused by a group of genetic errors in uric acid metabolism that all lead to hyperuricemia. Unlike most animals, man lacks uricase, so that uric acid is the end product of purine metabolism. Hyperuricemia resulting in secondary gout may be caused by increased nucleic acid turnover in hematologic diseases and in chronic renal disease. Neutrophils play a central role in inflammation of human gout by avidly phagocytizing urate crystals. Crystals are taken into phagolysosomes where they mechanically injure membranes, permitting hydrolases to leak into the cytoplasm to damage the cell. Crystals are released from the dead neutrophil to induce again a cycle of neutrophil uptake and degeneration.

ADDITIONAL READING

Harbison, M. L., and Godleski, J. T. Malignant mesothelioma in urban dogs. *Vet. Pathol.* 20:531, 1983.

Newsholme, S. J., et al. A suspected lipofuscin storage disease of sheep associated with ingestion of the plant *Trachyandra divaricata* (Jacq.) Kunth. *Onderstepoort J. Vet. Res.* 52:87, 1985.

Owen, C. A., and Ludwig, J. Inherited copper toxicosis in Bedlington terriers. *Am. J. Pathol.* 106:432, 1982.

Pawelek, J. M., and Korner, A. M. The biosynthesis of mammalian melanin. *Am. Sci.* 70:136, 1982.

Phillips, M. J., et al. Cholestasis. *Lab. Invest.* 54:593, 1986.

Pritzker, K. P. H., et al. Adrenal and hepatic calcium stearate crystal deposits in dogs fed a thiamine-deficient diet. *Am. J. Vet. Res.* 43:1481, 1982.

Tomlinson, M. J., et al. Urate nephrolithiasis in ranch mink. *J. Am. Vet. Med. Assoc.* 180:622, 1982.

Extracellular Substances

8

COLLAGEN FIBER DISEASE

Biology of collagen

Collagen forms the building blocks for connective tissue fibers and nonfibrous structures such as cartilage and basement membranes. Mammalian tissues produce at least five distinct types of collagen, each designed for different construction work outside the cell (Table 8.1). The common property of all types is the collagenous triple helix, a unique coil of three polypeptide chains that are wound together in a helix to form a rodlike molecule. Within each type of collagen, heterogeneity occurs since variations in hydroxylation, glycosylation, and cross-linking of the molecule are dependent on tissue type, age, and hormonal status. For example, collagen type I in the Achilles tendon is highly cross-linked, whereas that of the tail tendons is much less so.

Tropocollagen is the basic unit of collagen.

The functional form of collagen types I, II, and III is the collagen *fibril,* an ordered polymer visible by electron microscopy as a banded structure in the extracellular matrix of connective tissue. Collagen *fibers* are the ordered aggregates of fibrils seen by light microscopy. The basic structural unit, called *tropocollagen,* is a rod 300 nm long, one of the longest protein molecules known. Its peculiar amino acid composition allows for its stable conformation. Hydrox-

Table 8.1. Distinct collagen types in vertebrate animal tissue

Type	Form of Polymer	Formula for Chains of Triple Helix	Tissue Distribution
I	Fibrillar	$[\alpha1(I)]_2\alpha2$	Only collagen of bone and tendon Dominant collagen in skin and connective tissue Dentin
II	Fibrillar	$[\alpha1(II)]_3$	Cartilage, vitreous body of eye Nucleus pulposus of intervertebral disk
III	Fibrillar	$[\alpha1(III)]_3$	Reticulin fibers Blood vessels (10–50% of collagen) Skin (10% in adult; 50% in fetus) Granulation tissue
IV	Granular	$[\alpha1(IV)]_3$	Basement membranes of all epithelium and endothelium Lens capsule, Descemet's membrane
V	Granular	$A(B)_2$ or $(\alpha A)_3$ and $(\alpha B)_3$	Minor component of basement membranes of smooth and striated muscle, fibroblast surfaces
VI	Fibrillar	?	Microfibrils, in connective tissue
VII	Fibrillar	?	Anchoring fibrils in basement membranes
VIII	?	?	Endothelium

ylysine and hydroxyproline, rarely found in other tissue proteins, permit extensive cross-linking, and glycine, which makes up one-third of the tropocollagen molecule, allows a wide range of folding in the peptide chain.

Type I collagen is for strength.

Type I collagen accounts for about 90% of total body collagen. It is the collagen that forms large, well-organized fibrils and is the molecule present where tensile strength is important. Even in fibers containing only type I, the diameter and weave of collagen fibrils vary greatly, depending on the strength required. Type I collagen of tendon forms thick, uniform fibrils packed in parallel bundles, whereas type I collagen of bone is in contorted waves of finer fibrils.

Procollagen peptides are produced in fibroblasts.

Synthesis of collagen molecules begins with the production of polypeptide chains on the ribosome. These α chains (analogous to the α chains of fibrinogen) have a simple amino acid constitution: about one-third glycine, one-third proline and hydroxproline, and one-third other amino acids. Hydroxylation of proline causes the chains to become entwined to form a complex triple helix. These are transported to the Golgi complex, where carbohydrate subunits are synthesized and procollagen molecules are assembled. Procollagen is a large precursor molecule of tropocollagen. It has additional peptide chains at its amino and carboxy termini that prevent fibrillogenesis before it is released from the cell.

An enzyme cleaves procollagen to form tropocollagen.

As procollagen molecules are released from the fibroblast, they are acted on by the enzyme procollagen peptidase, which cleaves away the peptide chains at either end of the molecule to form tropocollagen. While still near the surface, tropocollagen molecules spontaneously assemble by linking together in an overlapping pattern to form the collagen fibril.

Tropocollagen is stabilized by cross-links.

Cross-links between lysine side chains stabilize the tropocollagen molecules after they are linked together. The importance of cross-linking in conferring mechanical strength is evident in lathyrism, a disease caused by ingestion of seeds of *Lathyris odoratus,* the sweet pea. The toxic agent is β-aminopropionitrile, which inhibits the transformation of lysyl side chains into aldehydes. Collagen in affected animals is extremely fragile.

Elastic fibers contain elastin.

Elastic fibers are branched globular or fibrous aggregates that have two components: *elastin,* which forms the bulk of the fiber, and glycoprotein *microfilaments.* Elastin is an insoluble protein with a soluble precursor, tropoelastin. Although chemically similar to collagen (with high glycine and hydroxyproline), the cross-links between peptide chains are by two unique amino acids, desmosine and isodesmosine.

Defective collagen degradation

In normal tissue, collagen fibrils are continually broken down and replaced by fibroblasts. Lysosomes in fibroblasts contain enzymes that degrade collagen, elastin, and proteoglycans. They release these enzymes into the interstitium both as free soluble enzymes and in specialized, membrane-bound matrix vesicles.

Macrophages secrete collagenase.

Macrophages secrete collagenase, elastase, and plasminogen activators that mediate hydrolysis of connective tissue proteins extracellularly. Local conversion of plasminogen to plasmin allows elastase easier access to its substrate, elastin. After the initial hydrolysis, macrophages endocytose protein matrix fragments that are completely degraded within lysosomes.

Fibrosis

Increase formation of collagen fibrils in connective tissue occurs in such diverse conditions as inflammation, healing, atrophy, and degeneration. Chronic progressive fibrosis may develop if collagenases and elastases are missing or abnormal. Fibrosis of the lungs, myocardium, and liver may in fact contribute significantly to disease and death. The point of irreversibility in *cirrhosis* of the liver has been correlated with disappearance of liver collagenase.

Hepatic fibrosis

Fibrosis in the liver occurs when collagen is laid down in the spaces of Disse. Although interstitial fibroblasts are credited with releasing much of the collagen, it is clear that hepatocytes can synthesize and release collagen. Type IV collagen (for basement membranes) is synthesized early while types I and III are produced later in hepatic injury. Fibroplasia in chronic liver injury is an important component of cirrhosis.

Cirrhosis is characterized by *diffuse fibrosis* and parenchymal *nodular regeneration* (hepatocellular necrosis, an antecedent to cirrhosis, is sometimes listed as a third component). Cirrhosis is the result of abnormal reconstruction of liver architecture and is usually a scarred end stage of chronic inflammation of the liver (if clinical features of hepatitis predominate, the diagnosis should be "chronic hepatitis with cirrhosis." Collagen fibers are deposited around the vascular sinusoids in connective tissue septa that link the portal and central zones. Thus fibroplasia is both a result of and a contributor to vascular obstruction. Because of postsinusoidal portal hypertension, there is increased hepatic lymph flow and portal lymphatics are dilated.

Pulmonary fibrosis

In *pulmonary fibrosis* that accompanies cardiac failure in the dog, ischemia, parenchymal cell degeneration, and hormonal factors combine to sustain progressive collagen deposition. Excess collagen fibrils and their associated connective tissue microfibrils and thickened basement membranes are characteristic. Basement membranes become attached to underlying collagen by specialized anchoring fibrils and to the plasma membranes of overlying pulmonary epithelium by hemidesmosomes. The final lesion is thus due to a complex interaction with collagen and glycoproteins of the interstitial ground substance.

Diffuse pulmonary fibrosis may result from inhalation or expiration of toxins. Prolonged low levels of noxious chemicals in inspired air produce slow progressive degenerative changes accompanied by extensive diffuse fibroplasia of the alveolar wall interstitium. Aerogenic toxicity involves vacuolation in pneumocytes and endothelium. Hyperplasia of granular pneumocytes occurs as a reparative process. If toxicity continues there is progressive deposition of glycosaminoglycans, basement membranes, and collagen.

Collagen is produced by interstitial fibroblasts and deposited in the proteoglycan-rich matrix of the alveolar septae. Macrophages are prominent in fibrotic alveolar walls, probably to degrade and recycle collagen and, in chronic microbial infections, to process antigens.

Chronic pulmonary fibrosis can also be produced by toxins that arrive in the lung hematogenously and are eliminated during exhalation. Bleomycin, an intravenously administered anticancer agent, produces damage to endothelium, movement of protein-rich fluid into the interstitium, and slowly progressive fibrosis of the alveolar septae.

Dermatosparaxis

Dermatosparaxis is an inherited disease characterized by loose fragile skin easily torn with minor trauma. It results from a deficiency of procollagen peptidase, the enzyme that cleaves the amino terminal nonhelical extension from the precursor procollagen molecules. Although procollagen has both carboxy and amino terminal extensions cleaved to yield collagen, procollagen with the amino terminus is the only precursor that accumulates in dermatosparaxis.

The degree of enzyme deficiency is a major species difference.

The degree of enzyme deficiency is a major species difference. Sheep have almost no collagen chains in skin and generally die at birth or within a few weeks. The defect is less severe in cats and calves, which have significant amounts of normal collagen chains. Newborn calves with dermatosparaxis have extremely fragile skin with large numbers of flat, twisted, unbanded collagen fibrils in disordered patterns. The striking deficiency of mature collagen fibers is demonstrable by their lack of birefringence under polarized light and abnormal X-ray diffraction patterns.

Dermatosparactic collagen fibers vary in size and shape.

Instead of the normal weaving of fibers, dermal collagen has a tangled organization of fibrils within the fiber and an abnormal weaving pattern (Fig. 8.1). The aberrant collagen molecules alter the structure of individual fibrils, the assembly of fibrils into fiber bundles, and the woven network in the reticular dermis of skin. In calves the abnormal fibrils are embedded in excess ground substance, which may be responsible for the jellylike touch of the skin.

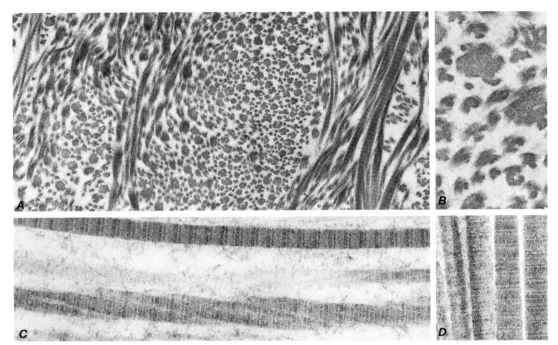

Fig. 8.1. A–C. Dermal collagen fibrils, cat with dermatosparaxis. A. Collagen fibers with fibrils in various planes of section. B. Bizarre shapes in cross section. C. Longitudinal section, loosely woven bundles of filaments that spiral around one another. D. Collagen fibrils, normal cat. (Photographs: K. Holbrook, *J. Invest. Dermatol.* 74:100, 1980, used by permission)

Other hereditary syndromes

Dermatosparaxis of calves, sheep, and cats is an autosomal recessive disease caused by a specific genetic enzyme deficiency. Cutaneous asthenia in dogs, mink, and cats is inherited in dominant manner and its mechanism is not known (Table 8.2).

Human syndromes of dermal fragility and hyperextensibility due to defective collagen metabolism are termed collectively Ehlers-Danlos syndrome. There are seven forms: three are dominant (types I, II, and III) and four are recessive. Recessive disorders are due to specific enzyme defects, but mechanisms are unknown for those inherited by dominant genes.

MUCOSUBSTANCES

Mucosubstance is a deliberately vague term used to denote the poorly characterized glycans and glycan-protein complexes of connective tissue. These substances occur as mixtures, and the histochemical staining reaction of a tissue is related to the dominant components in the mixture.

Connective tissue ground substance

Interstitial ground substance is the extracellular gel of mucosubstances and fluid in which connective tissue fibers are embedded. Its viscosity and gel nature are due to proteoglycans both free and attached to collagen and elastic fibers (Fig. 8.2). Proteoglycans are identified in tissue sections with alcian blue, which complexes with glycosaminoglycans.

Glycosaminoglycan is a modern term for mucopolysaccharide.

Glycosaminoglycans (GAGs) are those polysaccharides containing amino sugars (glucosamine, galactosamine) on their chains. Nearly all vertebrate GAGs also contain sugar groups with carboxylic acid units (glucuronic acid, galacturonic acid) and are referred to as acidic mucopolysaccharides. The major GAGs are hyaluronic acid, heparin, keratin sulfate, and the chondroitin sulfates. Strongly acid sulfate groups on GAGs bound to protein impart basophilia to ground substance. Other complexes carry large numbers of negatively charged groups along their molecules. Their polyanionic nature is responsible for staining with alcian blue. The carbohydrate chains, when coupled to protein cores, form large molecules called proteoglycans.

Ground substances contain mixtures of GAGs.

Dermatan sulfate is the most common molecule in skin, tendon, and gastric mucus. Hyaluronic acid is prevalent in synovial fluid, umbilical cord, and vascular walls, while chondroitin

sulfates dominate in cornea and cartilage. Enhanced synthesis or reduced degradation may produce excesses of GAGs in tissue, and this occurs in metabolic, inflammatory, and neoplastic diseases. The deposition and degradation of GAGs is markedly influenced by the anabolic steroid hormones.

Proteoglycan production is linked to connective tissue metabolism and fluid movement.

Although proteoglycans accumulate throughout the body, their significance in disease and tissue diagnosis lies chiefly in the production of subcutaneous swellings in skin, mucodegeneration in arteries, and distortion of cartilage and soft tissues of bones and joints. Marked increases in proteoglycans are seen in tissue in-

Table 8.2. Steps in the normal and defective formation of collagen fibers

Activity and Location in the Cell	Defect
Translation of mRNA, amino acid assembly into polypeptides (pro α chains) on the ribosomes of the fibroblast	Protein deficiency Starvation
Hydroxylation of proline (and other amino acids) by proline hydroxylase on ribosomes of the rough endoplasmic reticulum	Inhibition of proline hydroxylation Ascorbic acid deficit (scurvy) Corticosteroid therapy Dilantin therapy (from tie-up)[a]
Helix formation: aggregation of pro α chains into triple helix of procollagen in endoplasmic reticulum cisternae and Golgi complex by disulfide bonding	
Release of soluble procollagen by secretory granules at the cell surface	Inhibition of cell release Monensin (ionophore) Ehlers-Danlos (type IV) disease
Extracellular alignment of tropocollagen molecules from procollagen (pro α chains converted to α chains by procollagen peptidase, which cleaves away amino and carboxy terminal peptides	Procollagen peptidase deficiency (lack of procollagen to collagen conversion) Dermatosparaxis (calves, sheep, cat) Ehlers-Danlos (type VII) disease

Cross-linking of amino acids: formation of aldehyde end groupings in tropocollagen. Lysyloxidase converts peptidyl lysine to allysine (aldehyde). Lysyl hydroxylase converts hydroxylysine to hydroxyallysine	Lysyl oxidase deficiency
	β-aminopropionitrile poisoning (inhibition of lysyloxidase)
	Copper deficit[b]
	  Dietary deficiency
	  Menke's kinky hair syndrome
	  Enzyme deficiency in mottled (blotchy) mice
	Lysyl hydroxylase deficiency
	  Ehlers-Danlos (type VI) disease[a]
	Blockade of aldehyde groups
	  D-penicillamine toxicity
	
	Homocystinuria[a]
	Marfan's syndrome[a](?)

Defective fibrogenesis	? Ehlers-Danlos (man, types I, II, III) Cutaneous asthenia (dog, mink) Fibrillogenesis defect

[a]Reported only in man.
[b]Copper is essential component of lysyl oxidase.

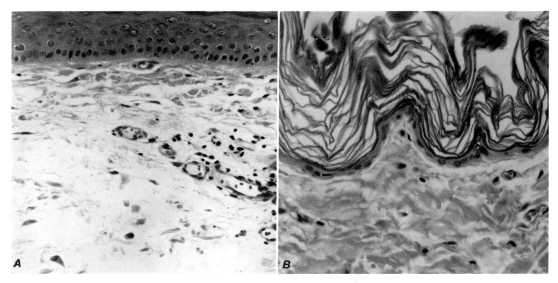

Fig. 8.2. A. Epidermal hyperplasia and dermal swelling with edema fluid and mucosubstances; perineal skin (sex skin), female rhesus monkey during estrus. B. Epidermal atrophy, decreased mucosubstances, inactive collagen. Skin, dog with chronic treatment with adrenocorticosteroid hormones.

jury and inflammation, endocrine dysfunctions, excessive lipolysis of starvation, and nutritional deficiencies (especially of copper and zinc). Zinc deficiency in pigs is characterized by diffuse dermatitis due largely to an abnormal increase in hyaluronic acid of skin, which makes this barrier more susceptible to bacterial invasion.

Hormones profoundly affect glycosaminoglycans.

Striking accumulation of GAGs in ground substance is associated with stimulation by sex hormones. Growth of the cock's comb under the influence of testosterone and swelling of the vulva due to progesterone are two examples. In some female monkeys, a striking "sex skin" develops that is an attractant to males. The edematous, red, moist skin is caused by subepidermal capillary dilation, accumulation of fluid, and massive deposition of GAGs. These phenomena are related to cell receptors, as mucosubstances are not increased in other tissues.

Adrenal corticosteroids also have a promoting effect on GAGs in ground substance. In massive doses they act on capillaries to decrease permeability and edema, thereby playing a significant role in suppressing acute inflammation.

Glycosaminoglycans accumulate in thyroid deficiency.

The role of thyroid hormones on ground substance is clearly seen in *myxedema,* the accumulation of GAGs, albumin, water, and mast cells in subcutis that accompanies hypothyroidism. Primarily a disease of adult humans, myxedema has also been reported in the dog. GAGs, as seen by staining with alcian blue, accumulate around capillaries and veins. Water and albumin leak into these areas. Accumulation of fluid is due partly to the great capacity of hyaluronic acid to bind to water and to the subsequent suppression of lymphatic drainage. Changes similar to those in skin occur throughout the body, including lung and intestine. Deposits of GAGs in skeletal and cardiac muscle cells predispose to weakness and cardiac failure. Affected renal glomeruli alter plasma filtration and enhance fluid and electrolyte problems. Soon after treatment with thyroid hormone, tissue fluids and GAGs return to normal amounts.

Glycosaminoglycans accumulate at sites of tissue injury.

In acute inflammation, GAGs are deposited as a prelude to collagen fibrillogenesis and healing.

Hyaluronic acid imparts high viscosity to ground substance and is important in restricting the spread of bacteria through fascial planes. Some of the most invasive bacteria produce hyaluronidases that degrade hyaluronic acid and facilitate the spread of bacteria through tissue (e.g., staphylococci and clostridia). Larvae of *Schistosoma mansoni* secrete proteolytic enzymes that facilitate their entry into venules and lymphatics of skin.

GAGs increase in areas of necrosis of connective tissue and provide a stimulus and focus for calcification; that is, certain GAGs play an initiating role for deposition of calcium salts in necrotic tissue just as they do in normal calcifying cartilage.

Glycosaminoglycans direct embryonic development.

Fetal mesenchyme contains massive amounts of proteoglycans. During early embryonal growth, extracellular collagen and proteoglycans direct mesenchymal and epithelial cell shape, motility, and differentiation. For example, corneal epithelium will not grow and differentiate in vitro if separated from its underlying matrix. When matrix material is added, epithelial growth resumes. This stimulation of cell activity occurs via connection of collagen-fibronectin complexes with specific receptor molecules in the cell surface and extension of those connections from the receptor to submembrane actin filaments.

Some neoplasms deposit glycosaminoglycans.

The mesenchymal tumor called a *myxoma* produces large amounts of GAGs. Adenocarcinomas of the uterus, nasal cavity, and urinary tract also produce complex mucins. In most neoplasms, the mucosubstances produced are normal, although polymerization and complexing with proteins may be abnormal.

Basement membranes

Basement membranes are extracellular, homogeneous-appearing sheets of dense granular material interposed between cell layers of different types. They are composed of collagen type IV, which is complexed with noncollagenous proteins (laminin and fibronectin) and GAGs. Heparin sulfate, which predominates in most basement membranes, imparts a filter action because it is a strong polyanion.

Basement membranes are synthesized by endothelium, epithelium, and myoepithelial cells, which produce predominantly (probably exclusively) type IV collagen. Type IV collagen fails to undergo conversion to typical fibrils, possibly as a result of glycosylation of its hydroxylysine residues.

Matrix glycoproteins: Fibronectin and laminin

The glycoproteins of basement membrane material are named for their location and action. *Fibronectin* (from the Latin *fibra,* fiber, plus *nectere,* to tie) promotes attachment of fibroblasts to collagen. It occurs as a polymer in basement membrane but also circulates in plasma as a small dimer. Fibronectin, which is associated with fibroblast surfaces, plays important roles in cell migration and adhesion, particularly of platelets to collagen during inflammation. *Laminin,* a similar glycoprotein, is a specific attachment factor for epithelial cells to type IV collagen. *Chondronectin* promotes attachment of cartilage cells to collagen.

Degradation of basement membrane material is inhibited in starvation.

Tissue atrophy of starvation is characterized by increased thickness of basement membranes in several organs, as well as excessive deposits of collagen and ground substance proteoglycans (see atrophy of starvation, Chapter 29). The mechanism is continued synthesis in the face of inhibited degradation and removal.

Production of basement membranes is excessive in diabetes.

Systemic thickening of capillary endothelial basement membranes underlies the chronic complications of *diabetic microangiopathy,* including blindness and renal failure. Hyperglycemia-induced glycosylation is the major pathogenetic factor in basement membrane thickening (enzymes involved in glycosylation have been shown to be increased in human diabetes). Hyperglycemia also produces nonenzymatic glycolysis of basement membranes, as well as hemoglobin, collagen, and lens crystallin.

Some neoplasms and congenital malformations have excess basement membranes.

Neoplastic epithelial cells often secrete large amounts of basement membrane material. Thick, irregular membranes that surround tumor cells are common in mammary gland tumors of dogs and in squamous cell carcinomas of most species.

Fibrous rings in the aortas of Newfoundland dogs with familial subaortic stenosis contain peculiar chondrocytelike cells that secrete large amounts of basement membrane material rich in GAGs. These lesions also have poorly developed elastic fibers and cross-banded collagen fibrils.

Mucopolysaccharidoses

The mucopolysaccharidoses are a group of genetic diseases characterized by storage of incompletely degraded GAGs in cells that normally degrade these substances (Table 8.3). Storage results from diminished activity of specific hydrolases (in lysosomes) required for degradation. Massive accumulation of giant lysosomes bearing GAG polymers causes marked distortion of the affected cells (Fig. 8.3). Different lysosomal hydrolases can be demon-

Table 8.3. Cell storage diseases: Mucopolysaccharidoses

Deposit	Enzyme Defect	Animal
Heparin sulfate Dermatan sulfate	α-L-iduronidase	Cat Dog Man
Heparin sulfate Dermatan sulfate	L-iduronosulfate sulfatase	Man
Heparin sulfate	Sulfamidase and other enzymes	Man
Keratan sulfate Chondroitin sulfate	N-acetyl hexosamine 4-sulfate sulfatase	Man
Heparin sulfate Dermatan sulfate	Arylsulfatase B N-acetyl hexosaminidase-6-sulfate sulfatase	Cat Man
Heparin sulfate Dermatan sulfate Chondroitin sulfate	β-glucuronidase	
Glycoprotein	?	Dog Man
Uncharacterized	?	Cow Goose

strated to be deficient or absent in fibroblasts cultured from skin of affected animals.

An α-L-iduronidase deficiency occurs in cats and dogs.

Mucopolysaccharidosis (type I), which results from an absence of α-L-iduronidase, has been reported in Siamese cats and Plott hounds. Affected cats have facial and bony deformities and clouded corneas. Diagnosis is confirmed at weaning by detection of excess GAGs (dermatan sulfate and heparin sulfate) in urine. Leukocytes have abnormal storage granules, and activity of the lysosomal enzyme α-L-iduronidase is less than 1% normal. Lameness is a prominent clinical sign in dogs and is caused by accumulation of mucopolysaccharides in chondrocytes and synovial villi.

Arylsulfatase B deficiency occurs in cats.

Siamese cats with mucopolysaccharidoses (type VI) from arylsulfatase B deficiency have cytoplasmic inclusions bearing dermatan sulfate in hepatocytes, bone marrow granulocytes, vascular smooth muscle, and fibroblasts of skin, cornea, and cardiac valves. Mild ventricular dilatation of the brain is often present.

Glycoprotein inclusions

Glycoproteins aggregate into bodies, both extra- and intracellularly, that are useful in diagnosis. Composed of irregular fibrous materials, they arise by polymerization of GAGs and vary in histochemical staining because they incorporate various substances such as components of collagen, basement membranes, and calcium salts.

Corpora amylacea

These large, round extracellular bodies are associated with secretory processes in brain, pineal, pituitary, and mammary gland. In the bovine mammary gland they are common in early lactation (Fig. 8.3). They occur in glandular acini, and as involution heralds the cessation of lactation, they begin to disappear and are found in interstitial areas in macrophages.

Mammary gland corpora amylacea arise from secretory proteins released by epithelial cells into the acinar lumen. They aggregate around necrotic neutrophilic leukocytes, probably attracted by enzymes released from dying cells.

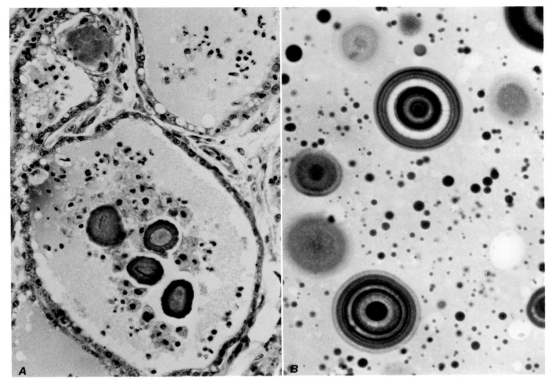

Fig. 8.3. Corpora amylacea. These calcified spherical bodies develop due to progressive layering of glycosaminoglycans. They sequester calcium salts and may be a storage form of calcium. A. Mammary acinus, cow in last stages of lactation. B. Yolk sac, 2-day-old turkey.

Progressive accretion of proteins produces laminae of fibrils and granules.

Lafora inclusions occur in old brains.

Glycoprotein inclusions are found as nonspecific inclusions in senile brains, and although useful in diagnosis, the relationship of inclusions to disease processes is unclear. Giant periodic acid–Schiff (PAS) staining inclusions in neurons are diagnostic for Lafora's disease of dogs and humans. They are also found in asymptomatic old dogs, especially over 8 years, and probably represent an age-related phenomenon accelerated by epilepsy.

AMYLOID

Amyloidosis is the disease resulting from deposition of amyloid in tissue. Amyloid (from the Greek *amylon,* starch) is most prominent in

spleen, liver, and kidney and, when present in large amounts, causes these organs to be large, pale, and waxy.

Amyloidosis is complicated in the terminal stages by two major events: (1) the effects of circulating amyloid precursors on the reticuloendothelial system (overloading it) and (2) the destruction of parenchymal cells and capillaries as amyloid masses progressively expand. Although amyloid deposits interfere with the normal function in any organ, the fatal effects occur in the kidney. Animals with systemic amyloidosis commonly die in uremia because of massive deposits of amyloid fibrils in the renal glomerulus.

A discrete cellular defect in protein metabolism always underlies amyloidosis. Instead of protein being processed normally, peptide units are assembled into fibrils. By some unknown redirection of lysosomal protease activity, the abnormal "amyloid cell" produces a preamyloid molecule that polymerizes into fibrils as it is released at the cell surface. Although uniform physically, amyloid fibrils may be composed of abnormal peptide segments of such diverse proteins as albumin, immunoglobulin, insulin, growth hormone, and an acute phase protein of inflammation called serum amyloid A.

Detection of amyloid

Amyloid was classically detected at necropsy by applying aqueous solutions of iodine to tissue surfaces, because iodine stains amyloid brown. Generations of light microscopists have defined amyloid as a homogeneous, extracellular glycoprotein, distinguished from other hyalin material by its specific sites of deposition, association with specific disease states, and staining with Congo red. A characteristic green birefringence is induced under polarized light because of the peculiar alignment of Congo red on parallel amyloid fibrils. Violet dyes (crystal violet) and fluorochromes (thioflavin T) are also useful, but staining is variable and nonspecific.

Amyloid fibrils are identified by electron microscopy.

Amyloid fibrils are 7.5–10 nm in diameter (Fig. 8.4). They are rigid, nonbranching, hollow-cored tubules of indeterminate length, since they crisscross into and out of the plane of section. When examined by X-ray diffraction, fibrils have a characteristic B-pleated sheet configuration. This macromolecular helix of 100-nm periodicity formed from two twisted B-pleated sheet micelles is responsible for the resistance of amyloid fibrils to proteolytic digestion and to dissolution. The implacable deposition of these inert fibrils leads to pressure atrophy and interference with tissue function.

Glycosaminoglycans give amyloid its carbohydrate character.

The iodine-staining characteristic of amyloid is imparted by glycosaminoglycans deposited in tissue coincidentally with protein AA. Amyloid-secreting cells, like some neoplastic cells, alter the connective tissue stroma and facilitate amyloid deposition; it is uncertain if amyloid acts as a trap for glycosaminoglycans or if glycosaminoglycans predispose to amyloid polymerization.

The *P component,* a tiny 8-nm-diameter, pentagonal, donutlike body, is also a component of amyloid. Chemically unrelated to the amyloid fibril, this glycoprotein is identical to an α_1-glycoprotein of normal serum (and both are related to complement component C1t and to C-reactive protein).

Amyloid is a spongelike scaffold.

Amyloid fibrils constitute pure amyloid. They are a matrix on which plasma protein and glycoproteins are absorbed. Variations in density and staining of amyloid results from differences in amounts of nonamyloid components that have attached to the fibrillar scaffold. Fibrin, collagen, complement, globulin, and glycosaminoglycans can all be present in amyloid. Histochemical techniques such as the PAS reaction may give positive results, chiefly because amyloid, depending on its stage of deposition, is contaminated with varying amounts of these substances. Vascular permeability is enhanced in blood vessels permeated by amyloid, which allows progressive deposition of plasma proteins on the underlying fibrillar framework.

Types of amyloid

The common denominator of all amyloids is that they are aggregates of proteinaceous, twisted, B-pleated sheet fibrils. Despite their physical homogeneity, the chemical nature of the fibrillar proteins is distinct; that is, the fibril is composed of repeated units of specific type of peptide. The peptide is identical (or highly similar) to normally occurring proteins and is the basis for classifying the different types of amyloid (e.g., amyloid A protein–derived amyloid, endocrine polypeptide–derived amyloid, and immunoglobulin–derived amyloid) (Table 8.4). The most common type by far in animals is the fibril composed of amyloid A that develops in chronic infections and sepsis.

Amyloid A–derived systemic amyloidosis

Amyloid A, a low-molecular-weight, single-chain protein, is the major component of fibrils purified from the amyloid of chronic sepsis (also called "secondary amyloid"). Amyloid A is *formed in macrophages* by proteolysis of antigenically related but larger molecules circulating in blood, serum amyloid A (SAA).

Serum amyloid A is an acute phase reactant of plasma present in normal animals (increasing during early phases of acute inflammatory processes). Plasma concentrations rise within a few hours after fever or infection and decline rapidly

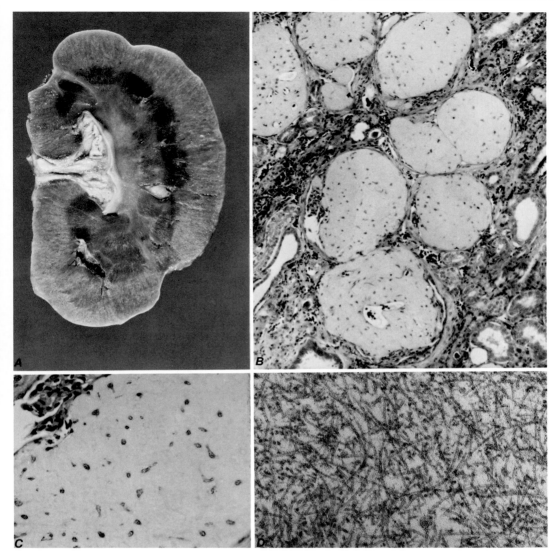

Fig. 8.4. Amyloidosis: 19-year-old collie with chronic enteritis treated recently with corticosteroids. A. Kidney, pallor of cortex. B. Massive deposition of amyloid in glomeruli. C. Enlargement of B: amyloid-producing stellate cells among delicate amyloid deposits. D. Ultrastructure of amyloid fibrils.

Table 8.4.   Classification of amyloid

Type	Precursor	Occurs in
Amyloid A (AA)[a]	Serum AA (SAA)	Lymphoid organs and viscera in chronic sepsis (e.g., osteomyelitis, metritis)
Endocrine	Endocrine peptides	Pancreatic islets (insulin), thyroid (calcitonin), pituitary (growth hormone)
Immunoglobulin	Ig light chains[b]	Lymphoid organs in animals with plasma cell neoplasia (plasmacytomas)
Senile	β-protein	Heart, brain, etc.

[a]Protein AA is an *N*-terminal degradation product of SAA.
[b]May be amino terminal fragments of monoclonal Ig light chains.

to normal values after recovery. SAA is markedly elevated in animals with amyloidosis. Normal monkeys have SAA concentrations of 40–65 ng/ml plasma, but monkeys with amyloidosis have levels of 1700–95,000 ng/ml. SAA is *synthesized in hepatocytes* (much like albumin or fibrinogen). It is transported in the bloodstream, associated with high-density lipoproteins, and may circulate as an apolipoprotein.

Immunoglobulin-derived systemic amyloid

Here, amyloid results from aberrant immunoglobulin production. Analysis of concentrated amyloid fibrils produced by purification of tissue amyloid reveals that amino acid sequences of the amyloid proteins are similar, if not identical, to immunoglobulin light chains and to the light chains excreted in the urine of plasmacytoma patients. Furthermore, fibrils can be synthesized in vitro from urinary immunoglobulin fragments (Bence Jones proteins) from human patients with plasmacytoma and amyloidosis. In vivo studies suggest that reticular cells produce amyloid by intralysosomal proteolytic digestion of circulating light-chain fragments.

Endocrine-derived local amyloid

Insulin-derived amyloid found in the *pancreatic islet* is the most common example. It is most often seen in old cats and nonhuman primates. In cats, islet amyloid may be associated with B cells but is formed by peculiar, stellate nongranular cells located around capillaries. Drs. Barry Yano, Kenneth Johnson, and David Hayden, at the University of Minnesota, have shown that there is an association of pancreatic islet amyloid and diabetes mellitus in cats.

Although rare, amyloid can also be formed from abnormal processes of proteins destined to become glucagon, calcitonin, growth hormone, and other hormones.

Pathogenesis of secondary amyloidosis

Secondary amyloidosis is found incident to long-standing, progressive infections or tissue-destructive processes. It is common in tuberculosis, malaria, leishmaniasis, and bacterial osteomyelitis. In these diseases, the clinical sequelae of amyloid deposits are often masked by the severity of the causal septic disease.

The relationship of secondary amyloidosis to persistent antigenic stimulation is clear, and the classic veterinary literature includes amyloidosis in horses given large amounts of antigen to produce antitetanus serum.

A familial pattern of renal amyloidosis has been reported in Abyssinian cats by Dr. John Boyce. Cats had marked medullary deposition of amyloid. Amino acid sequences of the amyloid protein isolated from kidneys suggested that it was amyloid A.

Amyloid deposition occurs in two phases.

Secondary amyloidosis begins with a long, clinically silent period. This *preamyloid* (initial) *phase* is characterized by an accumulation of reticular cells and macrophages in spleen and other lymphoid tissues and a rise in SAA and globulins in plasma. SAA synthesis in the liver is stimulated by a macrophage cytokine, possibly interleukin-1. The *amyloid* (second) *phase* is characterized by development of PAS-staining cells (filled with abnormal glycoproteins), amyloid deposition, and a decrease in peak SAA levels.

Transition from the initial phase to the amyloid phase is dependent on suppression of proliferating reticuloendothelial cells, either by exhaustion of the immune mechanism following protracted antigenic stimulation or by immunosuppressive drugs. Corticosteroid therapy markedly hastens the transition from preamyloid to amyloid phases.

Plasma protein abnormalities occur early in amyloidosis.

As amyloidosis develops, marked abnormalities are found in plasma proteins, especially in globulins. Synthesis of α_2-, β-, and γ-globulins is increased, and degradation of α_2-globulin is accelerated. Studies with gray collies with cyclic hematopoiesis illustrate that plasma changes occur long before amyloid is deposited in tissue (Fig. 8.5). Neutrophils in these dogs disappear from their bloodstream for 24 hours every 11 days. Affected puppies suffer recurring bacterial infections that correlate with neutropenic episodes. Gradual elevations in α_2-globulin occur early, and progressive increases in all plasma globulins characterize late disease.

Spleen is the primary site of amyloid deposition.

Amyloid first appears in atrophic lymphoid tissue at the periphery of the periarterial lymphoid sheath. This perifollicular amyloid causes

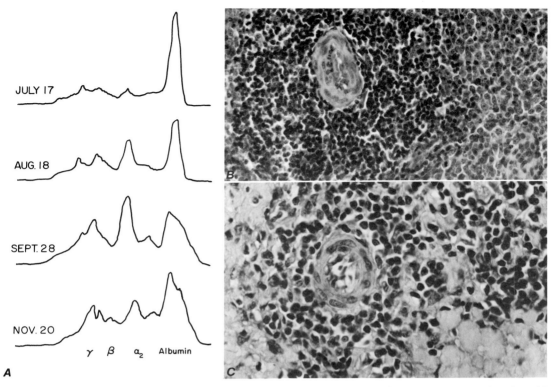

JULY 17

AUG. 18

SEPT. 28

NOV. 20

γ   β   α₂   Albumin

A

B

C

Fig. 8.5. Plasma protein changes and lesions in spleen biopsies, dog with progressive amyloidosis. A. Plasma proteins. B. Splenic histology on Sept. 28 is normal. C. Splenic histology on Nov. 20 shows loss of lymphoid cells and infiltrates of amyloid.

corpuscles to be large, gray, and translucent and to bulge from the cut surface to resemble grains of tapioca or sago. Even though rare, the "sago spleen" is a classic Virchovian lesion.

Histologically, amyloid accumulates in large masses around peculiar dendritic cells, and in early stages is free of contaminating collagen, fibrin, and other proteins. Amyloid also appears between adventitial and smooth muscle cells of the central artery; it is produced by the smooth muscle cell. In red pulp, amyloid occurs in discrete clumps, often associated with plasmacytes.

Renal amyloid can kill.

Kidneys with amyloid are pale, opaque, and yellow to orange-brown. Gray, translucent areas of amyloid occur as spots in the cortex and streaks in the medullary areas. Histologically, amyloid is deposited in the renal glomerulus, in and below basement membranes of the renal tu-

bules (pars recta), and in small arterioles.

Within the glomerulus, amyloid accumulates in the mesangial matrix, initially along the capillary basement membranes. It is formed in situ by mesangial cells (it can also be phagocytized locally by macrophages). Deposition may begin as small focal areas in one segment of the glomerulus and spread to progressively affect all areas of every glomerulus. Secondary damage to both glomerulus and tubule leads to proteinuria, hyalin casts in the tubule lumen, and tiny foci of necrosis.

Amyloid is deposited rapidly.

Although the preamyloid phase is usually long, actual deposition of amyloid may occur in a very short period. A splenic biopsy taken at 3 months from a collie with cyclic neutropenia had no amyloid but contained small lymphocyte sheaths with no germinal centers. At 4 months there were wide cuffs of large lymphoblasts but no amyloid. At necropsy at 6 months of age, marked splenic amyloid was present.

Amyloid is progressive.

Amyloid is inefficiently removed by the reticuloendothelial system. Fibrils are curiously resistant to phagocytosis and proteolysis and are not remarkably immunogenic, due to the large size of the amyloid molecules. When amyloid is incubated with neutrophils and monocytes experimentally, very little is phagocytized. However, if the molecules are slightly altered or distorted by adding antibodies, phagocytosis occurs readily. Neutrophils rapidly take up degraded amyloid, and further hydrolytic destruction occurs in phagolysosomes.

Even though phagocytosis and elimination can be demonstrated in vitro, the persistence of the underlying defect in animals with amyloidosis usually causes production to dominate resorption. If the cause of the underlying disease is removed, amyloid disappears from organs with active macrophages such as spleen but may not do so from the renal glomerulus.

Senile amyloid

The cerebral cortex of aged mammals develops tiny foci of degenerate axons and neurites surrounding a core of amyloid fibrils. Called *senile plaques* (or neuritic plaques), these foci are the hallmark of human Alzheimer's disease. Dr. Linda Cork, a veterinary pathologist at Johns Hopkins University Medical School, has collaborated with medical researchers to show that amyloid filaments in senile plaques of dogs, bears, monkeys, and man are similar biochemically. In man a gene for production of an amyloid fibrillar protein has been localized to chromosome 21 and a change in quantity (excessive) or quality (altered amino acid sequences) of gene transcription may underlie familial Alzheimer's disease.

ADDITIONAL READING

Boyce, J. T., et al. Familial renal amyloidosis in Abyssinian cats. *Vet. Pathol.* 21:33, 1984.

Haskins, M. E., et al. The pathology of the feline model of mucopolysaccharidosis. *Am. J. Pathol.* 101:657, 1980.

Hynes, R. O. Fibronectins. *Sci. Am.* 254 (6):42, 1986.

Keene, W. E., et al. Degradation of extracellular matrix by larvae of *Schistosoma mansoni*. *Lab. Invest.* 49:201, 1983.

Martinez-Hernandez, A., and Amenta, P. S. The basement membrane in pathology. *Lab. Invest.* 48:656, 1983.

Trelstad, R. L. Glycosaminoglycan: Mortar, matrix, mentor. *Lab. Invest.* 53:1, 1985.

Vos, J. H., and Gruys, E. Amyloid in canine mammary tumors. *Vet. Pathol.* 22:347, 1985.

Yano, B. L., et al. Feline insular amyloid. *Vet. Pathol.* 18:181, 1981.

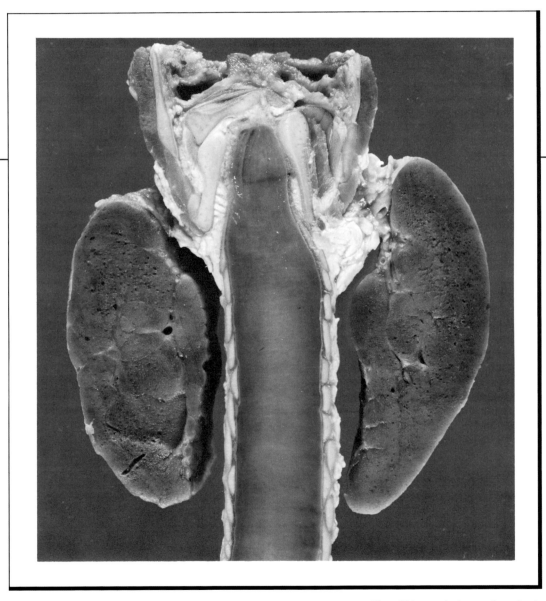

Thyroid hyperplasia, newborn lamb.

GROWTH DISTURBANCES

ABNORMALITIES of mitosis and growth lead to several categories of tissue change. These changes will be discussed under three headings: (1) abnormalities of *cellular growth,* which are either excesses (hypertrophy and hyperplasia), or decreases, such as developmental ones (agenesis and hypoplasia), or those acquired after full development (atrophy aplasia); (2) abnormalities of *cellular differentiation,* which includes metaplasia and the dysplasias; and (3) *neoplasia,* a markedly abnormal and uncontrolled pattern of cellular growth. The basic language used in growth disturbances has already been defined in Chapter 1. Here is explained the basic nature of these defects and how they occur. Because of the clinical importance of neoplasia and the current research effort on it, this group of diseases dominates this section.

An understanding of abnormalities of growth centers on the mechanisms whereby cells divide and differentiate. All cells in the body possess the capacity to undergo mitosis since all have the same genome as the zygote. Some cells divide with extraordinary speed, such as hematologic stem cells in bone marrow, progenitor cells in crypts of the small intestine, and basal epidermal cells in active hair follicles. Other cells such as neurons and cardiac myocytes do not effectively undergo mitosis. The controlling factors, which make only some cells divide, re-

side in the genome in the cell nucleus. These factors turn genes on or repress them so that the cycle of mitosis is closely regulated. Other soluble peptides secreted by cells (called *growth factors* and *chalones*) regulate the speed and activity of mitosis.

Cell growth is geared to these major events in the *cell cycle* (the period extending from one mitosis to the next): DNA synthesis, chromosome replication, and cell division. Factors that inhibit or enhance these events underlie both hypertrophy and atrophy. For example, specific mitosis-inducing factors are elevated in *hyperplasia.* Their action is enhanced by the neural and hormonal causes of hypertrophy, which act by influencing transcription and translation. In contrast, the decreased functional needs of *atrophy* lead to diminished amounts of mitotic stimulants. The metabolism of cells during hibernation, for example, are markedly suppressed; proliferation is blocked in the first resting phase of the cell cycle (G1), and cells cannot synthesize DNA.

Most growth abnormalities evolve into complex lesions. They develop over long periods from obscure beginnings, they often have cyclical patterns of development, and their tissue manifestations vary according to species and age of the host. Thyroid hyperplasia of young, iodine-deficient animals illustrates the progression from hypertrophy to hyperplasia (see facing page). Initially, deficiency of iodine leads to the diminished output of thyroid hormones and the compensatory increase in pituitary production of thyroid-stimulating hormone (TSH). Increased circulating TSH causes hypertrophy of thyroid epithelium. If iodine deficiency is sustained and excess TSH not fully compensatory, hypertrophy progresses to thyroid epithelial hyperplasia. Hyperplastic thyroid glands are enlarged and highly vascular. Follicular lumina are small because of encroachment of epithelium. In older animals the uniformly hyperplastic thyroid gland gives way to cystic and papillomatous growth patterns of "colloid goiter," an involutionary variant of thyroid hyperplasia.

Defects in Cell Growth

9

HYPERTROPHY

Hypertrophy is an increase in size of a tissue or organ without an increase in number of cells. Although it may occur in any tissue, it is seen in pure form only in tissues composed of cells that do not reproduce readily. The most common examples of hypertrophy arise form increased work load or from endocrine stimulation. In hypertrophic cells, increased metabolic activity is reflected in increased size of nucleus and cytoplasm and in increased numbers of organelles.

Muscle hypertrophies during increased work.

The size of muscle cells increases progressively with work (e.g., the large muscle masses and large heart of the racing greyhound). In hypertrophic skeletal and cardiac muscle cells, the contractile myofilaments are increased in length and number. The stimulus for increased protein synthesis to expand myofilaments is a growth factor that, when extracted from hypertrophic muscle, induces normal muscle to hypertrophy. Experimentally, tissue extracts of hypertrophied canine heart, when perfused through isolated canine hearts, causes myocytes to enlarge and begin synthesizing new proteins.

Kidneys have cycles of hypertrophy.

Renal hypertrophy and regression occur during normal diurnal and nocturnal cycles of urine secretion. Substances that stimulate renal metabolism (antidiuretic hormone, catecholamines, and adrenocorticosteroids) produce this subtle, transient hypertrophy.

Surgical removal of a single kidney because of neoplastic disease or congenital defects results in marked and rapid hypertrophy of the remaining kidney. When one kidney is experimentally removed from a dog, hypertrophy can be detected within a few days (Fig. 9.1). All parts of the renal tubule enlarge, including the glomeruli. As in myocardium, the stimulus for renal hypertrophy involves some circulating factor. Kidneys of a normal rat cross-circulated with blood from a nephrectomized rat show the same increase in mass and ribonucleoprotein as in the kidney remaining in a single rat after unilateral nephrectomy.

Hormones stimulate hypertrophy.

Hormones cause hypertrophy by increasing metabolism in cells bearing appropriate hor-

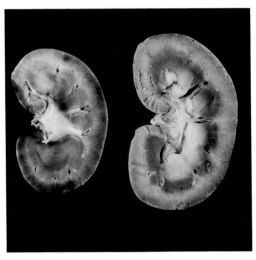

Fig. 9.1. Renal hypertrophy. Kidney removed by unilateral nephrectomy in dog (*left*) and the hypertrophic kidney (*right*) removed 14 days later.

mone receptors on their surfaces. *Thyroid hormones* have a general anabolic effect, manifested as increased oxygen consumption and activation of protein synthesis. Hyperthyroidism in most species is accompanied by cardiac hypertrophy, caused in part by general work load demands of the excessively active hyperthyroid animal but mostly by direct stimulation of protein synthesis in the myocyte.

The same hormone may produce different effects in different tissues. While the hyperthyroid animal has cardiac hypertrophy, it also develops atrophy of skeletal muscle and liver. This is possibly caused in part by generalized protein drain of gluconeogenesis, which drains amino acids more easily from skeletal muscle and liver, and by different effects that thyroid hormone has on muscle and liver through its stimulation of tissue-specific lysosomal hydrolases.

Adrenal corticosteroids stimulate cells by inducing production of enzymes crucial for mitochondrial oxidation, glycogen formation, and lipogenesis. In liver, small doses of cortisol induce hepatocyte hypertrophy. Large doses, as used in treatment of shock, produce massive glycogen deposits (see Fig. 6.2). Glycogen accumulation results from stimulation both of enzymes of glycogen synthesis and of enzymes that cause amino acid degradation and gluconeogenesis.

Androgens stimulate muscle growth.

Part of the body weight difference of males and females is attributed to testosterone-dependent muscle mass. *Androgenic steroids* are used as growth stimulants by weight lifters and other athletes to build muscle mass. Skeletal muscle cells contain specific receptors for androgens and show a selective response to these hormones.

Estrogens and genital hypertrophy

Some of the most striking examples of hypertrophy occur in glands when they are stimulated by the appropriate hormones. In females, for example, the acinar cells of the *mammary gland* undergo marked hypertrophy in late gestation under the influence of the steroid hormones of pregnancy and the pituitary peptide hormone prolactin.

Protein production in mammary epithelial cells is initiated when estrogens diffuse into the cells and combine with specific cytoplasmic estrogen receptor molecules. The *estrogen-receptor*

complex migrates to the nucleus, where it activates the gene with codes to produce specific proteins (prolactin stimulates genes for milk proteins). The activated gene produces mRNA, which migrates through nuclear pores to the cytoplasm where it joins ribosomes to initiate production of the appropriate protein.

Cycles of *uterine endometrial hypertrophy and regression* typify the mammalian estrous cycle. In the bitch, endometrial cells markedly enlarge under the influence of both estrogen and progesterone. At the end of anestrus, as serum estrogen rises, endometrial cells grow in the crypts and differentiate from glandular epithelial cells to well-developed, mucus-secreting cells. As estrogens decline and progesterones rise in metestrus, cells become hyperplastic and develop characteristics of absorptive and secretory cells. The uterine effects of progesterone are dependent on prior exposure to estrogen; that is, estrogen "priming" increases the concentration of progesterone receptors in the cytoplasm of endometrial epithelial cells.

Estrogens have an anabolic effect on the liver.

Estrogens have a pronounced general anabolic effect on liver. They increase protein synthesis and induce hypertrophy. Potent *anabolic steroids* with estrogenic activities are used as subcutaneous implants to increase growth rates of ruminant farm animals. They increase nitrogen retention in liver and promote protein synthesis. In sheep and cattle the hepatocyte partitions amino acids between the use of protein synthesis and deamination to yield substrates for energy production. In the latter case, amino groups are incorporated into urea by liver enzymes. Anabolic steroids reduce the urea entry rate in cattle and sheep, leading to more amino acids available for protein synthesis.

Injection of exogenous estrogen stimulates different hepatic proteins in different species. In avian liver, the egg yolk protein vitellogenin is stimulated. In mammals, plasma proteins and coagulation factors increase; the latter are particularly important in liver disease during human use of estrogenic contraceptive agents.

HYPERPLASIA

Hyperplasia is an increase in the number of cells in a tissue. As in hypertrophy, the hyperplastic cell and its organelles are not qualitatively abnormal. They are simply present in greater numbers.

One of the most common causes of hyperplasia is *chronic irritation.* Mechanical or toxic injury induces epithelial cells to proliferate and accumulate, and the thickened epithelium forms a protective barrier against the inciting causal agent. Parasite infestation of the skin, gut, respiratory tract, or urogenital system usually causes epithelial hyperplasia. A callus in the skin is due to hyperplasia of keratinocytes within the epidermis.

A syndrome of gastric hyperplasia develops in aged dogs with severe systemic disease. The gastric mucosa is thrown into thickened folds (Fig. 9.2), and there is an increase in HCl-producing parietal cells and in chief cells. Mucous hyperplasia of the fovea or neck regions of the gastric glands occurs, and dilatation deep in the gland creates a cystic appearance in the mucosa. The lesions seem to arise from the influence of hormones (chiefly gastrin) and by action of some of the epithelial growth factors.

Hyperplasia of endocrine origin

Tissues that are target organs of the sex hormones show cyclical growth and regression according to hormone levels in the bloodstream. The mammary gland undergoes hyperplasia during lactation. Rarely, excess production of mammary gland tissue occurs during nonlactating periods. A unique condition occurs as a rapid, benign growth of one or more mammary glands of young estrus-cycling or pregnant cats. It is called *fibroepithelial hyperplasia* because of its proliferation of stroma and mammary ductal epithelium.

In the bitch, *cystic endometrial hyperplasia* arises from an arrest in the estrogen-progesterone-induced cycle of endometrial hypertrophy and regression. Prolonged hormonal stimulation causes the uterus to expand with marked increases in secreting cells and accumulation of secretions in the lumen. The uterus becomes infected, usually with *Escherichia coli,* and is filled with pus. Inflammatory exudates block the ducts of hyperplastic glands to cause cysts in the endometrium. Lesions of endometrial hyperplasia can be induced experimentally by treating dogs with large amounts of progesterone or estrogen-progesterone combinations.

Prostate hyperplasia

In several species, prostate hyperplasia develops in intact males of advancing age. Epithelial cells increase in size and number, and fibromuscular tissue markedly expands the interstitium. Prostatic epithelial cells are filled with secretory granules, and there is reduplication of organelles involved in protein synthesis (Fig. 9.3).

Chronic prostatic hyperplasia, which is common in aged dogs, develops in the presence of a functioning testis and is produced by testosterone and its metabolites. Hyperplasia of prostate tissue regresses after castration, but can be restored by administration of androgens. The

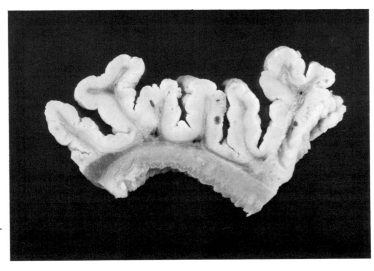

Fig. 9.2. Gastric hyperplasia, dog.

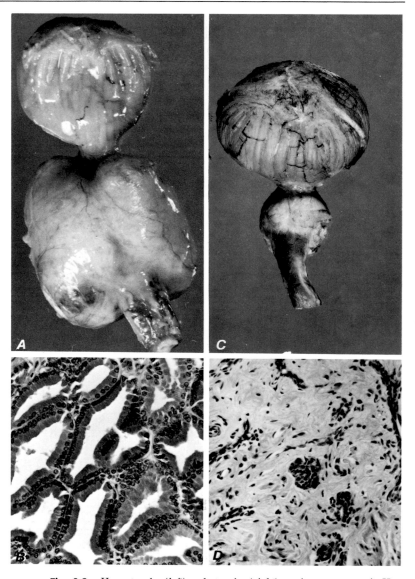

Fig. 9.3. Hypertrophy (*left*) and atrophy (*right*), canine prostates. A. Hypertrophic gland, aged intact dog. B. Tall columnar epithelial cells, little stroma. C. Atrophy of prostate gland, aged, castrated male dog. D. Small epithelial cells surrounded by masses of collagen and fibrocytes.

pathogenesis of canine prostate hyperplasia involves unbalanced testosterone metabolism and complex synergism with hormones. Circulating in blood, testosterone diffuses into prostate cells where it can act directly or be converted to other steroid that are more androgenic, estrogenic, or inactive on the reproductive tract.

Testosterone binds to receptors in the cytoplasm.

After testosterone binds to androgen receptors, the testosterone-receptor complex is conveyed to the nucleus, where it binds to chromatin and causes gene transcription. The new mRNA that is produced exits through nuclear pores into the cytoplasm where it initiates (in ribosomes) synthesis of new peptides for cell growth of the prostate epithelial cell.

The pathway that forms 5α-dihydrotestosterone (5α-DHT) is more important in males: testosterone −(5α-reductase)→ 5α-DHT → 5α-androstanediol. 5α-DHT amplifies the androgenic action of testosterone. Androstanediols are also androgenic, but their activities depend on back conversion to 5α-DHT. Both testosterone and 5α-DHT bind to the same androgen receptors, although 5α-DHT-receptor complexes are more efficient in action on the chromosome and hence more androgenic. In adult male dogs, production of 5α-DHT from testosterone occurs rapidly in the prostate, and when measured biochemically, prostate hyperplastic tissue contains 5 times more 5α-DHT than does prostate tissue of young dogs.

Estradiol is synergistic with androgens in prostate.

Estradiol arises via the enzyme aromatase and acts, after combining with specific *estrogen receptors,* either in the tissue where it is produced or at distant sites. In adults, the actions of testosterone on muscle and brain are mediated through its conversion to estradiol. In prostate, estradiol increases the number of androgen-receptor complexes in the nucleus and causes progesterone receptors to appear in the cytoplasm.

5β-androgens stimulate liver metabolism.

This metabolite of testosterone arises by action of the enzyme 5β-reductase. It has no growth-promoting effects on male reproductive tract, and thus is not a true androgen. It stimulates metabolism in liver and bone marrow and acts after combining in the cytoplasm with specific β-steroid receptors.

Steroid receptors and hyperplasia

Both androgen and estrogen receptors occur in canine prostate epithelium. With age, androgen receptors diminish and become unequally distributed. Hyperplastic prostates have proliferation of both androgen-receptor-bearing and receptor-free cell populations. When androgenic receptors are measured in cytoplasmic extracts of canine hyperplastic prostate tissue, total content is not diminished. In contrast, nuclear extracts show marked increases in androgen receptor complexes, possibly arising from estrogenic stimulation. Hyperplasia of fibromuscular components is an estrogen-dependent phenomenon.

There are also hypothalamic-pituitary alterations in prostate hyperplasia. Affected dogs have increased serum growth hormone and diminished prolactin. Hyperplastic prostate tissue has markedly increased numbers of cells bearing receptors for prolactin (which may explain the low amounts in serum), and prolactin is known to facilitate uptake of testosterone in prostate.

Virus-induced hyperplasia

Hyperplasia is induced specifically by some viruses. Pox, herpes, and other DNA viruses contain a curious preliminary hyperplastic response that precedes the degenerative changes typical of cytolytic infection. Papillomaviruses, however, induce massive hyperplastic responses with little cytolytic effect. Hyperplasia of the stratum germinativum of epidermis results in massive keratin formation (hyperkeratosis) with a very small number of virus-producing cells discretely placed at the superficial junction where keratinocytes are cornified. Papillomaviruses elicit two different processes. First, they stimulate increased cell activity, mitosis, and proliferation (i.e., papilloma formation). Later, selected cells are usurped to produce virus. Hyperplasia is initiated by contact of virus with cell nucleoproteins, which either directly stimulate mitosis or induce production of peptides that act as epidermal growth factors to enhance proliferation and differentiation of keratinocytes.

Control of mitosis

The *cell cycle* is the period extending from one mitosis to the next (Fig. 9.4). Cell activities are geared to the nuclear cycle of chromosome replication and segregation that define the four periods G1, S (for synthesis), G2, and M (mitosis). Control, regulation, and inhibition of cell replication are achieved by interruption of the nuclear cycle. The three major chromosomal events in cell division (reproduction, movement, and cleavage) all occur with strict continuity in the cycle. If one is blocked, the others do not occur (Table 9.1).

G1 is the resting phase: RNA and protein synthesis are necessary for cells to progress through it. The S phase is initiated by a new

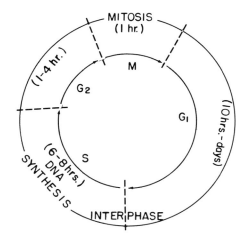

Fig. 9.4. Phases of the cell mitotic cycle.

protein that initiated DNA synthesis. Subsequent progress through the cycle is governed by a temporal sequence of genetic transcriptions held in sequence by the dependency of one on the next.

Primordial cells normally undergo mitosis to provide populations of differentiated cells. Epithelial cells of the epidermal stratum germinativum, crypt cell of the intestine, and stem cells in bone marrow undergo mitosis via influence from humoral substances (see erythropoietin, Chapter 17). Feedback control circuits exist between functions of the differentiated cells and proliferation of the primordial cells.

Growth factors and chalones

Decreased functional need (as in atrophy) leads to diminished amounts of mitotic stimulants. In hibernation, the kinetics and metabolism of cells in animals are markedly suppressed. Proliferating cells are blocked in the G1 phase, and they cannot synthesize DNA. Transcription and translation are suppressed, and permeability of plasma membranes is diminished. Shrunken mitochondria with only a few short cristae reflect the low metabolic activity of the cell.

Growth factors stimulate mitosis. Mitosis is maintained by tissue-specific peptide factors that promote or suppress the cell cycle (Table 9.2). Media used in cell cultures is supplemented with serum to promote growth; the serum contains a number of peptide growth factors that induce mitosis. Similar peptides are present not only in blood but in urine, tears, saliva, and colostrum. They are given names according to the system used in their study and detection (e.g., *epidermal growth factor,* or EGF, and *platelet-derived growth factor,* or PDGF). *Insulin* is also a growth factor. To function, growth factors bind to specific plasma membrane receptors, enter the cell, and assert their effect on the mitotic cycle. Their control is tightly regulated by gene action during their profound effects in the developing fetus. In contrast, their role in wound healing, hyperplasia, and neoplastic disease is determined by acquired characters; that is, their production can be turned on according to body needs.

Chalones are mitosis-inhibiting factors. Chalones permeate tissue and inhibit the cell at various points in the G phase of the cell cycle. In theory, chalones in the keratinocyte suppress mitosis and permit the cell to become cornified. In epithelial injury, chalones are missing, inhibition of the G1 phase is weakened, and cells enter the S phase. Chalones are studied only in

Table 9.1. Indices of mitotic activity

Term	Definition	Comment
Mitotic index	% of cells in a population in mitosis at a given time	Low mitotic index may indicate a few cells dividing rapidly or all cells dividing slowly
Mitotic time	Time from prophase to telophase	
Generation time	Prophase to prophase (mitotic time + interphase time)	
Turnover time	Time required for the production of number of cells equal to number already present	Does not equal cell cycle time unless all cells dividing
Labeling index	Number of cells taking up thymidine-H^3 over total number of cells	Analogous to mitotic index but greater, since DNA synthesis duration is greater than mitotic time

Table 9.2. Families of growth factors

Growth Factor (GF)	Source	Molecular Weight	Other Members
Platelet-derived GF	Platelet α-granule	30,000	Osteosarcoma-derived GF Fibroblast-derived GF Transforming protein of several viruses
Epidermal GF (EGF)	Urine (human) Saliva (mouse)	6,000	Transforming GF
Insulin	Pancreatic β cells	5,700	Somatomedin C

crude extracts of tissue and have not been adequately purified, so their activities have not been clearly identified in the living animal.

METAPLASIA

Metaplasia is the substitution of one type of fully differentiated adult cell in a tissue for another adult cell type normally found there. It represents replacement of vulnerable cells by cells more resistant to an inciting stress. Like hyperplasia, it is a form of controlled, abnormal cell growth. The change is orderly, and there is faithful reproduction of the new cell type. Squamous metaplasia of trachea, bronchioles, gallbladder, and glandular excretory ducts often occurs when these tissues are chronically irritated or inflamed. Vitamin A exerts a controlling influence on epithelial differentiation, and its deficiency leads to widespread squamous metaplasia throughout the body.

Metaplasia often occurs in organs undergoing atrophy. Long-term treatment of male animals with estrogens causes atrophy of the prostate with squamous metaplasia of prostatic glandular epithelium. Secretory cells shrink and disappear, and basal reserve cells proliferate and undergo squamous metaplasia.

ATROPHY

Atrophy is the decrease in size of cells that have gained full development. The muscle wasted in disuse, the mammary gland shrunken in old age, and the diminished size of genitalia after castration are all examples of atrophy. Atrophy represents adaption to a changed cellular environment. Cells shrink when their level of work is diminished or when their source of nu-

trition or stimulation is removed. Obviously, when large numbers of parenchymal cells shrink, the organ involved decreases in size commensurably.

Some examples in which cells decrease in size after once functioning in full capacity follow. The prefaces used indicate the various causes associated with the process but do not reflect the complex interplay that often exists between them. *Disuse atrophy* may result from inactivity or a limitation in movement. It is particularly important in muscle when limbs are restrained by casts or other mechanisms. *Neurogenic atrophy* is loss of innervation due to peripheral nerve injury or loss of central control due to brain or spinal cord injury. *Endocrine atrophy* results from lack of pituitary trophic hormones and decreased metabolism. *Vascular atrophy* is a consequence of loss of blood supply. *Pressure atrophy* comes from direct pressure on the cell; most instances involve pressure on the blood supply or blockade of a duct.

Senile atrophy is sometimes applied to changes that involve the slowly progressive loss of parenchymal cells with advancing age. The reproductive organs atrophy first, followed by muscles, bone, and later the nervous system. "Physiologic atrophy" is applied by some to the programmed disappearance of embryonic tissues that degenerate as part of their normal life cycle, a process here referred to as *necrobiosis*.

Atrophic cells are smaller than normal.

Organelles of atrophic cells are small and sparse. Appropriate stimuli for cell metabolism are lacking. The reduction in transcription, translation, and conjugation of secretory proteins results in loss of ribosomes, endoplasmic reticulum, and secretory granules. *Autophagy* (autophagocytosis), the process in which degenerating organelles are taken into lysosomes, is exaggerated so that atrophic cells are often filled with large secondary lysosomes called residual bodies. When prostatic epithelial cells are deprived of androgens by castration, they cannot produce secretory granules. The rough endoplasmic reticulum is strikingly diminished in volume.

Endocrine atrophy

In the natural cycling of sexual activities, the ovary and testis alternately become hypertrophic and atrophic. Changes are most striking in animals with seasonal breeding and sexual cycles. During involution, parenchymal cells shrink, interstitial spaces expand, and activated monocytes invade and differentiate to macrophages as they scavenge cell debris.

In the testicles of carnivores, blood vessels expand during the breeding season and regress during the long months of sexual inactivity (Fig. 9.5). Testicular atrophy in these species is governed by light-dark cycles. Exposure to darkness stimulates the pineal gland to release antigonadotropic substances that inhibit release or synthesis of hypothalamic-releasing hormones, luteinizing hormone (LH), and follicle-stimulating hormone (FSH).

Atrophy of cachexia

Wasting syndromes that occur in senility, nutritional deficiencies, and prolonged chronic infections often result in diffuse atrophy of skeletal muscle. In cachectic atrophy, muscles are small and pale. Myofibers vary considerably in size, and shrunken atrophic fibers are intermingled with normal fibers. As the myofiber diminishes in size, nuclei become pyknotic and persist in linear arrangement in the destroyed myofiber. Destruction of myoglobin incites lysosomes to develop in perivascular spaces and along sarcolemmal sheaths. Lipochrome pigments develop and persist in some myofibers, especially in the cow.

Fat atrophy

When lipid mobilization is excessive and extended over long periods, lipolysis induces characteristic changes in adipose tissue. These lesions are commonly present in starving hypoproteinemic animals, particularly in the very young and very old. Fat around the coronary band of the heart is prominently affected. The watery and translucent appearance of atrophic fat is responsible for the term *serous atrophy of fat.*

Microscopically, lipid locules of the adipose cell break up and decrease in size when fat undergoes atrophy. There is an increase in glycosaminoglycans, which is best seen as thickened basement membranes around adipocytes. In the interstitium, large mesenchymal cells appear that actively synthesize and release large amounts of collagen and basement membrane material. Glycosaminoglycan granules increase, and the tissue stains intensely with alcian blue for mucopolysaccharides.

HYPOPLASIA

Hypoplasia is the failure of organs or tissues to obtain full size. Hypoplastic organs are typically discovered in young animals. They are caused by events that occur in late stages of the developing fetus and neonate. Often the etiologic agent cannot be determined. Known causes of hypoplasia include (1) genetic mutations that alter the proper differentiation and migration of cells in the embryo and (2) deletion of critical cell populations by viruses and toxins that produce degeneration and necrosis.

Virus-induced hypoplasia

Congenital cerebellar hypoplasia occurs in young animals and is manifest as ataxia. Although no evidence of cause may be present at necropsy, viral infections during pregnancy clearly can cause cerebellar hypoplasia (e.g., feline panleukopenia virus, bluetongue virus in lambs and calves, and bovine viral diarrhea virus in calves).

In feline panleukopenia, fetal brains examined at the peak of febrile disease in utero show evidence of acute cytolytic disease, often with viral inclusion bodies. The actively mitotic cells of the external germinal layer are specifically destroyed and fail to migrate to form the definitive internal granular layer of the cerebellum. Cerebellar folia are stunted and fail to function properly.

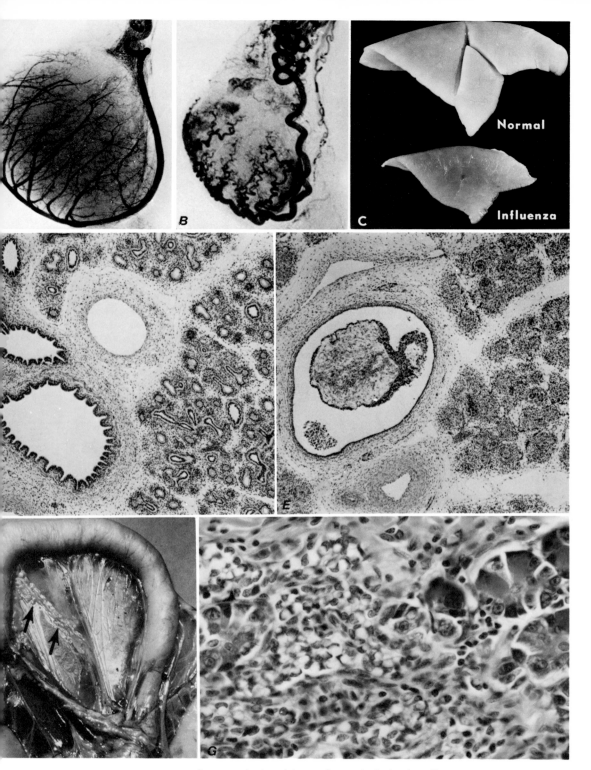

Fig. 9.5. A. Arterial tree, fox testis during breeding season. B. Arterial tree, testis during sexual inactivity. (Photographs: M. Joffre, *Anat. Rec.* 183:599, 1975, used by permission) C. Fetal lungs of normal and influenza virus–infected fetal pigs. D. Normal lung. E. Degeneration and necrosis of developing bronchiolar epithelium and primordial alveoli in influenza-infected lung. (Photographs C–E: Talmadge Brown, *Vet. Pathol.* 17:455, 1980) F. Pancreatic hypoplasia, dog. Only remnants of pancreatic tissue remain in the mesoduodenum. G. Hypoplastic and degenerate pancreatic acinar cells.

Hereditary hypoplasia

Hypoplasia of pituitary, thyroid, pancreas, and kidney occur spontaneously. Causes are not known but presumably involve a hereditary tendency. Pancreatic hypoplasia in the German shepherd leads to a complex of intestinal malabsorption, with wasting, polyphagia, and abnormal feces. Pancreatic tissue is rudimentary (Fig. 9.5), and although the dog may survive early life, it will succumb in early adulthood. During rapid growth of the young dog, the few remaining normal acinar cells progressively degranulate, leaving dark hypoplastic cells around an intact ductal system. Islet cell destruction and diabetes mellitus often accompany exocrine pancreatic failure.

Familial renal hypoplasia follows the same pattern. Pups may survive for a time with partial kidney function but succumb during the first crisis involving increased demands on renal excretion.

APLASIA

Aplasia is complete failure of an organ to develop. The organ may be totally absent (*agenesis*) or may be represented by a rudimentary structure composed of connective tissue. Thymic aplasia and gonadal aplasia are two clinically important examples.

Aplasia is most common and best understood in the reproductive organs, particularly in the male genital system. Chromosomal sex, established at the time of conception, directs development of the indifferent gonad to testis or ovary. The Y chromosome initiates testicular development; in its absence, ovaries form.

When testes are produced by action of the Y chromosome, two secretions are essential for the male reproductive organs: (1) *Mullerian-inhibiting substance* (from primordial spermatogenic tubules), which causes regression of the Mullerian ducts, and (2) *testosterone* (produced slightly later by the interstitial cells), which stimulates the Wolffian duct system. If these hormones are not produced, the fetal gonad secretes estradiol and promotes the female system (the castrated embryo develops as a female).

Aplasia may arise from defects in the primitive gonad: (1) defective synthesis of Mullerian-inhibiting substance by spermatogenic tubules and (2) defective testosterone production by in-

terstitial (Leydig) cells (Table 9.3). Several syndromes of testosterone deficiency occur in man, each with a defect involving an enzyme required for conversion of cholesterol to testosterone.

Single gene mutations can cause defective testosterone synthesis.

If testosterone synthesis is missing or suppressed in the developing fetus, the Wolffian duct system will not develop and there may be aplasia of the male genital tract. The epididymis, vas deferens, and seminal vesicles may be missing or rudimentary (Table 9.3).

Defects may occur not in the gonad, but in *testosterone metabolism* in the genital target tissue. Inside cells, testosterone can act directly or be converted by the enzyme 5α-reductase to dihydrotestosterone (see prostate hyperplasia). Although these two androgens are both bound to cytoplasmic androgen receptors, they do not uniformly affect the male genital primordia; that is, their effects are organ specific. Testosterone receptor complexes cause virilization of the Wolffian ducts. Dihydrotestosterone receptor complexes induce virilization of the urogenital sinus and external genitalia.

Persistent Mullerian duct syndrome

Male pseudohermaphroditism, the most common form of intersexuality in dogs, occurs in male miniature schnauzers with the persistent Mullerian duct syndrome. Mullerian duct derivatives persist, and there is unilateral or bilateral cryptorchidism. Affected dogs have normal male chromosome patterns (i.e., 38 pairs of autosomes, a large X chromosome, and a small Y chromosome). Biosynthesis of testosterone proceeds normally because affected males are masculinized and the Wolffian duct system is present. A genetic basis for this syndrome is likely since it is seen in siblings, but the mode of inheritance is not known.

DYSPLASIA

Dysplasia, meaning abnormal development, is a deliberately vague term used to describe tissues with cell populations that are affected by different processes and are improperly arranged. In most cases it is uncertain whether the condition is truly hypoplastic or has undergone a programmed degenerative change or at-

Table 9.3. Mechanisms of aplasia in fetal reproductive tracts

Defect	Phenotype	Mullerian Duct (oviduct, uterus)	Wolffian Duct (epididymis, vas deferens, seminal vesicles)	Urogenital Sinus (vagina, clitoris; penis, scrotum)
		GENETIC MALE		
Mullerian-inhibiting substance synthesis in spermatogenic tubules (persistent Mullerian duct syndrome)	♂	+	+	Penis
Testosterone synthesis in Leydig cells (various syndromes of incomplete virilization in man)[a]				
Severe form	♀	−	−	Vagina
Slight form	♂	−	±	Penis (hypospadius)
5α-reductase synthesis in genital tissue (absence of 5α-DHT)	♀	−	+	Vagina
Androgen receptor synthesis in genital tissue (testicular feminization [Tfm] mutation in man, rat, mouse)	♂	−	+	Vagina
		GENETIC FEMALE[a,b]		
Androgen exposure during fetal development (female virilization)	♀	+	±	Vagina, hypoplastic
Female born co-twin with male, fused placental circulation (bovine freemartin)	♀	−	±	Vagina, hypoplastic
Congenital adrenal hyperplasia, defect in 21-hydroxylation and cortisol synthesis with compensatory androgen production (man)	♀	±	±	Vagina, hypoplastic
Maternal androgenic tumors or androgen therapy	♀	±	±	Vagina

[a]Several single-gene mutations causing defective testosterone synthesis are known; no mutations have been identified that cause deficient estrogen synthesis or tissue resistance to estrogen action.

[b]Female embryos have same androgen receptor system in genital tissues as male; sexes differ only in gonadal production of hormones.

rophy induced by an abnormal genome. Dysplasia is most commonly used in reference to developmental defects in the eye, skin, brain, and skeletal system. By definition dysplasia applies to tissues malformed during maturation. For example, spermatozoa are dysplastic when the head and tailpiece are structurally abnormal or improperly aligned.

Classically although somewhat erroneously, dysplasia is also applied to disorganized tissues that have peculiar cells but are not clearly neoplastic. *Fibrous dysplasia* in bone indicates that fibrous connective tissue has replaced normal bone, but its growth will not progress in the manner of a tumor.

TERATOLOGY

Teratology is the study of congenital malformations. *Congenital* implies only that the disease was present at birth. *Malformations* involve a seemingly endless list of unrelated syndromes whose causes are found in the vague borderland between environment and genetics. Although some malformations are clearly associated with abnormal genes, many are acquired in utero when differentiating cells are destroyed by viruses or toxins.

Early in embryogenesis, cells become committed to specific developmental pathways. When genes are expressed sufficiently to alter cell structure or function, the cell has *differentiated.* Differentiation, which is usually irreversible, involves a change in genetic expression, not gene structure. Thus it seems that malformations can be acquired not only by deletion of critical primordial cells but also by drugs that influence genetic expression during early phases of fetal development.

Viral infections of pregnant females may cause fetal malformations.

Viruses that produce systemic infection and that cross the placenta to infect the fetus are often teratogenic, especially in the brain. Multiple organ systems are commonly affected (Table 9.4). Anomalies are caused by intracellular viral replication and necrosis of a specific group of cells. For example, in feline panleukopenia, an entire layer of the cerebellum is destroyed. Inclusion bodies, viral antigens, and other evidence of infection disappear by the time the animal is born; the only evidence remaining is a badly malformed brain.

Congenital cavitary anomalies of the brain appeared in the later 1960s after vaccination of pregnant ewes with bluetongue vaccines. *Hydranencephaly,* in which cerebral hemispheres are reduced to membranous, fluid-filled sacs

(the head is of normal size, in contrast to hydrocephalus), was common. Dr. Bennie Osburn, then at the Johns Hopkins School of Medicine, showed that these lesions were due to virus-induced necrosis (see Fig. 25.4). He injected bluetongue vaccine virus directly into fetal lambs at different stages of gestation. Lambs infected at 50–58 days developed severe necrotizing encephalopathy and by birth had severe hydranencephaly. Lambs infected at 75–78 days of gestation developed multifocal encephalitis, which presented at birth as porencephaly (discrete cystic defects). Lambs infected after 100 days of gestation developed only mild encephalitis and had no pathologic sequelae.

Influenza virus has been incriminated in congenital malformations of human fetuses whose mothers suffered infection during pregnancy. Although teratogenic effects have never been clearly confirmed in humans, influenza virus given to pregnant swine causes striking hypoplasia of the lungs (Fig. 9.5). Incriminating a particular virus after pregnancy is terminated is difficult, for the mother may not have exhibited clinical signs of viral infection. Hog cholera live-virus vaccines given to pregnant swine do not produce clinical disease yet may cause multiple fetal malformations including pulmonary hypoplasia, microencephaly, and liver nodules with ascites.

Plant toxins cause malformations at very precise fetal stages.

Ingestion of the plant *Veratrum californicum* by pregnant sheep between the 10th and 15th day of gestation induces *cyclopia* in the fetus. Before and after this period, there is little effect

Table 9.4.   Viral causes of malformation

Species	Virus	Malformation
Cat	Feline panleukopenia	Cerebellar atrophy
Pig	Influenza	Pulmonary hypoplasia[a]
Cow	Bovine viral diarrhea	Cerebellar hypoplasia, hypomyelinogenesis, arthrogryposis, porencephaly, retinal atrophy, hypotrichosis
	Akabane virus Bluetongue	Hydranencephalopathy, arthrogryposis
Man	Rubella	Cataracts, deafness, cardiac anomolies
	Varicella	Growth retardation, limb atrophy, neurologic and ocular defects
	Cytomegalovirus	Hearing loss
	Mumps	Placentitis and abortion[a,b]
	Influenza	Placentitis and abortion[b]

[a]Experimental evidence only; no clear evidence of naturally occurring defect.
[b]Loss of embryo or fetus; no malformations.

of the plant toxin on the developing ovine fetus. The teratogenic capacity of most plant toxins is not confined to such a narrow period. Calves born to cows that have ingested poison hemlock (*Conium maculatum*) during 40–70 days of gestation develop skeletal malformations. Coniine, the major toxic alkaloid in poison hemlock, is probably responsible for the defect, although γ-coniceine is also teratogenic. Piglets develop cleft palate (palatoschisis) when pregnant sows are fed poison hemlock during gestation days 30–45.

Drugs are important causes of malformations.

Drugs are only rarely associated with malformations in animals but are important human teratogens. The veterinary pathologist plays a significant role in prevention of human drug-induced malformations by testing and approving new pharmaceutical preparations. Widespread occurrence of *amelia* (absence of limbs) in human infants was traced to the drug thalidomide, given during pregnancy to prevent nausea. Thalidomide inhibits limb bud formation at a precise period of development.

Inhalation anesthetics were first incriminated as teratogens when operating room nurses were shown to have a high incidence of fetal malformations. Experimentally, exposure of pregnant rats to nitrous oxide causes fetal resorption and several types of malformations.

The teratogenic effects of drugs are not limited to pregnancy. Organs not fully developed at birth, such as brain, eye, and lung, are susceptible to damage in the neonatal period, especially to drugs that alkylate or interfere with DNA.

The etiologic factor in many congenital malformations remains unknown, especially for those diseases that permit survival. Because of the familial nature of these conditions, many are presumed to be of genetic origin. An environmentally caused disease, however, may masquerade as a Mendelian trait and only careful analysis can establish a genetic origin.

AGING

Increased age is inevitably accompanied by degenerative disease. Many aging changes are secondary to diminished function of supportive structure. Bone joints and connective tissues become increasingly rigid. Interstitial spaces are expanded by deposition of collagen and ground substance. The cardiovascular system has a diminished capacity to respond. Brain, muscle, and viscera suffer from the decreased perfusion by circulating blood. Neurons, myocytes, and other cells slowly accumulate metabolic products that remain in the cell. The progressing cycles of diminished function and structural change inevitably reach a point where tissue is more susceptible to injury. This in turn hastens the progression of tissue senescence.

In some specific diseases, the capacity of groups of cells to remain functional is related to factors of blood supply, innervation, endocrine stimulation, and combinations of these factors. If thyroid and adrenal hormones are diminished, so is the viability of the cells stimulated by these hormones.

Starvation is a common cause of death in aged animals. In some insects with short life spans, there is a genetically programmed loss of key enzymes in the digestive tract. In others, crucial mouthparts drop off during metamorphosis, and the insect dies after fat reserves are exhausted. These same mechanisms affect vertebrates, though less strikingly. Aged mammals, for example, may die from malnutrition brought about by loss of teeth.

Cell aging

Aging cells accumulate many abnormal gene products that can represent molecular mischief. Key enzymes (and the mechanisms for their production) become increasingly sluggish. Repair mechanisms for the major macromolecules DNA, RNA, and protein become less efficient, and the breaks that occur in these molecules are defectively repaired. In all of this the primary causes of aging are difficult to distinguish from secondary expressions of cell damage.

In addition to cellular damage, the relations within and between cells begin to break down, destroying the feedback mechanisms that orchestrate cell functions in the efficient multicellular organism.

Theories of aging
Error theories

Error theories, which involve errors in both DNA (somatic mutation) and protein synthesis, imply that cells accumulate nonlethal damage until reaching a threshold where biologic function ceases. The *somatic mutation theory* postulates a progressive accumulation, with age, of random errors in DNA of somatic cells, probably due to declining capacity for DNA repair. Evidence of defective protein synthesis can be readily detected in tissues of aged animals. Decreased quantities of crucial enzymes and of proteins that function as cell surface receptors are especially important in endothelium, macrophages, and leukocytes. Decreased activities of hydroxylases in fibroblasts cause production of collagen with abnormal ratios of α-chains. The diminished sensitivity to insulin associated with aging affects liver, muscle, and adipose tissue.

The immune system and aging

Lymphoid tissue dysfunction is implicated in aging. Death may be hastened because of progressive loss of the capacity to rid the body of unwanted protein antigens. Disappearance of the thymus and its hormone *thymosin* allegedly leads to loss of immunologic surveillance. Aging is also associated with abnormal antigens on cell surfaces that predispose to autoallergic disease and malignancy.

Neuroendocrine clocks control aging.

In some lower vertebrates, excess adrenal cortical activity is associated with senescence. Pacific salmon undergo an intriguingly rapid pattern of aging and death after their migration from the sea to freshwater rivers to spawn. After eggs are ejected and fertilized, the adults become increasingly sluggish and die within a few days. Adrenal cortical "toxicosis" has been reported to cause this rapid aging process. Changes that occur are associated with onset of sexual maturity; they include atrophy of the digestive tract, muscles, and viscera. Castration suppresses adrenal activity and allows an in-

creased life span in these fish. These findings relate to the common belief that the central nervous system mediates aging through the hypothalamic-pituitary axis. This genetically controlled neuroendocrine clock slows with age, and the loss of its hormonal direction deprives supporting tissues of stimuli to repair and reconstruct.

ADDITIONAL READING

Bolande, R. P. Developmental pathology. *Am. J. Pathol.* 94:627, 1979.

Bowden, D. M., and Williams, D. D. Aging. *Adv. Vet. Sci. Comp. Med.* 28:305, 1984.

Edwards, M. J. Congenital defects due to hyperthermia. *Adv. Vet. Sci. Comp. Med.* 22:29, 1978.

El Etreby, M. P., et al. Role of the pituitary gland in experimental hormonal induction and prevention of benign prostatic hyperplasia in the dog. *Cell Tissue Res.* 204:367, 1979.

Hayden, D. W., et al. Feline mammary hypertrophy/fibroadenoma complex. *Am. J. Vet. Res.* 42:1699, 1981.

Konno, S., and Nakagawa, M. Akabane disease in cattle: Congenital abnormalities caused by viral infection. *Vet. Pathol.* 19:246, 1982.

Leipold, H. W., et al. Bovine congenital defects. *Adv. Vet. Sci. Comp. Med.* 27:198, 1983.

Marshall, L. S., et al. Persistent Mullerian duct syndrome in miniature schnauzers. *J. Am. Vet. Med. Assoc.* 181:798, 1982.

Panter, K. E., et al. Induction of cleft palate in newborn pigs by maternal ingestion of poison hemlock (*Conium maculatum*). *Am. J. Vet. Res.* 46:1368, 1985.

Rowland, J. M., and Hendrickx, A. G., Corticosteroid teratogenicity. *Adv. Vet. Sci. Comp. Med.* 27:99, 1983.

Neoplasia

WE have defined *neoplasm* as a new, progressive, and uncontrolled growth of tissue (see Chapter 1), a broad definition left vague because of the wide range of neoplastic diseases. Like infectious disease, the term neoplasm includes lesions of varying causes and pathologic behavior. Furthermore, the current intense research effort in *oncology* (the study of tumors) renders a static definition almost immediately suspect. Since the term neoplasm should not appear oversimple, we retrace some definitions given by distinguished pathologists over the last century.

"Neoplasms are circumscribed atypical productions of tissue from a matrix of superabundant or erratic deposits of embryonic elements," Cohnheim, 1872. Early studies with the light microscope revealed the cellular nature of neoplasms and indicated that they grew independently. Classification schemes that were developed based on the correlation of histologic appearance and clinical behavior proved to have remarkable prognostic value.

The amazing success of microbiologists in transmitting infectious diseases at the end of the 1800s prompted similar attempts to discover a transmissible cause for neoplasms. Scattered reports of transmission occurred, but evidence pointed to accidental or fallacious interpretation; the consensus was that these attempts had failed. The singular success was that of the Russian veterinarian Novinsky, who in 1876 established the transplantability of the canine venereal tumor, one of the few truly transmissible tumors in nature. In the early 1900s, Jensen in Denmark passed tissue suspensions of mouse mammary tumors through several generations. His careful histologic examination established that transmission was effected by transplantation and not by inciting host cells to transform.

"A tumor is a new formation of cells which proliferates continuously and without control . . .," F. B. Mallory, 1914. Mallory's definition went on to state the tumor cells tended to differentiate toward their cell of origin, lacked an orderly structural arrangement, and served no useful function. In the early 1900s clues appeared that exogenous agents might cause cancer. Long-term exposures to X-radiation and coal tar were established as carcinogenic in animals, but these models related to only a few rare instances of naturally occurring neoplasms. Two highly significant discoveries were made at this time (even though they were largely ignored). First, Ellerman and Bang, in Denmark, showed that lymphoid neoplasms of the chicken were transmissible by cell-free filtrates. Second, at the Rockefeller Institute in New York, Rous readily transmitted a sarcoma of the chicken in a similar way and produced a rapidly expanding sarcoma in the recipient bird. Rous persisted for years with his chicken sarcoma and belatedly received the Nobel Prize in 1966.

"A tumor is an abnormal mass of tissue, the growth of which exceeds and is uncoordinated with that of normal tissue and persists in the same excessive manner after cessation of the stimuli which evoked the change," Willis, 1942. This definition attempts to incorporate the new knowledge of causal factors that began to emerge at the turn of the century. It is still practical, for it stresses the lack of *coordinated* growth. Subsequent revelations by studies on viruses and toxic chemicals, however, again transformed the definition of neoplasm.

"Neoplasia results from... somatic mutation and/or aberrant differentation," Prehn, 1971; and *"Cancer genes are normal essential genes run amok,"* Bishop, 1982. These two new definitions relate to our current views, as in the 1960s oncologists began to unravel ways in which viruses and toxins influence cell growth. Classes of agents were identified that specifically reacted with genetic material to cause mutation and neoplasm formation.

Before delving deeper into what neoplasms are, we look at two examples of tumors that represent the range of tumors that one might encounter. At one end of the spectrum are *benign* (from the Latin *benignus,* kind or friendly) neoplasms such as the sebaceous gland adenoma. Common in the skin of dogs, these neoplasms are well circumscribed, do not significantly invade or spread through tissue, and closely resemble their tissue counterpart (Fig. 10.1). In contrast, *malignant* (L. *malignans,* acting maliciously) neoplasms tend to become progressively larger and to result in death. Microscopically, malignant cells are distinctively abnormal,

and they invade and spread to other tissues. The squamous cell carcinoma of skin and other epithelial tissues is often highly invasive, and its cells are eventually disseminated throughout the host (Fig. 10.2).

GENERAL CONSIDERATIONS

The neoplastic process involves an intrinsic heritable abnormality in cells that gives rise to autonomous growth. Neoplastic cells do not behave as integrated, interdependent populations, as we expect in metazoan animal tissue. The regulatory mechanisms of mitosis, differentiation, and cell contact inhibition are defective. Cells grow in rapidly expanding masses that ultimately compromise host structure and function.

The capacity to undergo mitosis is inherent in all cells. Throughout life, mitotic activity is repressed or controlled in some way. Neoplastic cells lack this repression and must be considered cells unresponsive to the controlling mech-

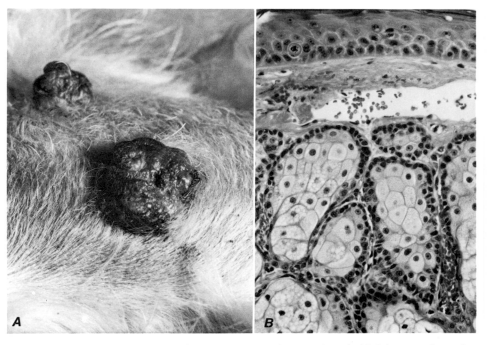

Fig. 10.1. Sebaceous gland adenoma, dog. A. Nodular growths project above skin surface. B. Large, lipid-filled sebaceous cells surrounded by small, dark germinal cells.

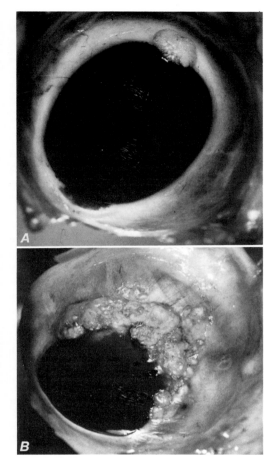

Fig. 10.2. Squamous cell carcinoma, eye, steer. A. Early lesion. B. Advanced lesion.

volved in early development," or as "misprogramming of gene function at any step of differentiation that leads to new gene expressions." These are all variations on the theme of *undifferentiation*. The search for causes for failure of differentiation in the 1970s directed attention toward two basic mechanisms, *genetic mutation* and *defective cell regulation*. It is now clear that these are poles in a spectrum of ways in which cells may become neoplastic and that there is a mutational basis for some neoplasms while others arise by nonmutational means. The crucial factor is *gene expression,* specifically of genes involved in growth and differentiation. These genes need not be abnormal (in the sense of directing faulty protein synthesis). Instead, control of gene expression may be defective, leading to synthesis of gene products in excess or at the wrong time.

Cancer is a chronic disease and begins many months before clinical signs first appear. The clinical phases of the disease represent only a fraction of the pathogenic process. Some epithelial lesions, termed *precancerous,* are known to smolder silently for months or even years before malignant foci of cells can be readily demonstrated.

Neoplastic cell transformation in many cases involves the development of a series of discrete cell populations. That is, the progressive development of a tumor is characterized by the evolution of successive clones of cells, each coming one step closer to the overt cancer cell type that proliferates to stop only with the death of the host.

Genetic instability underlies the sequential acquisition of biologic characteristics of neoplasms. Change in a previously normal cell may provide a selective growth advantage over adjacent cells. Neoplastic proliferation then proceeds as a result of uncontrolled mitosis in the expanding tumor population. While most variants die, due to metabolic or immunologic disadvantage, many cells survive. The surviving neoplastic population has a higher frequency of mitotic error and other genetic changes, and each cell division carries an increased risk of variation.

The growth rate of a tumor depends on several inherent growth characteristics: (1) the fraction of cells in a tumor undergoing mitosis, (2) the length of the cell cycle (i.e., the interval between mitosis and completion of subsequent mitoses in daughter cells), and (3) the number of

anism or in which the mechanism itself is imperfect.

Features that neoplastic cells have in common are (1) mitotic structures that are readily activated, (2) cell surfaces designed for movement and migration (at the expense of intercellular communication), and (3) simplified energy production via fermentation of glucose, with oxygen and the mitochondrial respiratory chain less effective. These are also characteristics of undifferentiated embryonic cells. Indeed, the common thread among cells of various malignant neoplasms is a failure of differentiation.

Experimental oncologists define neoplasia as "impairment of forward differentiation of stem cells," or as "selective reactivation of genes in-cells lost by death, exfoliation, and metastasis. The length of the tumor cell cycle is usually (but not always) shorter than that of its normal cellular counterpart.

Tumor growth also depends on the ability of the neoplastic cell to grow and move in its environment; that is, the new cell must move away from the expanding tumor mass, alter the connective tissue ground substance, and stimulate vascular growth. If new capillaries cannot nourish the tumor, necrosis results. There are differences in the capacity of various tissues and body regions to limit or permit neoplastic growth.

Classification of neoplasms

Classification is the means by which the pathologist communicates with the clinician who must provide a prognosis for the patient. Confrontation with enormous lists of neoplasms is overwhelming to the beginning student of pathology. Distinguishing between carcinoma and sarcoma or between adenoma and adenocarcinoma seems simple enough, but this is complicated by the capricious use of terms such as "mixed mammary gland tumor" or "transmissible venereal tumor" that have been established by precedent for neoplasms that do not fit comfortably within a rigid classification scheme based on histologic appearance. Even worse, the discipline of pathology is saddled with some confusing (and often humorous) eponyms such as "Sticker tumor" (canine venereal tumor) or "Wilm's tumor" (embryonal nephroma).

Benign neoplasms

Neoplasms that are well differentiated, grow slowly by expansion, and do not invade below basement membranes are called *benign*. A neoplasm is benign when its cellular characteristics are considered innocent. This implies that the tumor will remain localized and is removable by simple excision.

Benign tumors are often *encapsulated* (but lack of capsule does not imply malignancy). Benign tumors can cause serious disease by exerting pressure on ducts, arteries, or the nervous system. Parathyroid adenomas may be tiny and benign yet can generate lethal disease in the animal through secretion of hormones by the neoplastic cell.

Benign tumors are classified according to their histology (Fig. 10.3). They are designated by adding the suffix *-oma* to the cell type of origin. A benign tumor of epithelium is an *epithelioma,* of fibrocytes, a *fibroma,* and of chondrocytes in cartilage, a *chondroma.* In all of these, tumor cells closely resemble their normal counterparts. Benign epithelial tumors that produce glandular patterns are called *adenomas* (Table 10.1).

Malignant neoplasms

At the other extreme of tumor behavior are the *malignant* tumors, whose cells are anaplastic and which metastasize and invade. The aggressive neoplastic cells infiltrate and in some cases destroy normal tissues. Malignancy is a clinical concept (cells in culture cannot be considered malignant), and its determining character must relate to the growth of the neoplasm within the animal. A "cancer" is a malignant neoplasm. Those of ectodermal derivation are called *carcinomas* and those of mesodermal origin, *sarcomas.*

Preneoplastic lesions

The livers of aged dogs often contain multiple, discrete, well-differentiated nodules. These are considered "preneoplastic." Cells of the nodule do not replicate to form malignant tumors and are not neoplastic. Neoplastic cells do arise in these nodules, however, and dogs with nodular livers have a much higher incidence of hepatocellular carcinoma than do dogs with nonnodular livers. Preneoplastic lesions of this type precede several types of squamous cell carcinomas, transitional tumors of the bladder, and malignant melanomas of the skin and oral cavity.

Neoplasia-like malformations

Special terms are sometimes applied to malformations and tumors derived from them. A *hamartia* is a tissue defect of cells normally found in a particularly area; a *hamartoma* is a tumor of these components, that is, an excessive, focal overgrowth of mature cells in an organ of identical cellular elements. A *chorista* is a tissue defect of structures not found normally in the areas; a *choristoma* is a tumor of such structures.

Staging of neoplasms

Solid tumors are often categorized artificially into stages for use in surgical management and prognosis. Characteristics used to formulate

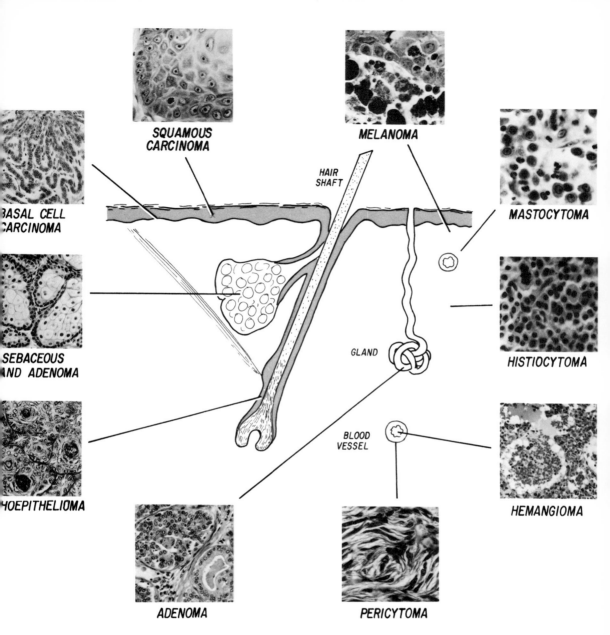

Fig. 10.3. Histogenetic origin of different types of skin neoplasms, dog.

each stage include appearance of the primary tumor, presence of tumor cells in the lymph nodes, and *metastasis,* the formation of tumor foci in a distant tissue. One system of staging is as follows:

Primary tumor:
T_0 = no evidence of tumor
T_1 = tumor confined to primary site
T_2 = tumor invades adjacent tissue
Lymph nodes:
N_0 = no evidence of tumor
N_1 = regional node involvement
N_2 = distant node involvement
Metastases:
M_0 = no evidence of metastasis
M_1 = in same cavity as primary
M_2 = distant metastases

Using these codes, variations on how a tumor may be staged include *stage I* = T_1, N_0, M_0; *stage II* = T_1, N_0 or N_1, M_1; and *stage III* = T_2, N_1 or N_2, M_2.

Table 10.1.   Classification of some neoplasms

Organ of Origin	Cell of Origin	Benign Tumor	Malignant Tumor
Epidermis	Squamous cell	Epithelioma	Squamous cell carcinoma
	Basal cell		Basal cell carcinoma
Adnexae	Hair follicle	Trichoepithelioma	Adenocarcinoma of
	Sweat gland	Adenoma of	Adenocarcinoma of
	Sebaceous gland	Adenoma of	Adenocarcinoma of
	Perianal gland	Adenoma of	Adenocarcinoma of
Other glands	Salivary gland	Adenoma	Mixed tumor
			Adenocarcinoma
	Mammary gland	Adenoma	Adenocarcinoma
			Mixed tumor
			Duct tumor
Neurectoderm	Melanoblast	Melanoma	Malignant melanoma
Connective tissue	Fibrocyte	Fibroma	Fibrosarcoma
	Adipose cell	Lipoma	Liposarcoma
	Undifferentiated cell	Histiocytoma	Reticulum cell sarcoma
		Myxoma	Myxosarcoma
	Mast cell	Mastocytoma	Mast cell sarcoma
	Schwann cells	Neurilemmoma	Malignant neurilemmoma
	Nerve sheath cell	Neurofibroma	Neurofibrosarcoma
Vascular tissue	Endothelium	Hemangioma	Angiosarcoma
		Hemangioendothelioma	Hemangioendotheliosarcoma
		Hemangiopericytoma	Malignant hemangiopericytoma
		Vascular leiomyoma	
Muscle tissue	Skeletal muscle	Rhabdomyoma	Rhabdomyosarcoma
	Smooth muscle	Leiomyoma	Leiomyosarcoma
Skeletal tissue	Cartilage	Chondroma	Chondrosarcoma
	Bone	Osteoma	Osteosarcoma
Other	Synovium	Synovioma	Synovial sarcoma
	Mesothelium	Mesothelioma	Mesothelial sarcoma
	Meninges	Meningioma	Meningioma, malignant

Incidence of neoplasms

Although occurrences of tumor types are similar among species, each species (and in inbred animals, each strain) has its own characteristic spectrum of tumors. The dog has a very high incidence of mast cell tumors in the skin (Fig. 10.3) whereas this is a rare tumor in most other species.

The incidence of each type of tumor usually has a characteristic distribution. For example, studies on squamous cell carcinomas in horses show that 43% occur on the head, eyes, and ocular glands; 45% are on male genitalia and 12% on female genitalia. Osteosarcomas in dogs tend to occur on the long bones of the limbs (Fig. 10.4).

THE NEOPLASTIC CELL

Certain features separate malignant tumors from their benign counterparts (Table 10.2). These features are not requisites of malignancy but are general characteristics of malignant tumors. *Differentiation* refers to the extent to which cells resemble the cells of their tissue of

Table 10.2.   Biologic characteristics of the malignant neoplastic cell

Metastatic – transferring to other tissues by blood and lymph

Invasive – cells not contained by barriers of connective tissue and basement membrane

Anaplastic – large nuclei and nucleoli; fewer mitochondria and other organelles; concerned with replication and not with normal cell metabolism

Mitotic – greater mitotic activity

Nondifferentiated – haphazard growth pattern, does not resemble normal tissues

Nonencapsulated

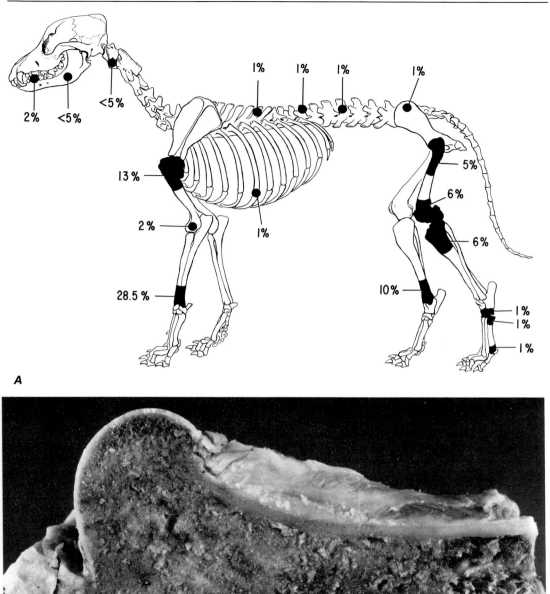

Fig. 10.4. Osteosarcoma, dog. A. Sites of origin of canine osteosarcoma. (Data from Brodey et al., *J. Am. Vet. Med. Assoc.* 143:471, 1963) B. Femur, Great Dane. This tumor has destroyed the growth plate, but there is no invasion of cartilage of the joint.

origin (in embryology, differentiation is used to indicate a change from a lower to a higher state of specialization). *Undifferentiation,* synonymous with *anaplasia,* refers to the loss of specialization and organization, with anarchic changes in cell organelles.

Neoplastic cell genesis

Cell differentiation, the derivation of specialized cells from less-specialized ones, is an expression of specific gene activity. As cells switch to differentiated forms, genes that control embryonic characters are switched off and genes for the more differentiated characters are activated.

In neoplastic cells, abnormal genes or normal genes expressed at abnormal levels favor proliferation over differentiation. In theory, then, causes of neoplasia may affect gene function by events either mutational or regulatory. That is, a neoplasm may arise from (1) *genetic mechanisms,* by mutation of somatic cells in which abnormal chromosomes or genes are reproduced to provide a stable, monoclonal population of cells, or (2) *epigenetic mechanisms,* in which the tumor cells have not lost any genetic information but are abnormally expressing genes related to cell growth (i.e., the genome of the cancer cell is normal although transcription and translation are abnormal).

Genes are altered in most neoplasms.

Most natural tumors probably arise by genetic mutation or by rearrangement of genes. The abnormal gene may act by producing a messenger RNA (mRNA) that directs ribosomes to begin hyperproduction of an abnormal gene product. The excess gene product might then diffuse throughout the cell to produce enzymatic or other reactions leading to cellular manifestation of neoplasia. The initiating gene change could occur either as a result of direct chemical or radiation damage to DNA or by insertion of viral cancer genes into host DNA that mimic normal growth-controlling genes.

Oncogenic viruses insert tumor genes into host cell chromosomes.

Rous sarcoma virus (RSV), the grandfather of all tumor viruses, carries four genes that enter fibroblasts of the chicken (its natural host) during infection. Three of these direct the production of new infectious virus, but the fourth

(*src*) gene induces fibrosarcomas (it also produces tumors in rodents and transforms fibroblasts in culture). The *src* gene is inserted into the host cell genome and can be passed for generations. When activated it causes the host fibroblast to produce an mRNA that initiates ribosomal production of a "*src* gene product," a peptide (kinase) that can phosphorylate proteins in a high degree.

Although the *src* gene product is present in small amounts, it floods the cytoplasm to reach substrates that normal cell enzymes cannot. In cells transformed in vitro, the *src* gene product is bound to the plasma membrane. It phosphorylates a tyrosine unit in vinculin, a protein in adhesion plaques at the cell surface. In theory, this disruption of adhesion zones would contribute to the ability of neoplastic cells to break away and metastasize.

Tumors also arise by nonmutational events.

Some tumors arise by epigenetic mechanisms (activation of genes that are normally turned off). Derepression of sections of the genome results in synthesis of specific proteins (enzymatic or structural) that characterize a particular tumor cell type. Epigenetic mechanisms can be oncogenic at two sites in the process of protein synthesis: during transcription of genetic information or during translation in formation of peptide chains. Neoplastic transformation appears to be a pathologic counterpart of normal differentiation, arising from a misprogramming of gene activity by these epigenetic mechanisms.

Neoplastic cells may contain normal genes.

Unequivocal evidence that neoplastic cells contain normal genes that are misprogrammed comes from studies on chimeric mice. Chimeric mice are produced by injecting tumor cells into normal embryonic blastocytes. These *allophenic* mice are produced experimentally by removing cleavage-stage embryos (of dissimilar genotype, for example, black and albino) from the uteri of pregnant females, lysing the zona pellucidae in pronase, and placing the embryos in contact at 35°C. Within 24 hours, cells aggregate and develop into a normal single blastocyst, which is then implanted surgically into the uterus of a foster mother, a female made pseudopregnant by being mated to a vasectomized male. Each newborn mouse thus has four parents and an incubator mother. They are fully immunocompetent to reject foreign proteins but fully tolerant to tissue of either mouse parent.

When single cells of a carcinoma (most studies use a teratocarcinoma, or "teratoma") are injected into blastocysts, they contribute to all major tissues of the chimeric mouse. Gene products used as markers for the teratoma cell include black melanin in epidermis, hemoglobin of erythrocytes, immunoglobulins, and liver isoenzymes. Male chimeric mice even produce sperm bearing only the genome of the teratoma cells. The teratoma cell can thus either differentiate normally or give rise to a tumor, depending on the environment into which it is injected. The malignant cells retain their neoplastic properties if left to themselves but revert to normal when closely associated with normal embryonic cells.

Tumors do not develop from end-stage cells.

For neoplasia to occur (for differentiation to fail) in adult animals, pluripotential stem cells must be present. Tumors do not arise from completely differentiated cells such as neurons or keratinized epithelial cells. These end cells do occur in tumors but only as a result of variance in differentiation as the tumor grows (Fig. 10.5).

Neoplastic cells do not "dedifferentiate" but fail to respond to normal signals for differentiation.

Neoplastic cell structure

Cellular anaplasia and invasion of tissue are the two most reliable hallmarks of malignancy (if the tumor has metastasized, there is no doubt). The characteristics of *anaplasia* are (1) pleomorphism (differences in cell size and shape), (2) large hyperchromatic nuclei with irregularities of the nuclear membrane, (3) increase in size and number of nucleoli, and (4) decrease in numbers of normal cytoplasmic organelles with the presence of many aberrant forms. There is usually a deficiency of mitochondria, endoplasmic reticulum, and other cell work–associated organelles. In summary, cells appear to function in reproduction and not in metabolic activity of other kinds.

Tumors are classified according to structure.

Histologic examination provides the basis for the *histogenetic classification* of neoplastic tissues. Cell structure and the architecture of cell

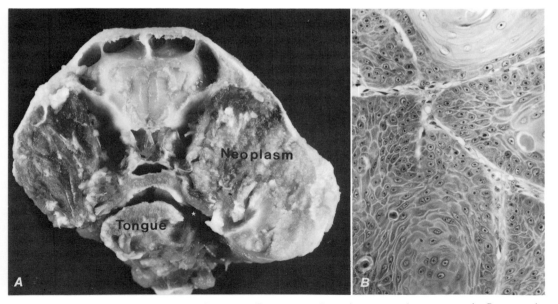

Fig. 10.5. Squamous cell carcinoma, oropharynx, cat. A. Cross section through posterior sinuses and frontal brain. The primary tumor originated in the right dorsolateral surface of the palate (*asterisk*) and spread through masseter muscles and salivary glands. B. Moderate differentiation of keratinocytes with keratin whorls.

arrangement in tumor tissue is matched to various normal tissue systems. In addition, the degree of differentiation is based on the relative resemblance to normal tissue. The well-differentiated mammary gland adenocarcinoma forms acini in which cells are tightly connected and contain secretory granules. In contrast, the anaplastic mammary adenocarcinoma shows great variation in size and shape, nuclei, and cytoplasmic organelles.

Specific proteins and inclusions can be identified histochemically and by immunocytochemistry. Undifferentiated cells can often be classified by staining for specific secretory components, such as hormones, melanin, and other proteins (e.g., techniques for casein have been used in the diagnosis of mammary gland carcinoma).

Ultrastructure analysis provides clues to the degree of differentiation. Cells of the squamous cell carcinoma have anaplastic characteristics that can be used to indicate the degree of malignancy: the cells are large and irregular, the nucleoli are massive, desmosomes are abnormal, and there is evidence of uncontrolled production of filaments and glycocalyx materials (Fig. 10.6).

Neoplastic cells lose contact.

One of the most important characteristics of malignant cells is the tendency to lose cohesiveness with neighboring cells. This decreased adhesiveness, representing a change in the plasma membrane, is manifested as the capacity of malignant tumors to spread by invasion of tissue, by implantation on new surfaces, or by metastasizing to new sites in lymphatics or blood vessels. Some of the changes seen in plasma membranes of tumor cells have been a more negative surface charge, a decrease in calcium content, the presence of abnormal glycoproteins and glycolipids, and the elaboration of humoral substances that enhance invasiveness. Negative surface charges reflect abnormal amounts of sialomucopeptides on the cell surface and tend to repel cells from one another.

In general, neoplastic transformation is associated with a reduction of cell surface glycoproteins. *Fibronectin,* which is present on surfaces of normal cells, is absent or diminished on many types of neoplastic cells. The failure of the matrix formed by aggregating fibronectin may destabilize the tumor cell population. Experiments with mouse melanoma cells show that fibronec-

tin suppresses invasiveness while laminin increases it. Cells with abnormal surfaces will be unresponsive to normal cell growth regulators.

Neoplastic cells lack contact inhibition.

When normal cells grow in vivo or in culture, there is inhibition of movement and mitosis when they contact each other. It is presumed that contact in some way allows the exchange of information and the establishment of gap junctions and desmosomes for maintaining contact. When tumor pieces are placed in culture, cells migrate away from the explant more quickly than do cells from normal tissue. They grow outward, not in organized radial strands but in random, haphazard patterns.

Cell junction defects are typical of neoplastic cells.

Alterations in *tight junctions* correspond with tumor differentiation but are not implicated in tumor growth promotion. They are a result, not a cause, of malignant changes. In epithelial tumors that produce basement membranes, hemidesmosomes may develop in a vain attempt to anchor the tumor cell.

Gap junctions are often broken in neoplasms; the absence of this direct communication between cells has significant effects on neoplastic growth. Gap junctions are freely permeable to small molecules and ions and provide a mechanism to share metabolites and control molecules so that cell systems can respond jointly to changing metabolic demands. When gap junctions are missing, the behavior of the tissue as a homogeneous unit is changed.

Some cancer cells have fewer gap junctions and an inability to send and receive signal molecules. This may promote uncontrolled growth, although cancer cells that have normal gap junctions may possess some internal defect in their ability to respond normally to transferred signal molecules. It has been hypothesized that vitamin A impedes development of epithelial neoplasms due to its ability to maintain epithelial differentiation and to block preneoplastic dedifferentiation by causing a significant proliferation of gap junctions.

The cell cytoskeleton is abnormal in many neoplastic cells.

There is evidence of cytoskeletal instability in many tumor cells. Abnormal microfilament or microtubule functions are reflected in both aber-

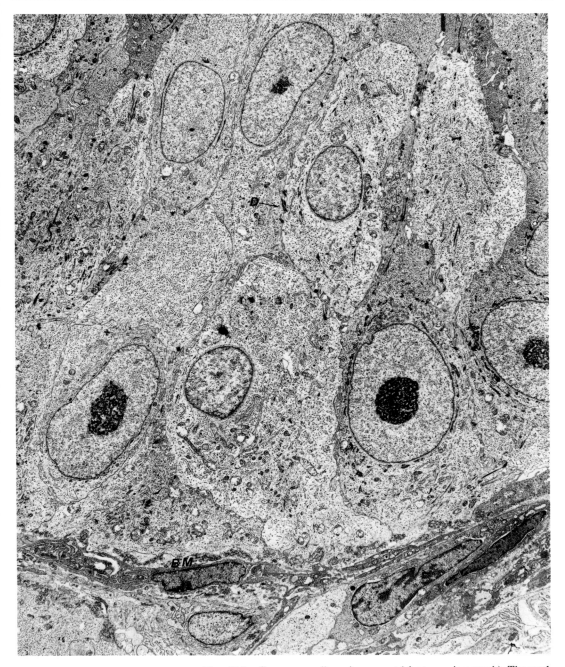

Fig. 10.6. Squamous cell carcinoma, cat (electron micrograph). The moderately differentiated tumor cells produce desmosomes (*D*) and basement membranes (*BM*).

rant cell movement and instability in chromosome movements via defective spindle formation. Normally concentrated at the cell surface, microfilaments of actin are found throughout the cytoplasm of highly malignant cells. Polymerization rates of actin are altered in malignant cells in vitro. *Microtubules,* which maintain normal cell shape, are also abnormal, and the irregular contours of transformed cells in culture have been correlated with abnormal polymerization of *tubulin* (the protein that makes up microtubules).

Mitotic figures are common in malignant tumors.

Microscopic examination of tumor tissue usually reveals an increase in the number of mitotic cells. The large cells with central aggregates of chromosomes are called *mitotic figures* (Fig. 10.7). The mitotic process, however, resembles that in normal cells. Replication and migration

of centrioles, appearance and disappearance of spindle tubules and kinetochores, and movement and replication of chromosomes can rarely be distinguished from normal. Nucleoli and some cytoplasmic organelles tend to persist during mitosis of neoplasms; they do not do this in normal cell cycles.

Mitotic defects involve abnormal chromatin.

DNA or DNA-histone complexes isolated from neoplastic cells commonly have behaved abnormally when analyzed chemically. In normal cells, genetic information is transcribed from DNA to a closely related single strand of RNA and, in turn, translated from that strand into a protein constructed of amino acids. It seems that the altering of DNA molecules, either by chemical oncogens or by insertion of viral material into the chromosome, would most readily explain the abnormal growth that occurs in neoplasms.

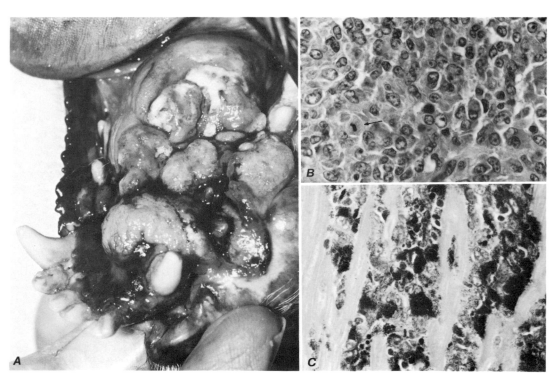

Fig. 10.7. Malignant melanomas, oral cavity, dog. A. Amelanotic type, gingiva, dog. Nodular white tumors are at the site of a biopsy of the primary tumor 3 months previously. B. Histology of A: highly undifferentiated plump cells with many mitoses (*arrow*) and no visible melanin granules. C. Histology of melanin-producing malignant melanoma.

In some cancer the DNA strand is certainly broken. Drugs such as dimethylnitrosamine break single strands of DNA, and the acetylaminofluorine compounds cause disruption of double-stranded molecules. Oncogenicity seems to be inversely related to the rapidity of strand repair in experiments in vivo.

Chromosome analysis may reveal physical abnormalities in specific chromosomes.

When examined by chromosomal analysis, malignant cells are usually *aneuploid* (having more or less than the normal diploid number) and have a variety of chromosomal defects. Most neoplasms have pathologic karyotypes (including chromosomal deletions, translocations, and other changes), and many have specific translocations that are faithfully reproduced in all tumor cells. It seems that chromosomal breaks and translocations correlate with cell type (more than with etiologic agent). If translocations occur in B lymphocytes (cells destined to produce antibody), breaks will occur at sites of immunoglobulin encoding regions, which in human B cells are on chromosome number 14 (Ig heavy chains), 2 (Ig kappa light chains), and 22 (Ig lambda light chains). Furthermore, the extent of translocation is related to the degree of differentiation of the B lymphocyte.

Neoplasms of leukocytes often have specific chromosomal defects.

Some tumors of B lymphocytes (the precursors of plasmacytes), when examined by karyotype analysis, have abnormal chromosomes containing genes for antibody production. Plasmacytomas of mice show translocation of segments of chromosome 15 to chromosome 12, which carries the genes for production of antibody heavy chains in mice. This suggests that rearrangement of chromosomal pieces may induce abnormal activation of otherwise normal genes for producing antibodies. During normal antibody formation, DNA breakage and reconnection occur as genes for light and heavy chains of the antibody molecule are assembled. A gene segment inserted into the host chromosome at this point could transform the cell.

Antibody genes may be transported to chromosomes with genes for growth.

Recent techniques using radiolabeled DNA probes are attempting to show that genes for producing antibody chains are translocated to chromosomes that bear genes associated with neoplastic growth. This has been done in cultured cells of human Burkitt's lymphoma, a neoplasm associated with infection with an oncogenic herpesvirus that transforms B lymphocytes. In about 90% of these patients, chromosomes 8 and 14 are abnormal and have translocated pieces of their long arms. In the process, DNA gene segments coding for the heavy chain variable regions are moved from their normal position on chromosome 14 to number 8. Other gene probes have shown this to be the location of another misplaced gene, designated *myc* (because it is similar to the *myc* gene of lymphoid leukosis of chickens). In the avian B cell lymphoma, an oncogenic viral sequence becomes integrated near a cellular *myc* gene, which then becomes activated. The expression of the *myc* gene is assumed to underlie neoplastic transformation.

Neoplastic cell metabolism

Normal regulation and flexibility of programmed protein synthesis is lost in neoplastic cells. Reprogramming of gene expression and messenger RNA translation in the cytoplasm is highly directed to (1) purine synthesis and utilization to supply requirements for mitosis, (2) altered mechanisms of energy production with dominance of glycolysis in the cytoplasmic matrix over mitochondrial respiration, and (3) altered plasma membrane components, especially defective sodium pumps (ATPases), skewed protein receptor molecules, and abnormal surface glycoproteins.

Much of our knowledge of metabolic shifts in neoplasia comes from studies of transplantable and carcinogen-induced liver tumors in rodents. Cells of these tumors are highly malignant and uniform in structure and metabolism. Fortunately, results from these models agree with studies on homogenates of natural hepatocellular carcinomas. Nonetheless, they do not entirely represent the spectrum of liver tumors that occur naturally in animals.

Enhanced glycolysis and glucose use typifies most tumors.

Warburg established in the 1920s that malignant cells have a high degree of glycolytic activity (both anaerobic and aerobic). Neoplastic cells produce large amounts of lactic acid from glucose, and this pathway is not markedly reduced in the presence of oxygen, as it is in normal tissue. From this it was theorized that malignancy is correlated with increased fermentation and decreased respiration. Currently, this metabolic defect is viewed as characteristic of tumor cells but not significant in the definition of cause.

In most experimental hepatomas there are increased glucose consumption and diversion of precursors into synthesis of purines, pyrimidines, RNA, and DNA. Gluconeogenesis and the urea cycle are diminished. The enzymatic imbalance responsible for this shift involves increased key glycolytic enzymes and decreased enzymes of gluconeogenesis. In addition, isozyme shifts replace normal enzymes with isozymes unresponsive to nutritional and hormonal regulation. This decreased dependence of the neoplastic cell on mitochondrial respiration confers a selective advantage to begin growth in the tumor mass, a poorly vascularized, oxygen-deficient environment (see Fig. 5.5).

Why do cancer cells develop excessive glycolysis?

One reason for excessive glycolysis may be that factors that damage genomic DNA also damage the self-replicating DNA of mitochondria. In fact, carcinogenic metabolites of benzopyrene that damage nuclear DNA have a much greater affinity for mitochondrial DNA. Recent studies, however, indicate that enhanced glycolysis is related to overproduction of inorganic phosphorus due to a high rate of ATP hydrolysis. In the early reaction of glycolysis, P_i is required to phosphorylate glucose to glucose-6-phosphate. The source of P_i is ATP hydrolysis; thus any system that needs the energy-requiring reaction $ATP \rightarrow ADP + P_i$, if markedly excessive, may stimulate glycolysis.

Abnormal enzymes on the cell surface may promote glycolysis.

The ATPase that operates as a sodium pump (Na-K-dependent ATPase) is inefficient in some tumor cells; several additional ATPs are required to pump out one Na^+. This produces an unusually large amount of ADP and inorganic phosphorus that could then stimulate glycolysis. Tumor ATPase may be abnormal because it is phosphorylated excessively by an abnormal protein kinase also found in tumor cells.

FOCUS

Melanoma

Tumors of melanin-synthesizing cells occur through all vertebrate species and have been reported in amphibians, reptiles, fish, and birds. The term *melanoma* often denotes malignancy ("carcinoma" and "sarcoma" are avoided because of the uncertainty concerning the derivation of the tumor cell). Malignant melanomas are vicious and capricious neoplasms.

Melanomas are common in dogs, where they occur in the oral cavity, skin, and the ciliary body and choroid of the eye. Pigmented breeds are especially affected; there is an increased incidence in the black cocker spaniel, Airedale, and Boston and Scottish terriers. Nonpigmented melanomas, called amelanotic melanomas, are common in the oral cavity of dogs. Cell type is determined by the content of tyrosinase. Tyrosinase oxidizes dihydrophenylalanine (dopa), which is added to the tissue section as part of the histochemical test (called the *dopa reaction*).

In horses, depigmented gray individuals are affected, especially the aged Percheron, which turns gray and white with age (although the skin remains black); melanomas are rare in horses of other pigmentations. About 80% of aged gray horses developed malignant melanomas, the most common location being the perianal region. It is theorized that there is failure of melanin synthesis, and the progressive loss of pigmentation stimulates melanoblastic activity associated with neoplastic transformation.

Why normal melanocytes become neoplastic is not known although in man there is a correlation of dermal injury such as sunburn with the incidence of malignant melanoma. Recently, a soluble growth factor has been identified in cultures of malignant melanomas grown in vitro that causes normal melanocytes to proliferate.

Transplantable melanomas have been widely studied as models. Mouse melanoma S91 arose from the tail of a mouse at the Jackson laboratory. It is strain-specific, and subcutaneous implants kill the host within 12 weeks, after metastasizing to the lungs and other viscera. S91 produces large amounts of melanin via the tyrosinase–dopa oxidase enzyme complex, and tumor cells are filled with melanosomes. An amelanotic variety arises when the tumor is implanted into albino mice. Cells of this neoplasm do not produce tyrosine or dopa oxidase and have few pigment granules.

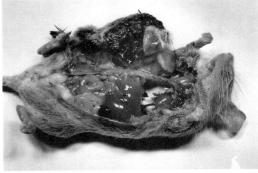

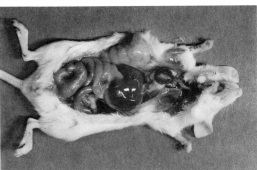

Melanomas of the swordtail platyfish are controlled by genes. Wild platyfish (*Xiphophorus* spp.) occur in different color patterns, depending on the distribution of macromelanophores in skin. Normal fish carry a macromelanophore gene, S_d, that is responsible for melanophore differentiation. In tumors, differentiation is blocked by abnormal genes. By combining appropriate hereditary patterns, melanotic or amelanotic tumors can be produced. Unpigmented fish that develop "albino" or amelanotic melanomas are killed by rapidly growing, undifferentiated tumors. The albino gene acts by inhibiting tyrosinase activity.

TUMOR SUPPORT TISSUES

Basement membranes

Neoplasms modify the interstitial ground substance in which they grow by (1) the synthesis of matrix components directly by the neoplastic cell, (2) increasing the synthesis of matrix by adjacent host mesenchymal cells, and (3) degrading the matrix components during invasion. In any malignant tumor, all three may take place in different regions of the tumor or one of these types may dominate.

Proteoglycans induce cell differentiation.

Proteoglycans and their constituent glycosaminoglycans influence cytodifferentiation in neoplasia just as they do in normal development. They induce both proliferation and migration of cells by forming structural links between cell and interstitial components. A role of chondroitin sulfate as a growth regulator is suggested by its stimulation of tumor growth experimentally; chemical analysis of human colonic carcinomas have shown a 12-fold increase in chondroitin sulfates compared with control tissue. The source of the sulfated proteoglycan was the host fibroblast adjacent to the tumor cells.

Collagen and basement membrane material are released by tumors.

These materials usually have normal molecular structure but fail to polymerize or aggregate properly once outside the cell. Well-differentiated tumors tend to produce more of these extracellular proteins than do highly anaplastic tumors.

Vascularity

The growth of a neoplasm is dependent on concomitant growth of a supporting vascular system. The probability of a neoplastic cell entering mitosis decreases with increasing distance of the cell from its nearest capillary. In the mouse mammary tumor, for example, the turnover time of endothelial cell populations lags behind that of the tumor cells. As the tumor expands, neoplastic cell proliferation is diminished, which is reflected in slowed growth in tumor size. When tumor cells are implanted into susceptible hosts experimentally, they grow to a diameter of a few millimeters and then lie dormant unless vascularization takes place.

Capillaries in neoplasms are abnormal.

New capillary growth within neoplasms is often more vigorous than capillary bud formation in the repair phase of inflammation. Endothelial cells are kinky and enlarged and have extensive contortions and surface projections of the luminal plasma membrane. In most cases, the blood vessels are not neoplastic (although true neoplasms of vascular tissue do occur) but are a host response induced in some way by the tumor itself. Tumor vascular systems are never normal, however, and the supply of oxygen, glucose, and other nutrients to the tumor is usually less efficient than in normal tissue.

The vascular pattern reflects tumor histology, not the tissue of origin. It can be revealed by perfusion with radioopaque substances and radiographic examination. By this method, tumor blood vessels are shown to be haphazard networks with a predisposition to form capillaries from arterial vessels of all sizes.

Tumor cells and blood vessels are interdependent.

In many cases, populations of neoplastic cells and host endothelial cells constitute an integrated system. The mitotic indices of one population depend on the other. Tumor cells stimulate endothelial cell proliferation, and vascularization has an indirect effect on tumor growth.

Diffusible soluble substances are released from tumor cells that act on host endothelium. New capillary buds are induced even when tumor implants are enclosed in filter chambers. Induction of DNA synthesis in resting endothelial cells of capillaries and venules can be demonstrated within a few millimeters of an implanted tumor. Mast cells accumulate at sites of tumor formation. They release the anticoagulant *heparin,* which can increase the migration of endothelial cells toward tumors.

Tumor angiogenesis factor is secreted by neoplastic cells.

This soluble factor, which has been extracted from animal neoplasms, is mitogenic for capillary endothelium (it is assayed in artificial subcutaneous air sacs in rats or in rabbit corneas). It is possible that growth of solid tumor might be deliberately arrested by blockade of angiogenesis factor and prevention of vascularization. Glucocorticoid hormones interfere with vascularization of tumors, and other hormones probably delay or facilitate tumor vascularity.

Necrosis occurs when tumors outgrow the vascular supply.

In highly malignant tumors, cell growth extends beyond that of the supporting vasculature, which causes *ischemic necrosis. Hemorrhage* and *calcification* are common in these foci. Necrosis may be accompanied by some decrease in tumor size, but the rapidly dividing malignant cells soon make up the loss.

Fibroplasia
Benign tumors often have a fibrous capsule at the periphery.

Many benign tumors contain a capsule derived in part from the fibrous stroma of the surrounding normal connective tissue and in part from the tumor itself (malignant tumors are almost never encapsulated). Encapsulation tends to contain the neoplasm as a discrete, palpable mass that can easily be removed by surgery. (Although a capsule is a characteristic of a benign neoplasm, lack of a capsule does not make a neoplasm malignant.)

Some tumors provoke fibrous proliferation within the tumor mass.

Fibroblast proliferation and deposition of collagen are the main components of fibromas and fibrosarcomas and are primarily involved in some of the rarer fibrous tumors such as fibrous histiocytomas. Marked fiber deposition also occurs in some epithelial tumors. These tumors are called *sclerosing* or "scirrhous" and are usually very firm and pale (Fig. 10.8). Some of these tumors secrete factors that stimulate fibroplasia. It may be that some lack the colla-

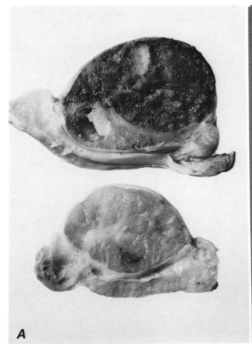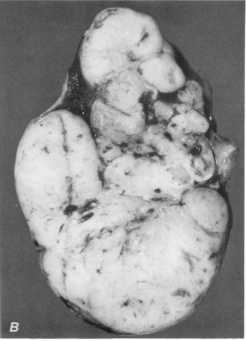

Fig. 10.8. Testicular tumors in the dog. A. Interstitial cell tumor. The tumor is the large, dark, bean-shaped area (*top*). Testis (*bottom*) is unaffected. Marked vascularity makes this tumor dark red instead of the tan/yellow usually seen in the interstitial cell tumor. B. Sertoli cell tumor: massive deposition of collagen makes this tumor very hard; it is termed "scirrhous" or "sclerosing."

genases and elastases that other tumors are known to secrete and that the scirrhous nature of the mass represent a host response that is repressed by collagenase in other tumors.

ADDITIONAL READING

Bostock, D. E. Prognosis after surgical excision of canine melanoma. *Vet. Pathol.* 16:32, 1979.

Croce, C. M., et al. Chromosome translocations and B cell neoplasia. *Lab. Invest.* 51:258, 1984.

Farber, E., and Sarma, D. Hepatocarcinogenesis. *Lab. Invest.* 56:1, 1987.

Folkman, J., et al. Angiogenesis inhibition tumor regression caused by heparin and a heparin fragment in the presence of cortisone. *Science* 221:719, 1983.

Grindem, C. B., et al. Cytochemical reactions in cells from leukemic dogs. *Vet. Pathol.* 23:103, 1986.

Iozzo, R. V. Proteoglycans: Structure, function, and role in neoplasia. *Lab. Invest.* 53:373, 1985.

Liotta, L. A., and Barsky, S. H. Tumor invasion and the extracellular matrix. *Lab. Invest.* 49:636, 1983.

Misdorp, W. Tumors in newborn animals. *Vet. Pathol.* 2:328, 1968.

Nowell, P. C., and Croce, C. M. Chromosomes, genes, and cancer. *Am. J. Pathol.* 125:8, 1986.

Russo, J., and Russo, I. H. Biological and molecular bases of mammary carcingogenesis. *Lab. Invest.* 57:112, 1987.

Schomber, G. J., et al. Neoplasms in calves (*Bos taurus*). *Vet. Pathol.* 19:629, 1982.

Squire, R. A., and Levitt, M. H. Report of a workshop on classification of specific hepatocellular lesions in rats. *Cancer Res.* 35:3214, 1975.

11

Clinicopathologic Effects of Neoplasia

LOCAL EFFECTS OF NEOPLASMS

Malignant neoplasms kill the host through a variety of effects. As neoplasms expand, they exert pressure on surrounding normal tissues to cause pain, interruption of vascular supplies and lymphatic blockade. Lumens and ductal systems may be obstructed. The squamous cell carcinoma in Fig. 10.5 caused dyspnea and hypoxia by obstructing the pharynx, diminished saliva production due to infiltration into the salivary gland, and anorexia from pain in muscles of mastication. Ductal systems and lumens of the lungs, intestines, and brain are especially susceptible to obstruction, usually with dire consequences. Obstructions of the urinary tract and biliary ducts are also important causes of death in neoplastic disease. Large tumors of the limbs may prevent foraging and cause inanition.

In the absence of overt causes of death, animals with cancer still progressively lose weight and die. Often, the mass of the neoplasm cannot fully explain death in mechanical terms; one must then turn to more subtle mechanisms that play major roles in killing the cancer patient.

SYSTEMIC EFFECTS OF NEOPLASMS

Cachexia

In terminal stages of neoplastic disease, animals develop anorexia (loss of appetite), lose weight, and become lethargic. Cachexia is due in part to anorexia brought on by depression of appetite centers in the brain. Many tumor-bearing animals are anorectic yet have tumors too small to directly affect appetite. Experimen-tally, when tumors are produced in one partner of a parabiotic pair of rats, both rats will show anorexia and weight loss. It is probable that some unknown humoral factor is released by the tumor that influences the hypothalamus.

Cytokines mobilize fat cell triglycerides.

Not all weight loss in cancer patients is due to anorexia. Some loss is associated with humoral factors secreted by tumor cells or by macrophages (indirectly affected by the neoplasm). Mobilization of triglycerides in adipocytes is associated with *cachectin,* a cytokine produced by activated macrophages. Cachectin causes decreased synthesis of lipogenic enzymes in adipocytes by suppressing a gene for enzymes that catalyze fat deposition.

Neoplastic cells act as an amino acid trap.

By virtue of tumor cell enzymes, neoplastic cells can irreversibly drain the host of essential amino acids. Skeletal muscles of animals with widespread metastatic cancer are thus in double jeopardy. They become atrophic, partially through the *disuse of lethargy* but also because of *metabolic defectiveness.* Spotty dropout of muscle fibers and degeneration of nerve branches occur. Later, muscle cells develop decreases in glucose uptake, insulin sensitivity, and activities of enzymes for energy production. The diminished glucose assimilation compounds the amino acid drain by the tumor mass.

The liver, pancreas, and other organs also regress in terminal cancer. Hepatocytes become small and their enzymatic composition more undifferentiated so that they resemble immature hepatocytes. Enzymes highly concentrated in fetal liver are the ones whose amounts increase (e.g., thymidine kinase and hexokinase).

Hypoglycemia

Hypoglycemia (blood glucose <70 mg/dl) is characteristic of tumors of the pancreatic islet cells (which produce insulin). Hypoglycemia also has been reported to occur in animals bearing various epithelial, mesenchymal, and hematopoietic neoplasms. In dogs, hepatic tumors are most often responsible, although hemangiosarcomas, melanomas, and salivary gland tumors have been accompanied by low blood sugar.

This type of hypoglycemia commonly occurs in the late stages of disseminated neoplasia but also can occur early as part of the initial clinical syndrome. Clinical signs of hypoglycemia are related directly to neuroglucopenic and adrenergic effects and include restlessness, weakness, tremors, and episodes of collapse and seizures.

Anemia

Anemia is common in metastatic neoplastic disease and is often responsible for a significant part of the clinical illness of the terminally ill patient. Major causes of anemia in cancer are (1) *hemorrhage* from erosion of normal tissues by the invading tumor (a common cause of death); (2) *decreased erythropoiesis* from invasion of bone marrow by the tumor and destruction of erythropoietic tissue; and (3) *erythrocyte fragmentation* as these cells pass through abnormal blood vessels of the tumor.

Highly vascular tumors are most likely to cause anemia by destruction of erythrocytes. In hemangiosarcomas of dogs, an *erythrocyte fragmentation syndrome* arises from "microangiopathic" hemolytic anemia. Fibrin erodes erythroctye surfaces, and the acantholytic erythroctyes are then sequestered in vascular spaces of the tumor.

Other contributing causes of anemia in cancerous animals may be (1) activation of the reticuloendothelial system with "hypersplenism," which excessively removes erythrocytes from circulation; (2) subtle iron-deficiency anemia associated with inflammatory disease in the cancer patient; (3) nonregenerative anemia associated with anticancer chemotherapy; (4) autoimmune anemia, which may develop in association with lymphoproliferative neoplasms; and (5) suppression of erythropoietin synthesis by the kidney.

In contrast to the suppression of erythrocyte production, tumor cells may produce *polycythemia* by secreting erythropoietin, although this has been reported only in human renal neoplasms.

Coagulation defects
Thrombocytopenia is common in viral leukemias.

Thrombocyte production is diminished in the viral leukemias and lymphoproliferative syndromes as a result of bone marrow suppression. In rare cases, thrombocytopenia may have an autoimmune basis.

Abnormalities of platelet utilization are also common in neoplastic disease. Platelet survival is reduced in nearly 40% of all dogs bearing local tumors and in 80% of dogs with metastatic tumors. Fibrinogen concentrations are increased in most of these dogs.

Thrombosis occurs in large tumors.

Local thrombosis in solid tumors arises from the combined effects of tumor-induced platelet adhesions and aggregation, release of procoagulant materials by the neoplastic cells, and incomplete endothelialization of tumor capillaries. Tumors that release large amounts of procoagulants may cause *disseminated intravascular coagulation,* with death due to thrombotic obstruction of renal glomeruli.

Any increase in viscosity of the blood tends to promote thrombosis. Cells of the plasmacytoma (multiple myeloma) secrete globulins causing *hyperglobulinemia.* In dogs the clinical features are a monoclonal immunoglobulin spike in serum, lytic bone lesions (sometimes with hypercalcemia), and fragments of globulin chains (Bence-Jones proteins) in urine. This all leads to a "stasis syndrome" in which thrombosis is promoted.

Hypercalcemia

Hypercalcemia is a complication in many cancers and lethal in some. It may arise by two mechanisms: (1) *osteolytic metastases* of solid tumors with excessive bone resorption and calcium release or (2) *tumor cell secretion* of peptides that mimic parathyroid hormone. Although osteolytic metastases may stimulate bone resorption and release of calcium that exceeds homeostatic capacity, this mechanism rarely produces serious disease. In contrast, tumors producing humoral factors that stimulate osteoclasts or parathyroidlike responses often produce serious complications.

Pseudohyperparathyroidism

This disorder results from secretion of peptides with parathyroid hormone activity. There is persistent hypercalcemia and hyperphosphatemia, hyperplasia of thyroid C cells, and atrophy of parathyroids (in response to hypercalcemia). Radiographically, only mild skeletal demineralization occurs, in contrast to severe bone changes in primary and secondary hyperparathyroidism of renal or nutritional origin. Diagnosis requires that there be no parathyroid tumor (or other parathyroid lesions) or bone metastases of other tumors.

Pseudohyperparathyroidism occurs in dogs and cats and has been associated with mammary gland carcinomas, fibrosarcomas, lymphosarcomas, and various adenocarcinomas. Gastric carcinomas in horses commonly induce this syndrome.

Pseudohyperparathyroidism is associated with adenocarcinomas arising from the anal sac apocrine glands in dogs. Dr. Donald Meuten, then at Ohio State University, studied 30 cases and showed that they occurred predominantly in aged females. The tumors develop as masses in the perirectal area ventrolateral to the anus and in close association with the anal sac (they are distinct from the more common perianal gland tumor).

Ectopic hormone syndromes

Nearly all cancer cells synthesize proteins, which are released into tissue spaces. When peptides are secreted with biologically active fragments that mimic hormones or neuropeptides, syndromes of clinical importance appear. Neuropeptides such as vasopressin are commonly involved. These peptides are synthesized as large chains bearing several hormone segments that must by cleaved away before release and activation. Similarly, tumor peptides may be large and abnormal and yet contain fragments resembling normal hormones closely enough to stimulate their target tissues.

At least 21 hormones or their precursors have been identified in human neoplasms. These vary from pituitary tumors that secrete ACTH to renal juxtaglomerular tumors that secrete renin.

In the latter, increased renin in plasma leads to hypertension, hyperkalemia, and hyperaldosteronism. Small cell carcinomas of human lungs have been shown to secrete the neuropeptide bombesin, which in turn releases an array of gastrointestinal hormones.

Zollinger-Ellison syndrome

This syndrome is associated with non-β cell tumors of the pancreas. Tumor cells secrete a polypeptide with activity similar to *gastrin,* which is normally secreted by "gastrin cells" of the gastric antrum and duodenal mucosae. Clinical signs involve diarrhea, vomiting, weight loss, hypersecretion of gastric acid, and hypergastrinemia.

These tumors have been studied by Dr. Ingrid van der Gaag, at the University of Utrecht, who has shown that the spectrum of changes includes ulcers in the stomach and esophagus, enteritis with villous atrophy, hypertrophy of gastric mucosa, and proliferation of C cells in the thyroid. Most canine tumors are malignant, and metastases are found in regional lymph nodes and in liver.

Diarrhea

Prolonged diarrhea unresponsive to routine therapy and not associated with known microbial causes may occur in disseminated neoplasia. First, intestinal bacterial and protozoal infections are associated with terminal cancer, particularly during immunosuppressive treatment. Second, primary tumors of the intestine may be accompanied by diarrhea, although this is unusual. Even rarer is a syndrome of diarrhea that accompanies some neurogenic tumors. Secretion of *vasoactive intestinal peptides* by the tumor cells are diarrheogenic and lead to a life-threatening loss of fluids and electrolytes.

Fever

Some tumor cells release pyrogens, and tumor-induced fever has been viewed as a natural antineoplastic mechanism. Fever is indeed common in patients with advanced metastatic neoplasms, but in most cases it is likely to result from complicating inflammatory or bacterial disease rather than a humoral factor of tumor origin.

SPREAD OF NEOPLASMS

Neoplastic cells spread within an animal by four basic mechanisms: (1) *invasiveness,* the growth though tissue planes; (2) *implantation on new surfaces,* particularly serosa; (3) *dissemination through the vascular system* by eroding veins or, in rare cases, arteries (Fig. 11.1); and (4) *dissemination through lymphatic vessels and lymph nodes.*

Invasiveness

The capacity to invade host tissue is an intrinsic property of the neoplastic cell. Extension of pseudopodia below basement membranes and between connective tissue planes involves changes in the cell surface. Some of these changes relate to increased negative charges, decreased calcium content, and uncontrolled cytoskeletal movements. More important, enzymes and soluble factors secreted at the tumor cell surface enable the tumor cell to dissect its way through normal tissues.

Some neoplasms release connective tissue–degrading enzymes.

Carcinomas invade tissues by elaborating enzymes that degrade connective tissue or by producing factors that cause the host cell to release proteolytic enzymes. Some basal cell carcinomas are directly *collagenolytic,* (that is, they produce a *collagenase* that degrades dermal collagen). Most tumors, however, invade without producing collagenase. Some release factors that stimulate host cells to release connective

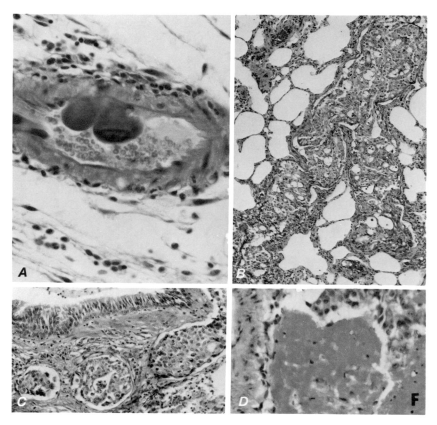

Fig. 11.1. Metastases. A. Metastatic carcinoma cells attached to arterial wall. B. Large collections of neoplastic cells in pulmonary veins, lung, canine mammary gland adenocarcinoma. C. Infiltration and growth of tumor cells in peribronchial lymphatics. D. Collections of carcinoma cells in pulmonary artery enmeshed in fibrin (*F*).

tissues degrading enzymes. Experiments with a squamous cell carcinoma in rabbits indicate that cathepsin B (a cysteine proteinase that degrades both collagen and proteoglycans) is stimulated in host fibroblasts and neutrophils by a humoral factor released from the neoplastic cell.

Lysosomal enzymes from neoplastic cells can kill host cells.

Lysosomal enzymes, secreted into connective tissues by neoplastic cells, often enhance invasiveness by killing host cells. Release of lysosomal hydrolases has been shown to be correlated with highly invasive mammary gland adenocarcinomas. The increased capacity of a transplantable melanoma of mice to metastasize has also been shown to be related to lysosomal enzymes of the tumor cell. Contact of the tumor cell with the normal cells may result in release of lysosomal enzymes and killing of the host cell. In some cases there is lysis of the tumor cell with liberation of a massive amount of lysosomal enzymes.

Metastasis

Metastasis is the hallmark of malignant neoplasms. All neoplasms that metastasize are malignant, although not all malignant neoplasms metastasize. Highly malignant tumor cells have relatively little tendency to adhere to one another and may be washed by lymph from the tissue spaces and enter the thoracic duct. Neoplastic cells may also directly erode vascular walls (Fig. 11.1).

Most cancer cells that enter the bloodstream die without initiating new metastatic foci. In a highly malignant tumor, however, enormous numbers of cells separate from the primary tumor and are swept into the blood and lymph vessels. Factors that influence whether tumor cells initiate new growths at sites distant from the primary tumor include (1) the way in which metastasis occurs (whether from single cells or from tumor emboli), (2) the intrinsic capacity of the malignant cell to lodge in and attach to host endothelial cells, and (3) the tissue environment at localization sites.

Systemic changes in the host that have been shown experimentally to enhance metastases include physical stress, extensive surgery, and halothane anesthesia. Tissue damage in an organ vulnerable to metastases may increase the deposition of tumor emboli. Treatment with the antineoplastic drug cyclophosphamide (which

may have an overriding beneficial effect) has also been shown actually to increase metastatic lesions in some tumors. Drs. Owen and Bostock, working in England, have shown that irradiation of the lungs of dogs with osteocarcinomas increases the incidence of lung metastases.

Tumor cells at metastatic sites usually resemble the cells of the primary tumor, although this is not always true. The remarkable variation that sometimes occurs may be due to formation of new clones of tumor cells.

Regional lymph nodes trap most malignant cells.

Lymphatic drainage to regional lymph nodes provides a common pathway for metastatic spread of many carcinomas. Adenocarcinoma metastases of the posterior mammary gland tend to be found in the inguinal lymph nodes; tumors in the anterior mammary gland drain anteriorly (Fig. 11.2). Spread via lymphatics should not be equated with vascular metastasis, for its result in the animals is not the same.

While most metastasizing tumor cells pass from lymphatic vessel to bloodstream, the reverse also occurs. Studies with radioactively labeled carcinoma cells injected intravenously in rats show that within 1 hour tumor cells can be recovered from lymph. Thus cells not trapped in the first capillary bed through which they pass may escape into the lymphatic system, probably in lymph nodes.

Lungs trap most neoplastic cells.

The distribution of tumor foci is determined largely by the anatomic characteristics of veins and lymphatic vessels draining the primary tumor site. In animals, most malignant tumors ultimately metastasize to the lung. In Misdorp's collection of 56 canine mammary gland carcinomas, the metastatic foci were 86% to lymph nodes, 72% to lungs, and 10–12% each to adrenals, kidney, liver, and bone.

Lung metastases occur because of the immense flow of blood through this organ and its large network of capillaries, through which circulation is slowed. The pulmonary capillary bed serves as a filter for aggregates of tumor cells that lodge in the vascular tree, insert pseudopodia between endothelial cells, and emigrate into the lung parenchyma. Lung metastases tend to have a peripheral distribution around bronchioles (Fig. 11.3).

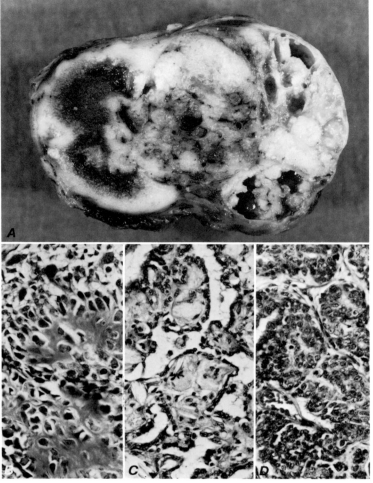

Fig. 11.2. Metastases to regional lymph node (superficial inguinal), dog with malignant mixed mammary gland tumor. A. Cross section of lymph node with areas that correspond to histology in B–D. B. Bony. C. Cystic. D. Solid.

Liver traps tumor cells circulating in the portal vein and hepatic artery.

The liver is highly vulnerable to metastases, particularly by carcinomas arising in tissues drained by the portal venous system. Most tumors, however, seed via the hepatic artery (often from secondary tumors lodged in the lungs). Diffuse lymphomatosis occurs in the liver of all species. In dogs, splenic hemangiosarcomas may be massively distributed throughout the liver.

Other organs where metastases are common include kidney and brain. Skin may be affected by carcinomas that enter the lymphatic system and creep along the subcutaneous lymphatics (Fig. 11.4).

The pathogenesis of metastases

Malignant tumors, as they expand, probably release cells into lymph or blood continuously. After murine mammary gland tumors reach a few grams, they release several million cells daily into the circulation. The overwhelming majority of these die very quickly; only a few survive the hostile nature of the bloodstream. Studies in which radioactively labeled mouse

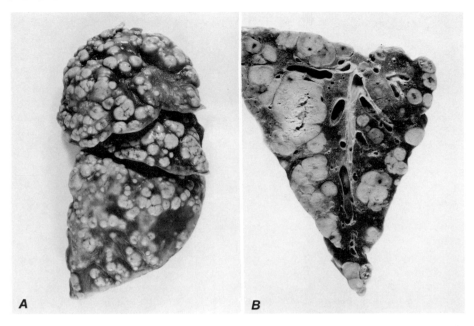

Fig. 11.3. Metastases to lung, dog with hepatocellular carcinoma. A. Large solid metastases in all lobes. B. Cut surface, caudal lobe. Metastases are within lung surface areas, and a few are around bronchioles.

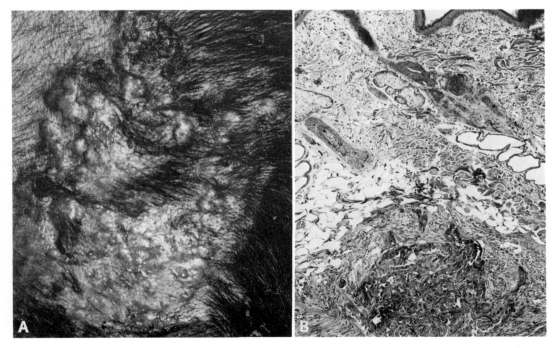

Fig. 11.4. Metastases to skin, dog with mammary gland adenocarcinoma. A. Massive nodular areas on abdominal skin. B. Small tumor mass in subcutis.

melanoma cells were injected intravenously showed that within minutes most cells were trapped in the lung. Only 1% remained alive after 1 day, and after 2 weeks, when metastatic lesions could be seen grossly, only 0.1% of the original cells were still alive.

Survival in the bloodstream is enhanced by several conditions. Clumps of tumor cells have a greater tendency to form metastases than do single cells. Thus tumor cells that adhere to each other by surface secretions are more dangerous. Furthermore, the larger the tumor cell clump, the more likely it is to be trapped in capillaries to form a new colony.

Some metastatic cells secrete procoagulant factors.

Neoplastic cell procoagulant factors may cause fibrinogen to polymerize on the tumor cell embolus. Some cancer cells activate clotting systems by shedding plasma membrane vesicles that carry procoagulant activity. The mesh of fibrin tends to protect the malignant cells from destruction, enabling them to proliferate.

Fibrin can clearly be seen histologically in tumor emboli, but it is quickly denatured by the fibrinolytic system and disappears during late stages of embolization. Some types of malignant cells in culture show increased production of *plasminogen activators,* which enhance the effectiveness of the fibrinolytic system. While this prevents the growth-promoting stabilizing effects of fibrin during metastasis and invasion, fibrinolysis enhances tumor growth in tissue once the metastatic focus is established.

Circulating cancer cells interact with platelets.

Some tumor cells contain surface materials that cause them to attach to platelets and to induce platelet aggregation. This interaction enhances the ability of tumor cells to adhere to vascular endothelium and to lodge in capillaries. The use of anticoagulant and antiplatelet therapy to reduce metastases of natural tumors has given inconclusive results. However, in studies with experimental murine melanoma B16, prostacyclin remarkably decreased the number of metastases to lungs, presumably through its potent inhibiting effect on platelet aggregation.

Once trapped in venules and capillaries, malignant cells adhere to endothelium and cause striking changes in adhesion of endothelial cells to their underlying matrix. Endothelial cells retract, leaving spaces through which the tumor cells can migrate into tissue (see Fig. 12.3). Once in the interstitium, the cell must induce alterations that promote further survival and replication. Again, fibrin deposited around the neoplastic cells provides a matrix for further development. Within tissue, tumor cells probably respond to chemotactic factors, but the role of these soluble substances in metastasis is not clear.

Metastasizing tumor cells are heterogeneous.

Metastatic foci are often composed of differing populations of cells. The mixed mammary gland tumor of dogs clearly contains both glandular and connective tissue components, and its metastases may be segregated in the draining lymph node (Fig. 11.2). The metastatic tumors include solid epithelial, cystic, and cartilagenous forms. Even tumors that at first examination by histology appear to be uniform are often composed of different cell types. Adenocarcinomas of the intestine may contain subtle mixtures of mucus and endocrine cells.

Metastatic cells are endowed with special characteristics for survival.

To survive in new tissue environments, the metastatic cell has probably developed new strategies. The B16 melanoma, which arose in a strain of black mice, is transplantable and will produce pigmented metastases in the lungs of recipient mice, with occasional tumor foci in ovaries, liver, and brain. After 10 cycles of experimental selection of cells from lung metastases, a variant malignant cell line was established with special affinity for lungs.

These adapted melanoma cells actually seek lung tissue. When injected into the tail vein, they are first trapped in lungs. When injected downstream from the lung, they may be trapped in other peripheral tissues but then detach and recirculate until they find the more desirable lung environment for growth. Specificity is shown more clearly when it is seen that the lung-prone variant is less likely to metastasize to brain or ovary. Furthermore, other variant lines have been established that prefer brain or ovary rather than lung. The reason for preferences resides in the plasma membrane. Each of the three variant lines shows different patterns of specific surface proteins. These tumor lines, like natural tumors, shed bits of plasma membrane–bound cytoplasm into the environment. When these tiny vesicles are harvested, purified, and transferred from the "lung line" to the "brain line," the preference of the treated cells is altered away from the brain.

Implantation

Because of their lack of cohesiveness, tumor cells growing on epithelial surfaces are prone to be shed into the surrounding spaces. Exfoliation of cells into fluids of the body cavities and respiratory and urogenital tracts is the basis for the cytologic examination of these fluids for cancer cells. Unfortunately, it is also the basis for massive implantation of cells and development of immense numbers of tumor cells on serosal surfaces.

This pattern of growth, called carcinomatosis, is characteristic of some glandular tumors. For example, pancreatic adenocarcinomas may seed through the peritoneal cavity to grow along the peritoneum; these lesions are referred to as *peritoneal carcinomatosis*. When the cavity is opened, massive growth of neoplastic cells may present the misleading appearance of an acute fibrinous peritonitis or, if in the pleural cavity, of pleuritis (Fig. 11.5). Tumor cell localization on the peritoneal membranes is enhanced when serosal surfaces are injured. Tumor cells adhere on exposed collagen fibrils and grow more rapidly. Peritoneal lymph drainage is blocked in carcinomatosis, and ascites is common.

Transplantation of neoplastic cells from contaminated surgical instruments and gloves is a significant potential hazard during cancer surgery. Although rarely reported in animal neoplasms, this is a well-documented sequel to cancer surgery in man.

RESTRAINT OF NEOPLASMS

Some malignant neoplasms grow rapidly from day to day, with death occurring in a few weeks. Conversely, some animals with cancer survive several years. These instances are extremes, and both are rare. It is usual for an animal with a malignant neoplasm to survive from 6 months to a year after the lesion is manifest as clinical illness. Many factors interact in the restraint of cancer. In addition to intrinsic properties of the tumor (cellular characters, vascular arrange-

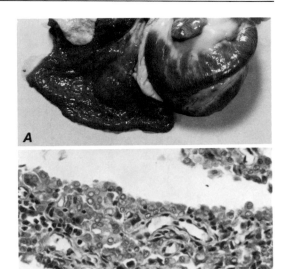

Fig. 11.5. Carcinomatosis: implantation of malignant cells (aortic body carcinoma) onto serosal surface, mediastinum. A. Neoplastic cells on mediastinal pleura (*bottom left*). Marked dilatation of right ventricle. B. Fronds of tumor composed of vascular and connective tissue supports on which tumor cells proliferate. Infiltration of lymphoid cells.

ment, and secretory properties), there are factors such as nutrition, endocrinologic status, and immunoreactivity that can be altered in the host.

Nonspecific lysis and phagocytosis

In most tumors, malignant cells are continuously removed by neutrophils and macrophages. The advancing edge of the expanding squamous cell carcinoma in Fig. 10.5 is surrounded by a zone of fibrovascular reactive tissue that contains monocytes and neutrophils. It is clear that these cells have not controlled the tumor and were probably functioning only to remove cells dying because of rapid growth in an environment of limited nourishment. In tumors of less malignancy, however, invading inflammatory cells may prove to be beneficial by inhibiting tumor expansion.

In vitro studies have shown that both macrophages and neutrophils are toxic to and can destroy tumor cells. On contact, macrophages insert cytoplasmic processes into the tumor cells and transfer lysosomal enzymes into the cytoplasm. Cancer cells have decreased peroxide catabolizing pathways (e.g., catalase and glutathione), which makes them highly susceptible to oxidative injury by macrophages.

Do neutrophils enhance tumor growth?

Although theoretical beneficial effects of neutrophils in killing cells in established tumors have been suggested, neutrophils clearly do not play a major role within the animal. Neutrophil enzymes may actually promote carcinogenesis in chronic inflammatory lesions. *Reactive oxygen metabolites* produced by the neutrophil's "respiratory burst" have proven to be mutagenic and may act to promote growth of a tumor.

Normal cell mechanisms against oxidation are important in preventing chemical carcinogenesis (e.g., rats given aflatoxin doses that induced hepatocellular carcinomas in 100% of cases, when treated with reduced glutathione, a harmless natural antioxidant, developed only irregular hepatic lobules). Liver cells had increased amounts of smooth endoplasmic reticulum, which synthesizes cytochrome-dependent monoxygenases known to be involved in detoxification of aflatoxin.

Nonspecific macrophage activity may inhibit tumor growth.

For a century, it has been suspected that natural tumors are suppressed by intercurrent inflammation, especially in lymph nodes and other reticuloendothelial tissues (Fig. 11.6). In the late 1800s William Coley, a New York surgeon, developed mixed bacterial "vaccines" that produced fever and chills and induced substantial regression of tumors in a few human patients. "Coley's toxins" acted as an immunopotentiator to enhance an otherwise inadequate host response. Experiments in this era showed that filtrates of gram-negative bacterial cultures produced striking hemorrhage and necrosis in experimental tumors.

Long overshadowed by other methods of treatment, new variants of this type of therapy are now used in hope that spread of tumors will by inhibited by stimulating macrophages nonspecifically. *Corynebacterium parvum* and an avirulent tubercle bacillus (bacillus Calmette-Guerin, BCG) are potent immunizing agents that are used as nonspecific adjuvants to stimulate the reticuloendothelial system. In some animal tumor models, macrophages so stimulated aggressively attack and cause degeneration of target tumor cells. Cows with ocular squamous cell carcinoma treated by intratumor injection of BCG vaccines had 71% regression; the untreated controls all developed progressive tumor growth with lymph node metastases. This treatment activates macrophages to delete susceptible and aged tumor cells and also potentiates tumor-specific immunity. Macrophages are intimately associated with specific lymphoid mechanisms of tumor immunity; their effect is to enhance the production of antitumor antibodies and lymphocytes. Unfortunately, macrophage function is depressed in the early phases of rapid tumor growth in natural neoplastic disease, possibly by some factor released by the tumor. BCG vaccine is now being used in human leukemias and melanomas but is credited with only limited success.

Even in most rodent models, malignant tumors progress unchecked despite their content of macrophages. It is probable that the lack of specificity in this form of cytotoxicity prevents macrophages from being effective. Dr. Stephen Russell, then at Scripps Research Institute, showed that monocytes recovered from regressing sarcomas in mice are cytolytic but, unlike T lymphocytes in similar studies, act to kill cells without antigenic specificity.

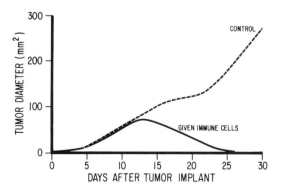

Fig. 11.6. Growth of experimental tumor in normal control mice and in mice given lymphoid cells taken from a mouse bearing a similar tumor. (Data from Reichert et al., *Lab. Invest.* 52:304, 1985)

Macrophages release antitumor soluble factors.

Activated macrophages release several soluble factors, some of which have been shown to produce antitumor activity experimentally

(Table 11.1). *Tumor necrosis factor* (TNF) is the prototype of a new family of antitumor factors. Secreted by macrophages, TNF causes necrosis in tumors by killing neoplastic cells. To be active, TNF activity requires a priming event to cause activation and proliferation of macrophages (such as *C. parvum* vaccine) and a second eliciting event, usually involving endotoxin or its purer form, a lipopolysaccharide from gram-negative bacteria. TNF has striking effects on subcutaneous tumor transplants in rodents but has not (to date) proven clinically useful.

Tumor immunology

The aberrant "precancerous" cell in transition to the neoplastic state undergoes biochemical changes that distinguish it from normal cells of the host. It often develops new proteins in its surface membranes that function as *tumor antigens* to distinguish the neoplastic cells from normal cells. These tumor antigens can evoke both antitumor antibodies and lymphocytes; specific, lymphocyte-mediated mechanisms may inhibit tumor growth.

Despite these exciting facts, hopes of effective tumor immunosuppression are clouded by the capricious and elusive nature of immune mechanisms against tumors and the difficulty of making them operable in living animals.

Tumor antigens

Naturally occurring animal tumor cells have specific antigens on their cell surfaces that are detectable by serologic tests (using appropriate antibodies). The *cytotoxicity test* is a highly sensitive assay; cells bearing a particular antigen are killed when incubated with antibodies specific to that antigen in the presence of complement.

Antigens used in diagnosis and analysis of tumors are of several types: *Fetal antigens* may reappear in the host when genes controlling their production are reactivated in dedifferentiated tumor cells. *Alpha-fetoprotein* is produced in the liver during fetal life but falls to undetect-

able amounts shortly after birth as its controlling genes are inactivated. As a consequence of neoplastic transformation, hepatocytes may again produce this fetal protein, and its detection in the bloodstream has been used in diagnosis of liver cancer.

Differentiation antigens arise only in cells following a particular pathway of cellular differentiation; that is, all lymphocytes derived from the thymus bear specific differentiation antigens as do lymphoid tumors arising from these cells.

Viral antigens related to the leukemia viruses appear on malignant lymphoid cells. In fact, expression of cell surface antigens of this type may by the only evidence for the presence of virus, since virions disappear when their genetic material is incorporated into the host cell DNA.

Lymphocytes and cytolysis

Specific tumor antigens can induce a selective, cell-mediated reaction that destroys malignant cells. This type of immunity can be transferred experimentally with lymphocytes (but not with serum). Some tumors contain lymphocytes in their stroma, and tumors with lymphocytes appear to have a better prognosis.

Experiments in mice suggest that immune lymphocytes are effective.

Experimental sarcomas produced in adult mice become infiltrated with mixtures of lymphocytes and macrophages. Whether these tumors progress or regress is influenced by the specificity of the invading lymphocytes for the tumor antigens and by the time in the course of tumor growth at which the immune response is initiated. When Stephen Russell injected mice with sarcoma cells, all mice were killed by expanding tumors that had little evidence of lymphocyte infiltration. When infiltrating cells were isolated from regressing sarcomas, the lymphocytes (of T cell lineage) were specifically cytolytic for the same sarcoma but macrophages were not.

Transfer of "immune" lymphocytes (lymphocytes obtained from mice given purified tumor

Table 11.1. Antineoplastic cytokines

Factor	Synonym	Source	Activity[a]
Tumor necrosis factor-α (TNF-α)	Cachectin	Macrophages et al.	Cytotoxic to some tumor cells
Tumor necrosis factor-β (TNF-β)	Lymphotoxin	Lymphocytes	Stimulate synthesis of other cytokines
			Activate endothelium and macrophages
			Synergistic action with interleukins

[a]TNF-α and TNF-β have similar activities.

antigens) into tumor-bearing mice clearly can lead to regression of the primary tumor.

Nonimmune lymphocyte cytolysis

Immunologic resistance to progressive tumor growth is attributed to mature, cytotoxic T lymphocytes specifically immune against tumor-associated antigens. Failure of T cell–deficient animals, such as nude mice, to develop a high incidence of natural malignant neoplasms suggests that other mechanisms are operative.

Natural killer cells kill some tumor cells.

Natural killer (NK) cells, a population of immature lymphocytes, arises in the late neonatal period and wanes with advancing age. NK cells bear Fc receptors on their surfaces that cause lysis of neoplastic and virus-infected cells that is initiated by means other than known B and T cell mechanisms. Experimentally, there is close correlation between NK cell activity and "antibody-dependent, cell-mediated cytotoxicity" (attributed to phagocytic cells resembling monocytes with surface complement receptors); in fact, these activities may be variants of the same cell type. NK activity if markedly increased in T cell–deficient animals and is diminished in some lymphoproliferative diseases.

Antibodies

Humoral antibodies are also important in some tumors. In virus-induced lymphosarcoma of cats, for example, a clear correlation has been established between humoral antibodies to virus-associated plasma membrane antigens and the failure of cats to develop progressive malignant tumors. How antibodies prevent tumor initiation or growth in vivo is not clear.

Why doesn't tumor immunotherapy work?

The immunoreactivity induced by the tumor is probably quantitatively insufficient to inhibit an already rapidly growing tumor. By continual antigen shedding, very large tumors could provide tumor antigens that would combine with immune cells or antibody sufficient to prevent them from reacting with neoplastic cells. There are several other theories about ineffective immunotherapy. (1) There is a close relation between oncogenesis and immunosuppression, and it may be that tumors develop in an already immunodefective host. (2) Humoral antibodies may even enhance tumor growth. It is proposed that they combine on the tumor cell surface and

block the effect of more potent immunotoxic mechanisms. Antigens on the cell surface may also be blocked by mucosubstances. (3) Prolonged exposure to tumor antigens may induce a partial or split state of tolerance in the host, in which immunoreactivity is ineffective (Table 11.2).

Immunologic enhancement

This concept originated in the field of experimental tumor immunology. During the early enthusiastic attempts to demonstrate the immunologic repression of tumors, it was unexpectedly found that the opposite results occurred; that is, an enhanced susceptibility of the host to the tumor graft developed. This was manifested as increased numbers of tumor "takes," increased size of tumors, and greater numbers of metastases.

Endocrine-dependent neoplasms

Neoplasms of the prostate and mammary gland are, to varying degrees, endocrine dependent. Growth is enhanced by the sex hormone appropriate to the host and inhibited by its absence or by therapy with opposing endocrine secretions. For example, prostatic carcinoma develops under the influence of testosterone. Orchiectomy inhibits growth, as does treatment with estrogens. Human carcinomas of the pros-

Table 11.2. Mechanisms whereby neoplastic cells escape immunologic destruction

Delayed immunostimulation
  The neoplastic cells may not stimulate immune recognition in early phases of tumor growth; the neoplastic population is too large for effect when the immunologic mechanism becomes established.
Antigenic modulation
  The neoplastic cell is stripped of bits of membrane bearing surface antigens by nonlethal immune reactions and does not react subsequently with antibody or lymphocytes.
Antigenic overload
  The host is flooded with tumor antigens that bind to antibodies or lymphocyte surfaces to prevent recognition and destruction of all neoplastic cells.
General immunodeficiency
  The host fails to respond to tumor cells; some viruses produce tumors only after injection into immunosuppressed neonates or adults; humans with immunodeficiency, either genetic or from transplantation therapy, have a higher incidence of neoplasia.
Specific immunodeficiency
  The host is normal immunologically except for the precise lack of immune response produced by genes required for recognition of particular tumor-specific antigens.

tate are enhanced and inhibited by testosterone and estrogen respectively. Dr. Irwin Leav, at Tufts University, has shown that the canine prostatic carcinoma is not as androgen-dependent as is its human counterpart. Neoplastic cells are more refractory to castration due to shift from a reductive to an oxidative pathway of steroid metabolism to reach an androgen-independent state.

Hormone receptors control estrogen or testosterone influences.

Quantitative biochemical assays for estrogen receptors in extracts of mammary carcinomas have proven useful in predicting estrogenic dependency of tumors. Steroid receptor molecules that bind estradiol have been found in the cytoplasmic fractions of extract of mammary gland and perianal gland tumors of dogs. Hormone receptors have also been localized in canine mammary tumors histochemically. In preneoplastic lesions of canine mammary gland, hormone secretion is dependent on estrogens but growth of cells is not.

The canine *perianal gland tumor* is androgen-dependent. Males show more than a 5-fold increased risk over females, and estrogens are conventional therapy for this tumor. Normal perianal glands are small at birth and enlarge until senility. Treatment of puppies with androgens induces adult-sized perianal glands in 2 weeks.

Nutrition and cancer

The nutritive status of an animal *may* play some role in susceptibility to neoplasia. Evidence favoring that premise is spotty, and it is difficult to apply statistics to incidence in naturally occurring tumors. In general, animals on very high calorie diets have a slightly increased incidence of tumors of some kinds. Most of this information comes from large colonies of rats and mice. It has been reported that when two groups of cattle were placed on high- and low-calorie diets and exposed to sunlight, there was a higher incidence of *squamous cell carcinoma* in the well-fed animals. In laboratory rodents, it even appears that transient caloric restriction

for periods during development has an inhibitory effect on tumor development.

After the appearance of tumors, high-calorie diets may also enhance neoplastic growth. Experimentally, fasting and starvation greatly prolong the G2 period of Ehrlich ascites tumor cells growing in the mouse peritoneal cavity.

Do dietary fats enhance intestinal neoplasia?

In some rodents, addition of unsaturated fatty acids to the diet significantly enhances the incidence of chemically induced tumors. Rats are more susceptible to aflatoxin carcinogenesis when fed high–fat diets deficient in lipotropes such a methionine and choline. These deficiencies depress hepatic enzymes required for aflatoxin catabolism. In contrast, dietary antioxidants such as vitamin E decrease tumor incidence, probably by regulation of hepatic enzyme levels. In addition to these effects on detoxification, other dietary deficiencies may lead to biochemical malfunctions that promote neoplasia.

ADDITIONAL READING

Dubielzig, R. R. Ocular sarcoma following trauma in three cats. *J. Am. Vet. Med. Assoc.* 184:578, 1984.

Durham, S. K., and Dietze, A. E. Prostatic adenocarcinoma with and without metastases to bone in dogs. *J. Am. Vet. Med. Assoc.* 188:1432, 1986.

Hall, G. A., et al. Thymoma with myasthenia gravis in a dog. *J. Pathol.* 108:177, 1972.

Kruth, S. A., et al. Insulin-secreting islet cell tumors. *J. Am. Vet. Med. Assoc.* 181:54, 1982.

Leifer, C. E., et al. Hypoglycemia associated with nonislet cell tumors in 13 dogs. *J. Am. Vet. Med. Assoc.* 186:53, 1985.

MacEwen, E. G., et al. Nonsecretory multiple myeloma in two dogs. *J. Am. Vet. Med. Assoc.* 184:1283, 1984.

Meuten, D. J., et al. Hypercalcemia in dogs with lymphosarcoma. *Lab. Invest.* 49:553, 1983.

Old, L. J. Tumor necrosis factor (TNF). *Science* 230:630, 1985.

Weiss, D. J., et al. Secondary myelofibrosis in three dogs. *J. Am. Vet. Med. Assoc.* 187:423, 1986.

Causes of Neoplasms

ALTHOUGH causal factors for naturally occurring tumors are nearly always elusive, the primary causes of certain cancers are known. Furthermore, the enormous amount of evidence about many others justifies presumptive statements as to their cause. In all tumors, however, the neoplastic process is multifactorial, and even though the cause is identified, there are always unidentified promoting factors that influence tumor development in capricious and undetermined ways. Neoplasms commonly arise from the combined effects of oncogens and chronic tissue injury.

The wide range of oncogens proven in laboratory rodents must be kept distinct from those agents actually shown to cause naturally occurring cancer in animals. Furthermore, as in toxicology, dosage and timing are critical. The use of massive doses of chemicals to test carcinogenicity renders some experimental results highly artificial, and such models should be placed in proper perspective. Even among the reliable models of carcinogenicity, there are only a few instances where the direct cause of cancer is determined and its mechanisms reasonably explained. In some of these, it has been suspected that the agent involved merely unmasks another oncogen that then exerts the primary oncogenic effect.

PHYSICAL AGENTS
Solar radiation

Cancer of the skin develops in nonpigmented animals exposed to intense sunlight for long periods. Heavily pigmented animals are practically resistant to this type of lesion. A great deal of epidemiologic evidence in man incriminates solar radiation. Skin cancer is more prevalent in (1) geographic areas where sunlight is most intense, (2) light-skinned races of man and animals, and (3) exposed areas of the body. The relation between solar radiation and carcinoma induction has been proven experimentally and the carcinogenic effect shown to be in the ultraviolet spectrum between rays of 2800 and 3200 Å.

Squamous cell carcinoma of the eye develops in white-faced Hereford cattle in the southern United States. The incidence of these tumors in black Angus cattle in similar localities is much less. The squamous cell carcinomas first appear at the corneal periphery in the medial and lateral aspect of the eyeball, areas not covered by the eyelid when the eyes are open.

Bovine ocular squamous cell carcinomas arise from nonmalignant precursor plaques (see Fig. 10.2). These lesions have been shown to contain papillomaviruses that may contribute to (but do not cause) the neoplastic process. It has also been reported that excessive ultraviolet irradiation stimulates suppressor T lymphocytes, and that this may aid the growth of oncogenic viruses.

Solar radiation induces neoplasia by causing damage to DNA. Ultraviolet radiation reaching the earth on sunny days generates pyrimidine dimers in DNA of exposed skin cells by linking adjacent thymine and cytosine. Once injured, DNA is repaired in normal cells by excision repair. Repair is never totally efficient, and some cells die. Others survive with DNA scars left by the process of mutation.

Evidence that DNA damage is a direct cause of squamous cell carcinoma comes from the human genetic disease *xeroderma pigmentosum*. These patients, because of defects in enzymes required for DNA repair, are extremely sensitive to sunlight and are susceptible to various kinds of skin neoplasms in childhood.

X irradiation

Since the early days of the use of X rays, it has been known that these forces can induce cancer. An enormous amount of evidence exists for local radiation-induced cancers in man. Pioneers in radiology were often affected by carcinomas of the skin overlying the hands and arms, areas the most exposed to radiation.

Whole-body radiation increases the incidence of neoplasms.

Epidemiologic studies indicate that even small doses of radiation delivered to the entire body increase neoplastic disease. Drs. Andras Fabry and Stephen Benjamin, at the Collaborative Radiobiologic Health Lab at Colorado State University, studied beagles given low-dose, whole-body, Co^{60} γ-radiation. There was an increased incidence of hyperplastic nodules of the liver (which are common in aged dogs) and a few cases of hepatocellular carcinoma.

The oncogenic changes resulting from whole-body radiation have been clearly illustrated in studies on human survivors of bomb fallout in Hiroshima and Nagasaki (see Fig. 26.2). Leukemia was more common in these populations, and the incidence of solid tumors also increased. Fallout of I^{131} has caused adenomatous change in thyroid of exposed humans. Similarly, young children irradiated in infancy for various reasons in the 1940s have returned several years later with adenocarcinomas of the thyroid. Radiation-induced bone cancer occurs in human adults irradiated for arthritis of the spine.

When dogs or other large mammals receive *large doses* of whole-body radiation, a spectrum of neoplasms occurs in ensuing years, including lymphosarcoma, reticulum cell sarcoma, and myeloid leukemia. The pathogenesis of these neoplasms is unknown although experiments in mice suggest that latent oncogenic viruses may be activated by the radiation.

Inhalation of radionuclides produces tumors in organs of deposition. Inhaled Sr^{90} goes to the skeleton where bone sarcomas evolve. Ce^{144} deposits in lung, liver, and spleen, causing carcinomas; hemangiosarcomas are common in some species. Long-range β-radiation emitters are more apt to produce neoplasms than are radionuclides emitting shorter radiation.

Radiation causes somatic mutation

The primary event in radiation-induced oncogenesis is the production of specific genetic alterations, that is, a somatic mutation. The dose rate and quality of radiation influence the frequency of mutation. Mutation occurs from direct damage to DNA. It may also occur by direct damage to the mitotic apparatus, by secondary damage to chromosomes, or by activation of latent oncogenic viruses. Additional damage to other enzymes of repair and detoxification probably amplify the cancerous transformation.

Trauma

In large breeds of dogs, osteosarcomas may develop at healed fracture lines of long bones. Fracture-associated sarcomas differ from other osteosarcomas in being diaphyseal rather than metaphyseal in location. The mean interval between fracture occurrence and tumor diagnosis is about 8 years.

Development of neoplasms at sites of tissue injury has been reported (very rarely) in dogs and man, usually on the limbs. Burn scar neoplasms are predominantly squamous cell carcinomas although basal cell carcinomas and sarcomas have been seen. Dr. Richard Dubielzig, now at the University of Wisconsin, reported anaplastic sarcomas in the eyes of cats several years after trauma to the affected eye.

CHEMICAL ONCOGENESIS

One of the earliest reports on a cause of cancer was the finding by Sir Percivall Pott in the 1700s that English chimney sweeps suffered a high incidence of carcinoma of the scrotum because of continual exposure to substances in soot. Although it was soon obvious that an oncogenic factor involved in scrotal cancer was present in soot, the substance was not identified for nearly 150 years. In 1915, Yamagiwa reproduced a squamous cell carcinoma similar to that in chimney sweeps by painting rabbits' ears with coal tar (Table 12.1). The precise chemical onco-

Table 12.1.   Milestones in experimental oncology

1838	Moller (Germany) demonstrates the cellular nature of neoplasms by examining tumor tissue with light microscope.
1858	Leblanc (France) establishes that animal tumors have similar cellular composition.
1876	Novinsky (Russia) demonstrates transplantability of canine venereal tumor.
1903	Jensen (Denmark) inoculates suspension of mouse mammary gland tumor into mice, reproduces tumors, and passes them serially.
1908	Ellerman and Bang (Denmark) discover transmissibility of avian lymphoid tumors.
1910	Rous transmits sarcoma of chicken by cell-free suspensions.
1910	Clunet (France) produces tumors experimentally by X radiation.
1912	Murphy shows that rat tumors will grow on chicken chorioallantoic membrane.
1914	Yamagiwa (Japan) proves carcinogenicity of coal tar by long-term application to skin of rabbits.
1924	Little and Strong develop inbred strains of mice for genetic analysis of tumors.
1932	Shope demonstrates viral nature of rabbit papilloma.
1933	Warburg shows high rate of anaerobic glycolysis in tumor cells.
1936	Lucke discovers virus-induced renal carcinoma of frog.
1936	Bittner discovers viral agent in milk causing mammary gland carcinoma of mice.
1943	Gross shows evidence for tumor-specific antigens by immunizing mice.
1947	Berenblum establishes two stages in chemical carcinogenesis: initiation and promotion.
1951	Gross isolates virus causing naturally occurring lymphoma in mice.
1962	Epstein and Barr isolate causal herpesvirus from Burkitt's lymphoma, shown later to cause infectious mononucleosis.
1964	Jarrett transmits lymphosarcoma to cats with retroviruses.
1969	Friedrich-Freksa shows early changes in liver chemical carcinogenesis are multiple foci of cells with abnormal enzyme patterns.
1974	Brinster and Minz inoculate teratoma cells into normal mouse blastocysts to produce normal but mosaic mice (showing that tumor cells lose malignancy and differentiate normally).

gen, dibenzanthracene (DBA), a polycyclic aromatic hydrocarbon, was identified in 1930 as the first known chemical carcinogen.

The polycyclic hydrocarbons, the most powerful chemical oncogens known, are present in tobacco smoke and in the urban atmosphere. Of these potent chemicals available to the experimental oncologist, the most widely used are DBA, 3-methylcholanthrene (MC), and 7,12-dimethylbenzanthracene (DMBA). By painting these carcinogens on skin, it is possible to produce epidermal carcinomas in most laboratory animals. In the respiratory tract, benzopyrene induces mucous cells to become metaplastic squamous cells, some of which transform to neo-

plastic cells. The same agents act directly to induce sarcomas when injected subcutaneously and to induce intestinal carcinomas when taken orally.

The clearest picture of chemical oncogenesis comes from studies involving the chronic application of oncogens to skin. When polycyclic hydrocarbons are painted on skin of laboratory animals, they accumulate in hair follicles and sebaceous glands and produce a necrotizing effect. After death of random cells, a transient hyperplastic reaction develops. Cells immediately above the germinal layer are enlarged and have large nuclei and nucleoli. Hyperplastic foci disappear within several days unless the oncogen is repeatedly applied. With each successive application, the epidermal cells show an increasing resistance to the toxic effect of the chemical, but hyperplasia becomes more intense. In time, anaplastic cells appear, and the tumor progresses to malignancy even if the oncogen is removed from the skin.

Initiation and promotion

The concept that multiple mechanisms may be involved in the chemical induction of cancer has given rise to a *two-stage theory of carcinogenesis*. Although the carcinogen induces an irreversible transformation in some of the epidermal cells, their neoplastic characteristics may remain unexpressed for the life span of the animal. The subsequent presence of a promoter will determine whether the neoplastic character is expressed.

In the rabbit–coal tar model, benign tumors induced in ears disappeared if painting was discontinued early. Rous could enhance carcinogenicity by punching holes (with a cork borer) in the ears of rabbits having received this minimal painting. After wounding, tumors began to grow along the edge of the wound. Thus tar *initiated* and wounding *promoted* tumor growth. Chronic inflammation may be a critical factor in promotion of natural tumors, and experimental promoters are often inducers of inflammation (Table 12.2).

If mouse skin is painted with a subcarcinogenic dose of methylcholanthracene, papillomas result from subsequent painting with croton oil (the reverse order does not elicit a tumor). Methylcholanthracene is the initiator, croton oil the promoter. The initiator converts normal skin cells to latent tumor cells, which persist until

Table 12.2.   Causes of naturally occurring neoplasms

Organ	Tumor	Species	Agent and Exposure
Liver	Hepatocellular carcinoma	Trout, man	Aflatoxin B_2 (contaminated feed)
		Man	Hepatitis B virus (chronic infection)
		Rat	*Taenia taeniaformis* (liver infection)
	Bile duct carcinoma	Man	*Clonorchis sinensis* (chronic infection)
	Angiosarcoma	Man	Vinyl chloride gas (aerosol, plastic industry)
Kidney	Renal cell carcinoma	Frog	Herpesvirus (infected water, via urine)
Bladder	Carcinoma	Cow	Bracken fern toxin (feeding)
		Man	Azo dye, or naphthalene (dye manufacturing)
			Schistosoma haemotobium (contaminated water)
Vagina	Adenocarcinoma	Man	Diethylstilbestrol (exposure of fetus)
Lung	Mesothelioma	Man	Asbestos (industrial worker inhalation)
	Carcinoma	Man	Cigarette smoke
			Nickel, or crystalline Ni_3S_2 (refinery worker inhalation)
Skin	Carcinoma	Man	Soot, or benzopyrene (chimney sweeping, scrotum)
		Many species	Ultraviolet irradiation (sunlight)
Mammary gland	Adenocarcinoma	Mouse	Oncornavirus (nursing, milk)
Tongue	Carcinoma	Man	Radiation from radium (licking contaminated brushes in watchmaking)
Esophagus	Sarcoma	Dog	*Spirocera lupi*
Rumen	Carcinoma	Cow	Bracken fern toxin (feeding)
Thyroid	Carcinoma	Man	Radiation from X rays (therapeutic radiation)
Hematopoietic	Granulocytic leukemia	Man	Benzene
	Malignant lymphoma	Chicken, mouse, cat, cow	Leukemia viruses
Connective tissue	Sarcoma	Man	Nickel subsulfide, or Ni_3S_2 (refinery workers)

activated by the promoter. From these experiments it is clear that (1) initiation is a rapid, permanent change in tissue, whereas promotion is a slow process consisting of a progression of reversible effects, and (2) initiation must take place before promotion, or it is without effect.

Mechanisms of chemical carcinogenesis

Chemical carcinogens induce cancer by altering DNA. Although some produce direct damage, most carcinogens require enzymatic conversion to strongly electrophilic reactants, which are the ultimate carcinogenic molecule (Table 12.3). This conversion is accomplished by soluble transferases in the *smooth endoplasmic reticulum*. For example, oxidases in the endoplasmic reticulum catalyze benzopyrene to products that bind covalently to DNA. The carcino-

genic potency of this and other polycyclic hydrocarbons correlates with the extent of their binding to DNA.

Mutation may result from mRNA template instability.

In some chemical carcinogenesis, somatic mutation results from direct injury to nucleic acids and the long time period required for the mole-

Table 12.3.   Models of initiation and promotion in experimental carcinogenesis

Initiator	Promoter	Tissue
Benzopyrene	Croton oil	Mouse skin
2-acetamidofluorene (AAF)	Phenobarbital	Rat liver
Methylnitrosourea	Saccharin	Rat bladder
Aflatoxin B_1	Methylsterculate	Trout liver

cule to reform. Loss of differentiation and control may depend on a defectiveness in messenger RNA template stability, that is, an altered capacity of mRNA templates to faithfully express cell differentiation. A new, altered set of mRNA templates, manifest as anaplasia, can be measured as a loss in control of enzyme synthesis.

Some of the azo dyes are potent oncogens of this type. For example, N-methyl-aminoazobenzene (MAB, or "butter yellow") has been widely fed to rats as a model of liver carcinoma. It requires conversion, during detoxification in the hepatocyte, to the oncogenic metabolite N-hydroxy-MAB. The metabolite induces foci of hyperplasia in the liver that progressively change to adenoma and, in turn, to adenocarcinoma.

The "industrial cancers" of the human bladder are caused by storage of urine containing oncogenic chemicals or their oncogenic metabolites. Bladder tumors, occurring in workers in the dye industry, are caused by three primary aromatic amines: 2-naphthylamine, benzidine, and 4-aminodiphenyl. These compounds are causally related to human transitional cell carcinomas and cause the same tumors experimentally in dogs.

Progression in carcinogenesis

Primary tumors of the liver usually occur in older animals with nodules of hyperplasia or other evidence of chronic liver disease (Fig. 12.1). Hepatic cancer has been linked to ingestion of toxic chemicals because of the liver's association with the portal venous system draining the intestine, its importance in detoxification, and proven cases of natural hepatocarcinogenesis that occur after ingestion of toxin (see aflatoxin, Chapter 27).

Chemical carcinogenesis develops in progressive stages.

Studies of liver have shown that chemical carcinogenesis occurs in stages of progressive development. Experimental feeding of carcinogens such as diethylnitrosamine leads to formation of *hyperplastic nodules* (regenerating nodules). These are preneoplastic lesions, within

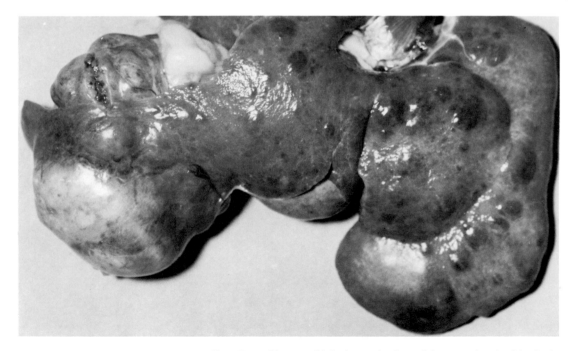

Fig. 12.1. Liver, multiple hyperplastic nodules associated with single, large hepatocellular carcinoma, aged dog.

which develop malignant *hepatocellular carcinomas,* providing that feeding is prolonged. If the carcinogenic diet ceases, hyperplastic nodules disappear and the cells are remodeled to become part of normal liver structure.

Enzyme cytochemistry detects the initial change.

Within 6 weeks after the start of a diethylnitrosamine diet, small foci of cells appear that show specific enzyme deficiencies. Affected cells appear normal by standard hemotoxylin and eosin staining, but when examined for glucose-6-phosphatase (in the Golgi complex) or ATPase (in canaliculi), they fail to react. These islands of cells have a higher rate of DNA synthesis than do normal hepatocytes. Furthermore, in a few islands, small groups of cells develop with extremely high rates of DNA synthesis and structure resembling carcinoma.

Chemical carcinogens trigger a chain reaction.

Carcinogens do not induce cancer in liver directly but initiate a sequence of events that ultimately results in autonomous neoplastic cells. Biologic evidence supports this concept: (1) virtually every chemical carcinogen is a toxic inhibitor of cell proliferation; (2) the proliferative responses that result from carcinogens given systemically are focal, not general, even though the carcinogen affects all hepatocytes; and (3) autonomous growth of initiated cells is a property acquired late in carcinogenesis (evidence of neoplastic growth does not appear until 4–5 months after dosage, and frank neoplasia is evident only at 7–8 months).

These facts suggest that one property of the focal responsiveness is a resistance to the inhibitory effect of the carcinogen. That is, hyperplastic liver nodules, the precursors of liver cancer, are resistant to cytotoxic properties of hepatocarcinogens. The resistant hepatocyte grows and thrives in an environment unfavorable for normal hepatocyte proliferation.

Carcinogens in food

Food supplies are major routes of exposure of animals to chemical carcinogens. A great many chemicals are intentionally added to foods during processing. Antioxidants, preservatives, and flavoring agents are potential carcinogens, as are dyes added to fruits and those used for labeling meats. Carcinogens may be present in food grains as unrecognized plant contaminants (e.g., *Senecio* sp. and *Crotalaria* sp.) or as spoilage molds on feed (e.g., aflatoxin). These oncogenic substances must be recognized and eliminated from food sources.

Food grains are often contaminated by chemicals during growth and processing. In general, these include the carcinogenic agricultural chemicals, pesticides, and mycotoxins. Contamination may be direct or may involve residues in plants and water supplies. In the past, concern has been translated into regulatory action when chemicals already in use have been found to produce neoplasms on testing in laboratory rodents. Thioacetamide and thiourea, used as fungicides on fruit, produce hepatomas in rats. Aramite, used to control mites on fruit trees, induces hepatomas in several species. The herbicide aminotriazole, used to control weeds in cranberry bogs, produces thyroid adenomas in rats. Release of this information to the press at the height of the holiday sales season produced disastrous results in the marketing of cranberries in the 1970s. The political furor that inevitably results from events of this kind can in turn adversely affect appropriate decisions based on real scientific evidence concerning the danger of carcinogens. Careless exploitation by journalists makes it difficult to place the valid scientific evidence of the true danger of these chemicals in perspective. Ignorance of which diseases are induced by long-term exposure often makes it impossible to provide an accurate prediction of oncogenicity.

Aflatoxin and hepatic carcinoma

Hepatomas were found to be widespread in fish farms and hatcheries in 1960. The cause was commercially pelleted cottonseed meal fish feed that contained the aflatoxins of *Aspergillus flavus.* Experiments promptly established that aflatoxin B_1 was the specific cause. Most species of trout were susceptible, but tumors developed more rapidly in fish reared commercially in waters of higher temperature. Dietary aflatoxin B_1 at 1–20 ppb induced hepatoma in trout in 3–6 months. When aflatoxin levels were high (1–15 mg/kg), fish died of acute hepatic necrosis and hemorrhage.

The trout hepatomas are well differentiated and grow by expansion. Metastases occur, although they are rare. Most tumors become fibrotic, cystic, and regressive. Tumor cells faithfully reproduce the structure of normal hepatocytes. Liver carcinomas have also been produced by aflatoxin in rats and monkeys.

Natural hepatomas occur in turkeys fed on feed contaminated with aflatoxin, and circumstantial evidence has incriminated aflatoxins in human carcinogenesis (as contaminants of peanuts and other feed grains). Chronic aflatoxicosis appears to be one factor in the high incidence of human hepatocellular carcinomas in Africa and Asia.

Bracken fern and bovine bladder tumors

Bovine enzootic hematuria is a disease of grazing cattle largely confined to woods and areas containing bracken fern (*Pteris aquilina*). This disease has been shown to be accompanied by carcinomas of the bladder in cattle and water buffalo in Turkey. Dr. Pamukcu of Ankara, working with Dr. Carl Olson in a nonenzootic area of Wisconsin, induced bladder carcinomas experimentally by feeding bracken fern. Tumors indistinguishable from natural lesions developed in cows that survived over 3 years on the feeding program. Bracken fern fed to sheep also produces bladder tumors and, after 3 years, will cause fibrosarcomas of the mandible.

Natural grazing of bracken fern in upland areas of Scotland promotes carcinogenesis in virus-induced papillomas of the alimentary tract. The chemical carcinogen in the fern is not characterized but is believed to be a metabolic breakdown product of a fern toxin. Fern toxins also produce intestinal and urinary tumors in rats, aplastic anemia in cattle, and leukemia and pulmonary tumors in mice.

Cycasid nuts and liver tumors

Nuts of the plant *Cycas circinalis* contain a carcinogenic glycoside termed *cycasin*. When flour from these nuts is fed to rodents, they develop renal, small intestinal, and hepatic carcinomas. Methylazoxymethanol, an aglycone moiety of cycasin, is cleaved away by intestinal flora that possess a β-glucosidase and is the active carcinogen. Experimentally, methylazoxymethanol causes early inhibition of DNA synthesis (as shown by decreased incorporation of thymidine into DNA), which leads to inhibition of protein synthesis.

Diethylstilbestrol is associated with human genital tumors.

Stilbestrol was widely prescribed in the 1940s for women threatened with abortion. It was shown in 1971 to have an association with vaginal adenocarcinomas reported in young women whose mothers had been treated while they were being carried in utero. Subsequently, diethylstilbestrol has been banned from beef production, where it was widely used to enhance the fattening of cattle. This synthetic hormone causes similar lesions in offspring of mice and monkeys treated during pregnancy. It induces mammary tumors in susceptible strains of mice at a level as low as 6.25 ppb and is therefore classed as a carcinogen.

Other carcinogens

There are many examples of carcinogens in animals and man in which the precise carcinogen is unknown even though the environmental circumstances are evident, such as lung carcinoma in human cigarette smokers, bladder carcinoma during human bilharzia infections, and lip cancer with betel nut chewing.

Carcinomas of the human esophagus, which have a high incidence in certain provinces of China, have been ascribed to the combined effects of dietary nitrosamines and fungal metabolites. *Candida* sp., found in metaplastic premalignant lesions in the esophagus, release metabolites that reduce the pH of the esophageal surface to induce production of carcinogenic nitrosamines.

Tests for carcinogenicity

Studies of large numbers of animals or man exposed to specific environmental factors have shown an association between exposure and onset of cancer. Arsenic, asbestos, benzene, and nickel are some of the chemicals classed as human carcinogens from epidemiologic studies (Table 12.4).

Effective regulation of toxic substances requires identification of carcinogens before human exposure. The veterinary pathologist is involved in this process, both identifying coincident animal populations exposed to environmental carcinogens and examining tissues from laboratory animals exposed experimentally to suspected chemicals. The conventional

Table 12.4. Classes of carcinogenic chemicals

Type	Mode of Action	Example
Genotoxic		
Direct acting	Electrophile organic compounds that interact with DNA	Ethylene imine
Procarcinogen	Requires conversion through metabolic activation	Aflatoxin Vinyl chloride Benzopyrene 2-naphthylamine Dimethylnitrosamine
Inorganic carcinogen[a]	Leads to DNA change by alteration of DNA replication	Nickel Chromium
Epigenetic		
Hormone[a]	Alters cell differentiation via endocrine imbalance; may be promoter	Diethylstilbestrol Estradiol
Immunosuppressor[a]	Stimulates viral, transplanted, or metastatic neoplasms	Azathioprine Antilymphocyte serum
Cocarcinogen[b]	Enhances effects of genotoxic agents when given at the same time	Ethanol Phorbol esters
Promoter[b]	Enhances effects of genotoxic agents when given subsequently	Phenol Bile acids Saccharin

[a]Not genotoxic.
[b]Not genotoxic or carcinogenic.

way to detect toxic substances is through long-term bioassays in animals, typically rodents.

Animal testing for carcinogens

Guidelines of the U.S. National Cancer Institute suggest a suspected chemical be tested in two animal types and in both sexes, with subgroups of 50 animals of one sex and one strain used for each experiment. The chemical should be administered by a route that closely approximates human exposure at a minimum of two doses. Treatment should be continued long enough to produce a maximum response, after which the animals are necropsied.

In general, these tests give results that agree with experience in man (although not all chemicals carcinogenic in animals produce human tumors). Advice for work in this area is available from the Federal Regulations Committee of the American College of Veterinary Pathologists, currently headed by Dr. Dawn Goodman. Major problems with animal tests are that they are expensive and there are too few sufficiently trained scientists to carry out such ambitious testing. To circumvent animal testing, several (less reliable) in vitro systems have been devised.

Bacterial tests for carcinogens

The standard, most widely used in vitro test is the *Salmonella*-mammalian liver assay (Ames test) for mutagenesis. The effectiveness of this test depends on the degree with which mutagenesis correlates with carcinogenesis. Mutant strains of *Salmonella typhimurium* that are unable to synthesize the essential amino acid histidine are exposed to suspected chemicals that, if mutagenic, correct this defect and allow bacteria to grow in a histidine-free medium. Most carcinogens act only after conversion to reactive forms; to overcome this problem, homogenates of liver cells containing enzymes that metabolize the test chemical are added to the system. The concordance between mutagenicity in the Ames test and carcinogenicity in animals is good for nitrosamines and highly electrophilic molecules such as nitrogen mustards but is low for some of the antimetabolites, polychlorinated compounds, and hydrazines (all of which have more complex metabolic routes).

A second test with bacteria is the Pol-A test based on mutant strains of *Escherichia coli* that lack a particular DNA repair system; chemicals that interfere with DNA kill the mutant bacteria.

VIRAL ONCOGENESIS

Naturally occurring tumors of animals are caused by DNA and RNA viruses. Both types interact with cellular DNA to cause neoplasia, but the basic differences between these two groups necessitate a different mechanism. RNA viruses that cause neoplasia are members of the family Retroviridae. DNA viruses known to cause or contribute to natural malignant neoplasms include herpesviruses, papovaviruses (especially the papillomaviruses), and the hepatitis B viruses of man and woodchucks.

Ultimately, all virus-induced neoplasms involve multiple contributing factors, only one of which may dominate as causal. These may be (1) a direct effect of a gene (called an *oncogene*) carried by the virus, (2) a viral factor that affects a host gene, (3) factors that incapacitate or delete "anti-oncogenes," and (4) genes that do not affect cell growth but influence the expansion, metastasis, or other behavior of neoplasms.

Retroviruses

Members of the family Retroviridae cause malignant tumors in three orders of vertebrates: mammals, birds, and reptiles. They are especially important as causes of malignant lymphomas and sarcomas of chickens, cattle, cats, and mice and are implicated in these tumors in dogs and primates (Fig. 12.2). The expression of oncogenicity of these retroviruses relates to the age of the host and to the character of the virus. The relatively rapid mitotic activity and the immaturity of the immune systems are important factors in the exceptional susceptibility of the young animal.

These viruses take the name *retrovirus* from their unique life cycle. When they infect cells, they reverse the usual biologic sequence of flow of genetic information. Their genetic code, carried on RNA, is transcribed "backward" into DNA. In neoplasia, this new viral DNA is integrated into the host cell chromosome in a sequence of units called a *provirus*. Later, the cell transcribes the proviral genes and synthesizes the proteins that they encode (which are assembled into new virions).

Retroviruses cause cancer by several different mechanisms.

Some retroviruses contain a single gene, called an *oncogene,* that is solely responsible for neoplastic induction. Retroviruses bearing oncogenes rapidly produce tumors in animals, and most can also transform cells in culture (Table 12.5). The *src* gene of Rous sarcoma virus (RSV) is the prototype oncogen. If the gene segment bearing *src* is isolated and transferred to cells in culture, it can cause cell transformation. After the *src* gene is heat-inactivated in vitro, it no longer causes neoplasia.

Other retroviruses, such as avian leukosis virus (ALV) of chickens, lack oncogenes but carry a viral RNA segment called a *long terminal repeat* (LTR) sequence at the end of the viral genome. The LTR sequence contains segments called "promoters" and "enhancers" that activate transcription of viral genes into mRNA. Viruses that lack oncogenes produce tumors slowly in animals and do not transform cells in culture.

Recently several viruses have been shown to produce cell transformation in vitro by a third mechanism. They contain proteins with the ability to *transactivate,* that is, to increase the expression of genes attached to viral control sequences (whether or not these genes are integrated into the cell gene); presumably a gene with the ability to stimulate viral gene expression also can stimulate expression of a similar cellular gene.

Retroviral genes are inserted into the host cell genome.

During the early hours of retroviral infection, the viral RNA genome is transcribed into DNA by a *reverse transcriptase.* The DNA copy of the viral genome is then integrated into the cell's genes and replicated along with other cell genes. In RSV infection at least three genes direct production of mRNAs that are translated into proteins for production of virions; the product of the *src* oncogene is not a component of the virion but remains in the cell.

In many cases retroviral infection is innocuous. Virions are manufactured and leave the cell without producing damage. This partnership goes awry when an oncogene is selectively activated (as in RSV tumors) or when a *provirus* inserted into the cell chromosome activates an adjacent normal cell gene for growth. ALV does not carry its own oncogene, for example, but the provirus is inserted in the vicinity of another gene known as *myc,* which is then greatly amplified and plays a role in neoplastic change.

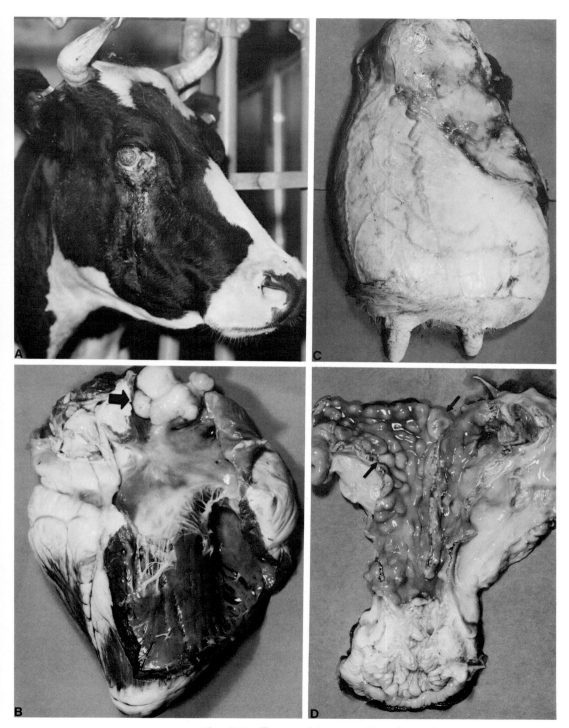

Fig. 12.2. Tumor nodules, cow with malignant lymphoma. There is damage to critical organs. A. Periorbital tumor tissue with marked panophthalmitis. B. Tumors in atrial wall. C. Supramammary lymph node with tumors (*top*) and lymph stasis in afferent lymphatics. D. Tumor invasion of placentome, uterus.

Table 12.5.   Mechanisms of retroviral oncogenesis

Action	Factor	Example	Mechanism
Direct	Oncogene	RSV	Oncogene contained in virion and directly causal in neoplasia
Indirect	Long terminal repeating sequence	FeLv AVL	Activation of cell proto-oncogene by insertion of viral long terminal repeating sequence adjacent to it
Transactivation	Protein factor	BLV Visna HTLV	Virus has gene for factor that increases transcription from viral promotor in long terminal repeating sequence

FOCUS

Abnormal genetic material leads to chromosome breakage in leukemia.

B cell leukemias involve proliferation of clones of lymphocytes each at a specific stage of differentiation. The malignant cells are the genetically identical progeny of an original transformed cell. Some have B cell surface markers, that is, immunoglobulins on their surfaces; the lineage of these neoplasms can be identified in vitro by demonstrating binding of fluorescent-labeled antibodies on tumor cells and by extracting immunoglobulins from tumor tissue. Monoclonal antibodies, with their remarkable specificity, permit more complex analyses and immunocytochemical techniques on frozen tissue sections. Although many lymphomas can be shown to be of B cell origin, others cannot be identified by the above techniques.

Recently, *gene rearrangement analysis* has revealed the key to the identity of proliferating tumor cells. DNA is extracted from tissue, purified, and then digested with several different restriction enzymes. A *restriction endonuclease* is an enzyme that cuts DNA at a specific set of nucleic acid-base pairs; by using several restriction endonucleases, the oncologist can isolate and examine the activity of DNA segments. The resulting fragments are separated by electrophoresis in agarose gels and transferred to activated nylon membranes – the Southern blot technique. Joining of Ig genes via DNA rearrangement early in B cell differentiation produces changes in locations of restriction endonuclease sites that are detectable on southern blots with DNA probes.

B cell precursor leukemias are tumors fixed in the developmental stage in which rearrangements of *heavy chain diversity* (D_H) segments to *joining* (J_H) segments is followed by addition of variable segments.

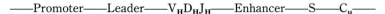
——Promoter——Leader——$V_H D_H J_H$——Enhancer——S——C_u——

This is a schematic model of the heavy chain gene. The variable region of the heavy chain is encoded by three elements: variable, diversity, and joining sequences. When a stem cell matures into a plasma cell, a DNA rearrangement joins V_k and J_k segments (the remaining intervening sequences are removed by RNA splicing). To the left (5′) side of the leader is the promoter, which together with the enhancer sequences, controls the rate of mRNA transcription.

Cells that enter the B cell lineage rearrange their immunoglobulin genes in a unique way so as to create antibodies with precise specificity. In the process of shifting genes, chromosomes appear to be inordinately susceptible to breakage. If an abnormal gene segment (say, a viral oncogene) has been inserted into the B lymphocyte genome, the chromosome may break and the subsequent translocation of chromosome pieces will occur. In human B cells one break is prone to occur at a chromosome bearing genes for immunoglobulin production, usually on chromosome number 14 at the site of heavy chain segment genes (breaks may also occur at chromosomes 2 and 22, the sites of kappa and lambda light chain genes). The second break occurs on chromosome 8 within a region where a gene for growth is located, in this case, the oncogene *c-myc*.

The translocation of pieces of chromosome 14 to chromosome 8 initiates expression of *c-myc* (it is turned off in normal cells), possibly by allowing a promoter or enhancer of the immunoglobulin gene to activate the *c-myc* gene.

Burkitt's lymphoma is an endemic tumor of human B cells that develops in several steps. Three gene systems are involved. (1) A herpesvirus called Epstein-Barr virus is highly transforming for B cells and inserts segments of its genome into that of the B lymphocyte. (2) Burkitt's lymphoma cells carry chromosome translocations, usually 14–8, which act by juxtaposing a gene for immunoglobulin chain synthesis to a protooncogene called *c-myc* (there is also evidence for activation of other oncogenes called *ras* and *Blym*). (3) There is also an environmental cofactor—in Africa, chronic malaria; in the United States, AIDS infection. One of the EBV gene segments called LT-1 (a lymphocyte surface marker) seems responsible for induced subsequent cell proliferation. Another segment may repress the viral lytic cycle, to permit cells to survive and replicate.

It is unclear how the Ig/*myc* translocation contributes to neoplasia. Current evidence suggests *dysregulation*; the *myc* gene juxtaposed to Ig genes comes under *cis* control by the active Ig region and behaves as if it were part of the Ig locus.

Gene analysis explains how viral genes cause some cancers.

Techniques of genetic engineering are used to show how neoplasia oncogenes might cause neoplasia. Viral DNA is cut into fragments at specific sites using a battery of enzymes called *restriction endonucleases*. Fragments are isolated, inserted into bacteria, grown within bacteria to large quantity, and reinserted into cultured cells where they express the gene carried by a partic-ular DNA fragment. Analysis has shown that one of these DNA segments, the *src* gene, is capable of encoding a single gene product that can transform cells in culture.

The *src* gene product is a protein kinase.

The protein encoded by the *src* gene (designated pp60$^{v\text{-}src}$ for phosphoprotein with MW of 60,000 daltons) is a protein kinase, an enzyme that attaches phosphate ions to amino acids by phosphorylation. Specifically, pp60^{v-src} attaches phosphate ions to tyrosine. This is typical of oncogene-encoded enzymes but differs from other protein kinases, which usually phosphorylate serine or threonine.

Oncogenes govern cell activity by phosphorylating proteins.

By phosphorylating several proteins, one enzyme could vastly alter cell functions. It might stimulate DNA synthesis, enhance mitosis, or render ATP inefficient. In cultured cells, the protein kinase generated by the *src* gene migrates to the plasma membrane where it phosphorylates a tyrosine unit in *vinculin,* a protein in normal adhesion plaques (where acting filaments are anchored to the plasma membrane). If it causes cell adhesion plaques to disintegrate, the kinase might contribute to loss of cell coordination and uncontrolled cell movement.

All cells possess *src*-like genes.

A striking fact to emerge from studies of RSV is that normal cells in all vertebrates possess a cell gene related to the viral *src* gene. Using radioactive DNA copies of *src* and nucleic acid hybridization techniques, it was found that the radioactive DNA would hybridize with DNA from uninfected birds and mammals. In addition, the cell gene was also active and produced small amounts of the protein kinase called pp60^{c-src}.

Of over 20 retroviral oncogenes identified, most have close relatives in genomes of normal cells. The normal cell counterparts are called *proto-oncogenes;* most contain codes for cellular growth factors (e.g., the *sis* proto-oncogene encodes one polypeptide chain of platelet derived growth factors, and the *erbB* proto-oncogene encodes one for epidermal growth factor). Thus retroviral oncogenes are viewed as copies acquired (during phylogenetic development) from genes of the vertebrate host in which the virus replicates. Cell genes from which the retroviral genes originate are themselves involved in neoplasia when activated by agents other than oncogene-bearing retroviruses.

Retroviruses native to the host are called endogenous viruses.

Endogenous type-C retroviruses are detectable in the DNA of animals by determination of nucleic acid sequences (comparable with those in the virion) and by detection of RNA in normal tissue expressed by these viral genes. Even though infectious viruses cannot be isolated, the transcription of their gene information can be identified. For example, nucleic acid sequences of type-C viruses isolated from baboons have been found in DNA of normal baboon tissue, indicating that they are endogenous, vertically transmitted viruses of baboons. In contrast, nucleic acid sequences of two type-C viruses from tumors of woolly monkeys and gibbon apes cannot be detected in their corresponding normal primate tissue but are found instead in DNA of normal mice, an indication that the viruses originated from viruses endogenous (or xenotropic) to mice.

Malignant lymphoma

One of the most common malignant neoplasms in the animal kingdom, malignant lymphomas kill large numbers of animals and man. They appear as solid, fleshy, white masses that destroy the architecture of lymphoid organs and develop in parenchyma of viscera (Fig. 12.2). The malignant cells vary from normal-appearing, small, lymphocytelike cells to large blastic cells (Fig. 12.3). When lymphoma cells disseminate through the bloodstream, the disease is called lymphoid *leukemia.* The white blood cell counts of leukemic animals may exceed 100,000 WBC/mm^3.

Some lymphoid tumors are leukemic, even though space-occupying lesions are not found. In contrast, some animals with large tumor masses never become leukemic. The pathogenetic factors responsible for release or peripheralization are not known.

Feline leukemia

Feline leukemia virus (FeLV) causes several neoplastic and nonneoplastic diseases in cats (Table 12.6). Persistent viremia precedes clinical evidence of disease, and FeLV antigens can be detected in circulating leukocytes with an indirect immunofluorescent antibody test. Cats showing antigens may be healthy or may have any of the FeLV-associated diseases. Resistance to and recovery from FeLV disease depend on two separate responses of the host: one toward the infecting virus, as antibodies to *viral envelope* antigens prevent viremia, and one toward tumor antigens, as antibodies against the *feline oncornavirus–associated cell membrane antigen* (FOCMA) correlate with resistance to oncogenicity.

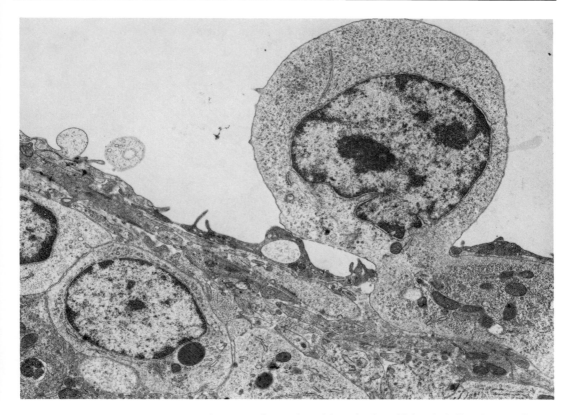

Fig. 12.3. Separation of hepatic sinusoidal endothelium by a malignant lymphocyte, chicken with lymphoid leukosis. Other lymphocytes are in intersinusoidal spaces (*bottom left*).

Feline leukemia is transmissible.

The first successful transmission experiments of feline leukemia were done by Dr. William Jarrett, in Glasgow, and were soon repeated in several laboratories. FeLV virions were identified in tumor tissue both extracellularly and

Table 12.6. Diseases associated with feline leukemia virus

Neoplastic diseases
  Lymphosarcoma (common)
  Erythroleukemia
  Erythremic myelosis
  Myelogenous leukemia (rare)

Nonneoplastic diseases
  Immunodeficiency (thymic atrophy)
  Anemia (nonregenerative)
  Glomerulopathy (immune complex)
  Abortion/fetal resorption syndrome
  "Panleukopenialike" syndrome

with cells, usually budding from the surfaces of cells. They were most prevalent in bone marrow, thymus, lymph node, and spleen. In cells of the circulating blood, virions occur on platelet surfaces. Megakaryocytes serve as a reservoir of virus. When young kittens are first infected, thrombocytopenia occurs as a direct effect of virus and may provide an early clue to the preleukemia states.

Experimental infection of germ-free kittens with FeLV results in persistent viremia. Kittens fail to produce an effective immune response to either FeLV envelope antigens or FOCMA and usually die from malignant lymphoma (although the resulting disease depends on the strain of FeLV inoculated). Dr. Edward Hoover, now at Colorado State University, showed that the pathogenesis involves progressive appearance of FeLV antigens in circulating monocytes, neutrophils, and platelets in both local and systemic lymphoid tissues and in bone marrow, cells, and (eventually) epithelium of the oropharynx and gut. When adult cats are inoculated with FeLV, 85% develop self-limiting infection with transient (or absent) viremia. Macrophages are especially susceptible to infection. Corticosteroids, silica, and some carcinogens suppress macrophages and render adult cats more susceptible to infection.

FeLV is most active in immunosuppressed cats.

Induction of leukemia in cats is related both to FeLV and to immunologic abnormalities in the host. When kittens are inoculated with FeLV, radiation increases the percent of animals that develop lymphoma. Predisposing factors involved in natural disease are largely those associated with immunosuppressive disease that occurs in kittenhood.

FeLV is itself immunosuppressive.

This attribute is necessary in the prodromal stages of infections for lymphosarcoma to develop. The marked depression of T-lymphocyte activity that occurs during FeLV viremia is caused by activity of an envelope protein of the virions called p15E. FeLV-induced immunosuppression also renders cats susceptible to other infectious agents. Cats with lymphosarcoma have a much higher incidence of severe anemia induced by *Hemobartonella felis* than do non-FeLV-bearing cats. In the preneoplastic phases of experimental disease, significant depression of cell-mediated immunoreactivity occurs and thymic atrophy is prominent.

Feline lymphoma occurs in clusters.

FeLV can be passed genetically from parent to offspring. One cat can infect another with this virus. When one cat in a household of several cats develops the disease, unrelated associates are apt to come down with it. By examining platelets for the presence of FeLV, Dr. William Hardy, at the Sloan-Kettering Institute, found that of almost 1500 healthy cats from disease-free households only 2 carried FeLV. In contrast, 177 of 543 cats from households with lymphosarcoma carried FeLV, and many of these subsequently developed the disease. These infected cats were followed for several months; it was found that 24% died with feline lymphosarcoma within the next 6 months. FeLV is present in blood, saliva, and urine, and cats spread the virus during fighting and mating (which involves biting and scratching). Grooming with the tongue and multiple use of litter boxes may also be involved in spread of the virus.

Feline leukemia involves mixtures of B and T cells.

Feline leukemia occurs in four variants, each with distinct sites of cell replication and routes of migration through lymphoid tissues (Table 12.7). The malignant cells are mixtures of B and T lymphocytes. In individual cats, the malignant cells may be predominantly lymphoblastic, prolymphocytic, histiocytic, or lymphohistiocytic. There is little correlation between the cell type and the clinical course of the disease.

Table 12.7. Types of feline lymphosarcoma

Form	Primary Involvement	Occurrence
Alimentary	Mesenteric lymph nodes	Most common
Multicentric	Generalized Lymph node, para-cortical areas	Common
Leukemia	Bone marrow Splenic red pulp	Uncommon
Thymic	Thymus Anterior mediastinum Lymph node, para-cortical areas	Least common

Myeloproliferative disease of cats

Poorly characterized neoplastic syndromes involving bone marrow proliferation occur in cats. The most common of the feline myeloproliferative diseases is *granulocytic* (myelogenous) *leukemia*. The proliferating marrow seeds the body with immature-appearing, malignant granulocytes (which contain small, dense granules typical of progranulocytes). The less differentiated cells are often associated with FeLV virions. In spleen, cells infiltrate the pulp cords, sparing germinal centers until late in the disease. This is in contrast to lymphoid leukemia, which involves the germinal centers first. In liver, periportal areas are first infiltrated, with subsequent replacement of parenchymal cells.

The other myeloproliferative diseases are *erythremic myelosis* (malignant transformation of the red blood cell series), *erythroleukemia* (a mixture of neoplastic granulocytes and erythrocytes), and *reticuloendotheliosis* (proliferation of primitive mesenchymal cells in bone marrow and spleen). Like granulocytic leukemia, these diseases are associated with severe refractory *anemia,* undifferentiated cells in the circulation, and infiltration of cells into tissues.

The etiology of the myeloproliferative diseases is not established. Although FeLV may be causal, other feline retroviruses have been implicated (Table 12.8). It probably bears the same relationship to feline neoplastic disease that RSV bears to lymphoid leukosis in chickens. A feline C-type virus, *feline endogenous virus* (RD114), has been isolated but not proven to be involved in neoplasia.

Feline fibrosarcomas are associated with viruses.

The *feline sarcoma virus,* which shares antigens with FeLV, is associated with solid tumors in cats. After inoculation of feline sarcoma virus into kittens, tumors arise in over three-fourths of the animals. Rapidly growing masses tend to have loose, myxomatous patterns of stellate cells with vacuolation and pleomorphic nuclei. The more slowly growing tumors are compact and have fusiform-shaped cells with elongate nuclei.

Lymphosarcoma of cattle

There are two forms of bovine malignant lymphoma: enzootic bovine lymphosarcoma and sporadic bovine lymphosarcoma (with thymic, cutaneous, and multicentric forms) (Fig. 12.2). The first is associated with bovine leukemia virus (BLV); infected cattle develop progressive lymphocytosis, which precedes development of lymphosarcoma, and carry antibodies to BLV. Animals with the second form do not have antibody to BLV.

BLV is an exogenous RNA oncogenic virus first discovered by Dr. Janice Miller, then at the University of Wisconsin. Its target cell is the B lymphocyte, in which proviral DNA is integrated into the host cell genome. After infection by BLV, cattle develop antibodies to at least four structural proteins of the virus. One of these, a glycoprotein of the virion envelope, provokes antibodies that neutralize viral infections.

BLV causes persistent lymphocytosis in calves.

Experimental infection of cattle with BLV produces persistent elevations in the lymphocyte count in about one-third of animals inoculated. The excess lymphocytes are a subpopulation of B cells that are transformed but cannot produce virus (they undergo spontaneous blastogenesis when cultured in vitro). The second, smaller population produces virus but is not involved in lymphocyte production. A strong genetic influence determines whether individual animals will develop persistent lymphocytosis. The development of lymphosarcoma after experimental infection is rare, and BLV is much more oncogenic in sheep; this was first seen in 1961 by Enke as enzootic lymphosarcoma in German sheep that had been vaccinated with bovine blood against piroplasmosis. Lymphosarcoma has been reproduced in sheep using various preparations containing BLV.

Lymphosarcoma in chickens is caused by two viruses.

Avian leukosis viruses (ALV) are a large group of retroviruses that induce various hematopoietic and mesenchymal tumors in chickens (of which *lymphoid leukosis,* a neoplastic disorder of T cells, is by far the most common). Host response is determined by both viral genome and

Table 12.8. Feline retroviruses

Group	Designation	Characteristics
Feline leukemia virus	FeLV	Chronic leukemogenic viruses; provirus is in genome of infected cat
Subgroup A		Grows only in cats
Subgroup B,C		Grows in cells of other species
Xenotropic endogenous feline retrovirus	RD114	Complete genome present in virus
Acute transforming	Sarcoma	Induce neoplasms with short latency period; transform cells in culture. Genomes contain FeLV-related sequences and transformation specific sequences (*v-onc*). Four different *v-onc* genes have been found in ATTR: *v-fms, v-fes, v-sis,* and *v-abl.*
Feline T-lymphotropic virus	FTLV	?

host cell. Marek's disease (MD) virus, a herpesvirus, induces lymphomas of T cells in chickens. Both viruses have a high incidence of infection but a low one of tumor development.

ALV-induced lymphosarcoma is characterized by foci of white, solid tumors in the bursae, liver, and spleen. Other organs are affected, and the clinical appearance is related to muscle wasting, anemia, and hepatosplenomegaly. Neoplastic lymphoid cells are large stem cells with large nucleoli and few cytoplasmic organelles. Malignant cells are of the B lineage, and large amounts of IgM may be produced. Virions may be found budding from the cell surfaces but are not readily detectable in natural tumors. ALV exerts its oncogenic effect by interrupting the switch from IgM to IgG that occurs in the cell of the normal bursa.

The *myc* gene is abnormal in lymphoid leukosis.

In tumor cells the cell locus *c-myc* has been interrupted by insertion of ALV DNA sequences; that is, a LTR with properties of a transcription promoter is inserted within the "normal" cell genome. The viral LTR causes an increase in expression of *c-myc* (and increased amounts of the *c-myc* gene product can be detected). A second locus *b-lym* is important in lymphoma development, but how it interacts with the *c-myc* gene is not known.

The bursa is the target organ of ALV.

When newly hatched chicks of a susceptible strain are inoculated with an oncogenic isolate of ALV, transformation of lymphoid cells in the cloacal bursa occurs at about 6–8 weeks of age. By 10–16 weeks transformed follicles are visible in nearly all birds, and metastasis from the bursa to viscera occurs around the time of sexual maturity at 20 weeks. Lymphoid leukosis is a neoplastic B cell transformation and requires the bursa for development.

The initial change in bursal follicles involves uncontrolled replication of B cells, which form isolated gigantic follicles. These compress and distort adjacent follicles and eventually spread to involve the entire bursa. The process is confined to the bursa for 2–4 weeks but then disseminates throughout the chicken (Fig. 12.4).

Bursectomy prevents dissemination of neoplastic B cells.

Obliteration of the cloacal bursa prior to transformation (by bursectomy, chemotherapy, or

lytic viral infection) destroys the capacity of the virus to induce lymphoid tumors (thymectomy has no effect on the disease). Even after the tumor has localized in the bursa, removal of this organ will suppress the dissemination of the tumor cells and the incidence of leukosis. In other words, a bursectomy at 12 weeks of age will prevent the occurrence of lymphosarcomas in the liver and spleen even though the neoplastic process has already been initiated within the bursa.

Virus replicates in female reproductive tracts.

ALV is transmitted to offspring vertically. In natural conditions, ALV passes from hen to chick via the egg. In the hen, virions are demonstrable in the ovary and oviduct. They bud from the plasma membrane of cells in direct contact with the oogonia and germinal epithelium. Large numbers of virions are also in the albumin-secreting glands of the magnum of the oviduct. They bud from surfaces of microvilli into the lumen, and the zygote is exposed to high concentrations of virus in the magnum while it is still a single cell.

When the chicken embryo is infected, the chick appears immunologically tolerant to ALV and does not develop antibodies. At hatching, most chicks are viremic, although a variable percentage will not have virus. Virions are demonstrable in most tissues, especially in liver and kidney.

In infected flocks, maternal antibody is present in newly hatched chicks, but it gradually disappears and is gone in 4–6 weeks. These chicks may become infected by carrier birds, but the incidence of tumors is suppressed by antibodies and by some unknown factor associated with aging of the chick.

ALV also causes sarcomas.

In natural lymphoid leukosis, the expression of viral infection depends on the availability of certain target cells and the degree to which the viral RNA is homologous to the long DNA sequences in host cells. The mode of transmission influences the availability of target cells. In *vertical* transmission (dam to offspring), viral DNA is uniformly distributed among most tissues of the neonate. *Horizontal* infection after hatching results in increased viral DNA only in tissues with many dividing target cells. The expression of oncogenicity may therefore involve (1) myeloblasts and their precursors that give rise

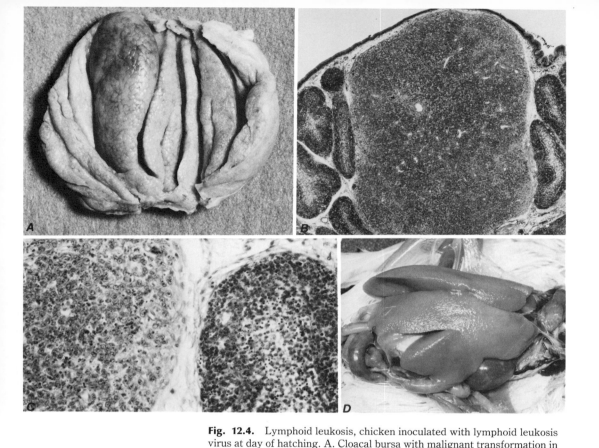

Fig. 12.4. Lymphoid leukosis, chicken inoculated with lymphoid leukosis virus at day of hatching. A. Cloacal bursa with malignant transformation in single focus at 6 weeks of age. B. Histology of A: malignant follicle expands into adjacent follicles, which are atrophic. C. Follicle with malignant cells (*left*) next to atrophic follicles with necrosis of central lymphocytes (*right*). D. Massive expansion of liver and spleen due to metastasizing cells 20 weeks after inoculation.

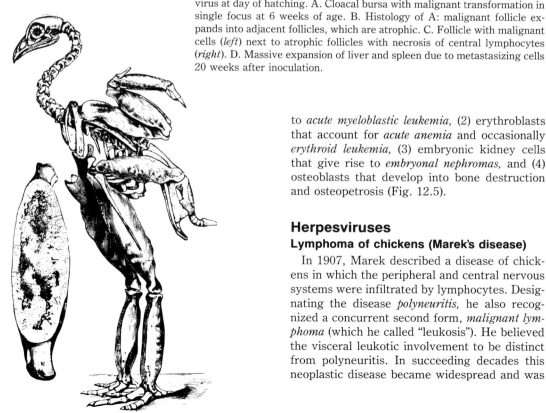

Fig. 12.5. Avian osteopetrosis, skeleton of chicken.

to *acute myeloblastic leukemia,* (2) erythroblasts that account for *acute anemia* and occasionally *erythroid leukemia,* (3) embryonic kidney cells that give rise to *embryonal nephromas,* and (4) osteoblasts that develop into bone destruction and osteopetrosis (Fig. 12.5).

Herpesviruses
Lymphoma of chickens (Marek's disease)

In 1907, Marek described a disease of chickens in which the peripheral and central nervous systems were infiltrated by lymphocytes. Designating the disease *polyneuritis,* he also recognized a concurrent second form, *malignant lymphoma* (which he called "leukosis"). He believed the visceral leukotic involvement to be distinct from polyneuritis. In succeeding decades this neoplastic disease became widespread and was a major cause of mortality in the domestic chicken until a vaccine using a nononcogenic turkey herpesvirus was developed.

When MD herpesvirus is injected experimentally, the first changes occur in lymphoid tissue and include lymphocyte destruction and atrophy, with subsequent infiltration of pale, large reticulum cells. Virus then replicates in epithelium of feather follicles and is transmitted from bird to bird by skin flakes in dust aerosols. Infected epithelial cells are hyperplastic and contain intranuclear inclusions composed of naked virions.

Some infected chickens develop minimal lesions in the nervous system; lesions do not progress but regress into an inflammationlike condition dominated by edema, with plasmacytes scattered throughout the spongy nerve tissue.

Frog renal carcinoma

Large, multilobular metastasizing renal adenocarcinomas occur in 2–5% of frog populations in some parts of North America. Large, dense nuclear inclusion bodies develop in tumor cells (composed of herpes virions). Tumors can be induced in susceptible frogs by injection of a suspension of tumor.

The renal adenocarcinoma herpesvirus infects frog eggs when they are developing in the water in spring. Carcinomas appear in the third or fourth summer of the frog's life. These "summer tumors" do not produce virus but contain viral genetic material. During the summer months the tumor grows and may expand to kill the frog. If it does not, tumor growth ceases at hibernation in the autumn. As the tumor cells cease their growth cycles, they become virogenic; that is, they produce infectious virions that lyse the tumor cell. Virus is excreted into the urine and, with the end of hibernation, is expelled into the pond water where it infects eggs and tadpoles during the spring season.

Growth of the frog herpesvirus is temperature-dependent. This has been shown in the laboratory, where tumor cells can be converted from a virus-free summer state (in which the viral genome is present but unexpressed) to a virus-containing state by merely lowering the environmental temperature of the host frog.

Malignant lymphoma in primates

Herpesvirus saimiri is indigenous and noncytopathic in squirrel monkeys (*Saimiri sciureus*). It originally grew out of degenerating primary kidney cells cultured from a healthy squirrel monkey. When injected into into other squirrel monkeys, no disease developed. However, a rapidly progressive malignant T cell lymphoma (of the reticulum cell type) developed when the virus was injected into other New World monkey species, such as owl (*Aotus* spp.), spider, and marmoset (*Saguinus* spp.) monkeys. The disease has a very rapid course of 13–28 days.

Drs. Ronald Hunt and Norval King, at the New England Regional Primate Center, have shown that the neoplasm produces extensive invasion of many organs. Lungs, liver, kidney, adrenals, and lymphoid organs are all affected. The fundamental change is proliferation and invasion of tissue by neoplastic reticulum cells. Herpesviruses cannot be seen in tissue even though the viral genome is present in infected cells. In recent studies on a *H. saimiri* variant virus that had lost its oncogenic potential, a region of the viral genome was identified that is required for oncogenicity (but not for viral replication).

Papovaviruses
Papillomas

Infectious papillomas (e.g., warts and verrucae) are virus-induced hyperplastic lesions of epithelium. They are not neoplasms. They regress naturally due to a systemic, cell-mediated immunologic reaction directed against the infected cells. Once regression begins, papillomas at all sites regress simultaneously. Regressing papillomas contain lymphoid aggregates, and regression is inhibited by immunosuppression.

Several animal species have multiple types of papillomaviruses (which are distinguished by restriction endonuclease cleavage patterns and degree of nucleotide sequence homology). The bovine papillomavirus types include types 1 and 2 in cutaneous fibropapillomas (widespread), type 3 in cutaneous papillomas (rare), type 4 in alimentary tract papillomas, and type 5 in teat papillomas. Papillomas of teats may also be caused by type 4, and it is probable that type 4 is transferred to the alimentary tract of calves by suckling of infected teats.

Because of a peculiar host cell–viral genome interaction, a small number of papillomas in cattle, rabbits, and man may undergo malignant transformation. The classic rabbit papilloma of Shope, when in natural infections of wild cottontail rabbits, contains large amounts of virus and rarely developed neoplastic changes. Conversely, experimental papillomas in domestic rabbits had much less virus but a greater propensity to undergo malignant transformation.

Alimentary tract papillomatosis of cattle

Widespread in the United Kingdom, this disease is associated with alimentary tract carcinomas in upland areas of Scotland. Cattle grazing bracken fern are affected by its toxins in a way that makes them susceptible to the oncogenic effects of bovine papillomaviruses.

Bovine papillomavirus causes equine sarcoid.

This locally aggressive connective tissue tumor of the dermis is composed of characteristic whorling patterns of fibroblasts (resembling neural sheath tumors of other animals). Its epidemiologic pattern suggests an infectious nature, and classically it was considered to have spread from horse to horse on harnesses. Equine sarcoids tend to recur after surgical excision; they can be transplanted from one site to another on individual horses but not between horses. In the 1950s Dr. Carl Olson suggested that this tumor was caused by bovine papillomavirus and produced sarcoids in horses by inoculating them subcutaneously with bovine papillomavirus. Recently, DNA sequences of bovine papillomavirus have been shown in natural sarcoids (although they are not integrated into the host cell genome).

SV_{40} virus is a potential primate oncogenic virus.

SV_{40} causes a natural infection of monkeys where it is associated with destruction of renal tubules and inclusion bodies. It is also oncogenic in laboratory rodents and is considered a potential human oncogenic virus. In the 1950s, when human poliomyelitis vaccines were prepared from monkey kidney cell cultures, SV_{40} was inadvertently given to millions of young children (see Chapter 25), but no tumors were ever associated with this episode.

SV_{40} is widely used by experimental oncologists to study the role of genes of DNA viruses in producing cancer (in particular, how viral genes might interact with normal cellular genes to produce tumors). SV_{40}-induced tumor cells produce a specific tumor antigen (*T-antigen*) on their surfaces (that is not associated with virion structural proteins). T-antigens are present on proteins encoded by SV_{40} genes during the infectious cycle. During conversion of normal to neoplastic cells, the segment of the viral genome that encodes the T-antigen proteins integrates into host cell chromosomes to become inherited genetic material.

Hepadnaviruses

These hepatotropic DNA viruses cause acute and chronic liver disease in man (hepatitis B virus), Pekin ducks (duck hepatitis virus), woodchucks (woodchuck hepatitis virus), and other rodents. In chronic persistent infections, there is an association with hepatocellular carcinoma. Dr. Lois Roth, at Cornell University, showed that of 15 woodchucks infected with WHV, 15 had chronic hepatitis and 13 of these had a primary hepatocellular carcinoma. There is a strong correlation between the presence of HBV antigens and incidence of human hepatocellular carcinoma. Viral antigens have been demonstrated in tumor cells. Integration of duck hepatitis virus into carcinoma cells has been established.

Possible virus-induced tumors
Pulmonary adenomatosis

This transmissible disease of sheep is characterized by slowly progressive respiratory distress and emaciation but no loss of appetite or orientation. Lungs are large, mottled, and frothy, and the condition is often complicated by secondary bacterial infection. Solid foci may be scattered over the surface as in typical pulmonary carcinoma. Histologically, the lesions of pulmonary adenomatosis consist of dense, disorganized collections of epithelial cells that distort the normal lung parenchyma and grow into and along the alveolar septa. Proliferating cells are derived from type 2 (granular) pneumocytes. The lesions are viewed as neoplastic on the basis of their structural resemblance to adenomas and because they expand progressively to kill the host. In rare cases, similar epithelial masses occur in the bronchial and mediastinal lymph nodes. Metastatic lesions have also been seen in skeletal muscle, kidney, and peritoneum.

Nasal adenocarcinoma of sheep

Adenopapillomas (or adenocarcinomas of the nasal cavity of sheep) have been reported as epizootics in various countries. They are composed of well-differentiated epithelial acini and villous projections. The tumors grow into the nasal cavity, the frontal sinus, and the pharynx. Extension to the cranial cavity has occurred due to pressure atrophy of bone. Metastases are not evident. In the 1950s the German veterinary pathologist Paul Cohrs transmitted this tumor by cell-free filtrates, but the nature of the agents involved has not been clarified.

Equine cutaneous histiocytoma

This rare disease of horses is characterized by large proliferative lesions composed of small lymphocytes and large macrophages (Fig. 12.6). It is classified as a malignant lymphoma of the reticulum cell type. The disease progresses to kill the horse, usually with no metastatic lesions. In all cases to date a peculiar coryneform bacterium has been isolated from these lesions. The pathogenesis of the disease is not known.

Tumors associated with parasites
Canine esophageal sarcoma and *Spirocerca lupi*

A correlation between the presence of sarcoma of the esophagus and infection with *Spirocerca lupi* has been established in certain geographical areas. This peculiar parasite encysts and causes granulomas in or near the esophagus of the dog. Elsewhere, highly destructive lesions may be responsible for aortic aneurysms and ossifying spondylitis. In a small percentage of cases, a sarcoma develops. The tumors are malignant and are often disseminated. Metastatic foci occur in lymph nodes and lung. The mechanism of tumor induction is not clear, but experimental work on a similar model in rats (liver sarcomas caused by infection with the larvae of *Taenia taeniaeformis*) show that secretions of this cestode cause fibroblastic hyperplasia and appear to be oncogenic.

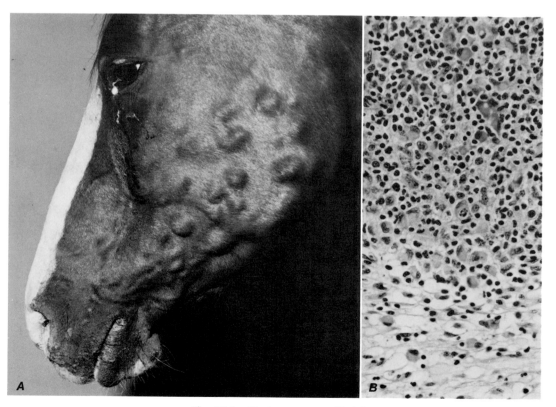

Fig. 12.6. Equine cutaneous histiolymphocytic lymphoma. A. Nodules in various stages of growth in dermis. B. Nodules are composed of malignant small lymphocytes and large numbers of histiocytelike cells.

ADDITIONAL READING

Ames, B. N. Dietary carcinogens and anticarcinogens. *Science* 221:1256, 1983.

Hoover, E. A., et al. Host-virus interaction in progressive versus repressive feline leukemia virus infection. *Cold Spring Harbor Symp.* 7:635, 1980.

Jarrett, W. F. H. Transformation of warts to malignancy in alimentary carcinoma. *Bull. Cancer* 65:1914, 1978.

Klein, G., and Klein, E. Evolution of tumors and the impact of molecular oncology. *Nature* 315:190, 1985.

Miller, J. M., and Van der Maaten, M. J. Bovine leukosis: Its importance to the dairy industry in the United States. *J. Dairy Sci.* 65:2194, 1982.

Pamukcu, A. M., et al. Lymphatic leukemia and pulmonary tumors in female Swiss mice fed bracken fern (*Pteris aquilina*). *Cancer Res.* 32:1442, 1972.

Snyder, R. L., et al. Chronic hepatitis and hepatocellular carcinoma associated with woodchuck hepatitis virus. *Am. J. Pathol.* 107:422, 1982.

Todd, G. C. Induction and reversibility of thyroid proliferative changes in rats given an antithyroid compound. *Vet. Pathol.* 23:110, 1986.

Waldmann, T. A., et al. Molecular genetic analysis of human lymphoid neoplasms. *Ann. Int. Med.* 102:497, 1985.

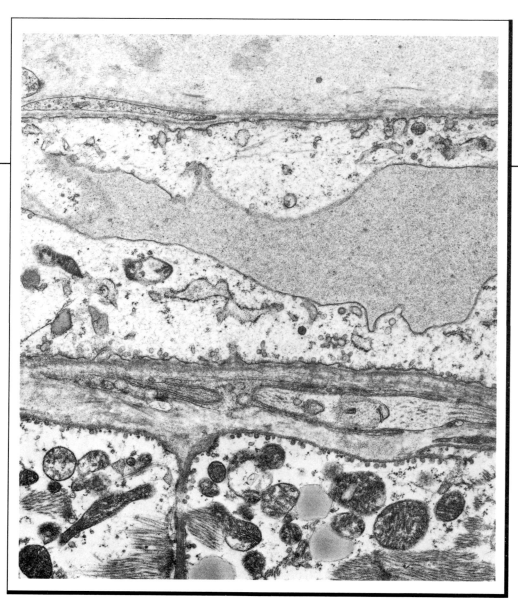

Capillary, heart, dog with congestive heart failure.

BLOOD AND THE VASCULAR SYSTEM

4

YOUR understanding of how fluids pass from tissue into the vascular system and back again will affect how well you understand disease and its treatment. Changes in blood vessels are associated with virtually every serious disease. Edema, heart failure, shock, thrombosis, and inflammation are life-threatening processes, and all are caused by or lead to alterations in endothelium and the vascular wall.

The enormous volume of the *capillary bed* is dwarfed by an even greater capacity to expand under the influences of the nervous system and of vasodilatory substances. Capillaries, which are not innervated and do not have encircling muscular layers, are sites where fluid exudes from circulating blood. In this section, how these tiny blood vessels react to injury is discussed in detail.

Endothelial cells constantly synthesize glycoproteins and secrete them onto their luminal surfaces. Lying like a blanket over the endothelium, these glycoproteins are exposed to flowing blood and act to inhibit clotting and to protect the delicate junctions between endothelial cells. When endothelium is injured, synthesis and release of these glycoproteins is diminished, causing defects in hemostasis and fluid transport. Just as injured epidermis fails to protect underlying subcutis, injured endothelium does not permit normal transport of needed substances into and out of tissue. If circulation of blood is altered, this endothelial defect may be the straw that breaks the camel's back by leading to ischemia and its attendant tissue injury.

In capillaries, substances are transported across the endothelial cell in three ways: (1) *direct diffusion* (e.g., ions, water, and very small molecules passively diffuse across the vessel wall); (2) *active transport,* which occurs via special protein ion pumps embedded in the plasma membranes at the cell surface (i.e., charged particles cannot pass the cell's plasma membrane and must be moved into and out of cells via membrane proteins that function as active pumps); and (3) *endocytosis* and *exocytosis,* in which tiny vesicles on the luminal surface of the endothelium take up materials, pinch off from the surface, and carry materials across the cytoplasm to exit at the basal surface (the capillary on the facing page, from a cat with cardiac failure, has a marked increase in plasmalemmal vesicles). In edema and other disturbances of fluid balance, *expansion of cell junctions* occurs to allow large molecules and fluids to pass into the interstitium.

Arterioles and venules regulate blood flow through the capillary bed. *Precapillary arterioles* contain small myocyte sheaths that are innervated and that contract to control blood flow. Pharmacologic manipulation of these arterioles is important in indirectly controlling the exudation of fluids in the vascular bed. *Postcapillary venules* are extraordinarily susceptible to some toxins and, along with capillaries, are sites of fluid exudation.

Regional differences in capillary permeability depend on structural variation in the vascular wall. Studies on transport kinetics show that permeability to macromolecules varies in limbs, intestine, liver sinusoids, and brain. Restricted transport in capillaries of the brain, the *blood-brain barrier,* is due to very tight intercellular junctions reinforced by covering of the capillaries by astrocyte foot processes. In contrast, the bone marrow sinusoidal endothelium is exceptionally open to passage of both soluble and particulate material.

Cyclic changes occur in vessels of some endocrinologically controlled organs. For example, endothelium of capillaries of the uterine mucosa are flattened and relatively structureless in sexually inactive females. They become markedly enlarged and filled with ribosomes on stimulation with progesterone during the mating season.

Blood pressure exerts an effect on passage rates of low-molecular proteins. When hypertension is induced experimentally, there is evidence that protein tracer molecules pass into tissue in massive amounts. This implies a loss of barrier function in endothelium under high pressure.

13

Disorders of Blood Volume and Fluid Balance

FLUIDS OF INTERSTITIAL TISSUE

Total body water consists of fluid of plasma, fluid of interstitial tissue spaces, and intracellular fluid. The distribution of fluids between these compartments is a carefully controlled homeostatic mechanism, and deviations from normal have profound effects on the body. Plasma fluid can be manipulated directly by intravenous fluid therapy, and thus both interstitial and intracellular fluid can be indirectly controlled.

Interstitial fluid, the "milieu interne" of Claude Bernard, is the intermediary through which all metabolic products pass to enter or leave the cells. It is in constant exchange both with plasma and with cellular fluids. Maintenance of its normal volume is the sum of two sets of forces having contrasting action (Fig. 13.1).

(1) Forces promoting passage of fluid from intravascular plasma into the interstitium: (a) hydrostatic pressure of the blood and (b) osmotic pressure of interstitial fluid.

(2) Forces promoting passage of fluid in the

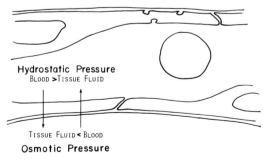

Hydrostatic Pressure
BLOOD >TISSUE FLUID

TISSUE FLUID< BLOOD
Osmotic Pressure

Fig. 13.1. Forces draining fluid from and into the capillary.

opposite direction, from interstitium to plasma: (a) osmotic pressure of blood and (b) hydrostatic pressure of tissue fluids.

These forces operate normally only when blood vessels and lymphatics are intact. Endothelium along with its underlying basement membrane permits free passage of water and ions but opposes passage of plasma proteins. It is the most vital element in the maintenance of blood volume.

In *healthy mammals* the hydrostatic pressure at the arteriolar end of the capillary bed is about 35 mm Hg. At the venular end it is 12–15 mm Hg. The oncotic pressure of the plasma is approximately 20–25 mm Hg (rising slightly at the venular end as fluid escapes in the arteriolar end and returns in the venular end). In *edema* there is expansion of interstitial fluid or accumulation of fluid in body cavities (e.g., the pleural and peritoneal cavities).

EDEMA

Edema (Gr. *oidema,* swelling) is the abnormal accumulation of excess fluid in interstitial tissue spaces or in body cavities. Edematous tissue, when examined grossly, is wet, gelatinous, and heavy. In several species, fluids are slightly yellow, especially if proteins have exuded. Microscopically, tissue spaces are distended by eosinophilic albuminous fluids. Hyperemia is often obvious, and lymph vessels are always dilated.

There are two major types of edema, inflammatory and noninflammatory (Table 13.1). This section concerns noninflammatory edema, in which fluids move into tissue spaces because of oncotic and hydrostatic pressure changes. Edema fluid closely resembles lymph. In this type of edema, the fluid is "protein poor," characterized as a *transudate;* that is, it has a low protein content and a specific gravity below 1.012.

In inflammatory edema, endothelial damage leads to increased capillary permeability. The transudate is rapidly converted to an *exudate* that is high in protein and specific gravity. The massive edema of the subcutis in severe burns and trauma are characterized by exudation of large amounts of albumin and fibrinogen.

Edema results when the forces that move fluid from the vascular lumen to the interstitium are augmented over those producing the reverse effect. Starling's law states that hydrostatic pressure in the vascular system (aided slightly by perivascular osmotic pressure) moves fluid out of the system (Fig. 13.1). The forces holding the fluid within the blood are osmotic pressure of the plasma proteins and, to a lesser extent, tissue pressure around blood vessels.

Local edema

Edema may be general or local. Local noninflammatory edema is nearly always due to *lymphatic blockade* or *impaired venous drainage*. The normal flow of interstitial fluid into lymphatics is prevented, and edema fluid accumulates locally. This type of edema is associated with lymphatics damaged by surgery, neoplasms, and in-

travascular parasites. Causes of generalized edema, such as chronic cardiac failure or reduced osmotic pressure of plasma, do not cause local edema.

Rare hereditary malformations of the lymphatic vessels occur in dogs, calves, and pigs. Because of blockade in the lymph vessels, the diseases are manifested as local subcutaneous edema of the limbs.

Generalized edema

Generalized edema occurs most often in one of two basic mechanisms: increased hydrostatic pressure of blood or decreased colloid osmotic pressure of plasma proteins. Decreased levels of plasma proteins are seen in chronic blood-loss anemia, in chronic renal disease (with loss of albumin in the urine), and in starvation. When protein levels in plasma fall below 5%, the potential for edema is present. Fluid is usually found in the subcutis of the cervical areas and around the legs. In large animals, several liters of fluid may accumulate in interstitial tissue spaces before edema is obvious clinically.

The sites of edema are important factors in both diagnosis and prognosis. In most tissues, fluid does not have immediate clinical significance to the patient. In lungs and brain, however, edema may rapidly produce severe disease and even death. Fluid in locations that relate to severe clinical affection often have special desig-

Table 13.1.   Causes of edema

Mechanism	Clinical Example
Inflammatory	
Increased endothelial permeability	Burns
	Trauma
	Surgery
	Infection
Noninflammatory, systemic	
Increased hydrostatic pressure	Congestive heart disease
	Pericarditis/myocarditis
	Severe liver disease
Reduced oncotic pressure of plasma	Malnutrition
	Gastroenteritis
	Glomerulonephropathy
Increased osmotic pressure of interstitial fluid related to sodium retention	Reduced renal perfusion
	Increased tubular resorption
Noninflammatory, local	
Lymphatic obstruction	Neoplasia
	Inflammatory scarring
	Congenital absence of lymphatics
Impaired venous drainage	Trauma

FOCUS

Plasma proteins and edema

The individual net charges of plasma proteins are used to separate them by electrophoretic migration. In the electrophoresis unit, a small sample of plasma is placed on paper wetted with buffer and migration is induced by opposing electrical charges at the ends of the paper strip. Proteins on the paper are then stained and the pattern is transposed to graphic form, the *electrophoretogram,* by a sensitometer. The percentage of each plasma protein can be calculated by partitioning the peaks on the electrophoretogram and calculating the various percentages from the total plasma protein concentration. For practical purposes, the protein most affected in edema and hypoproteinemia is albumin.

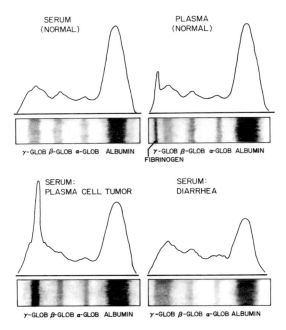

The albumin molecule, at 69,000 MW, is the smallest of the major plasma proteins. It regulates the exchange of water between blood and tissue and is a major factor in maintaining osmotic regulation; each gram percent of serum albumin exerts osmotic pressure of 5.5 mm Hg. Albumin also acts as a buffer because it is amphoteric and can combine with both acids and bases.

Albumin levels in blood do not rise above normal except during hemoconcentration or dehydration. Hypoalbuminemia is a common finding in edema and in other acute diseases such as glomerulonephritis and protein-losing diarrhea, in which the albumin molecules escape from the vascular system. Reduced plasma protein concentration is reflected in the lower peak of albumin in the electrophoretogram.

Albumin is synthesized in the liver and can be detected in hepatocytes by a specific fluorescent antialbumin antibody stain. Developed in late gestation, albumin production by hepatocytes peaks soon after birth. With growth, albumin production declines but in plasma protein–losing diseases such as cirrhosis and nephritis, all hepatocytes again convert to albumin production.

nations: *anasarca,* swelling of the subcutis due to severe generalized edema; *hydrothorax,* fluid in the thoracic cavity; *hydropericardium,* fluid in the sac around the heart; and *hydroperitoneum,* fluid in the peritoneal cavity.

Anasarca occurs in cardiac failure.

When edema is severe and generalized and causes diffuse swelling of all tissues, it is called *anasarca.* Anasarca is especially prominent in the subcutis of some species. In progressive cardiac failure, generalized edema is nearly always present. Fluid seeps into the body cavities and subcutaneous tissues, particularly in the limbs. Because the heart cannot pump the amount of blood received from the veins, venous pressure rises and is transmitted to the capillary bed, where fluid exudes.

Endothelial cells of capillaries and veins involved in stasis are swollen and cell organelles disoriented. Fluid and protein precipitates disrupt the basement membranes and pericapillary spaces. In the end stage of cardiac failure, capillaries of the myocardium are involved in edema; tiny vesicles accumulate at both sides of the endothelial cell and are evidence of the cell's attempt to increase the flow of fluid from interstitium to blood vessel (see the facing page to Part IV). In these final stages of cardiac failure, other secondary problems are superimposed on the capillaries. Retention of chlorides by the kidney aggravates the already existing edema. The continued escape of protein lowers the osmotic pressure of blood and raises that of tissue, enhancing fluid exudation.

Ascites

The intraperitoneal accumulation of fluid involves retention of sodium ions and water, hypoalbuminemia, and decreased colloid osmotic pressure. Ascites is not mediated solely by increased hydrostatic pressure in all species (e.g., experimental ligation of the portal vein in dogs does not cause remarkable accumulation of fluid in the peritoneal cavity).

Pulmonary edema

Pulmonary edema is accumulation of edema fluid in alveoli of the lungs. It is brought about by excessive amounts of plasma exuding into alveoli from the capillary bed of the lung. In the earliest phases, fluid accumulates in the interstitium of the alveolar wall, where it disrupts the

basement membranes of the endothelial cells and pneumocytes. The first histologic evidence of edema appears perivascularly. Fluid is rapidly drained along connective tissue fibers to perivascular cuffs leading to lymph vessels.

Two major mechanisms are involved in the causation of pulmonary edema: (1) *circulatory failure-induced changes in pulmonary hemodynamics,* which result in a slow exudation of fluid into alveoli, and (2) any sudden diffuse and direct *damage to pulmonary capillary endothelium.* The latter is usually a peracute stage of inflammation and, if the animal survives, is followed by pneumonitis. Both of the above conditions are associated with marked capillary dilation; the distinction between extreme hyperemia and pulmonary edema is often arbitrary.

Pulmonary edema associated with cardiac failure is inevitably chronic. Lymph flow increases, lymphatics enlarge, and the alveolar walls become thickened. Hyperplasia of granular pneumocytes is common, and these cells may line the alveoli. In long-standing pulmonary edema, collagen is deposited in the alveolar walls, diminishing the resiliency of the respiratory lobules (Fig. 13.2).

Edema of the brain

Edema of the brain is seen in trauma to the calvarium, obstruction of venous outflow, and intracranial infections (meningitis, brain abscess, and encephalitis). At necropsy, the brain is heavier than normal. Sulci are narrowed, and gyri are swollen and become flattened by con-

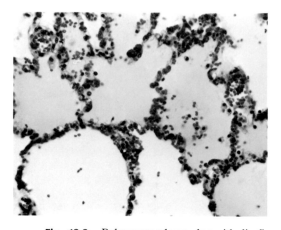

Fig. 13.2. Pulmonary edema, dog with dirofilariasis (*Dirofilaria immitis*).

tact with the skull. On section, white matter is gelatinous and appears softer than normal. The external layer of the gray matter is widened. Histologically, there is expansion of the perivascular (Virchow-Robin) spaces, which are seen as clear halos in the neuropil around blood vessels (Fig. 13.3).

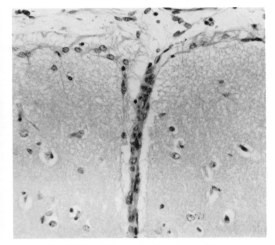

Fig. 13.3. Edema, brain, dog with acute encephalitis caused by *Escherichia coli* (see Fig. 1.6). Water accumulated in the neuropil makes the tissue section pale and causes spaces around blood vessels to expand.

SHOCK

Introduction

Shock is the syndrome resulting from a disproportion between *blood volume* and *volume of the circulatory system* that needs to be filled, that is, an acute generalized failure of the capillary bed. The fundamental disturbance is that blood volume is too small to fill the vascular system. The accompanying cell damage is due to *inadequate perfusion of tissue* that directly causes *hypoxia.*

Shock is most often due to one of three events: blood loss, reduced cardiac output, or loss of peripheral vasomotor control. Death may occur at any phase of shock; its attendant damage is due to circulatory failure in the central nervous system, myocardium, and other organs.

Loss of blood pressure is a common finding in shock. Arterial blood pressure is maintained normally by a proper amount of blood in the system, by adequate cardiac output, and by total vascular peripheral resistance. Shock may follow marked depression of any of these mechanisms. It is an ominous sign, often terminating in death, despite treatment.

Animals in shock are lethargic and unresponsive to external stimuli. Muscle weakness is a prominent sign. Body temperature is apt to be subnormal (because of lowered metabolism), and there is pallor and coolness of the skin. Heart rate is increased in most types of shock but may be slow and irregular. Depression of renal function and urine production often occur.

Because shock can be caused by diverse types of injury, the clinical appearances cannot be rigidly defined. Factors such as pain, cold, general anesthesia, hypoproteinemia, dehydration, and exhaustion do not cause shock directly but do augment the mechanisms that cause circulatory collapse. Trauma impairs thermoregulation, and in the presence of a cold environment, body temperature and oxygen consumption both fall, suppressing mechanisms that operate to overcome the shock state.

Cytopathology

Tissue lesions of shock are a result of hypoxia. As a consequence of inadequate peripheral circulation, there is decreased oxygen delivery. Hypoxia leads to decreased oxidative phosphorylation and ATP production in cells, and mitochondria degenerate. Pyruvate cannot enter the citric acid cycle; as a result cells are forced to obtain energy by anaerobic glycolysis. Lactate accumulates and leads to metabolic acidosis. Thus in the terminal stages of shock a metabolic disease accompanies the circulatory deficiency. Although hyperglycemia is characteristic of early shock (related to catecholamine release), hypoglycemia occurs in the later stages due to depletion of liver glycogen and hyperinsulinemia. During shock there is a prolongation of insulin half-life due to reduced peripheral utilization.

Pathogenesis

The brain and heart are highly susceptible to hypoxia generated by a fall in blood pressure; foci of necrosis and hemorrhage develop in these organs in most species. Tissues vary in the amount of oxygen removed during blood flow. While the average is approximately 25%, myocardium removes 75% of the oxygen of blood flowing through the capillaries of the heart. When cardiac output is diminished by one-fourth and blood oxygenation is reduced, as happens in shock, the total oxygen transported to the heart cannot meet the requirement of myocardial metabolism (Table 13.2).

Counterregulatory mechanisms are activated during shock regardless of the cause; they are evoked by low blood pressure and diminished cardiac output (via pressure receptors). These mechanisms stimulate the sympathetic nervous system to produce *peripheral vasoconstriction* and *tachycardia*. Hemodynamic alterations of the pulmonary circulation reduce the active ventilatory surface, resulting in hypoxic stimulation of respiratory centers in the brain. Catecholamine output, stimulation of the renin-angiotensin system, and activation of the sympathetic nervous system maintain blood flow to critical organs. Flow is increased to heart, brain, kidney, and lungs at the expense of reduced flow to peripheral tissues such as skeletal muscle and skin.

Progressive deterioration of the circulatory system occurs in massive burns and blood loss despite these compensatory mechanisms. The designation *irreversible shock* implies the refractory state of circulatory failure with inability to control the disease clinically. When blood is removed from a dog in sufficient quantity to produce shock and is not replaced for 4 hours, the dog will enter a shock state that cannot be reversed despite total restoration of blood volume. The infused fluid or blood seems to be seques-

tered in the peripheral capillary beds, suggesting that there is vasomotor paralysis of the microcirculation, caused in part by hypoxia.

Hypovolemic shock

This is shock due to loss of blood volume. A common cause is massive loss of whole blood during hemorrhage, called *hemorrhagic shock*. Loss of blood volume can also occur deceptively when large amounts of plasma exude into tissue, as happens in severe burns and crush injuries.

Extensive blood loss is required before animals develop hypovolemic shock. Healthy animals may lose one-fourth of their blood volume without showing immediate clinical signs, and loss of one-half the blood volume may be required to produce death. When much blood is lost, the arterial blood pressure drops and venous return to the heart decreases. The heart rate may increase, but stroke volume and cardiac output are diminished.

Vasoconstriction is a rapid response to hypotension.

Arterial vasoconstriction produces increased peripheral resistance, which shunts blood from the skin and viscera to the heart and brain. The interacting mechanisms that enhance vasoconstriction include (1) *lessened stimulation of baroceptors* in the aortic arch and carotid sinus, which decreases the afferent vasodilatory and

Table 13.2.   Lesions of shock in the dog

Organ	Gross Appearance	Microscopic Lesions	Mechanism
Liver	Congested Swollen	Hyperemia of sinusoids Serous exudation (in spaces of Disse)	Constriction of myocytes of hepatic vein and increase in portal venous pressure
Intestine	Hyperemia Hemorrhage (blood in feces)	Hyperemia of villi Subepithelial edema Necrosis and sloughing of villous tips	Elevated portal venous pressure
Stomach	Hyperemia	Mucosal erosions	Hypoxia, back diffusion of H^+
Heart	Hyperemia Subendocardial hemorrhage	Focal necrosis of cardiac myocytes	Hypoxia (also medial necrosis of aorta); inadequate coronary artery blood flow
Lung	Hyperemia Edema (rare)	Hyalin thrombi in capillaries	Vascular stasis, intravascular platelet aggregation or coagulation
Adrenal	Hyperemia Hemorrhage (rare)	Foci of necrosis and hemorrhage	?
Muscle	Pale	Foci of necrosis	Vasoconstriction, hypoxia

cardioinhibitory neural discharges; (2) *vagal and vasomotor discharge* from the medulla oblongata; and (3) *release of catecholamines* from the adrenal medulla. Norepinephrine constricts peripheral vascular beds; epinephrine constricts most of these and dilates the coronary arteries. Vasoconstriction initiated by the early outpouring of catecholamines is maintained by the renin-angiotensin system.

If arterial blood pressure is measured during and after extensive blood loss, two plateaus in the pressure curve occur (Fig. 13.4). The first, which begins during blood loss, is due to pressoreceptor reflexes. These produce strong sympathetic stimulation (and parasympathetic inhibition) to blood vessels when the arterial pressure begins to fall. The response is vasoconstriction and contraction of the spleen, spewing erythrocytes and platelets into the blood. These compensatory mechanisms are blocked by general anesthesia; animals whose reflexes have been so removed lose arterial pressure from the onset of blood loss. Another later and more powerful plateau is the central nervous system ischemic reflex. This reflex is activated when arterial pressure drops enough to cause brain ischemia.

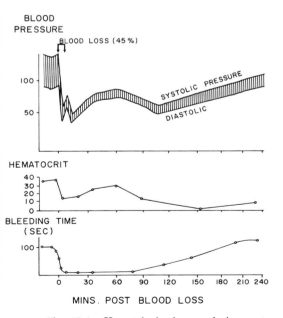

Fig. 13.4. Hematologic changes during acute hemorrhage.

Blood

Hemorrhagic shock causes slow capillary blood flow, which depletes oxygen and favors aggregation and sludging of erythrocytes. Slow flow instantly affects tissue pH, which may fall below 7.0 (even though lungs blow off CO_2 and tend to produce an early transient alkalosis). Severe capillary acidosis with endothelial injury and release of clotting factors may lead to immediate and striking *hypercoagulability* (Fig. 13.4).

Platelet surfaces become sticky in shock, so platelets tend to aggregate. Platelet-leukocyte microemboli are found in blood removed from dogs with hypovolemic shock. Although hemorrhagic shock produces hypercoagulable blood, intravascular coagulation does not occur unless clot-initiating factors are released. These factors are more common in shock involving bacterial toxins and the massive thromboplastin release in trauma and burns.

As blood is lost, tests on blood for the packed cell volume (*hematocrit*) show decreased values (Fig. 13.4). As blood cells are sequestered in the expanded pulmonary capillaries, there are also decreases in circulating leukocytes (*leukopenia*) and platelets (*thrombocytopenia*). Cell damage in hypoxic tissues is reflected in increased amounts of certain cellular enzymes in plasma; that is, β-glucuronidase, creatine phosphokinase, and other enzymes seep out of damaged cells into the circulation. There is a positive correlation of amounts of these enzymes with the severity of shock.

Lung

Dogs in hypovolemic shock have lungs that are wet, solid, and frothy, usually with tiny hemorrhages near the surface. Pulmonary edema and increased pulmonary vascular resistance occur because of trapping of platelets and leukocytes in the capillary bed (if trauma has occurred, megakaryocytes may also be found in capillaries of the lungs). As capillaries of the alveolar walls are obstructed, vascular endothelium swells and enhances the edema.

As platelets disintegrate within the pulmonary capillaries, they release vasoactive factors and chemoattractants. Neutrophils are attracted and degranulate at these sites to release lysosomal enzymes that damage tissue. *Platelet-leukocyte emboli* may detach from the capillary walls and be released into the circulation. Fibrin is not a major component of the microemboli, probably because of mast cell histamine release and the intense activation of the pulmonary fibrinolytic system that occurs in shock.

Liver

The liver is a prominent organ affected in shock of the dog. Constriction of veins within the liver raises the portal venous pressure and causes stasis in both the liver and intestine. Because of the hypoxia associated with stasis, hepatocytes degenerate, resulting in failure of effective detoxification. Kupffer cells fail to remove macromolecules. Bacteria, endotoxins, and split products of fibrinolysis, which arrive in the liver from the portal vein, are allowed to pass into the general circulation.

In shock, liver cells must adapt to hypoxia associated with decreased blood flow. The first few hours of massive blood loss are characterized by hyperglycemia, increased blood lactate, and decreased blood pyruvate, all evidence of the switch to anaerobic glycolysis by the hepatocyte. *Mitochondrial degeneration,* a result of hypoxia, is an early hepatocellular lesion of shock.

Kidney

The effects of extensive loss of blood volume produce profound changes in the kidney (Fig. 13.5). Renal vasoconstriction reduces perfusion and causes the juxtaglomerular cells to degranulate. Plasma renin concentration rises and activates the angiotensin system. *Angiotensin tends to raise the falling blood pressure* by causing peripheral vasoconstriction. It also stimulates the secretion of *antidiuretic hormone* (ADH, or vasopressin) by the pituitary, which acts to conserve water normally lost from the lower nephron. *Aldosterone* secretion by the adrenal cortex is augmented, leading to increased resorption of salt and water by the renal tubule. All these mechanisms conserve fluid and support blood volume.

Small amounts of dilute urine are produced in hypovolemic shock. The decreased glomerular filtration and oliguria (reduced urine output) are consequences of increased renal vasoconstriction. Loss of urine-concentrating ability is related to the decreased medullary sodium osmotic gradient.

Heart

Myocardial damage in hemorrhagic shock consists of two types of lesions: *subendocardial hemorrhage and necrosis* due to hypoxia (which mimics lesions produced by exogenous catecholamines) and *zonal lesions* deep in the myocardium caused not by hypoxia but by the heart beating strongly and rapidly at very low ventricular volumes. Zonal lesions of necrosis, unique to hypovolemic shock, are foci of supercontracted areas within myocytes that involve several sarcomeres, located adjacent to intercalated disks. They show severe sarcomeric narrowing, fragmented Z bands, dislocated mitochondria, and distorted myofibrils. Foci of myocardial necrosis is common in dogs with shock due to pooling of blood in the intestinal tract. Experiments in dogs have shown that zonal lesions are produced only in a hypovolemic situation with low end-diastolic volume, intense sympathetic stimulation, and increased force and rate of the heart.

Adrenals

Adrenals are markedly hyperemic. As blood loss becomes severe, epinephrine rises promptly in circulating blood. Degranulation of adrenalin-producing cells of the adrenal medulla occurs within a few minutes and progresses to total degranulation with vacuolar degeneration as hypotension becomes critical (norepinephrine-producing cells are little changed). If endothelial damage is superimposed on shock (as in septic or toxic shock), adrenal glands become hemorrhagic with foci of necrosis.

Gastrointestinal tract

Hyperemia and mucosal erosions occur throughout this tract in hemorrhagic shock (Fig. 13.6). As the intestine becomes hypoxic, it releases vasoactive serotonin into the portal circulation, which enhances alterations in blood vessels. Mucin biosynthesis is diminished by hypoxia, and loss of the mucosal barrier exposes mucosa to proteases that initiate erosions.

In severe shock, tips of intestinal villi may become necrotic because the villous countercurrent mechanism is bypassed; oxygen is shunted from the large central capillary of the villus directly to the descending peripheral capillaries and does not reach the villous tips. Although blood flow to the villi is not markedly changed, the villous tips become ischemic.

Skeletal muscle

Peripheral vasoconstriction induced by catecholamines such as adrenalin quickly leads to pale muscle. In prolonged hemorrhagic hypoten-

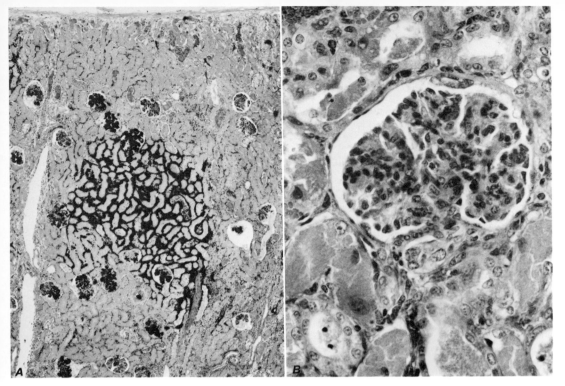

Fig. 13.5. Renal lesion in shock, sheep with anaphylaxis. A. Infarction with dark hemorrhages in infarcted zone. B. Necrotic tubules in infarct.

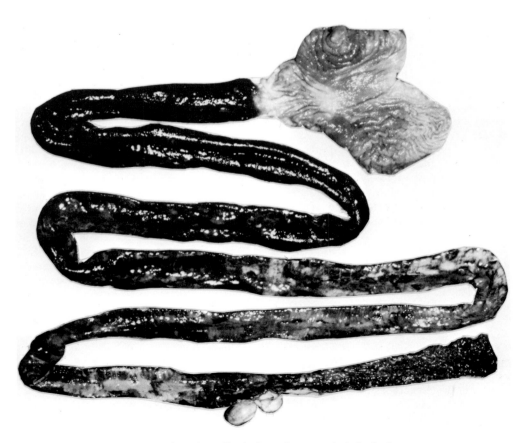

Fig. 13.6. Gut lesions of postsurgical shock, dog.

sion, skeletal muscles may vasodilate, chiefly due to hydrogen and potassium ions released into surrounding interstitial spaces after mild hypoxia. These ions stimulate capillary dilation.

Shock caused by pooling of blood

Expansion of the capillary bed beyond the capacity of blood to fill it results in shock. Vasodilation is a potent mechanism for reducing arterial blood pressure. When the splanchnic blood vessels are fully dilated, they have the capacity to accommodate nearly the total blood volume. If this occurred, blood pressure would drop to zero. Normally, continual vasoconstriction of the terminal arterioles prevents this from happening. However, toxins and other substances that cause peripheral vasodilation may lead to the shock state. This type of shock, common in animals, is seen particularly in septic conditions.

Toxic shock

Toxic shock is mediated by toxins released from damaged tissue, venoms, and microbial endotoxins that cause vascular paralysis. It commonly accompanies severe burns and intestinal gangrene. The mechanism is decreased cardiac output and arterial pressure secondary to sequestration of venous blood in the hepatosplanchnic bed. Severe injuries may be accompanied by release of hepatic lysosomal hydrolytic enzymes in a free, active form; elevation of acid phosphatase may accelerate the appearance of shock.

Major effects of *burn shock* occur in kidneys and lead to oliguria and dilute urine. As blood flow to the kidney is reduced, both glomerular filtration and tubular function are suppressed. This occurs within minutes after burn injury (before hypovolemia develops), initiated by nervous system control on renal function.

Gangrene of the gastrointestinal tract promptly leads to shock. In dogs, an important cause is gastric dilatation and volvulus. Release of vasoactive factors into the circulation from necrosis of gastric mucosa initiates pooling of blood and hypotension. Shock is enhanced by subsequent compression of the posterior vena cava and portal vein by the engorged stomach and by acidosis.

Experimental *tourniquet ischemia* shock is an example of a generalized vascular response to local tissue destruction. Products from ischemic tissue enter the circulation and cause circulatory collapse. Widespread vascular damage with release of kinins, prostaglandins, and histamine dilates blood vessels throughout the body. The systemic effect of local ischemia is confirmed in cross-circulation experiments in which a dog is traumatized by blows to the hindlimbs while a connected dog is not injured. The normal dog goes into shock and dies a few minutes before the traumatized dog.

Shock in bacterial disease

Lysis of gram-negative bacteria releases potent cytotoxic lipopolysaccharides of the bacterial cell wall called *endotoxins* (see septicemia, Chapter 21). Endotoxins adsorb to surfaces of endothelium, erythrocytes, leukocytes, platelets, and mast cells. They induce plasma membrane defects that cause both cell degeneration and release of biologically active substances that produce the clinical signs of endotoxic shock. These signs include, in addition to vasodilation and circulatory collapse, fever, coagulation, thrombocytopenia, and leukopenia. In contrast to hypovolemic shock, endotoxic shock is manifest by intense activation of the coagulation, fibrinolytic, kinin, and complement systems. The critical organ is the lung; lesions involve microthrombi and vascular leakage in both alveolar capillaries and bronchial veins. After the experimental intravenous injection of endotoxin, there is a precipitous decline in arterial blood pressure, with simultaneous elevation in portal venous return and cardiac output. Examination of the splanchnic veins 1 hour later reveals marked congestion and dilatation. Venous pooling plays a highly significant role in endotoxic shock. In dogs, pooling in the hepatic-portal system is responsible for a significant decrease in venous return of blood to the heart.

Slow capillary flow and release of thromboplastic substances from damaged endothelium trigger intravascular coagulation, and fibrin is deposited throughout the vascular system. The fibrinolytic system is activated, degrading fibrin into split products, which may prevent serious coagulation problems. However, if endotoxemia is severe and sustained, *disseminated* intravascular coagulation may develop. This disastrous condition has two important effects: depletion of coagulation factors, or "consumptive coagulopathy," and multifocal infarction caused by microthrombi in vessels of kidney, heart, and liver (see hemostasis, Chapter 14).

Platelet aggregation (with incorporation of neutrophils) has immediate and disastrous effects in the lung. Platelet-leukocyte-fibrin thrombi obstruct the capillary bed and induce hypovolemic shock. Endotoxin-induced leakage of bronchial veins augments the already serious interstitial edema. Acute death in shock of gram-negative septicemia is usually due to respiratory failure. In clinical cases treated with anticoagulant therapy, fibrin may not be deposited in large amounts due to the combined effects of heparin and naturally occurring fibrinolysis.

Pathologic changes in other organs may also lead to death. In *kidney,* the combined effects of hypotension and capillary injury may lead to necrosis (Fig. 13.5). Peritubular capillaries are particularly damaged and show acute tubular necrosis in the renal cortex. Endothelium of capillaries and venules of the *brain* often show severe extravasation. Early serious effects on the *heart* are complicated by edema of the heart valves.

In *liver,* sludged erythrocytes and microthrombi occlude and damage sinusoidal endothelium. Since sinusoids are further blocked by swollen Kupffer cells and endothelium, flow of blood may be reversed from the hepatic artery into the portal vein. Parenchymal cells of all these organs are affected by the metabolic defect in shock. After the initial period of hyperglycemia, the progressively developing hypoglycemia and hypoinsulinemia of canine endotoxic shock are associated with impending death.

It may be important to distinguish two pathways in which endotoxin produces injury: (1) gram-negative bacteremia, in which both circulating and phagocytized bacteria are killed, releasing cell wall fragments, and (2) endotoxemia, in which endotoxin, generated by intestinal bacteria, penetrates the mucosa to enter the portal venous system, producing an initial effect on the liver. (Because endotoxin is difficult to assay, this second mechanism is still hypothetical).

Septic shock (exotoxic shock) occurs in any overwhelming infection caused by cocci and other gram-positive bacteria. It is therefore essential that blood pressure be maintained in severe systemic infections. Blood viscosity increase is a factor that may reduce blood flow to the capillary bed.

Shock is likely in severe systemic viral disease.

Viruses that replicate in endothelial cells tend to be associated with severe, often fatal, systemic disease, and most of these viral diseases terminate in shock (e.g., simian hemorrhagic fever, epidermic hemorrhagic disease of deer, and equine viral arteritis). The collapse and death that characterize terminal stages of equine viral arteritis are due to a fatal sequence of events: capillary necrosis, increased vascular permeability, loss of intravascular plasma volume, hemoconcentration, and finally hypotension. Other factors such as thrombocytopenia, decreased prothrombin levels, adrenal necrosis, and lymphocyte depletion play roles in the process, but the hypovolemic shock is the most important factor in mortality.

Other types of shock

In addition to the two principal patterns of shock, there are less important ways in which shock syndromes occur. The varying adjectives applied to shock indicate the complexity of reactions leading to the final common pathway.

Neurogenic shock

Neurogenic shock occurs in animals with severe fright, pain, and trauma (without hemorrhage). It is commonly seen in restrained wild birds and mammals, especially in cold weather. Animals enter a shock state mediated by the nervous system, that is, nervous stimulation that induces peripheral vasodilation, which leads to loss of effective circulating blood volume.

Shock accompanying severe crush injury involves neurogenic shock. If tourniquets are applied to limbs crushed experimentally, external fluid loss is prevented but not circulatory collapse (if nerves remain intact). In contrast, sectioning of the nerves, even without the tourniquet, prevents shock. Neurogenic shock is true circulatory collapse and should not be confused with fainting.

Cardiac shock

Cardiac shock occurs due to the precipitous decrease in cardiac output that accompanies sudden extensive damage to the heart. Most animals succumb directly to myocardial inadequacy. In those rare animals that do not, shock may ensue because of pooling of the blood in capillary beds.

Anaphylactic shock

Anaphylactic shock is circulatory collapse accompanying the binding of antigens to cell-bound antibodies. It is mediated through the massive intravascular release of histamine, which induces increased arteriolar and venous dilation. Clinical signs are greatly reduced arterial pressure and venous return of blood to the heart. The syndrome may be complicated by immune complex–induced platelet aggregation, trapping of aggregates in the lung, and increased pulmonary vascular resistance.

ADDITIONAL READING

Crandall, E. D. Recent developments in pulmonary edema. *Ann. Int. Med.* 99:808, 1983.

Davies, A. P., et al. Primary lymphedema in three dogs. *J. Am. Vet. Med. Assoc.* 174:1316, 1979.

Meyrick, B. L., and Brigham, K. L. The effect of a single infusion of zymosan-activated plasma on the pulmonary microcirculation of sheep. *Am. J. Pathol.* 114:32, 1984.

Nordstoga, K., and Aasen, A. O. Hepatic changes in late canine endotoxin shock. *Acta Pathol. Microb. Scand.* [A] 87:335, 1979.

Pietra, G. G. New insight into mechanisms of pulmonary edema. *Lab. Invest.* 51:489, 1984.

Staub, N. C., and Taylor, A. E. *Edema.* New York: Raven Press, 1984.

14

Infarction, Circulatory Defects, and Ischemia

INFARCTION

Infarction is a local area of ischemic necrosis in a tissue caused by occlusion of the arterial supply or venous drainage. Infarcts are classified on the basis of color (white or red) and bacterial contamination (bland or septic). *White infarcts* lack blood (they are also called "anemic"); in contrast, *red infarcts* are filled with blood and usually contain hemorrhages. The amount of blood that escapes into the oxygen-deprived area is determined by age of the infarct, type of injury, and type of tissue. Most infarcts are hemorrhagic initially but become pale in a very short period. White infarcts usually have a red zone at the periphery, since capillaries at the border of the infarct undergo dissolution and blood seeps into the area of necrosis.

Most infarcts result from thrombosis or embolism. Viruses that produce endothelial damage commonly cause thrombi, which expand to block arterioles and to cause infarction in organs with end-arteries (kidney, heart, and spleen). Multiple causes are often involved; for example, an artery whose endothelium is injured by viral disease is more prone to be blocked by emboli arising from distant sources.

Infarcts tend to be wedge-shaped; the base of the wedge is at the periphery with the occluded vessel at the apex (Fig. 14.1). The margins of the infarct may be irregular, a reflection of the vascular supply from adjacent, nonaffected tissue. Initially, infarcts are ill defined and hyperemic (hemorrhage occurs in organs with loose parenchyma). By 48 hours, most infarcts become progressively paler. At necropsy, infarcts of the kidney are usually white (ischemic). In contrast, lungs usually develop red (hemorrhagic) infarcts.

Within the infarct, the parenchyma undergoes ischemic coagulation necrosis, providing that the animal survives for several hours (Fig. 14.2). All tissues are affected, including blood vessels, mesenchymal cells, and nerves; there is no regeneration. If the infarcts arise from septic emboli, the infarcted area may be converted into an abscess (which may not even be recognized as an infarct at necropsy). Ultimately, infarcts are replaced by scar tissue, which forms an indentation over the surface of the organ.

The consequences of a block in a muscular artery depend on a combination of several factors; that is, it determines whether infarction occurs and how serious that infarct will be for the host. The most important factor is the *degree of injury to the vascular supply*—whether a large artery is affected, whether the artery is totally blocked, and whether blood vessels surrounding the affected area can expand to supply the tissue. Other factors that affect infarction include the *rate of development* of the infarct, the *vulnerability of the cell types* involved, and the *oxygen-carrying capacity of the blood* at the time of infarction. Infarcts are larger in anemic animals than in normal animals.

Embolism

Embolism is the sudden blocking of an artery or vein by an obstruction that has arrived in the bloodstream. The consequence of an embolus is infarction. Emboli can be composed of many materials although the most frequent sources of emboli are thrombi. Many of the causes of thromboemboli and infarction are systemic infections in which endothelium has been injured; thrombi then form, and thromboemboli are discharged into the flowing blood.

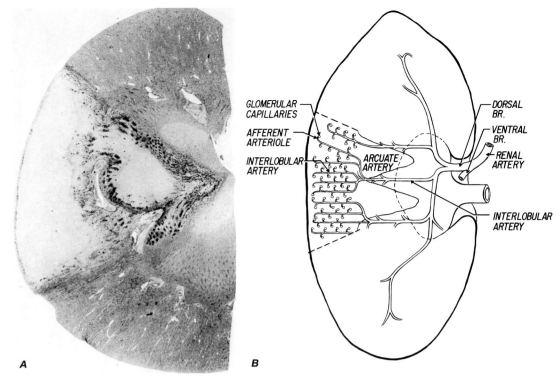

A

B

GLOMERULAR
CAPILLARIES

AFFERENT
ARTERIOLE

INTERLOBULAR
ARTERY

ARCUATE
ARTERY

DORSAL
BR.

VENTRAL
BR.

RENAL
ARTERY

INTERLOBULAR
ARTERY

Fig. 14.1. Infarction, kidney, pig. A. Pale infarct with hemorrhagic borders, infarct due to blockade of interlobular artery. B. Site of block in artery.

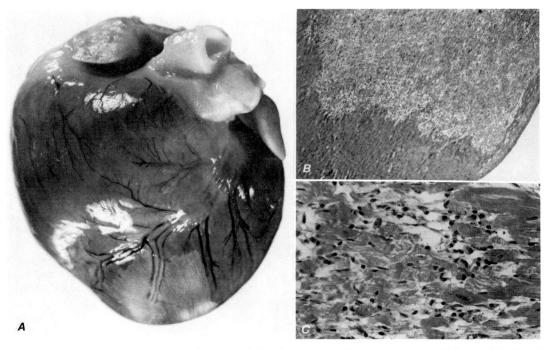

A

B

C

Fig. 14.2. Infarction, heart. A. Pale infarct at tip of left ventricle. B and C. Histology of infarcted area.

In cats, thromboemboli arising from valvular endocarditis lodge at the aortic bifurcation and in the origins of the iliac arteries. Clinical signs in cats with aortic emboli are cool and edematous limbs and lack of femoral pulse. If complete block of the arteries occurs, paralysis and shock are inevitable.

Parasite emboli commonly cause infarction.

Live and dead parasites that enter the bloodstream can cause infarction of the *lung,* as in the emboli caused by adults of *Dirofilaria immitis,* which reside in the right heart and pulmonary artery of the dog (see Fig. 13.2). These emboli may be dead adult parasites, groups of microfilaria, or thrombi that originate from parasite-induced erosions in the wall of the pulmonary artery. Ascarid larvae and other nematodes may lodge in the *brain* to produce foci of necrosis that end as abscesses containing dead parasites.

Infarction of the *intestine* is common in horses infected with larvae of *Strongylus* spp. These larvae invade, disrupt, and produce thrombi in endothelium of the mesenteric artery and its branches. Thrombi are the most common in the ileocecocolic branch of the cranial mesenteric artery; emboli arising from this site may be thrombi or emboli of parasitic larvae. Thromboemboli also lodge in the peripheral vasculature within the intestinal wall. Dr. Peter Little, at the Ontario Veterinary College, injected strongyle larvae into horses and found that aortic verminous thrombotic lesions gave rise to parasite emboli that lodged in blood vessels of the brain to produce *cerebral infarction.*

Fibrocartilagenous emboli cause spinal cord infarcts.

Infarction of the spinal cord caused by emboli of fibrocartilagenous material from ruptured intervertebral disks occurs in dogs, cats, horses, and man. Emboli lodged in arteries or veins of the leptomeninges and spinal cord cause a pattern of infarction and necrosis called *necrotizing myelopathy.* Material from the nucleus pulposus may herniate directly into venous sinuses or enter smaller arteries and pass back through the arterial system.

Fat emboli lodge in highly vascular tissue.

Fat emboli arise as a complication of bone fractures, prolonged surgery, or osteomyelitis. They seldom cause infarction. Although gross lesions are usually not obvious, capillaries in the lungs contain small masses of fat. The German pathologist Cohrs described retrograde embolism of fat (at slaughter) during the agonal period; when the jugular vein was opened for exsanguination, fatty tissue was sucked from the wound into the right atrium, inferior vena cava, and hepatic veins.

Fat emboli also lodge in the renal glomerulus, and in dogs, "lipid glomerulopathy" is a rare but fatal complication of trauma to fat tissue.

Systemic infections are associated with infarction.

Any disease that causes widespread damage to endothelium predisposes to infarction. Many bacterial diseases produce disseminated infection and septicemia in which vascular endothelium is damaged; thrombi obstruct the vascular system and tissue necrosis ensues (Fig. 14.3). In classic cases of hog cholera (swine fever), virus replicates in endothelial cells to produce marked vascular injury. Thrombi form at sites of viral injury in the arteries and arterioles and lead to occlusion of the blood vessel and infarction. Infarcts in hog cholera commonly occur in the spleen and intestine.

Obstruction of veins

Obstruction of veins is not apt to produce infarction but may cause slowly developing stasis with engorgement of the tributary venous system. The most serious effects result when the anterior or posterior vena cava is obstructed. The *vertebral vein system* is an alternate route for return of blood from body to heart, via anastomoses with anterior systemic veins and azygos veins that bypass the caval systems.

COLLATERAL AND COMPENSATORY CIRCULATION

Sudden total blockage of most any artery will produce infarction. If the block is incomplete, slowly progressive, or in an organ with anastomosing capillaries, however, collateral circulation will develop. When one *femoral artery* of the dog is experimentally ligated, transient lameness and edema may develop in the limb, but anastomosing vessels will enlarge and new channels will form to bypass the ligated artery. When the kidney is made ischemic by blocking

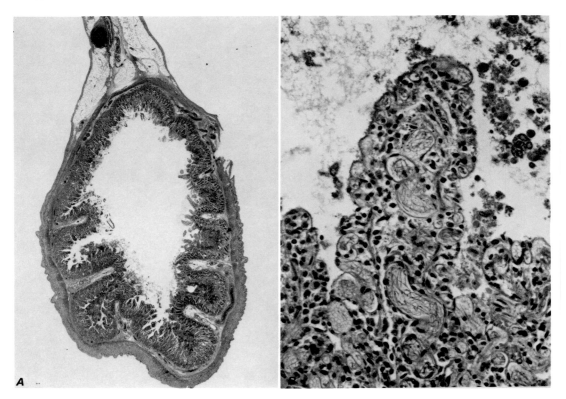

Fig. 14.3. Infarction, intestine, cow with *Corynebacterium equi* infection. A. Thrombus in mesenteric vein and necrosis of intestinal mucosa. B. Necrosis of intestinal villi with deposition of fibrin in capillaries. Epithelial cells have sloughed from the villous surface, leaving the capillaries of the tunica propria exposed.

the arcuate arterial system (intraarterial injection of latex beads is a common experimental model), new arterial channels develop from several neighboring vascular sources.

The greater the blood supply, the more rapidly collateral circulation develops. If the *right mammary* and *right external pudic arteries* are ligated in a young calf, circulation will be totally restored by adulthood. The vascular supply to gland tissue is completely supplied by surrounding vessels. At lactation, milk production in the right mammary glands will be identical to that in the left as the caudal branch of the left mammary artery fully restores the blood vessels of the right mammary gland.

Where alternative pathways of circulation exist, vascular blockage results in compensatory enlargement of what was a previously minor flow route. Bilateral blockage of the *common carotid arteries* of the dog shunts blood through vertebral arteries and also incites development of anastomotic connections of the internal carotid to the maxillary and ascending pharyngeal arteries.

Blockage of the portal vein

Blockage of the portal vein leads to infarction of the intestine. Animals with this condition rarely survive. In dogs, *gastric torsion* leads to striking obstruction of the portal venous system. Twisting at the pyloric and cardiac areas of the stomach blocks tributaries of the portal vein. Occlusion of the portal vein leads to severe venous congestion. Vascular stasis of the intestine causes ischemia, loss of endothelial integrity, and tiny hemorrhages along the veins at the mesenteric attachments of the gut wall (Fig. 14.4). Sudden complete block of the portal veins leads rapidly to shock.

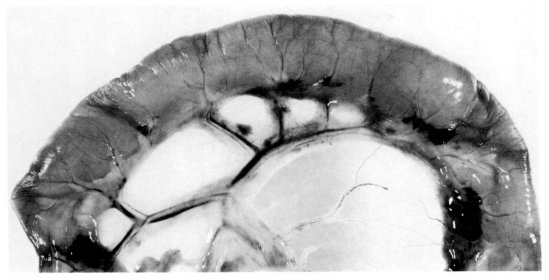

Fig. 14.4. Congestion and hemorrhage, small intestine, dog with gastric torsion. Intestine has hemorrhages along mesenteric border. Marked congestion of capillaries and venules of intestinal walls.

Blockage of the pulmonary artery

Obstruction of the pulmonary artery can accompany pneumonia, congenital heart disease, bronchiectasis, and parasite infestations. The pulmonary artery is commonly blocked in dogs with dirofilariases when dead worms lodge in the arterial wall, causing proliferative changes. In walls of affected pulmonary arteries, vasa vasorum are dilated proximal to and at sites of obstruction. As compensation, anastomoses develop between pulmonary artery and bronchial arteries (the bronchial arteries orginate from the 1st to 4th intercostal arteries and supply the hilar lymph nodes, vasa vasorum of the pulmonary arteries and veins, and bronchioles). In severe dirofilariases, the dilated tortuous bronchial arteries around the bronchial tree can be seen to terminate in branches in the periphery of lung lobes; this collateral circulation occurs most often in the right diaphragmatic lobe.

Blockage of the posterior vena cava

When the posterior vena cava is blocked (Fig. 14.5), blood is shunted into the azygos vein. In the dog, the single azygos vein begins at the

FOCUS

Gastric torsion

Torsion of the canine stomach leads to striking obstruction of the portal venous system by twisting at the pyloric and cardiac areas, resulting in blockage of tributaries of the portal vein (see the diagram). At the cardia, torsion of 180–360° occurs in a clockwise direction; the degree of torsion determines the extent of vascular obstruction. Although veins are obstructed, arteries often remain intact, leading to engorgement and stasis of the portal and vena caval systems.

▶

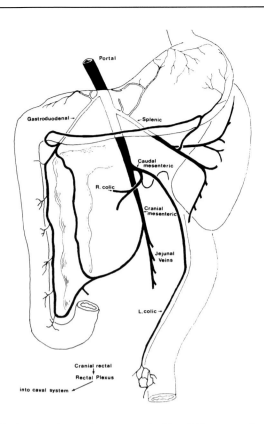

Gastric torsion is most common in Great Danes and other giant breeds (especially the males). It develops in the following progression: overeating → gastric dilatation → torsion of gastroesophageal junction → accumulation of fluid and gas. Early, the greater curvature moves ventrally (especially in deep-chested dogs), the gastrohepatic ligament becomes lax, and the pylorus is freed to move dorsally, cranially, and to the right—all preludes to *volvulus.* Gas accumulates largely from bacterial fermentation (stomach contents usually have the sweet odor of silage) although aerophagia and the action of HCl and H_2CO_3 also contribute.

Distension of the stomach has important secondary effects. (1) There is *direct pressure necrosis of gastric mucosa* due to vascular stasis, especially at the greater curvature of the fundus where small vessels anastomose with the left epigastric artery. The mucosa shows hyperemia, hemorrhages, edema, and necrosis (gangrene), probably due to histamine release and increased capillary permeability. (2) *Portal venous stasis* (Fig. 14.5) leads to hypoperfusion of viscera, causing release of prostaglandins and phospholipases. (3) Pressure on the thorax may precipitate *lung* dysfunction. (4) The *duodenum* is compressed. (5) The *spleen* is engorged from venous occlusion as it twists on its long axis.

Pressure on the *posterior vena cava* shunts blood through the vertebral veins, ventral vertebral sinuses, and azygos veins. Signs at this stage are extreme abdominal pain. Blockade of the gastroesophageal junction causes belching, retching (without vomiting), decreased venous return to the heart, and decreased cardiac output—a "slow-flow syndrome" that can precipitate intravascular coagulation.

third lumbar vertebra by confluence of intervertebral veins and has an anastomotic branch with the posterior vena cava (Fig. 14.6). It joins the precava at its termination in the right atrium opposite the third intercostal space. Although obstruction may cause edema of the limbs and engorged veins, many animals with extensive blockage of the posterior vena cava are asymptomatic. Enlargement of preexisting pathways gradually permits these vessels to compensate and normal tissue perfusion to occur.

VASCULAR SHUNTS AND FISTULAE

Portosystemic venous anomalies

Anomalous shunts between the portal vein and posterior vena cava are most commonly reported in dogs. When severe, the clinically important changes are central nervous sytem

signs, small liver, and high blood ammonia levels. Excretion of tracer dyes by the liver is delayed, and bile acids are increased in serum.

Reports of congenital venous anomalies in dogs in which portal blood bypasses the liver in its return to the right atrium include (1) persistent patency of the fetal ductus venosus; (2) atresia of the portal vein, usually with functional collateral portosystemic shunts; (3) anomalous connection of the portal vein to the caudal vena cava; (4) anomalous connection of the portal vein to the azygos vein; and (5) drainage of the portal vein and caudal vena cava into the azygos vein.

Hepatic injury leads to CNS signs.

In normal dogs the hepatic artery supplies about 25% of the blood to the liver; the remainder comes from the portal vein. In the 1870s Eck, experimenting with dogs, surgically shunted the portal blood into the posterior vena

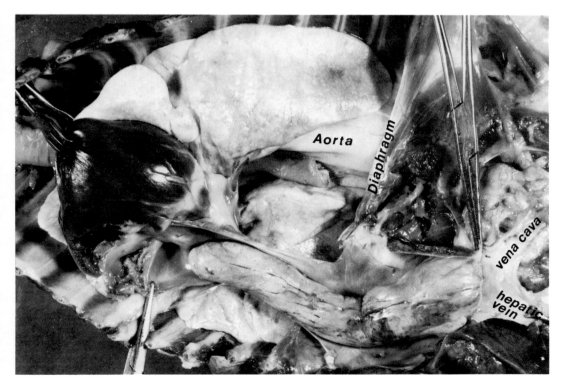

Fig. 14.5. Neoplasm obliterating lumen of posterior vena cava from emergence through diaphragm to entry into right atrium. The right ventricle is dilated, the left ventricle hypertrophic. The liver is massively enlarged, granular, and mottled.

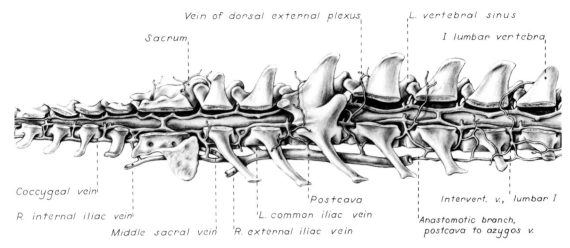

Fig. 14.6. Anastomotic branch of post cava to azygos vein, which markedly enlarges to permit survival in blockade of posterior vena cava. (Drawing: Karl Reinhard)

cava by creating a vascular fistula and ligating the portal vein at its entrance into the liver. He found that animals died within a few months with nervous signs and that there was an inverse relationship between the signs and the amount of food taken by the dogs. In the Eck fistula, the total hepatic blood flow is reduced to near 50% of normal despite a compensatory increase in hepatic arterial flow. The liver undergoes atrophy partly due to blood flow reduction and partly to loss of hepatotrophic factors (which arise from pancreatic and gastroduodenal sources) that are normally present in portal blood.

Hepatic encephalopathy is a disturbance in brain function associated with hepatic insufficiency.

The brain becomes progressively more sensitive to various exogenous and endogenous substances in chronic hepatic dysfunction. Affected animals are much more sensitive to hypoxia and electrolyte imbalance. Encephalopathy is associated with marked increases in blood ammonia, which arises in the colon. Normally NH_3 is absorbed and carried via the portal vein to the liver where it is incorporated into the ornithine cycle and converted into urea. In dogs with portal venous anomalies, serum NH_3 concentrations are from 2 to 11 times higher than normal. Methionine, amino acids, and short chain fatty acids have been reported as contributory to the CNS signs of hepatic encephalopathy.

Acquired portacaval shunts

During increased pressure in the portal venous system (portal hypertension), blood bypasses the liver and returns to the heart by various collaterals. As portal hypertension rises, blood begins to flow through channels that normally are not patent. For example, the *azygos vein* dilates and accepts blood from the portal system. Commonly, a complex of varices connecting the portal vein to the 13th intercostal vein (which drains into the azygos vein) can be seen in dogs with portal hypertension.

Varices between the cranial mesenteric vein and the caudal vena cava and the shunting of portal venous blood into the caudal vena cava via a patent ductus venosus can also be found in portal hypertension.

Portal hypertension arises from conditions such as carcinoma of the adrenal cortex growing into the caudal vena cava (Fig. 14.5), tumors of the right atrium of the heart, and liver disease, both posthepatic (obstruction of the hepatic veins) and prehepatic (obstruction of the portal veins).

Intrahepatic shunts
Portacaval shunts

Portacaval shunts occur when the portal vein ends in an aneurysmal dilatation in one of the liver lobes. Clinical signs are those of the portosystemic shunt further caudal, that is, high alkaline phosphatase, low blood urea nitrogen (BUN), and abnormal ammonia tolerance tests. Because the liver lacks glycogen, there is little or no rise in blood glucose after administration of glucagon (glucagon tolerance test).

Intrahepatic arteriovenous fistulae

Here there are communications between branches of the *hepatic arteries* and *portal venous radicles,* which result in retrograde flow into the portal vein. Most arteriovenous fistulae are congenital defects (resulting from failure of differentiation of embryologic analagen with persistence of many vascular communications). Other causes include trauma to the abdomen, rupture of an aneurysm of the hepatic artery, and as a sequel to surgery or diagnostic procedures of the abdominal vasculature.

Lesions are often found during angiography or surgery and include dilated, tortuous, pulsating vessels on the surface of the liver. On cross section, large cavernous vessels are found within the liver lobes. These make the liver large despite its reduced mass of hepatocytes. Microscopically, the arterial branches have foci of intimal hyperplasia and there is reduplication and splitting of the inner elastic membrane. Within the abnormal vessels there is evidence of thrombosis and recanalization.

Dogs with arteriovenous fistulae have evidence of *portal hypertension*: ascites, enlargement of the azygous vein, and extrahepatic portacaval venous shunts. Arteriovenous fistulae between *hepatic artery* and *hepatic vein* are very rare and are associated with rapid onset of cardiac failure.

Dr. Peter Moore, at the University of California, reported seven cases of congenital hepatic arterioportal fistulae in young dogs. All had sudden onset of gastrointestinal and neurologic signs and ascites (evidence of portal hypertension). Vascular walls were markedly altered, and dogs also had extrahepatic portacaval shunts.

LYMPHATIC BLOCKAGE

Blockage of lymphatic vessels leads to accumulation of lymph in tissue or in body cavities. When damaged by surgery, neoplasms, and intravascular parasites, the normal flow of interstitial fluid into lymphatics is prevented and edema fluid accumulates locally. Lymphatic vessels are enlarged, and if on the serosal surfaces lining body cavities, they may ooze fluid to cause ascites or hydropleura (Fig. 14.7).

Rare, hereditary malformation of lymphatic vessels in dogs, calves, and pigs are manifest as local subcutaneous edema of the limbs (see edema, Chapter 13).

Thoracic duct obstructions
Duct rupture leads to chylothorax.

Chyle, the milky fluid taken up by the lacteals from food in the intestine, is composed of lymph and triglyceride droplets. When the thoracic duct is ruptured, chyle flows into the thoracic cavity. The presence of effused chyle in the thoracic cavity is called *chylothorax* (also "chylopleura"). This syndrome is manifest by dyspnea and tachypnea on exertion and has been alleviated by ligation of the thoracic duct.

Chylothorax in dogs and cats is most often caused by trauma (such as surgery and the tearing that occurs in vomiting and chronic coughing). It can also accompany congenital defects, neoplasms, and granulomas such as blastomycosis and histoplasmosis. For example, *Histoplasma capsulatum* grows within lymph vessels to produce lymphangitis, blockade of the lymph vessel lumen, and rupture of the vessel wall (Fig. 14.8).

In dogs, the thoracic duct lies on the right side of the caudal thorax and crosses to the left side at the level of T6, the 6th thoracic vertebrae. In cats, the duct lies entirely on the left side of the mediastinum. There are marked individual variations in thoracic duct anatomy in normal cats and dogs.

Thoracic lymphangiectasia is a cause of chylothorax.

Partial or total obstruction of the thoracic duct can cause lymphangiectasia and chylothorax. Effusion of chyle occurs because fluid oozes from dilated lymphatics (in contrast to the more rapid flow when the thoracic duct is ruptured). Many of these lesions are malformations (e.g., lymphaticovenous anastomoses) and can only be diagnosed by radiography. Oil-based contrast agents are injected into hindlimb lymphatics to outline the thoracic duct.

ISCHEMIA

Partial (hypoxia) or total (anoxia) deficiency of oxygen in tissue may arise from three basic phenomena: (1) *systemic anoxia,* inadequate oxygen

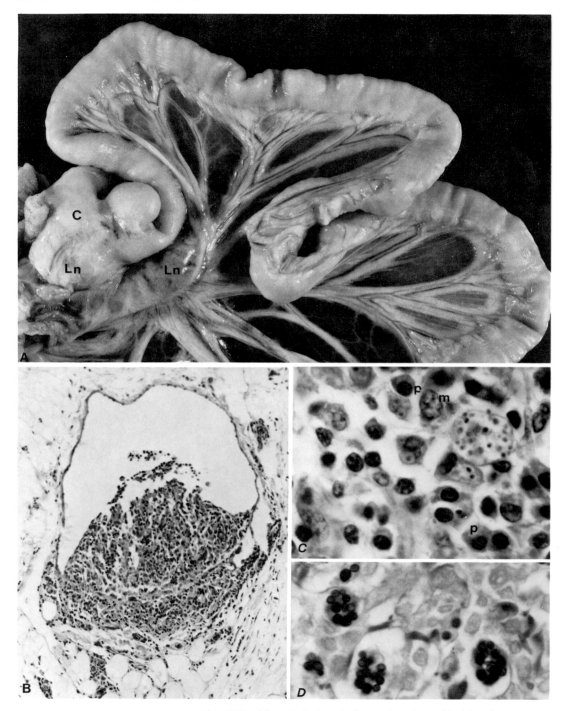

Fig. 14.7. Mesenteric lymphadenopathy, dog with histoplasmosis. A. Mesenteric lymph nodes are enlarged and meaty but do not exude milky fluid (as do lymph nodes affected by lymphoma). B. Granulomatous inflammatory tissue in lymph node. C and D. *Histoplasma capsulatum* in macrophages: Hematoxylin-eosin stain in C; Gomori methenamine silver stain in D.

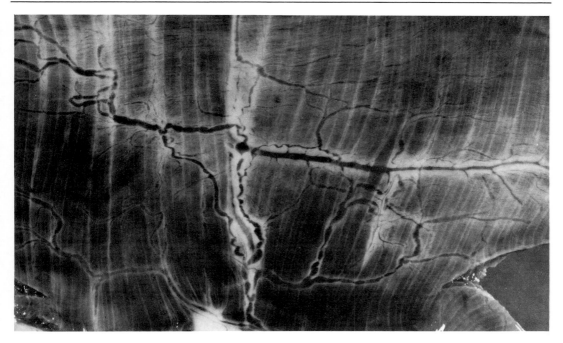

Fig. 14.8. Lymphatic dilatation, surface of diaphragm, dog with chronic histoplasmosis.

in the presence of an adequate blood supply, (2) *ischemic anoxia,* the decrease of arterial flow and pressure with stagnation and decrease in oxygen consumption, and (3) *cytotoxic anoxia,* interference with oxygen utilization by the cell. In this section we consider the ischemic variety. Ischemia is essentially a "localized tissue anemia." Failure of blood to circulate through tissue leads to a progressive, cascading series of events that ends in necrosis. If there is anoxia, cells quickly die from oxygen depletion and shutdown in ATP production (see infarction). Ischemia-induced pathologic processes are major causes of death in animals. They are also the major causes of death in humans, especially myocardial infarction and cerebral ischemia.

Before proceeding, we define several major processes involving the circulatory system. When used incorrectly, these terms can lead to misunderstandings of how circulatory system damage occurs.

1. *Anoxia*: absence of oxygen in tissue. The caveat "despite adequate perfusion of tissue with blood" does not apply, even though some veterinarians use it so.

2. *Hypoxia*: a reduction in oxygen in a tissue below normal amounts.

3. *Ischemia*: local deficiency of blood in tissue due to obstruction or constriction of a blood vessel.

4. *Hyperemia*: increased blood in tissue resulting in distension of blood vessels. *Active* hyperemia is due to dilatation of blood vessels, *passive* hyperemia to hindered drainage.

5. *Congestion*: an abnormal accumulation of fluid within the vessels of an organ. This is usually taken to mean blood, but the term occasionally is applied to mucus. Congestion is often equated with passive hyperemia but is a broader, less precise term.

Consequences of ischemia

The earliest change in ischemia is swelling and disintegration of mitochondria. Loss of energy in turn leads to cell membrane damage, which permits entry of water, electrolytes, and plasma proteins into the cells. Increases in cellular calcium lead to irreversible cytopathic changes and necrosis. Cellular enzymes are liberated into the interstitial fluids as the cell dies.

Ischemic injury develops in two phases.

Ischemic injury occurs in an *anoxic phase,* during which blood flow is shut down, and during a *postischemic phase.* as blood flow is begun again. In clinical situations in which animals survive an ischemic event, much of the tissue injury occurs during this reflow period.

Superoxide radicals are a major lethal factor in postischemic injury.

Oxygen deficiency enhances production of superoxide radicals from "leaky" sites in the mitochondrial electron transport chain in ischemia. A free radical is a molecule containing an odd number of electrons, and since a chemical bond consists of a pair of electrons sharing an orbit, it has an open bond with great reactivity (the odd electron is represented in formulas as a dot). If two radicals react, both are eliminated; if one interacts with a nonradical, another free radical is produced, enabling free radicals to participate in chain reactions.

A major source of superoxide in postischemic tissues is the enzyme *xanthine oxidase,* which is especially rich in intestine, lung, and liver:

xanthine + H_2O + NAD −(xanthine oxidase)→ uric acid + $2O_2^-$ + 2 H^+

In ischemic tissue there is conversion of the enzyme xanthine dehydrogenase to xanthine oxidase. This is initiated by a drop in cell energy. The cell fails to operate its membrane pumps, which maintain ion gradients across its membranes. Ions are redistributed, especially calcium, which is elevated in the cytosol and activates a protease that converts the dehydrogenase to oxidase. ATP is depleted, AMP accumulates, and AMP is catabolized to adenosine inosine and then to hypoxanthine. Hypoxanthine serves as an oxidizable purine substrate of xanthine:

xanthine (or hypoxanthine) + O_2 −(xanthine oxidase)→ O_2^-

In ischemia, there is a new enzyme (xanthine oxidase), a new substrate (hypoxanthine), and oxygen.

Intestinal ischemia

Ischemia of the intestine is a major cause of mortality in animals. The intestine becomes ischemic in three situations: (1) blockade of the portal vein, (2) shock, during which blood is shunted away from the intestinal mucosa to brain and myocardium (sometimes called "flow ischemia"), and (3) obstruction of a mesenteric artery. Horses are especially liable to intestinal ischemia; it arises from malposition of the gut or from strongyle larvae–induced thrombosis of the cranial mesenteric artery. In terminal stages of many equine diseases, low cardiac output accompanying low perfusion pressure of endotoxic shock perpetuates mucosal necrosis.

Ischemia of the gut is "multifactoral."

Mucosal damage causes decreased intestinal net fluid and electrolyte absorption. Three factors are implicated in intestinal lesions of ischemia: (1) *hypoxia at the tips of villi* (extravascular short-circuiting of oxygen in the villous countercurrent exchanger underlies the hypoxia present in villous tips, while intraluminal administration of oxygen experimentally prevents the mucosal lesions of shock); (2) *superoxide radicals* released during reflow of blood (damage is ameliorated by superoxide dismutase treatment); and (3) *pancreatic proteases* acting on mucosa when the ischemic mucosa ceases to produce protective mucus. The epithelial lining becomes vulnerable to luminal enzymes, particularly trypsin and chymotrypsin (intraluminal application of protease inhibitors prevents mucosal damage).

Blood is shunted away from villous tips.

In all species, intestinal ischemia induces inhibition of epithelial transport, bleeding from the mucosal capillaries into the lumen, and loss of epithelial cells from the villi. In the villi there is shunting of blood from central arteriole to peripheral capillaries. Thus blood bypasses the tips of the villi, which become hypoxic and slough into the intestinal lumen.

Bleeding is especially common in dogs, in which blood diarrhea is a sequel to shock. The first sign of ischemic mucosal damage is subepithelial spaces at the tips of the villi. This space expands, and the epithelial layer is lifted from the lamina propria. If ischemia is prolonged, this process continues down the side of the villus, which becomes denuded of epithelial cells (Fig. 14.3). Even with severe mucosal damage, the deep layers of the intestine are relatively normal.

Bacteria leak into lymphatics and portal vein.

Ischemia results in an imbalance of gut bacterial flora and usually leads to an increase in anaerobes (*Clostridia* spp. and *Bacteroides* spp.) and decrease in aerobic bacteria. *Clostridia* spp. and *Bacteroides* spp. increase in most species with intestinal ischemia. There is a progressive leak of bacteria into the portal vein and peritoneal lymphatics, thus creating a tendency to septicemia when intestinal ischemia occurs.

Ischemia of the small intestinal mucosa is much more lethal than colonic ischemia. Absorption of bacterial toxins, fermentation products, luminal enzymes, and products of necrotic tissue (i.e., peptides, lysosomal enzymes, and membrane fragments) leads to irreversible shock, then to thrombosis, and finally to intestinal infarction.

Vasospastic ischemia

This nonocclusive ischemia, or "abdominal angina," which arises from severe constriction of intestinal blood vessels, is comparable to that in coronary arteries of the heart. Excessive tension in smooth muscle of arterioles, the major control sites of blood flow in the intestine, causes release of cardiotoxic factors, which circulate and predispose to shock and infarction.

Evaluation of gut ischemia can be done during surgery.

Evaluation of intestinal viability is important in resection of necrotic portions of the intestine. It is done visually during surgery. Spontaneous peristalsis is the best index of intestinal viability. Other criteria include color of the serosa, reflex motility, refill following blanching, and inspection of the mucosa via enterotomy. These are not reliable, and some surgeons resort to special manipulations for a more precise analysis of the extent of ischemia, such as intravenous injection of sodium fluorescein. Fluorescein given intravenously is rapidly distributed to all perfused tissues. Intestine with a blood supply fluoresces under ultraviolet light; areas with reduced circulation show less or no fluorescence.

ADDITIONAL READING

Bennion, R. S., et al. The role of gastrointestinal microflora in the pathogenesis of complications of mesenteric ischemia. *Rev. Inf. Dis.* 6:S132, 1984.

Center, S. A., et al. Evaluation of serum bile acid concentrations for the diagnosis of portosystemic venous anomalies in the dog and cat. *J. Am. Vet. Med. Assoc.* 186:1090, 1985.

Christie, B. A. Collateral arterial blood supply to the normal and ischemic canine kidney. *Am. J. Vet. Res.* 41:1519, 1980.

Clendenin, M. A., and Conrad, M. C. Collateral vessel development after chronic bilateral common carotid artery occlusion in the dog. *Am. J. Vet. Res.* 40:1244, 1979.

Cornelius, L. M., et al. Anomalous portosystemic anastomoses associated with chronic hepatic insufficiency in six young dogs. *J. Am. Vet. Med. Assoc.* 167:220, 1975.

Hayes, M. A., et al. Acute necrotizing myelopathy from nucleus pulposus embolism in dogs with intervertebral disk degeneration. *J. Am. Vet. Med. Assoc.* 173:289, 1978.

Hochachka, P. W. Defense strategies against hypoxia and hypothermia. *Science* 231:234, 1986.

Liu, S.-K., et al. Pulmonary collateral circulation in canine dirofilariases. *Am. J. Vet. Res.* 30:1723, 1969.

Miller, L. M., et al. Ataxia and weakness associated with fourth ventricle vascular anomalies in two horses. *J. Am. Vet. Med. Assoc.* 186:601, 1985.

Moore, P. F., and Whiting, P. G. Hepatic lesions associated with intrahepatic arterioportal fistulae in dogs. *Vet. Pathol.* 23:57, 1986.

Parks, D. A., et al. Ischemic injury in the cat small intestine. *Gastroenterology* 82:9, 1982.

Scavelli, T. D., et al. Portosystemic shunts in cats. *J. Am. Vet. Med. Assoc.* 189:317, 1986.

Sheffield, W. D., et al. Cerebral venous thrombosis in the rhesus monkey. *Vet. Pathol.* 18:326, 1981.

Suter, M. M., et al. Primary intestinal lymphangiectasia in three dogs. *Vet. Pathol.* 22:123, 1985.

Cardiovascular System

15

CARDIAC ENLARGEMENT

Introduction

The heartbeat is controlled by the cardiac conduction system.

The *sinoatrial node,* or "natural pacemaker," initiates myofiber contraction. Located at the confluence of the precaval and atrial orifices in dogs, it is richly innervated by both *sympathetic* (which quickens the heartbeat) and *parasympathetic* (which slows the heartbeat) divisions of the autonomic nervous system. The specialized cells of the sinoatrial node are smaller than ordinary cardiac muscle fibers. They are embedded in dense connective tissue and, microscopically, are difficult to distinguish from fibroblasts.

Impulses generated in the sinoatrial node pass rapidly to the *atrioventricular node* in the atrial septal wall and into the *atrioventricular bundle,* which courses downward into the ventricular septum. The atrioventricular bundle subdivides into a complex network of conducting fibers called *Purkinje fibers,* which ramify over the subendothelial surfaces of both ventricles.

The cardiac conduction system is rarely implicated as a factor in heart disease. Hemorrhages around the atrioventricular bundle are common in some vascular diseases and may contribute to cardiac failure. Degenerate Purkinje cells are associated with the late stages of endocardial fibroelastosis of Burmese cats.

Fibrosis and fatty infiltration in the cardiac conduction system occurs with aging, especially in some large breeds of dogs. Studies by Dr. George Sandusky and colleagues on the cardiac conduction system of 40 large-breed dogs over 5 years of age at Ohio State University revealed loss of conduction fibers, infiltration by fat, and increased fibrous connective tissue. Meierhenry

and Liu, at the Animal Medical Center in New York City, found similar lesions in dogs to be associated with sudden death and episodes of viciousness.

Actin and myosin filaments interlock and move to cause contraction.

The performance of the heart as a pump is dependent on the contractile function of the *cardiac muscle cell* (or myofiber). Within this cell two filaments interact to produce the heartbeat. During contraction, ends of thin *actin filaments* slide deeply between thicker *myosin filaments.* Actin filaments are anchored at specialized lines, called *Z-lines*; the Z-lines demarcate the contractile unit of cardiac muscle, the *sarcomere.* As the two filaments interact during contraction, Z-lines are drawn together, shortening the myofiber. During relaxation, actin filaments are withdrawn from the myosin filaments, and the myofiber is lengthened.

An ATPase in myosin filaments drives hydrolysis of ATP for energy.

At the molecular level, actin and myosin filaments interact at cross bridges that emerge at regular intervals from the myosin filaments. These are the sites where contractile forces are generated. Contraction results from actin and myosin filaments actively sliding over one another. Sliding is produced by an adenosine triphosphatase (ATPase) located in myosin. Energy derived from ATP hydrolysis drives the cyclic association-dissociation of actin and myosin that causes filament sliding.

Contraction is controlled by calcium.

Within the myofiber the concentration of calcium ions (Ca^{++}) controls contraction. Membranes of the sarcoplasmic reticulum sequester Ca^{++} during rest and release it on arrival of a nerve impulse. The action of Ca^{++} is actually mediated by specialized calcium-binding proteins called tropomyosin and troponin, which are embedded in thin filaments within the twisted chain of the actin molecules.

Heart muscle is well protected against both hypo- and hypercalcemia. In contrast, defects in calcium regulation within the cardiac myofiber are commonly life-threatening.

Excess work load leads to cardiac enlargement.

The capacity of the heart to deal with transient increases in work load is enormous, provided that adequate intervals occur for recovery of nutritive and electrolyte levels. Permanent elevations in work load that produce changes in the heart include a wide variety of events that result in increased peripheral resistance to the outflow of blood from the heart (Table 15.1). Compared with direct injury to the heart, many of these diseases are complex and produce their effects on the heart by several different mechanisms.

Diffuse lung disease profoundly influences the heart.

The force required to pump blood through a pneumonic lung markedly increases heart work. For example, *acute* diffuse purulent pneumonia may directly cause acute heart failure and death; it is common for animals with a large percentage of lungs blocked by exudate to die in sudden heart failure. In contrast, heart damage caused by *chronic* diffuse lung disease is more

Table 15.1. Cardiac failure: Mechanisms of myocyte damage

Myocyte destruction (direct)
Myocarditis: inflammation of heart muscle
Myocardiopathy: primary myocyte degeneration (nutrition, genetic disorders)
Vascular disease: ischemia (acute or chronic)

Excessive work load (indirect)
Anoxia: anemia, lung disease, high-altitude disease
Chamber obstruction: heartworms, valve lesions, tumors
Obstructive lung disease: pulmonary fibrosis, embolism
Constrictive lesions: pericarditis, hydropericardium, hemopericardium
Congenital heart defects: septal defect, patent ductus, etc.

complex because increased work load is accompanied by secondary hypoxic effects.

Anemia contributes to heart work load.

Anemia causes an increased work load for the heart because of the decreased oxygen-carrying capacity of blood. Thus the body's reaction to anemia includes hyperventilation and increased cardiac output. Severe anemia not only predisposes the myocardium to ischemic injury but can be a direct cause of lesions in the heart muscle (even though they are commonly overlooked).

Hemoglobin below 50% endangers the myocardium and results in clinical signs of weakness, dyspnea, tachycardia, and electrocardiographic changes. Long-standing anemia of this type is accompanied by cardiac hypertrophy. If untreated, it may develop into dilatation with fatty degeneration and tiny foci of necrosis in the myocardium.

Hypertrophy and dilatation

The cardinal sign of heart disease is cardiac enlargement. If the heart works against a sustained overload, it eventually becomes unable to deliver the required output of blood. With development of myocardial fatigue, a slight dilation of the heart occurs due to stretching of individual myofibers. The myocardium responds to this early dilatation by *myocyte hypertrophy,* that is, by enlargement of individual myofibers (the number of myocytes remains nearly the same, even though ventricular weight and thickness increase).

Hypertrophied myocytes provide increased energy (although less efficiently) for production of the necessary output of blood from the heart. Hypertrophy may enable the heart to maintain sufficient work without further dilation, and in hearts examined during this stage the chambers appear relatively normal in size. Histologically, early hypertrophy is equally subtle and is usually detected only by quantitative studies on cell size.

Multiple cycles of dilatation and hypertrophy occur.

In time the hypertrophied myocardium still under an increased work load fails a second time. This again produces dilatation, leading to more hypertrophy, and so on until the cycle is unable to compensate for increases in work load. The chain of events involved in dilatation-hypertrophy may be accelerated or prolonged, depending on the severity of damage to the heart. In some instances, marked hypertrophy is present with little dilatation, particularly in the left ventricle. In others, little hypertrophy is seen, but there is remarkable dilatation with an enlarged, flabby heart.

Hypertrophied hearts are prone to hypoxia and failure.

In the normal heart, each myofiber is accompanied by a capillary. In cardiac enlargement hyperplasia of capillary endothelial cells occurs, but as fiber size increases, the vascular supply does not do so accordingly. Thus the *relative* amount of blood that can circulate within the heart decreases progressively with hypertrophy. The metabolizing mass of the myofiber enlarges markedly, but the cell membrane and its relation to the capillary does not. When the hypertrophied heart reaches a critical size, there is overgrowth beyond capillary supply and unseating of the heart valves, and in chronic hypertrophy the heart is set up for hypoxic injury.

Heart weight:body weight ratios increase in cardiac enlargement.

Normal heart weight:body weight ratios in dogs range from 1:5 to 1:11, depending on the breed. Racing greyhounds in good condition may exceed this range. One of the most striking alterations in heart weight:body weight ratios occurs in *racing-induced cardiac failure.* This syndrome develops in large males under 4 years of age, especially in hot climates, due to acute increases in work load in a hypertrophic heart compromised by heat stress.

Mitochondrial reduplication develops to provide added energy.

Myocardial hypertrophy caused by increased cardiac work has been studied experimentally in three models: (1) production of aortic stenosis by placing a band around the ascending aorta, (2) chronic swimming experiments in rodents, and (3) production of renal hypertension. Progressive hypertrophy of heart muscle caused by aortic stenosis in dogs shows that the ratio of mitochondria to myofilament decreases in waves. Dogs (whose normal ratio is 0.42) show increased values at 3–6 days postsurgery. Decreased ratios develop and persist until the 25th week, when elevated values are again found.

Biochemical data support the structural changes; that is, ATP values recover and relapse in concert with mitochondrial structural changes as seen in the electron microscope.

CARDIAC FAILURE

When the myocardium is no longer able to compensate for increases in work load, chambers of the heart dilate. Degeneration of cardiac myocytes occurs, but the pathologic changes vary according to the causal mechanism involved. In the slowly failing heart, secondary factors such as ischemia, aging, and endocrine imbalances may be superimposed on the primary structural alterations. In ventricular walls a spectrum of change from relatively normal myocytes to total fibrosis may exist. Degenerate myocytes may alternate with bands of fibrous interstitium.

The two sides of the heart usually do not fail together. In early heart disease, distinct syndromes of right or left failure occur, although failure of one cannot exist long without producing excess strain on the other.

Right heart disease

Obstruction of blood flow through the lung results in selective hypertrophy of the right ventricle. In the dog, a major cause of right heart failure is dirofilariasis. Lesions of the right atrioventicular valve and diffuse lung disease are also important causes of right heart disease (Fig. 15.1).

Cor pulmonale: Right ventricular change produced by diffuse pulmonary disease

Diseases such as chronic emphysema, pneumonia, and pulmonary fibrosis notably affect the right heart. Cor pulmonale also results from pressure atelectasis caused by tumors. Classic hypoxic cor pulmonale occurs in *high-altitude disease* of cattle in the mountains. Cattle transferred too quickly from low to high altitudes without time to adjust to low atmospheric oxygen develop edema in the subcutis, giving rise to the name "brisket disease." In the 1960s Dr. Arch Alexander, at Colorado State University, showed that hypoxia caused hypertension and hypertrophy of the right ventricle and, in turn, congestive cardiac failure.

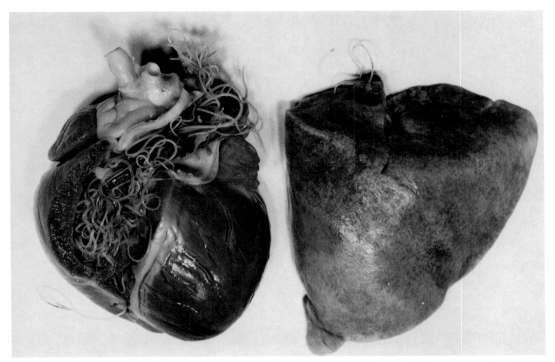

Fig. 15.1. Cardiac hypertrophy, dog. Right ventricle is filled with masses of adult *Dirofilaria immitis.* Lung is solid with nematodes in bronchi.

FOCUS

Dirofilariasis is a cause of cardiac hypertrophy in dogs.

Mechanical obstruction of the right ventricle and pulmonary artery by the heartworm *Dirofilaria immitis* leads to marked enlargement of the heart. Dirofilariasis is an insect-born disease. Microfilaria sucked from the blood of infected dogs by mosquitoes are transmitted as larvae to other dogs, where they develop to adult worms within the right ventricle and pulmonary artery.

Clinical signs in affected dogs (weakness, anorexia, and respiratory difficulty) are progressive. Clinical pathologic examination in early stages reveals microfilaria in the blood. Radiologic examination shows a markedly enlarged heart with dense areas distributed throughout the lungs. At necropsy, myocardial walls are thickened and chambers are enlarged. Lungs are large, pale, meaty, and do not collapse. Fluid is usually present in the abdominal and thoracic cavities.

Pathologic diagnoses include (1) *cardiac hypertrophy* with obstruction of the right ventricle and pulmonary artery, (2) *chronic multifocal*

granulomatous pneumonitis due to embolization of adult parasites and microfilaria in the capillary bed of the lung, (3) *bronchiectasis* with mucous hyperplasia of bronchial epithelium, and (4) *centrolobular fatty degeneration* of the liver with foci of necrosis and fibrosis.

In canine heartworm disease, disastrous increases of work load on the right heart occur by several mechanisms. First, there is mechanical obstruction of blood flow by adult parasites. Second, pulmonary arterial vascular lesions develop and shed thromboemboli into the pulmonary capillary bed. This leads to chronic inflammatory disease of the lung with hemosiderosis, alveolar wall fibrosis, and focal granulomatous lesions. Last, live microfilaria are shed into the pulmonary capillary bed. These factors, when combined, initiate the cycle of pulmonary edema–heart failure. Fluid accumulates in the alveolar wall, and fibrosis and emphysema develop. These, in turn, increase the heart work load. The failing right heart cannot pump sufficient blood to the lung. Death may occur during cardiac hypertrophy due to sudden embolization of microfilaria and thrombi, or it may not occur until cardiac failure and severe dilatation have developed.

Left heart disease

The heart's more powerful force is generated by the left ventricular myocardium, and the clinical signs that accompany disease of the heart are more readily apparent with its failure. Diffuse heart disease is therefore generally manifest as left side failure. The marked thickening of the left ventricular wall influences the position of the fibrous rings sealing the heart valves (Fig. 15.2).

End-stage heart disease

Congestive heart failure is the clinical syndrome resulting from the inability of cardiac output to keep pace with venous return. It is the final common pathway for several types of heart disease. Retention of water and sodium ions (from decreased renal blood flow and adrenal cortical mechanisms) may result in overhydration with increased blood volume. This distends

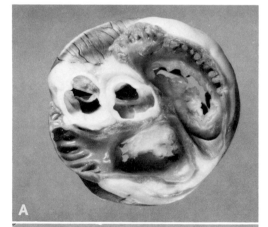
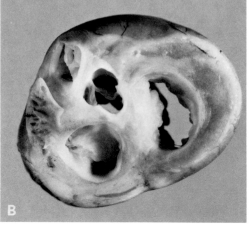

Fig. 15.2. Changes in seating of the heart valves in left ventricular hypertrophy, dog. A. Normal dog. B. Marked hypertrophy with thickened ventricular wall and enlarged valve openings.

the venous bed so that the heart chambers cannot keep up with the amount of blood delivered. The venous bed is distended further, and fluid begins to accumulate in the tissues.

Signs of congestive heart failure are due to the secondary effects of stasis and congestion. Lesions are extensive in the lungs and liver. They are rare in kidneys, brain, and subcutis, although lesions of anoxia and fluid exudation occur in these organs.

Dogs with congestive heart failure commonly develop edema, anemia, emaciation, and progressive deterioration. In those that die, there is massive enlargement of the heart with extreme distension of the vena cavae and atria (Fig. 15.3). Fluid is present in body cavities. Liver and spleen are enlarged, and the bone marrow is often red throughout.

Histopathologic diagnoses usually include (1) myocardial degeneration with edema and hyperemia of the capillary bed, (2) centrolobular degeneration of the liver with fibrosis and hyperplasia of Kupffer cells (due to erythrophagocytosis), (3) engorgement of the splenic red pulp, and (4) pulmonary fibrosis with fluid in alveoli.

Lung

Blood backs up in lungs of dogs with cardiac failure, and the increased pressure in the pulmonary veins is transmitted to the capillaries. Fluid accumulates in the alveolar wall and overflows into alveoli (*pulmonary edema*). Lesions seen postmortem include capillary dilatation (hyperemia), hemorrhage into scattered alveoli, and eosinophilic granular debris in alveoli. In long-standing cases, there are collagen fibers in the alveolar wall and iron-laden macrophages (called "heart failure cells") in alveoli. These result from erythrophagocytosis due to stasis in the capillary bed (Fig. 15.4).

Liver

Backing up of blood in the liver produces hepatomegaly and striking lesions of the parenchyma. "Nutmeg liver" results from congestive, red accentuation of centrolobular areas surrounded by pale, fatty hepatocytes. If heart failure is sudden and severe, the sinusoids become engorged with blood, resulting in sinusoid rupture with hepatocyte necrosis, a pattern called *hemorrhagic cardiac necrosis*. If portal hypertension is high, erythrocytes pass into the intersinusoidal spaces (of Disse). In many cases, large numbers of basophils lodge in these spaces, probably to release histamine (to sustain vascular permeability) and heparin (to prevent coagulation of blood in the slowed hepatic circulation).

In chronic heart failure, the centrolobular

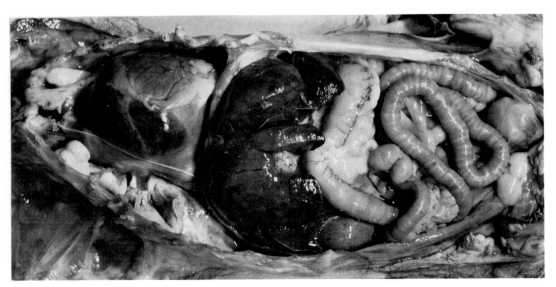

Fig. 15.3. Cardiac failure, dog. Late stage with heart stopped in diastole. Massive enlargement of heart with blood-filled right atrium and vena cava. Liver markedly enlarged, mottled, and granular.

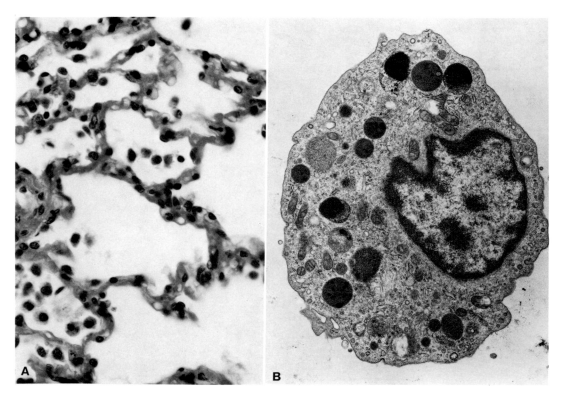

Fig. 15.4. Consequences of chronic heart failure. A. Lung: alveolar walls are thickened. Note the capillaries projecting into the alveoli. B. Macrophages in the alveoli ("heart failure cells") contain iron pigments.

areas slowly become fibrotic. These lesions are called *cardiac sclerosis* or cardiac cirrhosis. Abnormalities of portal system congestion are also responsible for *ascites.*

OXYGEN DEFICIT CARDIOMYOPATHY

Most tissues remove about 25% of the oxygen in blood during flow through the capillaries. Myocardium removes 75% and is exquisitely sensitive to oxygen deprivation. Myocardial cells will degenerate from oxygen deficit brought about by a variety of conditions, such as asphyxiation, severe anemia, severe hypotension, or any vascular lesion causing myocardial ischemia. The extent to which hypoxia affects the cardiac myocyte depends on the type, severity, and duration of oxygen deficit.

Metabolism of cardiac muscle cells

After hypoxia of any cause, amounts of high-energy phosphate compounds (ATP, ADP, and creatine phosphate) fall quickly in myocardial cells. In response, *anaerobic glycolysis* is stimulated via (1) increased glucose uptake due to greater activity of hexokinase, the enzyme that converts glucose to glucose-6-phosphate, and (2) accelerated glycogenolysis via activation of phosphorylase kinase. These processes augment glycolysis and contribute to cell viability and continued function of the hypoxic myocardium.

In anoxia caused by ischemia, there is also a burst of accelerated glycolysis, but it is brief. Because blood flow is stopped, the glycolytic rate falls rapidly and intracellular lactic acid increases. Accumulation of lactate and hydrogen ions causes a drop in pH within ischemic cells and inhibits glycolysis by suppressing enzymes of glycolytic pathways involved in glucose utilization and glycogenolysis. Thus the ischemic cell is prevented from using substrates even when they are available.

Fatty degeneration characterizes the hypoxic cardiac myocyte.

Normal myocardium derives most of its energy from oxidation of fatty acids. This process declines rapidly in ischemia because of suppression of carnitine palmityl coenzyme A (CoA), the mitochondrial enzyme catalyzing oxidation of fatty acids. As a result, long-chain fatty acid acyl-CoA esters accumulate and inhibit predecessor pathways in the cytosol. Free fatty acids accumulate and, if the cell survives, are shunted into triglycerides, which accumulate as lipid globules. This conversion increases the oxygen requirement, which in turn affects the mitochondrial oxidation process.

Plasma enzymes rise if heart muscle cells are killed.

Cell membrane changes in injured myocytes permit enzymes such as the transaminases to leak out of the cell. Enzymes appear in high levels in circulating blood, and the ischemic myocyte may be shown to be enzyme-deficient histochemically. After experimental myocardial infarction in dogs, lactic dehydrogenase (LDH) is abnormally elevated in plasma within 24 hours. This enzyme can be separated into five distinct components, or isozymes, according to speed of migration in an electrophoretic field. Myocardium contains predominantly LDH_5. LDH is not specific, however, and is also elevated in skeletal muscle necrosis, liver necrosis, neoplastic diseases, and some hematologic disorders.

Serum *creatine phosphokinase* (CPK) is more reliable in diagnosis of acute myocardial necrosis in most species. Abundant in skeletal muscle and brain, it includes an isozyme specific for myocardium. It is highly concentrated in myocardial cells and released only after injury has become irreversible. If blood samples for CPK determinations are obtained at 1-hour intervals for 24 hours after necrosis occurs, the resulting time-concentration curve of CPK permits a quantitation of the necrotic area. The CPK disappearance curve can be predicted with accuracy from values obtained during the first 5 hours in dogs. From this data, a predicted infarct size can be calculated.

Mitochondria are sites of immediate change in myocardial ischemia.

Mitochondria in the acutely hypoxic cardiac myocyte are swollen. When examined by electron microscopy, their matrix is clarified and their cristae fragmented. ATP, the energy currency of the cells, declines, and most cellular functions rapidly diminish. The most crucial damage occurs in the plasma membrane, which becomes leaky and permits water, electrolytes, and plasma proteins to enter the cell. Calcium plays the leading role in causing cell death.

Hypoxic disease

Oxygen-deficit cell damage occurs in one of two major ways: *hypoxia in the presence of adequate blood supply* and *ischemia,* which involves decreased arterial flow with stagnation and decreased oxygen.

Asphyxia following experimental clamping of the trachea rapidly leads to cardiac dilatation, heart stoppage, and death. As seen in movies of the living heart in rabbits, this acute hypoxic cardiac dilatation begins in the atria within seconds and spreads to the ventricles. If oxygenation is permitted, the ventricle rapidly returns to normal size. The cardiac dilatation correlates with a hypoxia-induced mitochondrial degeneration and a fall in ATP and high-energy phosphate concentrations in heart muscle homogenates. On regression of dilatation, mitochondria and their electron-transfer systems return to normal.

Focal necrosis results from severe hypoxia.

Severe *hypotension,* which characterizes the shock state following extensive hemorrhage, causes small *disseminated zonal lesions* throughout the myocardium. Certain individual cells are destroyed, allegedly because of their particular stage of metabolic activity at the time of injury. If hypotension is intense and prolonged, the process becomes irreversible and zonal lesions develop into large segmental areas of necrosis. If hypotension is transient, the myocardium returns to normal and the necrotic cells are broken down and processed by leukocytes and sarcolemmal cells. Dead cells accumulate calcium, and foci of necrosis may heal, leaving tiny areas of mineral within a connective tissue scar. These calcified areas are commonly found in ventricles of mammals but occur in the anterior heart more commonly in fishes and birds.

Tiny foci of necrosis associated with hypoxia are analogous to the focal lesions in man that are relics of angina pectoris. Hypertrophied hearts that have outgrown their vascular supply, which is apt to occur in shock and severe anemia, are particularly prone to this pattern of heart necrosis. Dogs that suffer prolonged *epileptic seizures* with interruption of breathing contain these small disseminated necrotic foci throughout the ventricular myocardium.

In dogs, these lesions have been produced experimentally. A large quantity of blood was removed, sufficient to result in severe systemic oxygen debt. After 8 minutes, the blood was replaced. Although the dogs recovered normally, foci of necrosis were present in the heart when the dogs were killed 4 days later.

Cardiac vascular (ischemic) disease

When the lumen of a coronary artery is narrowed, the myocardium supplied by its ramifications is affected. Depending on the extent of vascular narrowing, the consequence may be infarction and necrosis or fatty degeneration and diffuse fibrosis. As dogs age they become increasingly susceptible to arterial disease and its associated lesions of the myocardium (Fig. 15.5).

Coronary artery ligation: A model for myocardial ischemia

Biochemical events in the myocardium that follow restriction of coronary flow in this model are oxygen consumption depressed 45%, glucose consumption increased 91% (glucose extracted from heart muscle is increased 500%), and lactate increased in the venous outflow. It is clear, therefore, that myocardial ischemia is accompanied by accelerated glycolysis.

There is a shift to anaerobic glycolysis.

Anaerobic glucose breakdown (the glycolytic cycle) is insignificant as an energy source in the normal cardiac myocyte. When energy supplied by oxygen utilization in the mitochondria is insufficient, however, the myocyte oxidizes glucose to pyruvate and lactate, which provide a supplemental source of energy. In myocardial ischemia, this augmentation may generate enough energy to be of critical importance.

FOCUS

Atherosclerosis

Atherosclerosis is the accumulation of lipids in larger arteries in the form of elevated, lipid-filled plaques called *atheromas*. Necrosis and fibrosis follow the deposition of lipid and result in progressively enlarging lesions that expand the arterial wall. The consequences of severe atherosclerosis are often fatal. *Ischemia* and *infarction* develop in affected organs because of the encroachment of the vascular lumen. Less commonly, *aneurysms* develop from weakening of the arterial wall. *Rupture* of the artery with hemorrhage into surrounding tissue can be fatal.

Canine atherosclerosis is uncommon. Drs. Liu and Tappe reported 21 cases in a 14-year period at the Animal Medical Center in New York City. Eight of the cases were males and there was a preponderance for miniature schnauzers, doberman pinschers, and Labrador retrievers. Severe systemic atherosclerosis is most often seen in dogs with *hypothyroidism,* which leads to hypercholesterolemia and indirectly to atherosclerosis. Lesions are prominent in the media as well as intima of large muscular arteries of the heart, kidney, intestine, bladder, and other organs. Lipids fill the cytoplasm of myocytes, and lipid-laden *foam cells* distort the media of the vessel wall.

▶

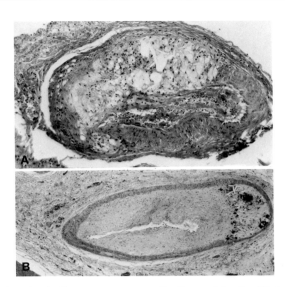

Atherosclerosis. A. Coronary artery, media distorted by fat-filled myocytes and macrophages, dog with hypothyroidism. B. Coronary artery, vessel wall contains evidence of acute and chronic changes, human female with diabetes mellitus.

In aged humans, atherosclerosis is an extremely common lesion and disease. The aorta, iliac, and coronary and cerebral arteries are most often affected. Because atherosclerosis can progressively or abruptly occlude these blood vessels, it often causes death by myocardial infarction or stroke.

The characteristic lesions of human atherosclerosis are fatty plaques in the large arteries. Smooth muscle cells are prominent, and macrophages and leukocytes are trapped in the dense matrix of the plaque. Collagen, glycoproteins, elastin, and fibrin are present in smaller amounts. Lipoproteins are both intra- and extracellular. Deep in the lesions are debris from dead cells and large amounts of lipid and cholesterol. Plaques often occlude arteries and predispose to thrombosis, which completes the blockade of the arterial lumen.

Studies in man have clearly shown that plasma lipids, elevated blood pressure, and cigarette smoking strongly influence the development of clinical disease; but data on the finite pathogenesis of the lesions indicate that the atheroma begins as an intimal lesion that progressively extends into and affects the media.

As constructed from serial examination of naturally occurring lesions, this involves (1) endothelial injury, (2) seepage of plasma lipids and lipoproteins into the intima, (3) invasion of the intima by circulating monocytes that transform into macrophages and then phagocytize lipids, (4) myocyte migration through fenestrae of the inner elastic membrane, (5) proliferation of myocytes in foci within the intima, and (6) accumulation of lipids within the cytoplasm of the vascular smooth muscle cell.

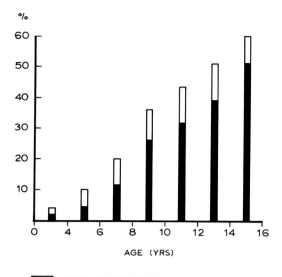

□ Hyalin or Amyloid in Arteries
■ Necrosis or Fibrosis in Myocardium

Fig. 15.5. Incidence of heart disease. (Data from Jönsson, *Acta Vet. Scand.* [Suppl.] 38:1, 1972)

Glucose decreases the severity of myocardial infarction.

In dogs, infusion of glucose-potassium-insulin solutions 30 minutes after experimental coronary artery ligation reduces the extent of myocardial necrosis. Infusion provides a quick source of utilizable energy, reduces circulating free fatty acids (which complicate the lipid defect of ischemia), and restores intracellular potassium. Myocardium can also be spared by inhalation of oxygen-rich gas, which enhances diffusion of oxygen by increasing the gradient between normal and ischemic heart muscle. This, when superimposed on oxygen deficit, has profound effects on heart function.

Extent of myocardial infarction depends on the balance between oxygen supply and utilization.

Factors that increase myocardial oxygen consumption also increase the extent of heart muscle injury. *Anemia* and *hypoxemia* increase ischemic injury after coronary artery ligation because both depress the delivery of oxygen to myocardium. *Hypoglycemia* augments ischemic injury by withholding glucose as the myocardium shifts to anaerobic glycolysis. *Hyperthermia* impairs myocardial performance through its

stimulation of oxygen consumption and heart rate.

Adrenal catecholamines, which stimulate B receptors of myocardium and conducting tissue, enhance function of the normal myocardium but have a deleterious effect on ischemic myocardium. Large doses of epinephrine alone may directly cause foci of necrosis that resemble infarcts. The potent inotropic and chronotropic properties of the sympathomimetic amine isoproterenal, when given to dogs with experimental infarction, cause an increased size of infarcts. Myocardial function improves in the normal and moderately ischemic zones but deteriorates severely in ischemic zones.

Recovery may be complicated by progressive myocardial fibrosis.

Morphologic studies of early changes in ischemic myocardium show swelling of capillary endothelium and interstitial edema. Abnormal fluid retention, although it improves cell recovery, severely inhibits myocardial contraction. Fluids are drained efficiently into cardiac lymphatics, so it is essential that these channels remain patent for recovery.

After coronary occlusion in dogs, cell death occurs first in subendothelial myocardium. A wave front of cell death then spreads across the heart wall to subepicardial zones. The size of the infarct is largely determined by subepicardial collateral blood flow. The capillary bed is irreversibly damaged within a few hours of infarction; its patency at infarct margins is important in limiting the size of necrotic zones. After infarction, neutrophils invade endothelium in infarcted areas and cause sloughing of endothelial cells, leaving only denuded basal laminae where the capillaries once were.

Chronic vascular obstruction of the myocardium slowly but progressively constricts the arterial supply to produce atrophy. There is disappearance of myocardial cells with concomitant fibroplasia of the interstitium. The end result is diffuse scarring of the myocardium and markedly altered function. Obstruction of lymphatics augments these chronic changes, and (in dogs) leads to endomyocardial fibrosis and mucodegeneration of heart valves.

ARTERIES AND HOW THEY CONTROL BLOOD PRESSURE AND FLOW

Muscular arteries and arterioles control blood flow and blood pressure. Normally, in a state of contraction called "tone," their contraction and relaxation occurs by action of smooth muscle cells of the arterial media, cells regulated both by humoral factors and by vasoconstrictor and vasodilator nerves of the autonomic nervous system. Local effects also influence the contractile ability of the blood vessels (e.g., increased temperature and increased carbon dioxide induce vascular relaxation).

Like cardiac muscle cells, vascular smooth muscle cells contain actin and myosin filaments. These filaments are not arranged in sarcomeres, and the vascular smooth muscle cell contracts much more slowly.

Pharmacological influences include catecholamines, histamine, acetylcholine, serotonin, angiotensin, and prostaglandins; most are mediated by calcium influx or release. The site of action in the arterial wall of neural and humoral factors is the myofilaments of the smooth muscle cell. *Epinephrine* acts directly on this cell to induce vasoconstriction. Angiotensin II, a powerful vasoconstrictor, induces widespread structural changes in both endothelium and smooth muscle cells. There are increases in the number and size of pinocytotic vesicles and widening of intercellular spaces in endothelium.

Neurologic control of the vascular wall

Direct stimulation of perivascular nerve fibers with microelectrodes clearly demonstrates the neural control of arterioles. Unmyelinated nerve axons ramify along the exterior layers of the terminal arterioles and penetrate the tunica media to lie in close apposition to vascular myocytes. In the terminal vascular bed, only those vessels with smooth muscle cells receive direct motor innervation. There is no evidence that nonmuscular capillaries have either efferent or motor innervation.

Most arteries and veins are supplied solely by fibers of the sympathetic nervous system which are responsible for tone. Activation of the sympathetic system enhances vascular resistance. In contrast, parasympathetic nerves decrease vascular resistance but innervate only a small part of the blood vessels, mainly in certain viscera.

Carotid sinus and aortic arch baroceptors

Vagal sympathetic stimulation to blood vessels causes vasoconstriction of terminal arterioles. This vasomotor discharge arises in the medulla oblongata and produces a systemic *pressor* (tending to increase blood pressure) effect. The vagal response is initiated by baroceptors in the carotid sinus and aortic arch, which sense a drop in blood pressure due to lessened cardiac action. Decreased stimulation of the aortic arch and carotid sinus baroceptors decreases the afferent vasodilatory and cardioinhibitory neural discharges.

Juxtaglomerular apparatus: A renal pressor system

The juxtaglomerular apparatus is activated by lowering of blood pressure and blood sodium. Arterial pressure drop, as sensed by the arteriole, is transmitted to the granular cells; action is initiated by their release of the enzyme *renin* into the bloodstream (Fig. 15.6).

Renin catalyzes formation of angiotensin.

Renin is a carboxyl protease that specifically cleaves leucine-leucine bonds in its circulating substrate, the plasma protein *angiotensinogen* (which, like other plasma proteins, is secreted by the liver). Reaction with renin transforms angiotensinogen to angiotensin I, which, as it circulates through the lungs, is acted on by *angiotensin converting enzyme* to form the most active product, angiotensin II (Fig. 15.7).

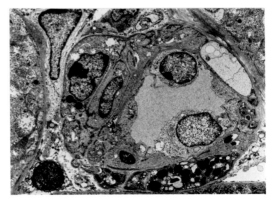

Fig. 15.6. Juxtaglomerular apparatus, kidney. Renin-secreting granular cells surround an arteriole at its entry into the renal glomerulus.

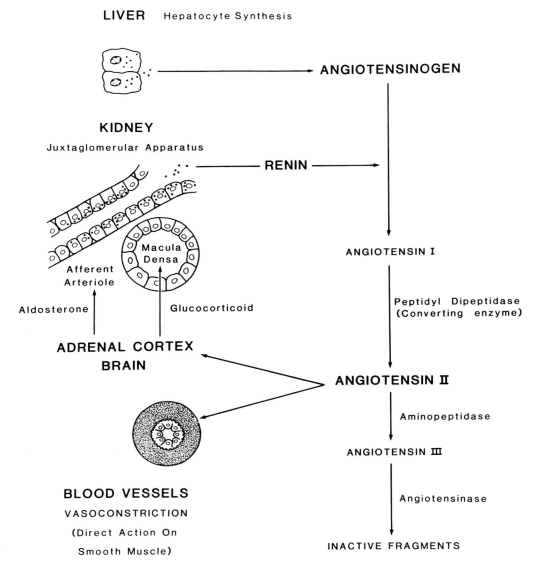

Fig. 15.7. Angiotensin metabolism.

Renin release is controlled by several mechanisms.

Renin secretion is controlled by (1) the renal vascular receptor in the glomerular afferent arteriole, which responds to changes in wall tension; (2) the macula densa receptor that detects changes in rate of delivery of sodium (and probably chloride); (3) the brain, which affects renin release directly via renal nerves and indirectly by stimulating secretions of the adrenal medulla and posterior pituitary; and (4) negative feed-back effects on juxtaglomerular cells of circulating angiotensin.

Angiotensin-converting enzyme converts angiotensin I to II.

Although this enzyme occurs in blood vessels, it is concentrated in lungs, along the luminal surfaces of pulmonary capillaries and venous endothelial cells. In addition to converting angiotensin I to II, it also is an important regulator of other circulating vasoactive peptides. Also known as kininase II, it inactivates bradykinin. This ability to activate a hypertensive factor and to deactivate a hypotensive kinin indicates its important role in blood pressure homeostasis.

Angiotensin II is one of the most potent pressors known.

This enzyme regulates blood pressure through vasoconstriction of precapillary arterioles and, to a lesser extent, postcapillary venules. It has a direct action on vascular smooth muscle, and its strongest vasoconstrictive effect is on viscera, skin, and kidney (brain is less affected and skeletal muscle even less so). The second major function of angiotensin II is to act directly on the brain to increase blood pressure via sympathetic and parasympathetic pathways (including vasopressin release and ACTH secretion). Angiotensin II also stimulates aldosterone secretion, which affects salt and water balance.

Low blood pressure

Angiotensin II, important in raising blood pressure by peripheral vasoconstriction, is effective in hypovolemic shock. When large amounts of blood are lost in the dog, blood pressure begins to drop. Levels of plasma renin rise as a compensatory reaction (Fig. 15.8). Elevated renin levels are also seen in dogs having cardiac failure with edema.

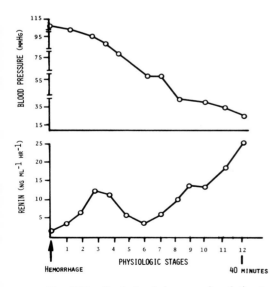

Fig. 15.8. Renin levels in serum in relation to blood pressure during hemorrhage in the dog. (Data modified from Hembrough)

Low plasma sodium

The secretory nature of the cytoplasmic granules of juxtaglomerular cells was first established in experiments showing increased cell content of granules in renal ischemia, adrenalectomy, and low sodium intake. *Hyponatremia* (decreased plasma sodium) increases renin synthesis and release, and *hypernatremia* diminishes them. High plasma renin values may be predicted, therefore, in low-sodium diets and during use of diuretics. The amount of sodium absorbed at the macula densa determines renin release. Dogs on sodium-restricted diets for 10 days have plasma renin activities 12 times normal and plasma aldosterone values 60 times normal. Their juxtaglomerular cells become progressively hyperplastic although they are rarely granulated.

Carotid and aortic bodies and chemoreception

Carotid and aortic bodies are small, difficult to find, and rarely examined at necropsy. They function as chemoreceptors by virtue of connection with the central nervous system. Although no secretion is demonstrable physiologically, they contain dense, secretory granules within their cells. Cytochemical staining indicates that they are sites for synthesis and storage of substances such as serotonin or epinephrine. These bodies are chemoreceptors for CO_2 in blood, and degranulation in response to changes in blood CO_2 occurs. Afferent innervation of the cells is prerequisite to this chemoreceptor hypothesis.

Carotid bodies of animals maintained at high altitudes undergo hyperplasia and have increased numbers of light chief cells. Tumors occur in the aortic and carotid bodies although tumor cells are not known to secrete biologically active peptides.

Atrial natriuretic factor

Atrial natriuretic factor (ANF), a peptide hormone produced in cardiac muscle cells of the atrial wall, is an important regulator of blood pressure and blood volume. Its hormonal effects were first shown when suspensions of homogenized atrial muscle were injected into rats and produced a rapid, massive, short-acting diuresis and natriuresis.

Inside the atrial muscle cell ANF is stored in secretory granules. Granules are released under the stimulus of low sodium and/or increased pressure in the atria (e.g., in congestive heart failure). Atrial myocytes are markedly granulated in animals fed diets low in sodium.

ANF is secreted from the myocyte in inactive form (as a much larger peptide) and released into the coronary vein and thence into the general circulation. In the kidney, ANF binds specifically to tubular epithelial cells, stimulates cyclic guanosine monophosphate (GMP), and induces natriuresis (excretion of sodium) and diuresis (excretion of water). ANF also directly inhibits the renin-angiotensin-aldosterone system.

Plasma atrial natriuretic factor increases in heart failure.

In experiments in dogs, an acute increase in cardiac filling pressure results in enhanced release of circulating ANF and degranulation of atrial myocytes. Clinically, the elevated cardiac filling pressure in congestive heart failure also leads to an increase in blood concentrations of ANF.

ADDITIONAL READING

Barajas, L., and Salido, E. Juxtaglomerular apparatus and the renin-angiotensin system. *Lab. Invest.* 54:361, 1986.

Buergelt, C. D., el al. Endocarditis in six horses. *Vet. Pathol.* 22:333, 1985.

Burnett, J. C., Jr., et al. Atrial natriuretic peptide elevation in congestive heart failure in the human. *Science* 231:1145, 1986.

Jönsson, L. Coronary arterial lesions and myocardial infarcts in the dog. *Acta Vet. Scand.* [Suppl.] 38:1, 1972.

Liu, S.-K., et al. Hypertrophic cardiomyopathy and hyperthyroidism in the cat. *J. Am. Vet. Med. Assoc.* 185:52, 1984.

———. Clinical and pathologic findings in dogs with atherosclerosis: 21 cases (1970–1983). *J. Am. Vet. Med. Assoc.* 189:227, 1986.

Meierhenry, E. F., and Liu, S.-K. Atrioventricular bundle degeneration associated with sudden death in the dog. *J. Am. Vet. Med. Assoc.* 172:1418, 1978.

Muir, W. W., and Weisbrode, S. E. Myocardial ischemia in dogs with gastric dilatation-volvulus. *J. Am. Vet. Med. Assoc.* 181:363, 1982.

Rooney, J. R., et al. Congenital cardiac anomalies in horses. *Vet. Pathol.* 1:454, 1964.

Sandusky, G. E., Jr. Morphologic variations and aging in the atrioventricular conduction system of large breeds of dogs. *Anat. Rec.* 193:883, 1979.

Van Vleet, J. F., and Ferran, V. J. Myocardial diseases of animals. *Am. J. Pathol.* 124:98, 1986.

Hemostasis

16

I N vertebrates, elaborate devices have evolved to prevent blood loss after injury. Despite species differences, these basic mechanisms of hemostasis are remarkably similar. They include (1) *vasoconstriction,* an immediate but transient response that is effective in reducing blood flow; (2) *platelet aggregation* at sites of endothelial injury, which loosely covers the defect; (3) *coagulation,* the polymerization of fibrin from fibrinogen, which forms a clot and firmly binds it to the platelet mass; and (4) *pressure of blood* accumulating extravascularly, which prevents further extravasation. The crucial reaction in stanching blood flow in wounds is the interaction of platelets and coagulation factors within the vessel lumen to form thrombi.

The initial event in clot formation occurs when circulating platelets (or nucleated thrombocytes in nonmammals) adhere to collagen and other fibrous materials exposed at sites of endothelial injury. As platelets aggregate to cover the vascular defect, they are stimulated to release their granules. Various soluble factors in platelet granules are spewed into the plug to recruit new platelets to the mass, to enhance vasoconstriction, and to initiate the process of coagulation.

Surfaces of activated platelets serve as an assembly area for an enzyme cascade of coagulation factors that produce the protein-cleaving enzyme *thrombin.* The target of this protease is *fibrinogen,* a large protein circulating in plasma. When attacked by thrombin, fibrinogen molecules undergo a remarkable polymerization, linking together to form *fibrin,* a large thread-like polymer. Fibrin strands form a network in the vicinity of platelets (because that is where

thrombin is generated), giving the clot stability (Fig. 16.1).

The fibrin clot is only a transitory device, rapidly formed and soon dismantled by fibrinolysis. The fibrinolytic system is a distinct group of enzymes that degrade fibrin into split products. It acts to prevent excessive coagulation that might otherwise kill the host. It also operates to dismantle large clots, thus permitting the permanent repair system of fibroplasia and endothelial regrowth gradually to cover the wound.

PLATELET AGGREGATION

Circulating platelets, or thrombocytes, are necessary for maintenance of normal vascular integrity. As endothelial cells age and detach, platelets extend long pseudopods that attach to subendothelial collagen and cover the defect. After attachment, they release soluble factors that induce them to aggregate with other platelets. When mammalian blood is devoid of platelets, capillaries and postcapillary venules develop fenestrations and are extraordinarily susceptible to hemorrhage.

Platelet structure

Mammalian platelets originate from bone marrow megakaryocytes. Platelet formation is initiated by focal invaginations of the megakaryocyte plasma membrane that rapidly spread inward to dissect the cell (along fissure lines that originate in the endoplasmic reticulum). Disintegration results in production of 3000–4000 platelets per megakaryocyte. When platelets

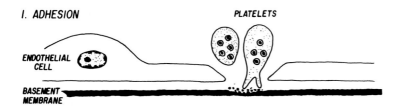

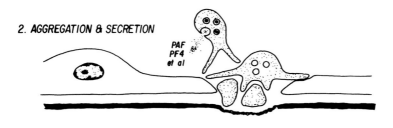

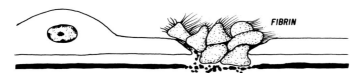

Fig. 16.1. Phases of hemostatic plug formation.

are decreased in circulating blood, megakaryocytes undergo hypertrophy and form increased demarcation lines. They may be spewed into the circulation but are trapped in the lung and rarely found in venous blood.

Platelet surfaces are highly reactive.

Platelet surfaces are covered by an amorphous layer of carbohydrate-rich glycoproteins that make the surface highly reactive and negatively charged. This *glycocalyx* is made of glycoprotein molecules embedded in the plasma membrane. These molecules serve as receptors for procoagulant molecules that either circulate in the bloodstream or are produced by the platelet. By this receptor-mediated attachment, the platelet readily absorbs clotting factors and fibrinogen, giving platelets an extreme tendency to aggregate when in contact with rough surfaces (Figs. 16.2 and 16.3).

In response to interactions with thrombin and subendothelial collagen, platelets release prostaglandins (PGs), which mediate many actions of platelets. The first step in PG synthesis is the release of fatty acid arachidonic acids from deg-

radation of phospholipids within the plasma membrane. Liberated from phospholipid molecules by phospholipases, arachidonic acid is utilized to form specific PGs that constrict vascular smooth muscle and induce platelet aggregation: thromboxane A_2, PGG_2, PGE_2, and PGH_2.

Storage granules contain potent aggregation factors and procoagulants.

Platelets contain two types of granules that are important in thrombosis, α-granules and a variable-sized granule often called a "dense granule."

Alpha-granules contain a variety of proteins that are synthesized in the megakaryocyte, including platelet-specific proteins, *β-thrombospondin, platelet factor 4* (which counteracts the anticoagulant effect of heparin), and *platelet-derived growth factor* (a potent mitogenic stimulant). Alpha-granules also contain fibrinogen, fibronectin, and cationic proteins that mimic those of neutrophils (although with much less effect) in attracting granulocytes from the circulation and increasing vascular permeability.

Dense granules contain surface reactants, most

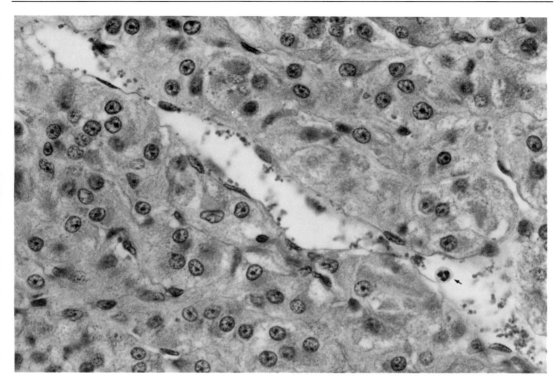

Fig. 16.2. Platelets adhering to veins in the adrenal medulla, sheep with hemorrhagic shock. A neutrophil (*arrow*) is shown in the venous lumen.

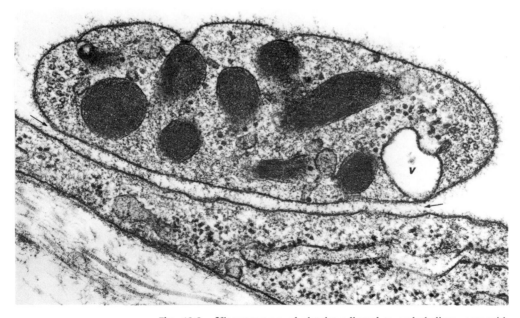

Fig. 16.3. Ultrastructure of platelet adhered to endothelium, cow with viral enteritis. Adhesion of glycocalyx of platelet to glycocalyx of endothelium. Platelet α-*granules* are large and dense; *dense granules* in the cow are electron-lucent with a small, dense, eccentric core.

of which are absorbed and taken into the platelet from plasma. These include amines (serotonin and 5-hydroxytryptamine), calcium, and a metabolically inactive nucleotide, ADP. ADP, when released, induces rapid aggregation of other platelets.

The platelet release reaction

This is the secretion of platelet granules. The process whereby platelets transform from tranquil, discoid bodies to spiked, sticky aggregates discharging their granules is initiated when platelets contact connective tissues of the damaged vascular wall. The contact of platelet with collagen and other thrombogenic substances below damaged endothelium causes a change in the platelet's plasma membrane. Adhesion is mediated by formation of an enzyme-substrate complex between galactosyl hydroxylysine groups of collagen and transferases located in the platelet surface.

Receipt of these "coagulation signals" at the platelet surface induces several striking surface changes. Some of the molecular events include movement of surface proteins, exposure of fibrinogen receptors and anionic lipids, activation of membrane-bound enzymes (such as phospholipases), and alteration of subsurface cytoskeletal fibrils, all of which lead to movement of the platelet surface.

Platelets transform after adhering to collagen.

Platelets change shape from disks to swollen spheres, extend spikelike pseudopods, and progress through a series of changes during the platelet release reaction. The lentiform shape of the normal platelet is maintained by a *marginal band* of microfilaments and microtubules at the periphery. Under stimuli, microtubules depolymerize and reassemble and are important in forming pseudopods and releasing granules. During the release reaction the marginal band contracts forcing organelles to the cell center. Contents of dense bodies and α-granules are extruded form the platelet; the released substances promote aggregation of other platelets.

Fibrinogen is a cofactor in platelet aggregation.

Activated platelets develop new receptors (binding sites) for fibrinogen on their surfaces.

Subsequent contact with fibrinogen leads to enhancement of platelet aggregation. This was first noted when stimuli that aggregated platelets from normal humans failed to do so in plasma from patients with hereditary afibrinogenemia. In vitro, washed platelets suspended in defibrinated plasma fail to aggregate in response to stimuli such as ADP or epinephrine, but addition of fibrin supports aggregation. Both stimuli are required; neither a single external stimulus or fibrinogen can cause platelet aggregation.

Other peptides are involved in strengthening platelet-fibrin binding. *Thrombospondin,* a recently discovered large glycoprotein, is secreted by platelets upon activation. It binds to receptors on the platelet surface (fibrinogen may be a platelet-bound receptor for thrombospondin) and enhances the rate and firmness of fibrin binding. At least one *coagulation factor* (von Willebrand factor) is required for platelets to firmly adhere to subendothelial collagen. Also present in α-granules, von Willebrand factor binds to collagen and to receptors on the platelet surface.

Platelets are phagocytic.

Platelet aggregation can also occur without defects in endothelium. When circulating platelets contact bacteria, bacterial mucopeptides, or cell debris, they are capable of phagocytosis. As phagocytic vacuoles form in the cell, degranulation and aggregation occur. Platelets are only mildly phagocytic and are deputized in inflammatory reactions, especially when neutrophils are missing or defective. This commonly occurs in the terminal stages of severe systemic infectious diseases. In blood smears, abnormal platelets contain distorted granules and intracellular microorganisms.

Hypoalbuminemia enhances platelet aggregation.

Albumin inhibits the platelet release reaction by binding platelet products that would otherwise enhance platelet aggregation. In dogs, the availability of these platelet substances inversely correlates with the amount of albumin in plasma. Dogs with hypoalbuminemia arising from renal disease may show increased platelet aggregation responses. Thrombosis, a common complication in these dogs, probably is due to low albumin in plasma. Increased release of platelet products may enhance the primary

renal defect and lead to a vicious cycle of albumin loss → platelet hyperaggregation →
platelet release reaction in glomeruli →
enhanced glomerulopathy.

Hyperlipidemia enhances platelet aggregation.

Elevations in plasma concentration of lipids
and cholesterol are associated with thrombosis
in various diseases. Hypercholesterolemia alters
the lipid content of platelet surface membranes
and endothelial cells (which is the more important is not clear), and platelets become hyperre-
sponsive to substances that stimulate the platelet release reaction.

Platelet aggregation can be quantitated in an aggregometer.

Blood is centrifuged so that leukocytes are removed, leaving the lighter platelets suspended
in plasma. When placed in the path of a light
beam and stirred, the diffuse cloud of platelets
scatters the light and prevents much of it from
reaching a photocell on the other side of the
glass tube. When an aggregating agent is added,
the platelets clump together, allowing more light
to pass through the suspension. A tracing of the
amount of light reaching the photocell provides
a record of aggregation.

Thrombocytopenia

Thrombocytopenia is a drop below 100,000
platelets/ml circulating blood. In most species, a
drop below 50,000/ml is accompanied by abnormal bleeding tendencies. In dogs, bleeding occurs when platelets drop below 30,000/ml. Vascular perfusion experiments clearly demonstrate the perpetual function of these cells in
maintaining a closed vascular system. When an
organ is perfused with platelet-poor plasma it
develops hemorrhages; organs perfused with
platelet-rich plasma do not.

The diagnosis of platelet deficiency is based
chiefly on three criteria: a history of bleeding,
low platelet counts, and increased bleeding
time. The history should include a tendency for
bleeding because it is impossible for platelet deficiency to exist for even brief periods without
affecting hemostasis. The platelet count should
be low, but platelet deficiency can also exist
when platelets themselves are abnormal (the
count may be normal and even elevated, but the

platelets do not function normally). To confirm
the diagnosis of platelet deficiency, the establishment of an abnormal bleeding time is essential.

Mechanisms of thrombocytopenia include (1)
deficient formation of platelets in bone marrow
(e.g., estrogen toxicosis); (2) excessive utilization, which occurs in any disease with widespread endothelial damage; and (3) premature
destruction, either by intravascular lysis or by
removal by the reticuloendothelial system. *Acquired thrombocytopenia* may occur in systemic
infectious disease, in acute radiation injury,
during drug treatment, and as part of some immunologic diseases involving antiplatelet antibodies (Table 16.1). When known mechanisms
of thrombocytopenia are not identified as causes
of bleeding, the condition is referred to as
idiopathic thrombocytopenic purpura.

Viruses cause thrombocytopenia by several mechanisms.

The widespread hemorrhagic diatheses that
characterize several peracute viral diseases are
due to diffuse virus-induced *endothelial damage*
(e.g., infectious canine hepatitis, hog cholera,
African swine fever, simian hemorrhagic fever,
and epidemic hemorrhagic disease of deer).
Thrombocytopenia is severe because platelets
attach to sites of endothelial injury throughout
the body (Fig. 16.4). When platelets are de-

Table 16.1. Platelet defect diseases

Defect	Association
Thrombocytopenia	
Platelet production	Neoplasms
	Estrogen therapy
	Hypothermia
Platelet destruction	Antiplatelet antibodies
	Viral diseases
	Uremia
	Drug toxicity
Thrombocytopathy	
Adhesion	von Willebrand's disease
	Thrombopathy (Bernard-Soulier syndrome)
Aggregation	Afibrinogenemia
	Thrombasthenia (Glanzmann's disease)
	Aleutian mink
Granule factors	Chediak-Higashi syndrome
Secretion	Aspirin and other nonsteroid drugs

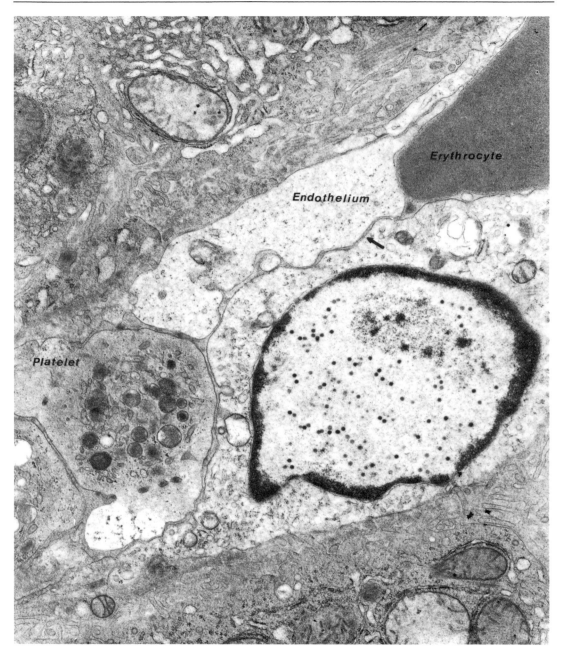

Fig. 16.4. Platelet trapping, liver sinusoid, infectious canine hepatitis (canine adenovirus-1). Marked swelling of sinusoidal endothelial cells with obliteration of lumen (*arrow*). Platelet apposed to endothelial cell surfaces is in early phase of release reaction: α-granules have pale areas, smaller dense granules at periphery.

pleted and sites of endothelial injury cannot be covered, hemorrhage occurs.

In most viral hemorrhagic diseases, thrombocytopenia results from the combined effects of direct viral injury to platelets and endothelium (e.g., the petechial and ecchymotic hemorrhages in the skin and below serosal surface in acute hog cholera). Dr. John Edwards, then working at the Plum Island Animal Disease Center, showed that thrombocytopenia is a major force in hemorrhages of African swine fever.

Bleeding into submucosal and subserosal areas is characteristic of terminal phases of *infectious canine hepatitis*. The occurrence of erythrocyte extravasation correlates with the lowest points in the thrombocyte count curve (Fig. 16.5). Although the liver is injured and decreased prothrombin and fibrinogen concentrations in plasma have been detected, these factors are less significant in promoting bleeding. They merely exaggerate the tendency to hemorrhage. Examination of liver lesions in early disease reveals the nature of the thrombocytopenia; platelets are trapped in hepatic sinusoids by

damaged endothelium to such a great extent that they disappear from circulation.

Thrombocytopathy: Defective platelet function

Acquired thrombocytopathy is common (usually subclinical) as a side effect of therapy with aspirin and phenylbutazone. Aspirin causes a primary release defect that irreversibly acetylates and inactivates the enzyme cyclooxygenase, thus inhibiting secretion mediated by prostaglandins and thromboxane. Aspirin prolongs bleeding time only slightly in normal animals but drastically in animals with other disorders of platelet function.

Congenital platelet defects

Hereditary thrombocytopathy is more severe than the acquired forms (Table 16.1). Rare specific congenital platelet defects are termed *thrombasthenia* (weak platelets) or *thrombopathy*. These have been seen in otter hounds, basset hounds, Simmental cattle, domestic cats, Aleu-

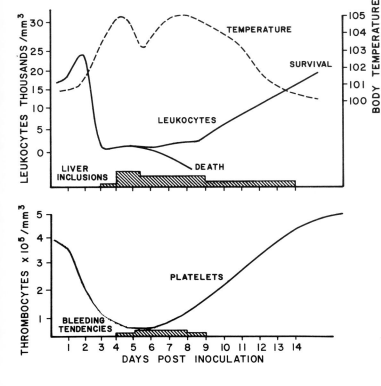

EXPERIMENTAL INFECTIOUS CANINE HEPATITIS

Fig. 16.5. Pathogenesis of infectious canine hepatitis: relation of platelet deficiency to bleeding.

tian mink, and fawn-hooded rats. In blood smears, severe structural distortions of platelets are present, and most affected animals have defective platelet granules. Platelets of some thrombasthenia patients lack platelet surface glycoprotein receptors and do not bind fibrinogen, and they do not aggregate normally.

Several genetic diseases with major problems in other tissue systems also have defective platelets as an accompanying abnormality. Platelets of mice, cattle, and mink with Chediak-Higashi disease are deficient in dense granules, serotonin, and ADP, and affected animals have prolonged bleeding times.

Platelets decrease in hypothermia and hibernation.

A decrease in circulating platelets accompanies some physiologic changes, particularly body temperature. Significant depressions in platelets, coagulation factors, and leukocytes occur in dogs made *hypothermic* by body surface cooling. These alterations serve as a protective mechanism to inhibit thrombosis under conditions of retarded blood flow.

Thrombocytopenia and prolonged clotting time (due to deficiency of coagulation factors VIII and IX) occur during *hibernation*. The striking decrease in platelet numbers is due to sequestration in the cords and red pulp of the spleen. The low body temperature induces the platelet's peripheral microtubules to contract, which changes the shape of the platelet and promotes its retention during passage through the spleen.

Platelet dysplasia occurs in megakaryocytic leukemia.

Megakaryoblastic leukemia is a very rare disease characterized by circulation of undifferentiated megakaryoblasts and infiltration of neoplastic megakaryocytes and their blast forms in bone marrow and viscera. In dogs, spontaneous bleeding may complicate the disease. In the circulation, there are many giant agranular platelets in addition to the leukemic megakaryoblasts.

BLOOD COAGULATION

Clotting (blood coagulation) results when blood vessel walls are injured, especially when endothelium is destroyed. The clot is formed by an enzymatic cascade, a series of zymogen activations in which an activated form of one coagulation factor catalyzes the activation of the next. Only small amounts of early factors are needed because of the catalytic nature of the process.

Coagulation (the formation of fibrin) is initiated when activated factor X (X_a) cleaves the circulating protein *prothrombin* into two fragments. One fragment is no longer functional in coagulation and is released into blood; the other is *thrombin,* a proteolytic enzyme that converts plasma fibrinogen to fibrin:

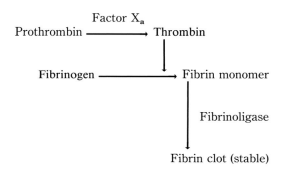

Two distinct enzyme pathways, intrinsic and extrinsic, cause activation of factor X. The end products of both pathways are proteolytic enzymes that initiate the final common pathway of fibrin formation shown above.

Extrinsic pathway

This pathway occurs outside the vessel wall when shed blood contacts tissue debris. Clotting is thus triggered by substances not normally in blood. Trauma to blood vessels releases membrane fragments into tissue. *Tissue factor* is a glycoprotein embedded in membranes of most cells. Also called thromboplastin and coagulation factor III, it modifies the enzyme proconvertin (factor VII) which in turn acts on factor X to initiate the common pathway of fibrin formation. The extrinsic pathway can be demonstrated by adding a few drops of a dilute suspension of brain tissue extract to normal plasma; clotting is rapidly induced as follows:

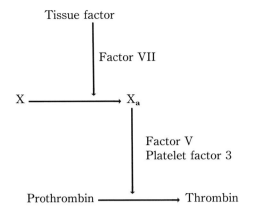

Intrinsic pathway

Intrinsic coagulation is triggered by the effects of abnormal surfaces on components normally present in blood. All the factors of the intrinsic system are present in normal plasma. In the 1860s, Lister demonstrated that blood remained fluid when placed in the excised vein of a cow but rapidly clotted when removed and placed in a glass tube; the glass surface triggered coagulation of components in the blood. In vivo, clotting usually involves a mixture of intrinsic and extrinsic mechanisms.

The intrinsic pathway involves a cascade of complex enzymic reactions, each of which activates the next until factor X is activated:

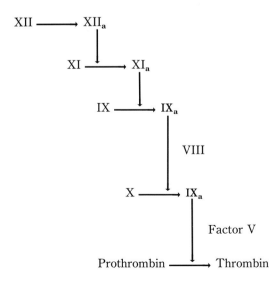

Factor XII is activated on platelet surfaces.

Commonly, factor XII is activated by contact with negative charges on the surfaces of aggregating platelets. When the blood vessel wall is disrupted, subendothelial collagen, basement membrane material, and other connective tissue elements are exposed to plasma. Free carboxyl groups of the exposed collagen activate factor XII, which then initiates the rapid, complex sequence of clotting that terminates in cleavage of prothrombin and ultimately in fibrin polymerization (Table 16.2).

In addition to activation on platelet membranes (or solid phase activation), factor XII is also cleaved in fluid phase by proteolysis to yield fragments active in fibrinolysis and kinin release (see Fig. 19.2). Thus, plasma deficient in factor XII not only clots abnormally but shows reduced ability to generate fibrinolysis.

Common pathway

Activated factor X (X_a) is produced by proteolysis of factor X, which occurs at the terminus of both intrinsic and extrinsic coagulation pathways. X_a is a prothrombinase complex that converts prothrombin to thrombin. Factor X may also be activated by a calcium ion (Ca^{++})-dependent activation on platelet surfaces.

Prostaglandins released by damaged endothelium are intimately associated with coagulation, that is, tissue injury → endothelial PGI_2 release → factor X activation → coagulation. Factor X_a is a potent inhibitor of thromboxane A_2 synthesis in platelets and prostacyclin (PCI_2) synthesis in endothelial cells. PGI_2 inhibits platelet aggregation but does not significantly affect coagulation.

Prothrombin is a zymogen for thrombin.

Prothrombin is synthesized in hepatocytes and released into the bloodstream by the liver. At one end of the prothrombin molecule is a string of carboxylated glutamates. These peculiar amino acids, arising by the carboxylation of terminal glutamates by a vitamin K–containing series of enzymes, are strong chelators of Ca^{++}. By binding Ca^{++}, prothrombin is anchored to phospholipid membranes derived from platelets, bringing it in close proximity to factors X_a and V, which accelerate prothrombin cleavage. During activation of prothrombin, the terminal Ca^{++}-binding fragment is cleaved away, leaving

Table 16.2.   Blood coagulation factors

Factor	Common Name	Deficiency
I	Fibrinogen (I_a = fibrin)	Congenital afibrinogenemia in goats, man, and borzoi dogs
II	Prothrombin (II_a = thrombin)	Acquired deficiencies common; congenital deficiencies in English cocker spaniels
III	Thromboplastin	Tissue product; concentrated in brain and lung
IV	Calcium	If plasma Ca^{++} is bound by oxalates or citrates, clotting is stopped
V	Proaccelerin	Deficiency not recognized in animals
VII	Proconvertin	Hereditary deficiency in beagles
VIII	Antihemophilic factor A	Classic hemophilia in cats, cattle, swine, horses, dogs (in males, sex-linked)
IX	Antihemophilic factor B	Hereditary deficiency, rare, in cats and dogs; depressed by coumarin-type drugs
X	Stuart factor	Deficiency hereditary or acquired; depressed by coumarin-type drugs
XI	Plasma thromboplastin antecedent[a]	Hereditary deficiency in Holstein cattle and English springer and Great Pyrenees dogs
XII	Hageman factor[a]	Hereditary deficiency in cats, standard poodles, German shorthaired pointer
XIII	Fibrinoligase	Strengthens clot network once fibrin is formed

[a]Activity not established in lower vertebrates.

active thrombin free on the membrane surface to activate fibrinogen.

Thrombin cleaves peptides from fibrinogen.

Fibrinogen is a soluble plasma protein with a molecular weight of nearly 340,000. The molecule is nodose and consists of three beads held together by a thin strand of protein (Fig. 16.6). Running throughout the molecule are three different chains (α, β, and γ) interconnected by disulfide bonds. There is an excess negative charge on the molecule with a disproportionate amount on the central region.

The triggering event for transformation of fibrinogen to fibrin monomer is the thrombin-catalyzed removal of small polar peptides (called fibrinopeptides A and B) from the central regions of the α and β chains. Cleavage of fibrinopeptides reduces the negative charge on the central region, so the fibrin monomer assumes

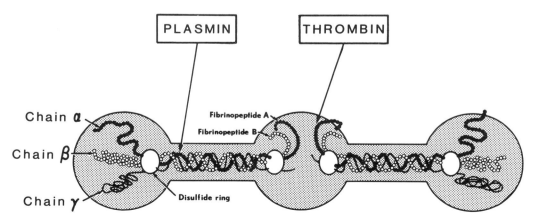

Fig. 16.6   Fibrinogen molecule: sites at which plasmin and thrombin exert their effects.

an overall positive charge. Since the terminal regions retain a negative charge (interchain areas are neutral), the fibrin monomers spontaneously polymerize in overlapping, staggered patterns that give the typical periodicity to fibrinogen in electron micrographs.

Fibrin is stabilized by an enzyme (factor XIII).

Establishment of covalent bonds between fibrin monomers by the enzyme factor XIII (fibrinoligase, or "fibrin stabilizing factor") strengthens fibrin strands and stabilizes the fibrin gel. Factor XIII is activated by thrombin from a precursor in plasma and in platelets. The enzyme stitches neighboring fibrin monomers together by forming a peptide bond between side chains to form cross-links (it catalyzes formation of amide bonds between glutamine and lysine).

Factor XIII not only cross-links fibrin-fibrin but also fibrin-collagen, fibrin-fibronectin, and fibronectin-collagen. Thus, the clot is firmly anchored into place in the tissue.

Coagulation disorders

Absence or defectiveness of any of the clotting factors may result in inadequate blood coagulation. Alternatively, coagulation may be impaired by inhibitors or by the proteolytic action of plasmin. The clinical signs of these diseases involve hemorrhage. In general, large hematomas suggest a coagulation disorder whereas chronic bleeding from a mucosal surface indicates a platelet deficiency. An accurate differential diagnosis is largely a laboratory exercise. It is usually necessary that the coagulation time, bleeding time, partial thromboplastin time, prothrombin time, and platelet count be determined (Table 16.3).

When an abnormal clotting mechanism is suspected because of prolonged clotting times and abnormal partial thromboplastin and prothrombin times, the specific coagulation factor deficiency can be determined. Dr. Jean Dodds, at the New York State Department of Health, has made a lifelong study of bleeding disease of animals and is the international authority on these conditions.

Hereditary deficiencies in coagulation factors

These disorders are discovered after excessive bruising, hematoma formation, and continued bleeding after minor trauma or surgery. In severe cases there may be melena, lameness due to periarticular hemorrhage, or prolonged estral bleeding.

Hemophilia is the bleeding diathesis resulting from a lack of procoagulant proteins in plasma. Affected animals develop localized hemorrhages in various tissues, particularly in joints. The defects are temporarily corrected by transfusions of normal plasma. Laboratory findings include prolonged clotting time and secondary bleeding time; platelets and prothrombin times are usually normal.

Hemophilia B is caused by factor IX deficiency.

Also a sex-linked recessive disease, hemophilia B is more rare than factor VIII deficiency. Most cases have less than 1% factor IX. It has been reported in 12 breeds of dogs: coonhound, St. Bernard, cocker spaniel, bulldog, Alaskan malamute, Shetland sheepdog, and cairn, Airedale, and Scottish terriers. It also occurs in cats. Blood tests are similar to factor VIII deficiency but the activated partial thromboplastin time defect is corrected by addition of normal serum

Table 16.3. Coagulation tests in dogs

Test	Normal Value	Definition
Coagulation time	1–5 sec	Time for blood to coagulate in vitro after withdrawal from vein
Bleeding time	<6 min	Time for bleeding to stop after puncture wound with periodic removal of blood with filter paper
Prothrombin time (PT)	<15 sec	Time required for clotting of oxalated plasma by addition of calcium (in presence of excess thromboplastin)
Activated partial thromboplastin time (APTT)	45 sec	Measurement of intrinsic and common coagulation systems

(because serum contains factor IX activity but not factor VIII coagulant activity).

Hemophilia A (classic hemophilia) is caused by factor VIII deficiency.

Hemophilia A is the most common severe hereditary coagulation defect of animals and has been reported in most breeds of dogs and in cats, Hereford cattle (in Australia), and in standardbred and thoroughbred horses. Hemophilia is a recessive, sex-linked disease; that is, it is carried by the female and manifest by the male. In dogs, hemophilia A may be mild, moderate, or severe.

Factor VIII is produced in the liver. After activation by trace amounts of thrombin, it accelerates the rate of factor X activation by factor IX. In circulating blood, factor VIII is carried by a large adhesive glycoprotein called von Willebrand factor (vWF). This *factor VIII complex* thus has two components: VIII ("antihemophilic factor") and vWF. It plays roles in both clot formation and platelet adhesion, and two of the most common bleeding disorders of animals are a result of a deficiency in the activity of one or the other of these components.

von Willebrand's disease is factor VIII component deficiency.

In plasma, von Willebrand factor is a huge multimere of several molecules. It is an adhesive glycoprotein synthesized by endothelial cells and megakaryocytes and serves as a carrier for factor VIII. By binding to platelet surfaces and to subendothelial collagen, it promotes shearing-dependent platelet adhesion to blood vessel walls.

In von Willebrand disease (VWD), this endothelial component is deficient (hemorrhages can be corrected by giving the patient plasma from factor VIII–deficient hemophiliacs). The von Willebrand factor is assayed with the antibiotic ristocetin, which agglutinates platelets suspended in normal plasma but not platelets in plasma from VWD.

This is the most common mild hereditary bleeding disorder of animals. It is an autosomal trait with two forms of genetic expression: an autosomal *recessive disease,* in which individuals are homozygous for the VWD gene and have two asymptomatic heterozygous parents, and an autosomal *incompletely dominant disease* with variable expression, in which both homozygotes and heterozygotes can have bleeding disease (homozygosity is usually lethal).

The incompletely dominant disease is common and occurs in over 28 breeds of dogs. Scottish terriers have a high prevalence of gene frequency. The recessive disease has been reported in Poland China swine, Scottish terriers, and Chesapeake Bay retrievers.

VWD presents as a bleeding diathesis involving mucosal surfaces and is often associated with physical stresses or other diseases. Signs include gastrointestinal hemorrhage, recurrent hematuria, epistaxis, and bleeding from gingiva, vagina, penis, and nose. Affected dogs may bleed to death after surgery. They have long bleeding times, abnormal platelet retention (in vitro), and variable factor VIII-C levels. In dogs, bleeding diathesis becomes less severe with age and during pregnancy. The disease may be silent, despite prolonged bleeding times, abnormal prothrombin consumption, and reduced platelet adhesiveness.

Acquired deficiencies of coagulation

Acquired deficiencies of coagulation accompany many severe diseases, often with serious consequences. There may be transitory depression of factor synthesis, excessive utilization for hemostasis, or consumption of factors during pathologic intravascular clotting. Factor deficiency may cause prolonged coagulation and prothrombin times even though the thrombocyte count is normal.

Acquired disorders may be general or specific. Severe *trauma* or deep *burns* produce consumption of most coagulation factors. In contrast, some snake venoms and plant toxins precisely affect only one coagulation factor.

Liver failure is associated with low coagulation factor levels.

The liver is the important site of synthesis of many coagulation factors, and acute destruction of hepatocytes or chronic liver disease may result in bleeding tendencies; for example *hypoprothrombinemia* secondary to liver failure can be responsible for the clotting disorder. Other causes are heparinemia (as in anaphylaxis) and poisoning with dicoumarin.

Hemorrhage is severe in vitamin K deficiency.

Vitamin K is required for synthesis of coagulation factors. Its deficiency, either dietary or due to malabsorption, is accompanied by defects in clotting. Vitamin K acts at the translational level of protein synthesis in the hepatocyte to regulate biosynthesis of prothrombin and other factors.

Abnormal prothrombin is synthesized in the absence of vitamin K or in the presence of vitamin K antagonists such as dicumarol. Although its amino acid sequence is normal, the carboxyglutamate amino terminus that binds Ca^{++} is defective because vitamin K is an integral part of the enzymes that carboxylate the glutamate residues. Cattle fed dicumarol (which occurs naturally in lush sweet clover) produce this abnormal prothrombin that cannot bind Ca^{++}.

Anticoagulating rodenticides are usually derivatives of 4-hydroxycoumarin (warfarin, dicumarol) or of indan-1,3-dione (diphacinone, pindone). These drugs inhibit coagulation by suppressing hepatic synthesis of coagulation factors II, VII, IX, and X. There is no effect on circulating coagulation factors so that a latent period of 24 hours occurs between consumption and clinical signs; in this period circulating coagulation factors are depleted.

The rat poison *warfarin,* a coumarin derivative, inhibits the hepatic enzyme system responsible for synthesis of coagulation factors. Poisoned dogs have pallor of mucous membranes, petechiae or ecchymoses, epistaxis, and hemoptysis. In severe cases hemorrhages in pulmonary and enteric tracts occur. Poisoning is characterized by progressive lowering of plasma concentrations of factors VII, IX, X, and II, leading to a hemostatic defect with prolonged bleeding times. Treatment with vitamin K corrects the deficiency and will produce reversal of hypoprothrombinemia within one hour. Coumarin derivatives produced by toxigenic fungi growing on clover cause similar bleeding diseases in animals eating contaminated hay.

Viruses cause hemorrhage by depressing coagulation factors.

Several of the viruses that attach endothelium produce clinical signs of hemorrhage that are a result, in part, of excessive consumption of coagulation factors. For example, hog cholera virus replicates in endothelium, platelets, and leukocytes and induces degeneration and cellular death. One of the consequences of the widespread endothelial damage is the exhaustion of coagulation factors in attempt to repair the vascular endothelium. The hemorrhages that typify the terminal stages of hog cholera, therefore, are due not only to the direct virus-induced dam-

FOCUS

Dicumarol and sweet clover poisoning

When it was discovered in the early 1900s that sweet clover (*Melilotus* spp.) would grow on marginal land, this plant became a popular crop among early settlers in the northern Midwest and upper plains area of Canada. Simultaneously, "outbreaks" of a new hemorrhagic cattle disease began to appear. Cattle were prone to bleed to death after castration or dehorning. Pregnant cows aborted, and newborn calves bled during the first few days of life.

Dr. Frank Schofield, the veterinary pathologist at the Ontario Veterinary College at Guelph, first recognized that this disease occurred only in cows that had eaten moldy sweet clover silage. He showed that feeding the spoiled sweet clover to rabbits caused them to bleed and that at the time of bleeding the clotting time of the blood was prolonged. He also noted that transfusions of clotted, defibrinated blood briefly stopped the hemorrhage and shortened the clotting time. Dr. Lee Roderick of Fargo, North Dakota, confirmed this work in 1929 and added that the plasma prothrombin level was depressed in cattle with sweet clover poisoning.

▶

The disease persisted wherever sweet clover was harvested and allowed to turn moldy in silos. In 1938, a second crucial link was put into place. A farmer strode down the corridors of the University of Wisconsin sloshing unclotted blood from a pail onto the floor. He wanted action because his castrated and dehorned cattle were bleeding to death. Biochemists shortly identified the toxic substance: two coumarin molecules linked by formaldehyde.

Called dicumarol, this compound was quickly developed as an anticoagulant in man. Shortly thereafter it appeared as a rodenticide called *warfarin* (for Wisconsin Alumni Research Foundation). Poisoned rats bleed from body orifices, especially into tissue around the eyes. Death results from massive bleeding into the abdominal cavity.

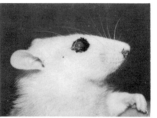

Warfarin markedly decreases the prothrombin concentration in circulating blood. Serum from poisoned rats has a pronounced depressant effect on prothrombin convertability. Dicumarol acts primarily by inhibiting the conversion factor and only secondarily by depressing prothrombin.

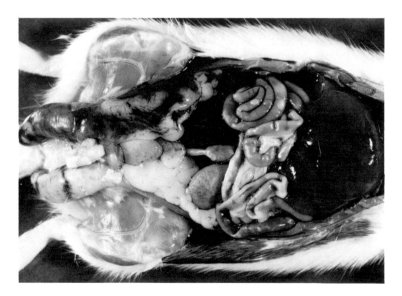

age to capillaries and platelets but to the superimposition of coagulation factor deficiency and exhaustion thrombocytopenia. The same process is true for infectious canine hepatitis and several other systemic viral infections.

PREVENTION OF COAGULATION

When activated within the vascular system, the combined effects of platelet aggregation and activation of the coagulation system would, if uncontrolled, lead to disastrous accumulation of fibrin thrombi within blood vessels. To prevent disseminated intravascular coagulation from following even minor wounds, three potent mechanisms of resistance to thrombosis are present: (1) *thromboresistance* of endothelial surfaces, (2) *thrombin inhibition* by antithrombin III and heparin, and (3) *lysis of fibrin* by the fibrinolytic system in circulating blood. Thus normal vascular patency appears to depend on an equilibrium between coagulation and fibrinolysis.

Thromboresistance of endothelium

Normal endothelium is resistant to thrombosis because (1) α_2-*macroglobulins* in the glycocalyx coating the lumenal surfaces of endothelial cells inhibit proteases of the coagulation, fibrinolytic, and kinin systems that operate extracellularly, (2) enzymes within endothelial cells convert endoperoxides to *prostaglandins* (particularly PGI_2 and PGE_1), which prevent or reverse platelet aggregation, and (3) protein C activation of *thrombomodulin,* a protein on the surface of endothelial cells that binds to thrombin, (a) decreasing its ability to catalyze clot formation and (b) increasing its ability to activate protein C. These powerful surveillance systems cooperate to prevent thrombosis during normal body functioning. PGI_2 (prostacyclin) inhibits platelet functions in all species of animals, including secretion of granules, release of arachidonic acid metabolites, and expression of fibrinogen receptors on platelet surfaces.

Protein C, which is a zymogen of a serine protease, is a potent anticoagulant that selectively inactivates factors V_a and VIII. Produced in the liver, it is activated at endothelial surfaces by thrombin, activating thrombomodulin. Protein C also stimulates fibrinolysis.

Antithrombin III and heparin inhibit thrombin action.

Activated clotting factors are short-lived because they are diluted by blood, removed by the reticuloendothelial system, degraded by proteases, and inactivated by specific inhibitors. *Antithrombin III,* a plasma protein that inactivates thrombin (by irreversibly complexing with it), also inhibits other clotting factors. Its inhibitory action is enhanced by *heparin,* which acts as an anticoagulant by increasing the formation of the irreversible complex between thrombin and antithrombin III. Treatment of an animal with heparin suppresses coagulation and induces a prolonged activated partial thromboplastin time (APTT).

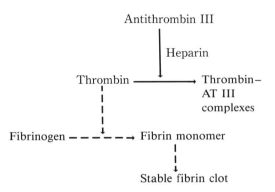

Fibrinolysis

Once a platelet-fibrin clot forms over a wound, endothelial cells bordering the wounded area release materials that activate fibrinolysis. The fibrinolytic mechanism is the biologic converse of the coagulation mechanism. The process begins when a circulating plasma protein is activated to form the fibrinolytic enzyme *plasmin* (sometimes called "fibrinolysin"). The end product of coagulation, fibrin, is the substrate for plasmin; that is, plasmin degrades fibrin and releases fibrin breakdown products into the circulation.

Plasmin, a relatively nonspecific serine protease, degrades not only fibrin but, to a lesser degree, several circulating proteins, including fibrinogen and other coagulation factors. Breakdown of fibrinogen produces fibrinogen fragments that are also anticoagulant.

The detection of plasmin is not clinically

meaningful in animal blood because the stress of collection tends to give faulty data and because detection in plasma is difficult due to the immense amount of antiplasmin in plasma. This, unfortunately, allows only limited knowledge of how plasmin functions in disease.

Plasmin is formed from circulating plasminogen.

Plasmin is formed by the action of an "activator" on an inactive precursor, *plasminogen,* a β-globulin present in normal plasma. Plasminogen activators convert plasminogen to plasmin chiefly on the surfaces of thrombi; although usually not detected, conversion also occurs in circulating blood.

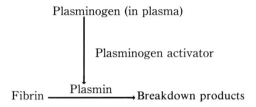

Plasminogen activator is synthesized by endothelial cells.

Plasminogen activator is distributed in tissues unevenly and is detected by a quantitative extraction and assay method or by a histochemical fibrin (substrate) slide technique. In the latter, a section of frozen tissue is placed on a slide containing a thin layer of fibrin rich in the fibrinolytic proenzyme plasminogen. Holes develop in the fibrin showing where fibrin has been digested by activated plasminogen.

Although fibrinolytic activity is most prominently associated with vascular endothelium, it also occurs around leukocytes and some epithelial cells. Macrophages that enter inflammatory sites produce large amounts of plasminogen activator, for example, and the secretion of this enzyme enables them to transect fibrin barriers encountered during migration. In severe, acute bacterial infections, increased amounts of activators of plasminogen can be detected in plasma.

Increases in plasminogen activators also occur in plasma during ischemia, shock, and disseminated neoplastic disease. Some neoplastic cells produce large amounts of plasminogen activators, which may promote tumor invasion.

Biochemists suggest that the plasminogen ac-

tivator circulating in plasma is slightly different from that found in tissue. The *tissue plasminogen activator* (which can be purchased commercially) is more specific than most plasminogen activators; it has a low affinity for circulating plasminogen and has been called "clot specific." Used experimentally as a thrombolytic agent to study removal of clots injected intravenously into animals, it has been used recently in human clinical trials to remove intravascular thromboemboli. Tissue plasminogen activator lacks the side effect of hemorrhage that accompanies the more commonly used urokinase or streptokinase.

Exogenous substances also activate plasminogen.

There is a direct relation between vasoactive change and fibrinolytic activity. Injections of histamine and adrenalin also induce enhanced fibrinolysis in dogs. Exogenous activators of plasminogen include the bacterial products streptokinase and staphylokinase. Vampire bat saliva is a potent source of fibrinolytic activity, enabling these predators to feed on the blood of cattle and other mammals.

THROMBOSIS

The solid mass of blood constituents that forms within blood vessels (or endothelium of the heart cavities) is called a *thrombus* (Fig. 16.7), and the process of its formation is *thrombosis.* The two inseparable mechanisms that induce thrombosis are platelet aggregation and fibrinogen polymerization. Any agent that extensively damages endothelial surfaces of blood vessels will cause thrombosis. Infectious agents are important causes. They include viruses that replicate in and destroy endothelial cells and bacteria and fungi that cause tissue lesions that erode through blood vessel walls.

Morphologically, thrombi must be differentiated from clots that form extravascularly and from clots that form in vessels after death (postmortem clotting). In addition, the presence of multiple thrombi suggests the possibility of disseminated intravascular coagulation.

Thrombi can be fatal if they occur in blood vessels of visceral organs, particularly lung, heart, and intestine. Partial obstruction of large arteries is one of the more common types of thrombosis, particularly in horses, in which thrombosis of the major arteries is associated

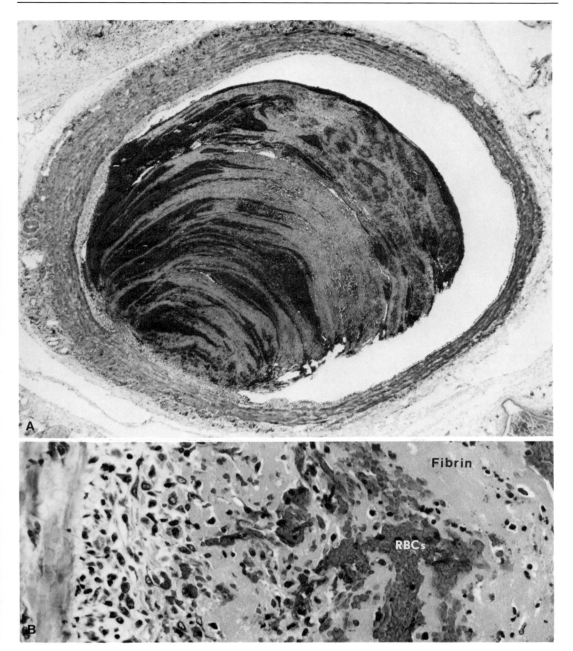

Fig. 16.7. Venous thrombosis, dog with histoplasmosis. A. Thrombus attached to wall of vein draining hepatic lymph node. B. Enlargement of A: Thrombus contains fibrin and entrapped leukocytes and erythrocytes (RBCs). Fibroblasts are at the site of attachment to endothelium (*at left*).

with strongyle infestation (Fig. 16.8). When thrombosis occurs in the splanchnic arteries, the intestine is at risk of gangrene and colic is an early sign. When the aorta is markedly involved, signs include exercise-induced hindlimb lameness, which disappears on rest (even if aortic lesions are severe). The affected limb is cool, fails to sweat during exercise, and has diminished arterial pulse and decreased filling of saphenous veins. Studies of thrombosis of the terminal aorta and iliac arteries of horses by Dr. Grant Maxie, at the Ontario Veterinary College, suggested that organization of strongyle-related thromboemboli were the cause of lameness.

Thrombus formation
Thrombosis involves suppression of natural vascular thromboresistance.

As platelets adhere to an injured vessel wall, a plug forms and enlarges by aggregation of other circulating platelets. The two systems of thromboresistance are overwhelmed by the great facility with which platelets synthesize the opposing prostaglandins that initiate aggregation (thromboxane A_2 and PGE_2). As the fusing platelets discharge granule factors and thromboplastin into the plug area, fibrin polymerization is initiated. Platelet stimulation by ADP, epi-

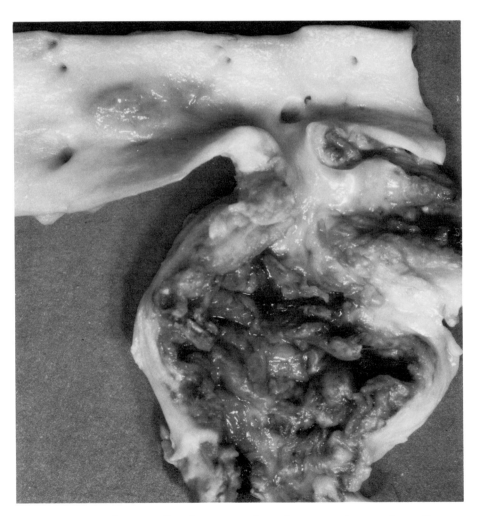

Fig. 16.8. Pseudoaneurysm of anterior mesenteric artery, horse. Rugose endothelial surface and thrombosis are due to invasion by the parasite *Stongylus vulgaris.*

nephrine, and thrombin exposes binding sites specific for fibrinogen on the platelet surface, where the large, intact, symmetric fibrinogen molecules immediately bind the platelets together in a stable thrombus.

Experimental thrombosis has been studied by placing a silk suture in the carotid artery of pigs. Within 1 hour, a thrombus of densely packed platelets is present. The subsequent formation of alternating bands of fibrin and platelets may impart a laminated appearance to the thrombus. With time, the platelets disintegrate and the thrombus appears as a friable, heterogeneous mass of fibrin. Anticoagulant drugs such as *heparin* have little effect on the platelet component but can effectively depress the deposition of fibrin.

Arterial and venous thrombi differ.

Thrombi are heterogeneous structures, and their heterogeneity is a reflection of both the site where they are formed and their age. Thrombi that develop in slow zones of blood flow such as veins are composed of fibrin strands with entrapped erythrocytes, since the dominant mechanism of formation is coagulation. In contrast, arterial thrombi are generally due to endothelial injury, and the initial thrombus is composed of aggregated platelets (Fig. 16.9). As arterial thrombi grow, however, flow patterns adjacent to the thrombi cause fibrin to be deposited and the platelet mass that persists is transformed into a fibrin mass. Fibrin strands

polymerize between the separating and degenerating platelets.

Neutrophils stick to thrombi.

When the fibrin around a platelet thrombus becomes fully polymerized, circulating platelets no longer adhere to it readily. Neutrophils stick to the fibrin-platelet mass via chemotactic factors produced by plasmin-fibrin interaction and the release of platelet factors that interact with complement. The invading neutrophils are important in dissolution of the thrombus.

Contraction occurs as thrombi age.

The contractile property of platelets resides in microfilaments and in microtubules (which contain a contractile protein called thrombosthenin). Organization proceeds as condensed bands of fibrin and platelets attach to the vascular wall and become overgrown by endothelium.

Recanalization of thrombi permits blood flow.

If significant occlusion of the blood vessel has taken place, recanalization permits blood to again flow through the vessel. This occurs by invasion of the thrombus mass by newly formed capillaries, which then anastomose.

Stasis promotes thrombosis.

During immobilization (as in surgery), procoagulant materials circulate and become trapped in areas of stasis. If stasis is prolonged,

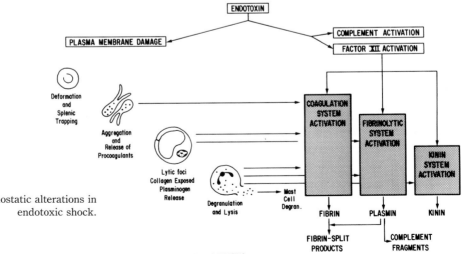

Fig. 16.9. Hemostatic alterations in endotoxic shock.

coagulation reactions may proceed to completion and form small intravascular clots. In normal animals these small thrombi fail to enlarge (to form significant venous thrombi), probably because of clotting suppression by inhibitors in plasma such as antithrombin III. Microthrombi are removed by the liver as they circulate.

Disseminated intravascular coagulation

Coagulation within the intact vascular system accompanies some severe systemic diseases in which clotting mechanisms are activated. During this widespread coagulation disorder, the blood is depleted of platelets and coagulation factors; the syndrome is sometimes called *consumption coagulopathy*. Fibrinogen polymerizes within the capillary bed, and although the fibrinolytic system is activated it cannot effectively deal with the large deposits of fibrin.

Animals with disseminated intravascular coagulation (DIC) have bleeding tendencies. The findings by the clinical pathologist are thrombocytopenia, hypofibrinogenemia, deficiency of prothrombin complexes, and depletion of factors V and VIII; there are also excess split products of fibrin in the blood (due to fibrinolysis). The first three deficiencies are required for the diagnosis.

The clinical consequences of disseminated intravascular coagulation are generalized hemorrhages and dysfunction of critical organs such as kidney and lung due to circulatory interference by fibrin thrombi. Fibrin-filled neutrophils are trapped in the capillary bed of the lungs, causing fatal interference with respiration.

The development of disseminated intravascular coagulation indicates a severe disease process of rapid progression. Deposition of fibrin is occurring at such a high rate that the fibrinolysin system cannot degrade it. Experimentally, when small amounts of thrombin are injected IV, aggregates of fibrin form in the blood and are removed by circulating neutrophils. These fibrin-filled cells lodge in the liver, spleen, and lung, and fibrin is readily detected in their phagosomes. The fibrin is degraded, and no signs of disease occur.

Intravenous thrombin produces DIC.

Thrombin, in addition to being the enzyme that polymerizes fibrinogen, is one of the most important activators of platelets (it can induce

the platelet release reaction directly). When large amounts of *thrombin* (or thromboplastin) are quickly injected IV, the circulating blood clots rapidly and the animal dies. The explosive induction of thrombin sets off intravascular clotting and fatal interference with circulation. When the same quantity of thromboplastin is injected slowly, the animal survives. The slower and more incomplete formation of fibrin is removed rapidly enough by the reticuloendothelial system that survival is possible. The animal is depleted of fibrinogen in the process, and its blood is incoagulable. Under the influence of thrombin, the platelets aggregate and the circulating platelet count drops. There is often activation of the intravascular plasminogen, and the plasma proteolytic enzyme plasmin may be detectable. As fibrin is degraded, fibrin split products are removed by the kidney, in which they can be detected histochemically.

DIC arises from tissue necrosis + abnormal coagulation.

Diseases characterized by large amounts of tissue destruction plus suppression of coagulation are prone to lead to DIC. Thus DIC commonly occurs in severe burns, widespread metastatic tumors, systemic viral disease, heatstroke, and shock. In dogs, it may also accompany severe pneumonia, congestive heart failure, and heartworm disease. Dogs so affected bleed from the nose and gingiva because of thrombocytopenia and depletion of factors V, VIII, and X, and fibrinogen.

Burns are associated with DIC.

Severe local lesions induce consumption of coagulation factors without evidence of DIC. Intense but local thermal injury is accompanied by marked, prolonged consumption within the wound of platelets, fibrinogen, and plasminogen. Later, hyperfibrinogenemia, thrombocytosis, and elevated split products occur in circulating blood, which is evidence of local intravascular coagulation in the burn wound rather than of DIC.

Tissue necrosis

Embolization of necrotic tissue during septic disease may induce coagulation. Disorders associated with *parturition* are common examples. Sepsis during abortion, intrauterine retention of dead fetuses, and the embolism of amniotic fluid and epithelial cells may be associated with a hypofibrinogenemia secondary to intravascular clotting.

Heparin treatment suppresses DIC and, experimentally at least, has a striking preventative effect in diseases involving tissue necrosis (which release thromboplastin); for example, heparin decreases mortality in carbon tetrachloride toxicity by inhibiting the sequence: necrosis → thromboplastin release → intravascular coagulation → tissue hypoxia.

Neoplasia

Neoplastic cells are the source of procoagulant factors in some types of vascular tumors and in leukemia. Metastasis of solid tumors may be accompanied by intravascular coagulation, but the direct cause is not known.

Snake venoms insert their effects into the coagulation scheme.

Snake venoms are mixtures of up to 30 different peptides, most of which are toxic. All poisonous venoms contain phospholipase A_2 (which has direct lytic action on plasma membranes of platelets and erythrocytes) and hyaluronidase (which cleaves glycosidic bonds of glycosaminoglycans and facilitates toxin spread). Venom of the tiger snake behaves as an activated factor X, while venom of the copperhead clots fibrinogen directly. The end result in both cases is defibrination with intravascular clotting. DIC is enhanced by the direct platelet damage caused by phospholipases.

Not all defibrinating syndromes lead to DIC. Crotalase, an enzyme fraction of rattlesnake venom, converts fibrinogen to an abnormal fibrin that is ineffective in clotting; the result is hemorrhage rather than DIC. Some venom toxins specifically block removal of fibrinopeptides from fibrinogen by thrombin. Reptilase (a toxin of *Bothrops atrox* venom) blocks removal of fibrinopeptide A. Enzymes in *Agkistrodon contortrix* venom block fibrinopeptide B removal. Other venom peptides have antithromboplastin activity (see snake venoms, Chapter 27).

Viruses that damage endothelium lead to disseminated intravascular coagulation.

Endothelial loss exposes subendothelial matrix to attract platelets, and the degenerating endothelial cells are a source of tissue thromboplastin and other procoagulant factors. Hemostatic defects of acute *infectious canine hepatitis* include thrombocytopenia, abnormal platelet

function, prolonged prothrombin times, depressed factor VIII activity, normal thrombin times, and increased circulating fibrin degradation products. This suggests the mechanism to be DIC. The reduced number of platelets reflects both increased consumption (to repair virus-induced endothelial injury) and direct damage to platelets by viruses. Depressed factor VIII levels are probably due to consumption caused by vascular lesions.

Although most cases of DIC in viral disease are due to liberation of procoagulant factors from tissue necrosis, immunologic reactions may contribute. Cats with *feline infectious peritonitis* (FIP) develop widespread thrombosis accompanied by thrombocytopenia, hyperfibrinogenemia, and increased fibrin degradation products in plasma. When FIP virus is experimentally inoculated, kittens with antibody develop more rapid and more severe disease than do kittens infected for the first time. Viral antigens and immunoglobulins are present in fibrinonecrotic lesions, which suggests an immunologic process.

Protozoal disease can cause DIC.

Endothelial damage occurs in parasitemic phases of malaria and other protozoal diseases. In massive infection, DIC may lead to death. In cattle, the intraerythrocytic parasite *Babesia* spp. causes alterations in fibrinogen catabolism and in coagulation and kinin systems. There is no evidence of fibrin deposition of fibrinolysis and little evidence that the disease progresses to DIC.

In the late 1970s studies by Dr. V. E. O. Valli and C. M. Forsberg showed that *trypanosomiasis* in calves caused by *Trypanosoma congolense* led to marked thrombocytopenia and hypofibrinogenemia. There was ineffective thrombopoiesis and increased megakaryocyte mass, which indicated that in chronic disease there was a partially compensated DIC.

Septicemia often involves DIC.

Widespread vascular damage occurring when pathogenic bacteria circulate is the most common cause of DIC. Intact bacteria initially activate Hageman factor, and bacterial endotoxins produce endothelial damage that both increases vascular permeability and sustains the intravascular coagulation defect. *Septicemic salmonellosis* in swine is frequently accompanied by vascular necrosis in renal interlobular arteries and afferent glomerular arterioles, with widespread thrombosis in glomeruli. Similar lesions occur in epidermal capillaries. *Leptospirosis* is characterized by thrombocytopenia, increased fibrinolytic split products in blood, and endothelial injury. Damaged endothelium releases plasminogen activators, which stimulate the fibrinolytic system.

Bacterial endotoxins activate both extrinsic and intrinsic systems of coagulation. Hageman factor (XII) is activated, and monocytes are induced to release factors that activate factor VII. Furthermore, endotoxin has a direct action on platelets that leads to aggregation and platelet release reactions (Fig. 16.9). Factor VII plays a key role in development of endotoxin-induced DIC. Infusion of endotoxin into factor VII–deficient dogs results in greater fibrin deposition and focal tissue necrosis than in normal dogs. Corticosteroids make blood vessels very sensitive to endotoxin by inhibiting catechol methyl transferase, thereby promoting α-adrenergic stimulation.

Platelets disappear rapidly after intravenous endotoxin and are trapped in capillary beds of lung and liver. Using ^{51}Cr-labeled platelets in dogs, thrombocytopenia has been shown to be biphasic, that is, a rapid drop in circulating platelets is followed by partial recovery and then a second drop. The initial rapid drop requires participation of *complement,* especially in dogs and cats whose platelets contain immune-adherence receptors.

Endotoxin DIC can be suppressed by deleting circulating platelets or neutrophils or by injecting heparin to prevent coagulation. DIC is induced with one endotoxin injection if lysed neutrophil granules are given simultaneously. Neutrophenic animals are fully susceptible to endotoxin but do not develop some of the lung damage that normal animals do.

Although deposition of fibrin thrombi are most prominent in the kidney and lung during endotoxin-induced disseminated intravascular coagulation, progressive microthrombosis also occurs in the splenic red pulp and hepatic sinu-

FOCUS

Experimental endotoxin reactions

The classic local endotoxin reaction as produced in skin by Shwartzman in 1932 was a result of an intradermal injection of *Salmonella typhosa* culture filtrate followed in 24 hours by an intravenous injection of the same filtrate. Severe hemorrhage and necrosis occurred at the dermal (preparatory) site of injection. This reaction was not immunologic, for it lacked specificity (it could be produced with other bacilli in the second injection) and the time interval between preparatory and eliciting reactions was too short. The preparatory injection produces tissue damage that remains subclinical due to clearance by macrophages. It evokes a granulocyte release from bone marrow, however, that exaggerates injury induced by the second injection where the damage has already been produced.

The *generalized Shwartzman reaction* is the experimental counterpart of endotoxin-induced disseminated intravascular coagulation. The reaction is dependent on two spaced injections of endotoxin with a given time lag. After the primary injection all the events occur, but lesions are slight because of fibrinolysis and phagocytosis. If the second injection is given within 20 hours, the reticuloendothelial system is sufficiently blocked so that the classic reaction develops, with thrombi in the kidney, lung, adrenal, and other viscera.

soids. Impairment of phagocytic function in these organs adds to the severity of endotoxic injury.

ADDITIONAL READING

Baker, D. C., and Green, R. A. Coagulation defects of aflatoxin intoxicated rabbits. *Vet. Pathol.* 24:62, 1987.

Bertram, T. A. Quantitative morphology of peracute pulmonary lesions in swine induced by *Haemophilus pleuropneumoniae. Vet. Pathol.* 22:598, 1986.

Casey, H. W., and Splitter, G. A. Membranous glomerulonephritis in dogs infected with *Dirofilaria immitis. Vet. Pathol.* 12:111, 1975.

Cramer, E. M., et al. Absence of tubular structures and immunolabeling for von Willebrand factor in the platelet α-granules from porcine von Willebrand disease. *Blood* 68:774, 1986.

Doolittle, R. F. Fibrinogen and fibrin. *Sci. Am.* 245:127, 1981.

Edwards, J. F., et al. Megakaryocyte infection and thrombocytopenia in African swine fever. *Vet. Pathol.* 22:171, 1985.

Esmon, C. T. The regulation of natural anticoagulant pathways. *Science* 235:1348, 1987.

Feldman, B. F., et al. Disseminated intravascular coagulation: Antithrombin, plasminogen, and coagulation abnormalities in 41 dogs. *J. Am. Vet. Med. Assoc.* 179:151, 1981.

_____. Hemorrhage in a cat caused by inhibition of factor XI (plasma thromboplastin antecedent). *J. Am. Vet. Med. Assoc.* 182:589, 1983.

Green, R. A., et al. Hypoalbuminemia-related platelet hypersensitivity in two dogs with nephrotic syndrome. *J. Am. Vet. Med. Assoc.* 186:485, 1985.

Meyers, K. M. Pathobiology of animal platelets. *Adv. Vet. Sci. Comp. Med.* 30:131, 1985.

Momotani, E., et al. Histopathological evaluation of disseminated intravascular coagulation in *Haemophilus somnus* infection in cattle. *J. Comp. Pathol.* 95:15, 1985.

Morris, D. D., and Beech, J. Disseminated intravascular coagulation in six horses. *J. Am. Vet. Med. Assoc.* 183:1067, 1983.

Schulman, A., et al. Diphacinone-induced coagulopathy in the dog. *J. Am. Vet. Med. Assoc.* 188:402, 1986.

Slauson, D. O., and Gribble, D. H. Thrombosis complicating renal amyloidosis in dogs. *Vet. Pathol.* 8:352, 1971.

Williams, D. A., and Maggio-Price, L. Canine idiopathic thrombocytopenia. *J. Am. Vet. Med. Assoc.* 185:660, 1984.

17

Anemia

NEMIA is a deficiency of circulating erythrocytes. Most often a reduction of erythrocyte numbers, it may also be due to a decrease in erythrocyte volume. The clinical consequences are the same: impaired delivery of oxygen to cells. The decrease in oxygen-carrying capacity of blood (hypoxemia) occurs when circulating erythrocytes are lost beyond the ability of storage sites in the spleen and bone marrow to replace them.

In severe anemia the blood becomes thin and watery, and as a result, mucous membranes around the eyes, mouth, and genitals become pale. The diagnosis of anemia is confirmed in the laboratory by a decrease in hemoglobin concentration or in erythrocyte numbers per cubic millimeter of blood. The packed cell volume (PCV), determined by centrifuging to sediment erythrocytes from plasma, is a good index of erythrocyte numbers and volume. Laboratory tests must be interpreted with regard to *dehydration,* which causes a decrease in plasma, that is, an increase in erythrocytes per volume of fluid.

As anemia progresses, compensatory mechanisms operate to combat the decreased oxygen-carrying capacity of the blood: (1) hyperventilation of the lungs, (2) increased cardiac output, and (3) reduction of hemoglobin-oxygen affinity. The decreased affinity of hemoglobin for oxygen permits an increased release of oxygen to tissues. These are only borderline adjustments, allowing the anemic animal to appear normal at rest but not overcoming the demands of exertion.

Anemia may be caused either by excessive loss of erythrocytes or by abnormal erythropoiesis (insufficient production) (Table 17.1). In practice, many anemias involve several mechanisms. Anemia of chronic blood loss (say from infesta-

Table 17.1. Classification of anemia

Mechanism	Example
Blood loss	
Acute	Blood vessel damage: surgery, trauma
Subacute	Endothelial defects: thrombocytopenia; poisoning with warfarin, clover, etc.
Chronic	Internal loss: blood-sucking parasites, hematuria, neoplasms, gut ulcers
	External loss: fleas, ticks, mosquitos
Erythrocyte destruction	
Erythrocyte lysis	
Hereditary	Defective enzymes or membrane proteins
Acquired	Physical, chemical, microbial toxins
Hemoglobin defect	
Hereditary	Defective proteins: heme
Acquired	Toxins: CO, nitrates, etc.
Erythrophagocytosis	Hypersplenism: splenic hypertrophy
Deficient production	
Erythrocytes	Bone marrow depression: viruses, drugs, toxins, hormones
Hemoglobin	Dietary deficit: iron, copper, cobalt

Note: Classification based on pathogenesis; other classifications are based on *size and hemoglobin content* (normo-, micro-, and macrocytic), and on *bone marrow response* (regenerative and nonregenerative).

tion with bloodsucking parasites) is primarily caused by the slow *loss of erythrocytes*; superimposed on this mechanism, however, is a progressively developing *iron deficiency* that depresses erythropoiesis. Anemia that accompanies ostertagiosis of calves results also chiefly from blood loss, but *bone marrow hypoplasia* also occurs, due to toxic products of the parasite. Similarly, infection with leptospires causes a destructive hemolytic anemia augmented by a toxic effect of the organisms on bone marrow. In anemia that occurs in complex diseases such as uremia, hypothyroidism, chronic infectious diseases, and neoplasia, it is often difficult to sort out the dominant cause.

Anemia is commonly due to events that are secondary to a primary disease process. Even though erythrocyte destruction occurs in many infectious diseases because of the direct effects of microbes, anemia may also be a nonspecific side effect of fever. Transient periods of high fever are followed by short periods of decreased PCV values and increased reticulocyte counts. The mechanism of anemia is related to elevated body temperature rather than to the primary cause of fever.

ERYTHROCYTE BIOLOGY
Erythrocyte Surface

The discoid shape of the normal erythrocyte belies the capacity of this cell to deform as it passes through tiny capillaries (Fig. 17.1). Changes that occur during circulation (as well as after injury) are determined by the three components of the cell surface: *plasma membrane, glycocalyx* (or external coating of carbohydrates), and subsurface filamentous *cytoskeleton.* The glycocalyx receives signals and the cytoskeleton translates those signals into cell change. The membrane itself provides the supportive framework in which all these actions occur. Within the membrane, molecules of phospholipids and cholesterol are methylated and shifted to control how membrane proteins can be moved about to conduct the reactions of the surface to injury (see Fig. 5.9).

Surface glycocalyx receives molecular signals.

The glycocalyx covering the erythrocyte surface is composed of carbohydrate molecules attached at their bases to proteins embedded in

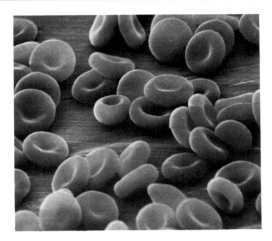

Fig. 17.1. Normal erythrocytes, sheep (scanning electron micrograph).

the plasma membrane. The sugar units act as receptors and cause selective attachment of signal molecules that circulate in the bloodstream. Most of the sugars are on large *transmembrane proteins* that extend through the cell membrane and are attached to cytoskeletal filaments just below the cell surface. By this arrangement, chemical instructions received at the surface (from hormones, enzymes, antibodies, toxins, and microorganisms) are then translated into movement and shape changes by filaments of the subsurface cytoskeleton. Anionic sites on neuraminic acid and other components of the glycocalyx are responsible for the net negative charge of the erythrocyte surface that normally prevents cell-to-cell contact.

Subsurface cytoskeleton translates signals into action.

Underlying the plasma membrane is a meshwork of actin microfilaments and a specialized protein, *spectrin.* Spectrin is attached to proteins embedded in the plasma membrane by another binding protein called ankyrin. It is the anastomosing network of spectrin and actin molecules that makes the erythrocyte sufficiently pliant to pass splenic and capillary channels less than half its diameter yet sufficiently durable to withstand turbulent passage through the heart.

The ability of erythrocytes to deform while circulating is essential because their shape must be constantly altered during passage through capillaries. Deformability is especially important in circulation through the spleen. There is marked distortion of the cell as it passes through endothelial fenestrae, and the normal shape is resumed as the cell enters the sinus. The pathologically rigid cell that cannot change shape is predisposed to lysis and erythrophagocytosis.

Spectrin determines whether an erythrocyte is rigid or fragile.

Subsurface polymers of spectrin control surface conformation. If spectrin polymerizes to form a rigid network at the cell surface, the erythrocyte becomes bumpy, or "spiculated." At the other extreme, if spectrin tetramers disaggregate and detach from the cytoplasmic face of the plasma membrane, the erythrocyte becomes fragile and loses its discoid shape. These two pathways of shape change are clues to different disease processes (Fig. 17.2).

Fragile erythrocytes swell and become round.

In most types of injury, spectrin-actin complexes become nonpolymerized, leading to excessive erythrocyte fragility. As erythrocytes swell, they become round (with greater volume but less total diameter). If swelling is limited, the central depression of the normal discocyte becomes flattened and remains visible as an oval-shaped area of central pallor in erythrocytes on the blood smear; these cells are called *stomatocytes*. If swelling is severe, the erythrocyte becomes a small, round, microcyte that lacks central pallor; these erythrocytes are called *spherocytes* (Fig. 17.3).

Drugs may cause stomatocytosis.

Different effects on erythrocyte membranes are caused by differences in where drug action occurs. Anionic phospholipids that make up the membrane are distributed asymmetrically, that is, in inner and outer parts of the lipid bilayer. Cationic drugs produce stomatocytosis, while anionic drugs cause crenation. Dr. Joseph Smith, at Kansas State University, has shown that because the inner, cytoplasmic layer of the membrane is most negative, cationic compounds locate there preferentially and expand the membrane to cause stomatocytosis.

Rigid erythrocytes have knobby surfaces.

Poikilocytosis is development of abnormally shaped erythrocytes. *Spiculocytes* (also called "acanthocytes" or "spur cells") are common poikilocytes and are formed by excessive polymerization of the spectrin-actin mesh. The crenated cell surface arises because the plasma membrane becomes excessively rigid.

Spiculocytes develop from focal defects in the plasma membrane.

Spiculocytes form when there are abnormal cholesterol:phospholipid or sphingomyelin:lecithin ratios, which decrease membrane fluidity and cause erythrocyte surfaces to develop folded or scalloped contours. Some drug-induced spiculocytes have very rigid membranes with knobby surfaces. On routine blood smears, these crenated erythrocytes may develop as artifacts caused by damage during preparation, but they also are bona fide examples of pathologic change. They are especially common in uremia (Fig. 17.4).

Elevated plasma lipids cause spiculocytosis.

Erythrocytes (and platelets) do not have enzymes necessary for synthesis of cholesterol and phospholipids and do not catabolize these sub-

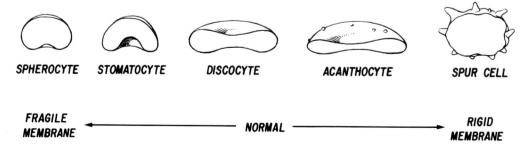

Fig. 17.2. Erythrocyte shape changes: erythrocyte swelling is associated with membrane fragility that leads to *spherocytosis;* erythrocyte crenation is associated with membrane rigidity that leads to *echinocytosis.*

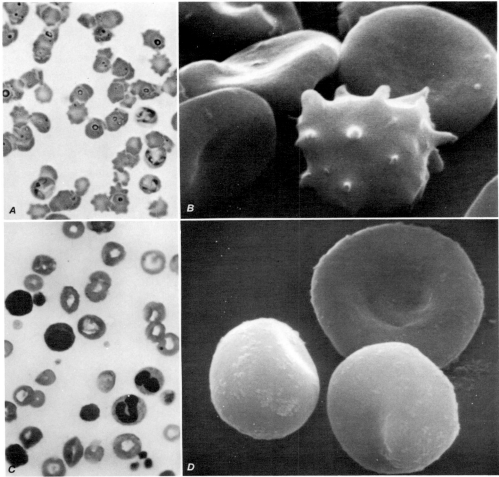

Fig. 17.3. Erythrocyte surface pathology. A and B. Echinocytosis, sheep with phenylhydrazine toxicity. Knobby protuberances on erythrocyte surfaces in B are evidence of plasma membrane rigidity. C and D. Spherocytosis, dog with autoimmune hemolytic anemia. D. Normal erythrocyte (*top*) and early and late phases of spherocytosis (scanning electron micrograph).

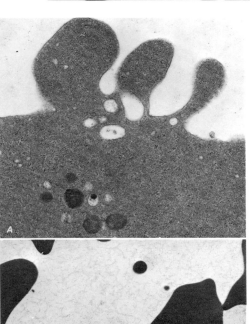

Fig. 17.4. Erythrocyte surface abnormalities. A. Pseudopod formation with vesicles and internalization, cortisol therapy for lymphosarcoma, cat. B. Fragmented erythrocytes, dog in terminal stages of uremia. Parts have pinched away from the cell.

stances. Characteristic spiculocytes develop in animals with hepatocellular disease and anemia and are associated with a diminished affinity of serum lipoprotein receptors on erythrocyte surfaces. In dogs, "spur cell anemia" develops when lipoproteins of hepatic origin rise markedly in chronic liver disease (experimentally, spur cell anemia can be produced by cholesterol-rich atherogenic diets).

Intravascular trauma causes erythrocyte fragmentation.

A shearing effect of mechanical damage occurs when erythrocytes are excessively fragile. This appears as fragmentation and pseudopod formation and is a common finding in uremia. It also occurs in severe illness such as heatstroke, plasma electrolyte imbalances, chemical toxicities, and neoplasia.

Hemoglobin: Heme + globin

Hemoglobin is a combination of the simple histone protein *globin* with *heme,* a porphyrin molecule containing an iron atom in its center. All vertebrate hemoglobins have the same molecular configuration. The globin, about 97% of the molecule, is a tetramer of two pairs of dissimilar polypeptide chains: two α and two β chains ($\alpha_2\beta_2$). The molecule dissociates into two symmetrical dimers: $\alpha_2\beta_2 \rightleftharpoons 2\alpha\beta$. The tendency to dissociate varies among species; for example, cat hemoglobin forms subunits much more readily than does dog hemoglobin.

Erythrocyte survival demands that intracellular hemoglobin remain in solution. To do so, the molecule must maintain its rigid, tertiary structure (the fold of chains within the molecule). Each coiled chain of hemoglobin must have an external, polar, charged layer of hydrophilic amino acids and an internal layer of nonpolar, noncharged hydrophobic amino acids. Disruption of the α-helix, replacement of polar with nonpolar amino acids, or disruption of the binding to heme results in the hemoglobin molecule becoming insoluble within the erythrocyte.

Heinz bodies are precipitates of hemoglobin.

Precipitation of unstable hemoglobin within the erythrocyte is manifested as aggregates of dense, irregular structures called Heinz bodies. Aggregates of granular hemoglobin attach to and deform the cell surface membrane, and this renders the cell susceptible to erythrophagocy-

tosis. Denaturation of hemoglobin is prevented largely by the presence of glutathione (reduced), which scavenges toxic oxygen radicals. Glutathione is maintained in the reduced state by the hexose-monophosphate pathway (see Fig. 19.6).

Fetal hemoglobin switches to adult hemoglobin at birth.

Ontogenetically, several types of hemoglobin (Hb) are produced. Mammalian erythrocytes change rapidly at birth from a content of fetaltype hemoglobin (Hb-F) to an adult-type (Hb-A), which differ in β chain amino acid sequences. Transition from Hb-F to Hb-A is abrupt; fetal hemogobin does not recur except in some specific types of anemia. In fetal sheep and goats, an intermediate hemoglobin type occurs called Hb-C. In blood loss anemia, Hb-C is again produced. The changes from Hb-A to Hb-C is mediated by an active globin-mRNA in the reticulocyte.

Hemoglobin differs sufficiently among species that its substructure can be used as a guideline of phylogenetic development (see forensic pathology, Chapter 3).

Anisocytosis is change in erythrocyte size.

Mean cell volume (MCV) expresses the average volume of individual erythrocytes. It is calculated: MCV = packed cell volume × 10/ erythrocytes (million/mm³). MCV is important in detecting microcytic anemia, wherein erythrocytes are smaller than normal, often as a result of deficiencies of hemoglobin synthesis. Erythrocyte numbers are not reduced to the same degree as hemoglobin, and the total red cell count does not truly reflect the severity of anemia. Formulae for determining hemoglobin include *mean cell hemoglobin* (MCH): MCH = Hb × 10/erythrocytes (in millions), and *mean cell hemoglobin concentration* (MCHC): MCHC (in 4g/dl) = Hb × 100/PCV.

Intraerythrocytic metabolic pathways

The normal erythrocyte is defended against colloid osmotic lysis by a membrane relatively impermeable to free ion movement.To balance the slow, continual, passive leak of potassium and the intake of sodium, an energy-utilizing pump operates actively to push sodium out and pull potassium in.

Energy in the form of ATP is supplied by oxidation of glucose to lactic acid (*glycolysis*). The erythrocyte has lost mitochondria including enzymes of the citric acid cycle; 90% of glucose enters the anaerobic glycolysis pathway, which converts glucose to lactic acid, generating ATP. ATP that is formed is used to maintain osmotic balance and hemoglobin. Glycogen is not produced, and erythrocytes are dependent on acquisition of glucose from plasma.

Erythrocyte swelling develops if pumps are inactive.

Deficiencies in erythrocyte metabolic pathways lead to water intake and osmotic hemolysis. When the sodium-potassium pump is destroyed, there is equalization of cell and plasma cations (sodium accumulation and potassium loss), intake of water, cell swelling, and lysis. If there is excess potassium loss without corresponding sodium gain, cell contraction develops.

Energy production declines as erythrocytes age.

As the erythocyte ages, the enzyme components maintaining energy output gradually wane. There is a concomitant decrease in ATP. Membrane function is affected, the normal biconcave shape becomes spheroidal, and the cells have an increased susceptibility to osmotic lysis. In passage through the splenic filter, aged erythrocytes are removed from the circulation and the component parts are processed by splenic macrophages. Any space-occupying defect in the cell membrane makes the erythrocyte less flexible and highly liable to erythrophagocytosis. *Pitting,* the removal of defective pieces of the cell surface membrane, may occur as the cell squeezes through the endothelial lining of the splenic venous sinuses. The mechanical trauma of excessively fragile erythrocytes may also result in intravascular *fragmentation* or in *hemolysis.*

Erythropoiesis

Mature erythrocytes originate from a pool of self-perpetuating bone marrow stem cells. They develop from large nucleated stem cells by almost imperceptible gradations of an orderly sequence. Different cells in this series are arbitrarily divided on the basis of structure and staining into pronormoblasts, normoblasts (basophilic, polychromatic, and orthochromatic), reticulocytes, and mature erythrocytes. The time required from stimulation of pronormoblast production to release of mature erythrocytes from bone marrow sinusoids is approximately 5 days in most mammals; this rate is markedly altered in anemia, especially in dogs.

During maturation the nucleus increasingly contracts, becomes pyknotic, and (in mammals) is ejected from the cell. *Erythroblastic islets* in the bone marrow are large pleomorphic reticulum cells surrounded by a ring of developing erythroblasts. They serve as nurse cells and transfer their cytoplasmic ferritin to erythroblasts, which accept it by endocytosis. Iron is also transferred to developing erythroblasts by *transferrin,* the plasma glycoprotein that transports iron in its ferric state. Transferrin attaches to immature red cells and gives up its iron to them but is not itself incorporated into the cell.

Howell-Jolly bodies are remnants of nuclear chromatin.

In anemia with intense erythropoiesis, nucleated erythrocytes appear in the blood prematurely. Some denucleate but dense remnants of chromatin persist in the cell as Howell-Jolly bodies. These stain intensely with nuclear dyes and are characteristic of certain types of anemia.

Anemia leads to bone marrow hyperplasia.

When animals become anemic, they respond by releasing erythrocytes from storage sites in spleen and bone marrow, by increasing cardiorespiratory function, and by changing the hemoglobin-oxygen association. For the long term, the most significant effect is induction of bone marrow hyperplasia (in severe anemia *extramedullary hematopoiesis* also develops in spleen and liver). When these occur, they are reflected in changes in some important clinical pathologic tests. As the body responds to anemia, there are increases in (1) bone marrow erythroid cells (decrease in myeloid:erythroid ratios), (2) reticulocyte counts in circulating blood (except in horses), and (3) serum iron levels (also in plasma iron turnover as measured using Fe^{59}).

Erythropoietins are soluble factors that enhance erythropoiesis.

Dormant reserves of erythrocyte precursors are triggered into action by humoral substances called *erythropoietins.* Erythropoietins are produced or activated in response to low tissue oxygen levels. Transient elevations are detectable during hypoxia, while sustained levels are often present in severe anemia (Fig. 17.5).

Erythropoietin can be measured by bioassay methods and by a radioimmunoassay technique. To date, these are insufficiently sensitive to measure erythropoietin in plasma directly and have not been regularly used in clinical evaluations.

Several hormones also influence erythrocyte production. In general, *androgens* stimulate and *estrogens* inhibit erythropoiesis. *Thyroid hormones* may increase the need for erythrocytes by increasing body metabolism.

Kidney is the chief site of erythropoietin production.

In anemic sheep, erythropoietin has been localized in epithelial cells of the renal glomerulus. It exists in precursor form as erythrogenin, which reacts with serum to give erythropoietin (Fig. 17.5). Experimentally, renal ablation in rats markedly inhibits their capacity to respond to hypoxia. Most anephric animals continue to produce new erythrocytes because erythropoietin is also produced at other sites.

ANEMIA DUE TO BLOOD LOSS
Acute

Immediate and remarkable increases in *hemoconcentration* and blood *coagulability* occur after major hemorrhage. Coagulation becomes highly efficient, and erythrocytes are rapidly spewed into the circulation by release from spleen and bone marrow. This is manifested as a rise in the PCV that develops immediately after the transitory drop accompanying actual blood loss. Peripheral blood shows an increased number of platelets initially but this soon drops as platelets are used in coagulation.

The stored erythrocytes are normal cells; no pathologic changes are detectable when blood is examined microscopically. The volume of lost blood is compensated for by the drawing of interstitial fluid into the vascular system, and hemodilution slowly begins to restore the PCV to normal. The neural and humoral factors that affect cardiac output and blood pressure are activated, and in spite of the loss of large amounts of blood, animals may remain conscious and appear normal clinically.

Indices of enhanced erythrocyte production (reticulocytosis and polychromasia indicate erythrocyte immaturity) are present in smears of circulating blood 48 hours after acute blood loss. The hemogram returns to normal within 1 to 2 weeks after hemorrhage.

Major blood loss causes shock.

Most animals can lose one-third of their total blood volume without evidence of disease. The consequence of acute blood loss is not anemia but hypovolemic shock. If increased heart rate, hyperventilation, peripheral vasoconstriction, and the shift of water from tissue to blood are unable to compensate, shock develops and death follows.

Chronic anemia

Internal hemorrhage (such as intraperitoneal blood loss) may also cause chronic anemia; but blood components, especially iron, are recoverable. Bleeding into the intestinal lumen or to the exterior causes loss of iron, and iron-deficiency anemia is superimposed on chronic blood loss.

Slow, insidious blood loss due to parasites is a

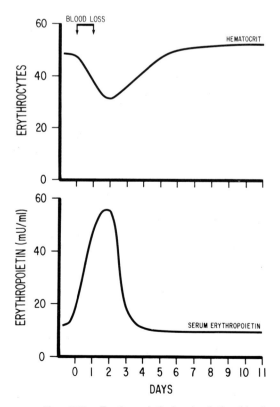

Fig. 17.5. Erythropoietin in circulating blood during hemorrhage.

frequent cause of death in animals. Bloodsucking intestinal parasites and external parasites such as fleas are frequent causes. These anemias are associated with a hypocellular but functional hyperactive bone marrow.

Haemonchus contortus is an important bloodsucking nematode of sheep. It causes blood loss both by sucking blood from the intestine and by causing tiny bleeding ulcers in the abomasum. The continual blood loss leads to an iron deficiency that in turn leads to diminished hemoglobin formation. When weanling lambs are infected with large numbers of larvae, their blood will have reduced amounts of hemoglobin in about 7 days and by 21 days anemia may be so severe that death occurs (Fig. 17.6). Erythropoiesis is stimulated at about 7 days after infection, but young lambs do not have adequate reserves of iron to withstand the severe blood loss caused by the parasite. Hemoglobin concentration is a more sensitive test for anemia in early infection. The erythrocyte count may be within normal limits because erythrocytes carry decreased amounts of hemoglobin per cell.

ANEMIA DUE TO ERYTHROCYTE DESTRUCTION

Erythrocyte destruction generally occurs via action at the cell surface, either by (1) *intravascular lysis,* which occurs when the erythrocyte's plasma membrane is ruptured, or by (2) *erythrophagocytosis,* as cells with damaged surfaces pass by phagocytic cells in the spleen and liver.

Hemolysis

Hemolysis arises either from direct damage to the membrane, or indirectly when the membrane is damaged as a result of abnormal hemoglobin or osmotic equilibrium (Table 17.2). If extensive damage produces overt lysis intravascularly, hemoglobin is liberated into the circulating blood. This *hemolytic anemia* is typical of drug-induced anemia, leptospirosis of cow and dog, clostridial infections of sheep and cow, copper poisoning of sheep, immunologic hemolysis in suckling newborn animals, and infection with intracellular parasites such as *Anaplasma* spp.

Hemoglobin is secreted into urine.

During a hemolytic crisis, the binding power of plasma haptoglobulin is exceeded and hemoglobin is excreted by the renal glomerulus. It dissociates ($\alpha_2\beta_2 \rightleftharpoons 2\alpha\beta$), and the dimer of about 32,000 MW is readily excreted by the renal filter. Hemoglobin is absorbed by the proximal convoluted tubule, but when the absorptive capacity is exceeded, *hemoglobinuria* results. The extent of hemoglobinemia and subsequent hemoglobinuria are indices of the severity of the disease process.

Erythrophagocytosis

Less explosive types of erythrocyte damage may not induce lysis but do sufficiently alter the erythrocyte so as to markedly enhance erythrophagocytosis of large numbers of cells in the spleen, liver, and bone marrow. Diseases associated with anemia of this type include those infections in which microorganisms replicate within the erythrocyte, uremia, some of the immunologic types of anemia, and metabolic diseases.

Removal of damaged or senescent erythrocytes is a function of the macrophages of the reticuloendothelial system. Enormous numbers of erythrocytes are destroyed each day; it is estimated that in normal man 9 million cells die each hour. In most normal mammalian species, phagocytosis is most effective in the spleen; but in anemia it may reach significant proportions in the liver, bone marrow, lung, and lymph nodes. In normal birds and lower vertebrates, the liver and bone marrow are highly effective in erythrophagocytosis.

Autologous antibodies (IgG) in serum of healthy animals bind to senescent erythrocytes and enhance their removal by phagocytes. As hemoglobin begins to denature, it forms hemichromes that cross-link the major erythrocyte transmembrane protein (band 3) into clusters.

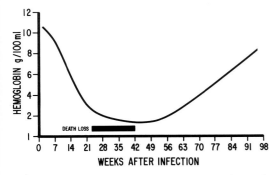

Fig. 17.6. Hemoglobin loss in experimental haemonchosis, sheep. (Data from Silverman et al., *Am. J. Vet. Res.* 31:841, 1970)

Table 17.2. Mechanisms of erythrocyte destruction

Site Mechanism	Example
Cell surface membrane damage—leads to hemolysis	
Enzymatic digestion	Rattlesnake venom (phospholipase), clostridial toxins
Viral replication	Feline leukemia virus
Bacterial adherence	*Haemobartonella* spp.
Immune lysis	Isoimmune (transfusion reaction) and autoimmune hemolytic anemia
Dietary deficiency	Vitamin E deficiency, hypophosphatemia
Mechanical damage	Uremia; microangiopathy in tumor vessels
Osmotic Lysis—leads to hemolysis and erythrophagocytosis	
Bacteria	*Anaplasma* spp. (anaplasmosis)
Protozoa	*Plasmodium* spp. (malaria)
Hypotonic solutions	Low sodium chloride
Enzyme abnormality	Pyruvate kinase deficiency (hereditary); aspirin toxicity (acquired)
Plant toxicity	Onions, red maple leaves, rye grass
Chemicals	Phenothiazine, acetaminophen, benzocaine
Hemoglobin abnormality—leads to hemolysis and erythrophagocytosis	
Abnormal globin	Hemoglobinopathy
Abnormal heme	Porphyria
Methemoglobinemia	Nitrate poisoning
Denaturation of Hb	Copper, phenylhydrazine toxicity

These clusters provide recognition sites for antibodies directed against the senescent cell.

Bilirubin forms from degraded heme.

When the erythrocyte is phagocytized, hemoglobin is released within the macrophage, inducing lysosomal enzymes that are specific for erythrocyte degradation. The hemoglobin molecule is rapidly broken down, and its component parts are metabolized separately. Protein and iron are returned to their respective "pools," and the porphyrin fraction is not reused.

Bilirubin is formed in macrophages of the reticuloendothelial system from ruptured heme and is shed into the plasma, where it is transported to the liver for conjugation with glucuronic acids. Bilirubin glucuronide is secreted by the biliary system into the duodenum. It is degraded by intestinal bacteria to several compounds termed collectively *fecal urobilinogen.* The differentiation of free (unconjugated) and conjugated bilirubin is important because during hemolysis free bilirubin is elevated. Bilirubin can directly predispose to hemolysis because it interacts with the outer half of the lipid bilayer of the erythrocyte plasma membrane.

The spleen selectively removes abnormal erythrocytes.

The spleen is anatomically adapted to remove circulating erythrocytes. Red cells pass from the arterial to the venous system through reticular cell networks beset by macrophages and must finally squeeze through the endothelial lining cells of the venous sinuses. Phagocytosis along this route may involve the removal of erythrocytes intact, or by fragmentation or pitting. Nuclei of erythroblasts are also selectively removed during passage through the marrow sinuses.

To enter the venous sinuses, erythrocytes, which in most mammals are near 7 μm in diameter, must pass through endothelial gaps of not more than 3 μm. To do so, considerable deformation of the erythocyte must be possible. Splenic blood is highly viscous; that is, its hematocrit is high, while levels of oxygen and glucose are low. These factors favor *spherocytosis,* the formation of less biconcave and more spheroid cells. Abnormal erythrocytes, which lose flexibility, cannot pass the splenic filter. They are retained in splenic sinuses and impede circulation. In the passage of abnormal cells through endothelial gaps, selective pitting occurs and small abnormal pieces of the erythrocytes are removed.

Hypersplenism

This vague syndrome of anemia, splenomegaly, and bone marrow hyperplasia accompanies a highly overactive spleen. Blood flow in the enlarged spleen is markedly retarded ("congestive splenomegaly"), allowing sequestration of erythrocytes. Slowing and stasis of blood result in excessive erythrophagocytosis.

Protozoal infections
Malaria

A bite by an infected female mosquito introduces sporozoites of *Plasmodium* spp. into a vertebrate host to initiate the first, *extraerythrocytic phase* of infection. In mammals the liver is usually involved, in birds the reticuloendothelial system. During this phase the organism goes through several asexual reproductions. Sporozoites transform to trophozoites, to multinucleate schizonts, and finally to mature schizonts. From this immense host cell, unicellular merozoites are released to invade new cells and repeat the extraerythrocytic cycle or to begin the *erythrocytic phase* by infecting erythrocytes. The periodic fever of malaria results from synchronous release of merozoites and toxic peptides from infected cells.

Encounter with erythrocytes leads to the attachment of the merozoite to sialic acids on carbohydrate moieties that project from transmembrane proteins. Penetration is initiated on contact of the specialized attachment structure of the merozoite (called a conoid) with the erythrocytic plasma membrane. Tight junctions form between membranes of the anterior merozoite and the erythrocyte. Junctions form by aggregation of intramembrane protein and alter to form a constricting ring (a spectrin-free focus) at the point of merozoite entry. A surface depression is created that develops into a cavity, eventually enclosing the parasite without disrupting membrane continuity. Within the red cell, the membrane-bound merozoite promptly begins its transformation and dedifferentiation (Fig. 17.7).

Plasmodial parasites feed on hemoglobin.

Hemoglobin is taken into the parasite by phagocytosis and enters its food vacuole directly. Some species have a specialized cytosome on the pellicle that actively ingests host cell cytoplasm. *Malarial pigment* (hemozoin) is the residue of hemoglobin digestion that accumulates in host tissues.

As new merozoites bud from mother schizonts, the erythocyte becomes irregular and pale. Debris, ferritin, and pigment are strewn through

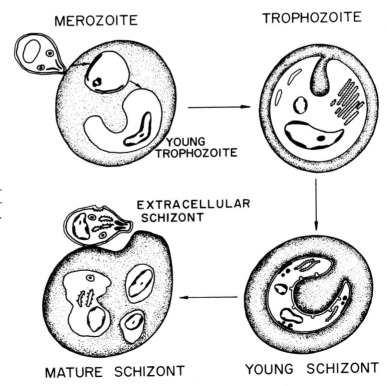

Fig. 17.7. Pathogenesis of intraerythrocytic replication of plasmodia.

MEROZOITE

TROPHOZOITE

YOUNG TROPHOZOITE

EXTRACELLULAR SCHIZONT

MATURE SCHIZONT

YOUNG SCHIZONT

the cell. Daughter merozoites feed by lysis of erythrocyte proteins, probably by secreting a lytic substance that disrupts the electrolyte-maintaining mechanisms of the plasma membrane.

Plasmodia alter erythrocyte surfaces.

Plasmodia alter the erythocyte surfaces in two ways: by shifting phospholipid molecules in the lipid bilayer so they are more accessible to phospholipases and by causing small knobby protuberances on erythrocyte surfaces that attach to venular endothelial surfaces, on which the erythrocytes stick until the parasite matures. Sequestration of infected erythrocytes in venules promotes the disease because parasitized cells are protected from removal during splenic circulation and because parasites appear to grow better in the hypoxic venular environment.

Babesia spp. lyse erythrocytes by replicating intracellularly.

Babesia spp., members of the suborder Piroplasmidae, destroy vertebrate erythrocytes by intracellular replication. Organisms replicate by modified schizogony; the pleomorphic offspring range from round to cigar-shaped forms, with central or peripheral nuclei. Erythrocyte destruction occurs by the direct action of the parasite, but the resulting anemia is often out of proportion to the number of parasitized red cells, possibly due to a late destructive immunologic reaction.

Bovine babesiosis (Texas cattle fever), caused by *Babesia bigemina,* was the first protozoan parasite infection shown to be arthropod-transmitted. Control of the tick vector eliminated the disease from the United States. This is a severe hemolytic disease accompanied by fever and hemoglobinuria. Infected female ticks feed on cattle, injecting sporozoites into the bloodstream. These enter erythrocytes and change into ring-shaped structures, then progressively transform into ameboid trophozoites. They multiply by budding to produce two pyriform bodies that are attached at one end (but later separate).

Parasitemia occurs when organisms break out of red cells. They infect others to initiate succeeding asexual cycles of schizogony. Parasitemia and relapse occur at irregular and unpredictable intervals. During relapses, phagocytosis of erythrocytes and trophozoites by monocytes occurs, but this does not significantly affect the life cycle of the parasite.

Bacterial infections

Two important groups of bacteria in the order Rickettsiales infect erythrocytes of vertebrates: Hemobartonellae and *Anaplasma* spp. As with other bacteria, these prokaryotic organisms lack nuclei and defined organelles such as mitochondria and endoplasmic reticulum.

Hemobartonella spp. attach to erythrocyte surfaces.

Hemobartonella spp. exist in deep, grooved infoldings on erythrocyte surfaces; they appear to be inside cells on casual examination of stained blood smears (Fig. 17.8). Anemia, the only known manifestation of infection, is due to increased rigidity of the cells and excessive erythrophagocytosis (not to overt damage to the erythrocyte).

Most infections with hemobartonellae are asymptomatic. The exceptions are very young animals or those with acquired immunologic deficiencies. Splenectomy is an established method for inducing parasitemia and clinical disease in individuals with inapparent infections.

Eperythozoon spp. are closely related members of the family Bartonellaceae that also exist indented into erythrocyte surfaces. They occur in coccoid, rod, or ring forms with diameters smaller than those of the hemobartonellae.

Anaplasma spp. enter and replicate inside erythocytes.

Anaplasma spp. are transmitted by ticks and other insects and enter the erythrocyte by in-

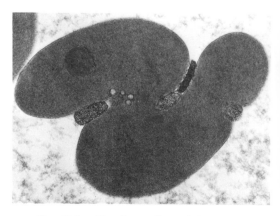

Fig. 17.8. *Hemobartonella canis* indented into surface of canine erythrocytes. (Photograph: John Venable, *J. Parasitol.* 54:259, 1968, used by permission)

vaginating into the cell surface. After penetration they occur as single initial bodies bound by a membrane at the erythrocyte periphery. Replication of the initial body by binary fission leads to two to eight bodies within the vacuole, the marginal or *inclusion body* that is diagnostic in Giemsa-stained blood smears of infected animals.

Erythrocyte metabolism is not markedly altered in infection, but because of the damaged cell surface, erythrocytes are rapidly removed by the phagocytic cells of the spleen. Anemia peaks 1–6 days after the peak of parasitemia (Fig 17.9). In the latter stages of anemia it is also alleged that an autoimmune process may contribute to red cell destruction. In chronic infection, bone marrow exhaustion contributes to

severe disease and death. The excess bilirubin formed by erythrocyte destruction is excreted, but animals dead of anaplasmosis are icteric and have splenomegaly and gall bladder enlargement.

Leptospires excrete a hemolysin.

Leptospirosis is an infectious disease caused by spirochetes of the genus *Leptospira*. Best identified by examining blood under dark-field illumination, these microorganisms produce bacteremia before localizing in kidney, liver, placenta, and other organs (Fig. 17.10). Hemolytic anemia occurs during bacteremia and, in its early phase, is due to a hemolysin produced by the leptospires. This toxin adheres to erythrocyte surfaces; those erythrocytes that are not lysed by this event remain susceptible to an immunologic form of lysis. In late stages of anemia antibodies with hemagglutinating activity appear in the plasma of infected animals and contribute to intravascular hemolysis.

Clostridia are bacteria that also cause erythrocyte destruction. They release potent exotoxins that digest lecithins in the red cell plasma membrane; anemia occurs in clostridial diseases such as blackleg and malignant edema of cattle, but extensive tissue damage (especially to skeletal muscle) preempts any clinical effects of anemia.

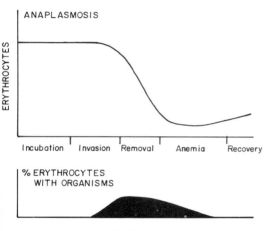

Fig. 17.9. Anemia in anaplasmosis.

Viral infections

Mild, transient anemia is common in severe systemic viral infections. The mature erythrocyte lacks metabolic pathways to support viral replication, and anemia is almost never due to

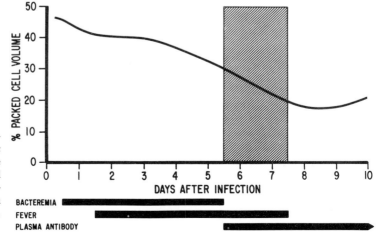

Fig. 17.10 Anemia, sheep experimentally infected with *Leptospira pomona*. Shaded area indicates time of hemolytic crisis. Antileptospiral antibody was determined by a microscopic agglutination test. (Data from Decker et al., *Am. J. Vet. Res.* 31:873, 1970)

direct erythrocyte destruction. Instead, viruses replicate in erythrocyte precursors in the bone marrow and depress erythropoiesis. Anemia that is clinically significant is largely limited to those viral infections in which platelet production is also suppressed, such as hog cholera (swine fever), infectious canine hepatitis, canine distemper, avian Newcastle disease, and duck plague. Bleeding that results from thrombocytopenia coupled with suppressed erythropoiesis may cause overt anemia.

Anemia commonly accompanies blood cell neoplasms.

Anemia is a usual response to leukemia virus infection. It occurs in the preleukemic period; that is, *feline leukemia virus* (FeLV) produces a normochromic, normocytic anemia with a low reticulocyte count soon after infection (long before lymphatic leukemia appears). The anemia is complex and due to varying mechanisms, one involving intravascular hemolysis and another bone marrow hypoplasia.

In 1975, Dr. William Jarrett and co-workers in Glasgow inoculated kittens with different isolates of FeLV. All kittens developed anemia, despite the paradox of having bone marrow hyperplasia and increased erythropoiesis. With one field isolate of FeLV, kittens died of severe anemia; they had developed *aplastic anemia* with depletion of erythroid tissue.

Toxicity

Chronic copper poisoning is most common in sheep, where it is manifest as anemia and neural and hepatic lesions. Reserves of copper are stored in the liver, and copper is transported in plasma as ceruloplasm, a complex of copper with globulin. Release of excess amounts of copper into the bloodstream by the overloaded liver is associated with forms of stress such as nutritional deficiency, strenuous exercise, or transport stress. It leads to acute crises of intravascular hemolysis; as many as 60% of circulating erythrocytes may be destroyed. Hemoglobinemia and hemoglobinuria are severe.

Immunologically mediated injury

Antibodies produced against certain erythrocyte surface antigens specifically react with those same glycoproteins embedded in the plasma membrane of circulating erythrocytes.

Antigen-antibody complexes on the erythrocyte surface attract complement components circulating in plasma (see Fig. 5.10). Activation of complement sequences on the erythrocyte surface leads to insertion of complement proteins into the red cell membrane, which produces discrete 100-nm pores and leads eventually to lysis of the cell (Fig. 17.11).

Equine infectious anemia is a viral infection of horses characterized by progressive debility, intermittent fever, and normocytic, normochromic anemia. Acute intravascular hemolytic episodes are associated with accumulation of complement on circulating erythrocytes, and the mechanism of anemia is thought to be immunologic. Stimulation of the reticuloendothelial system is a major event, and erythrophagocytosis and accumulation of abnormal monocytes occur in spleen and liver.

Drug-induced hemolytic anemia can develop after prolonged therapy, particularly after penicillin (although this type of anemia is rare). Propylthiouracil, used for treatment of hyperthyroidism in cats, can cause hemolytic anemia. Clinical signs appear after 20 days of treatment, and cessation of therapy leads to disappearance of anemia. Most drugs are not antigenic alone but act as haptens; by covalent bonding to a host protein, the hapten-carrier complex induces an immune response.

Hemolytic disease of the newborn

The fetus, by virtue of inheritance from the father, produces erythrocyte membrane proteins called *isoantigens* that are not present on erythrocytes of the mother. When fetal red cells gain access to the mother's bloodstream they induce antibodies, and if these antibodies are returned to the newborn via colostrum, hemolysis is induced. Absorption of antibodies occurs via milk in horses, calves, and piglets; in primates, transplacental transfer of antibody leads to a similar disease called *erythroblastosis fetalis.*

Hereditary defects
Enzyme deficiencies

Specific deficiencies of enzymes of glucose metabolism lead to anemia (Fig. 17.12). Although rare, they have led to a better understanding of erythrocyte function. The most common human red cell enzyme deficiency is that of glucose-6-phosphate dehydrogenase; the clinical syndrome of anemia is precipitated when af-

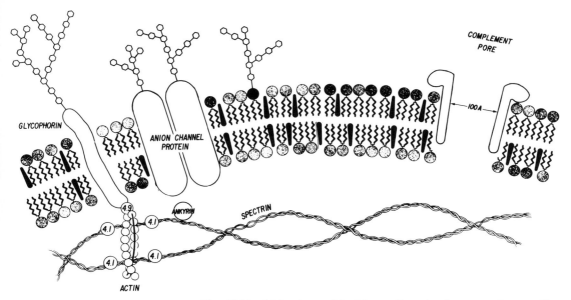

Fig. 17.11. Molecular model of the erythrocyte plasma membrane with transmembrane proteins and subsurface cytoskeleton. Complement-induced pores are formed by insertion of the final attack sequence of complement components (C5–C9) into the membrane.

fected patients take the antimalarial drug primaquine.

In dogs, three familial types of hemolytic anemia are known: pyruvate kinase deficiency in the basenji, membrane cation channel defect in Alaskan malamutes, and an idiopathic anemia in poodles.

Pyruvate kinase deficiency

Absence of enzymes of glycolysis may lead to reduced ATP formation and erythrocyte fragility. In the late 1960s, Drs. John Tasker, Gene Searcy, and D. R. Miller studied pyruvate kinase (PK) deficiency in erythrocytes of basenji dogs. This defect causes recurring episodes of *hemolytic anemia*. Affected pups, which are detected at about 8 weeks of age, have PCV and hemoglobin values 60–70% of normal. There is a 10- to 20-fold increase in circulating reticulocytes, and the erythrocyte half-life is greatly shortened during anemic phases. Erythrocytes show normal osmotic fragility and lack spherocytosis but develop hemolysis after a 48-hour incubation (which is not prevented by glucose).

PK deficiency disrupts the glycolytic cycle, resulting in altered plasma membrane energy sources. PK catalyzes the conversion of phos-

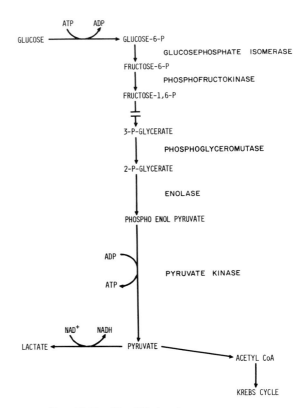

Fig. 17.12. Simplified pathway of glucose metabolism.

phoenolpyruvate to pyruvate. When this reaction becomes rate-limiting, the conversion of glucose to lactate (Embden-Meyerhof pathway) is impaired and leads to ATP deficiency and an increase in glycolytic intermediates in the anaerobic pathway proximal to the PK reaction.

Defects in membrane channel protein

A plasma membrane defect is involved in a mild hereditary hemolytic anemia with *stomatocytosis* that occurs in Alaskan malamute dogs affected with chondrodysplasia. Enlarged erythrocytes have a diminished mean corpuscular hemoglobin (30%) that is responsible for the reduced hemoglobin concentration, low red cell count, and normal PCV. Erythrocytes have increased Na^+ and water. Their survival time is shortened, and both red cell osmotic pressure and fragility are increased.

Defective heme

The porphyrias are a group of diseases of heme synthesis in which excessive amounts and abnormal types of porphyrins accumulate in tissue, blood, and feces. They include both hereditary and acquired forms and are grouped into two major categories, *erythropoietic* and *hepatic,* based on the tissue in which the metabolic defect is expressed.

Congenital erythropoietic porphyria

This defect of the heme part of hemoglobin involves overproduction of type I porphyrins caused by an enzymatic defect in the conversion of porphobilinogen to uroporphyrinogen. These porphyrins cannot be used for hemoglobin synthesis and interfere with erythropoiesis as the abnormal porphyrin forms in the immature developing erythrocyte.

Congenital erythropoietic porphyria has been seen in pigs, cattle, cats, and fox squirrels. Deficiency of the enzyme *uroporphyrinogen II cosynthetase* has been identified in erythrocytes of cattle and man with porphyria. Affected animals are unable to use the porphyrin isomers to synthesize protoporphyrin and heme.

The consequences of erythropoietic porphyria depend on which porphyrins accumulate and where they are deposited. There are (1) hemolytic anemia, usually with hemosiderosis of spleen, liver, and lymph nodes; (2) renal failure due to glomerulopathy and tubular disease, which in some animals leads to uremia and death; and (3) photosensitivity, sunlight exciting the uro- and coproporphyrins in the capillaries of the skin and eliciting molecular changes that cause degeneration, necrosis, erythema, and edema. Photosensitizing properties increase in this order: protoporphyrin, coproporphyrin, uroporphyrin.

Dr. Ellis Giddens, in studies on porphyric Siamese cats at the Washington Regional Primate Center, found severe macrocytic hypocychromic anemia; elevated porphyrins (type I isomers of uroporphyrin and coproporphyrin) were present in blood, feces, teeth, bones, and most viscera. Porphyrins are deposited in teeth and bone because of their affinity for mineral. The cats had hepatomegaly, splenomegaly, and renal glomerular lesions and became photosensitive.

Protoporphyria is a recessive trait in cattle.

Protoporphyria with extensive cutaneous lesions and high protoporphyrin concentrations in erythrocytes and feces was first identified in cattle by Dr. George Ruth, at the University of Minnesota. Even though affected calves tried to avoid sunlight, they developed dermal lesions of erythema, edema, and necrosis on the snout, ears, and back. Protoporphyria is associated with a marked decrease of *ferrochelatase* (heme synthetase) in liver and other tissues. This painful photosensitivity disease occurs without the discoloration of urine or teeth that characterizes bovine erythropoietic porphyria.

Acquired diseases of porphyrin metabolism

These diseases may arise from liver damage with suppression of porphyrin degradation. Porphyrins are commonly present in plants and fungi. When large amounts are ingested and absorbed, they are activated in skin to produce photodynamic dermatitis. Buckwheat (fagopyrum) and St. John's wort (hypericin) are noted for producing edema and necrosis of white hairless areas of the skin of herbivores. Sulfoxides of phenothiazine are excreted in tears, producing corneal edema and keratitis.

Phylloerythrin accumulates in hepatogenous porphyria.

Liver damage with obstruction of bile ducts leads to accumulation of phylloerythrin, a photosensitizing degradation product of plant chlorophyll. Severe photosensitivity has been seen in Turkey in humans who have consumed wheat seeds treated with hexachlorobenzene-containing fungicides. Griseofulvin, a drug that inhibits mitochondrial chelatase, causes diminished incorporation of protoporphyrin into heme and its accumulation in erythroblasts.

Acquired disorders of hemoglobin

Acquired defects in the hemoglobin molecule are only rarely responsible for erythrocyte destruction. Drugs such as phenylhydrazine induce oxidative denaturation of hemoglobin that precipitates as Heinz bodies. Aggregates of insoluble hemoglobin then render erythrocytes susceptible to lysis and erythrophagocytosis by altering the plasma membrane.

Carbon monoxide forms carboxyhemoglobin.

Carbon monoxide (CO) has an affinity over 200 times that of oxygen for hemoglobin. Binding is irreversible, and since hemoglobin conjugated with CO cannot carry oxygen, affected animals die with anoxia. The blood is bright red. Lethal effects occur in the brain, which is edematous, often with tiny hemorrhages. Neurons are killed, although this is difficult to demonstrate histologically.

Pet animals and piglets kept in closed houses heated by petroleum fuels are most often affected. CO passes the placenta and can poison the fetus. Dr. Mark Dominick studied pregnant sows made toxic with CO and showed that abortion is directly related to the dose of CO. Brain lesions of fetuses were similar to those in poisoned adults.

Nitrates form methemoglobin.

Methemoglobin, formed when ferrous iron of hemoglobin is changed to ferric iron, cannot transport oxygen. In animals, methemoglobinemia is due to oxidizing toxins such as nitrates, chlorates, and phenacetin. In *nitrate poisoning* of ruminants (nitrate is acquired in fertilizers, plants, and stagnant water), ingested nitrates are converted in the rumen to nitrite, which is absorbed. Nitrite may also be acquired by exogenous sources. Death from nitrate/nitrite poisoning also involves a vasodilatory effect of nitrite (nitrites are used pharmacologically in man to dilate the coronary artery) and the general effect of nitrites on iron-containing enzymes in the electron transport chain.

Hereditary disorders of hemoglobin

Two major types of inherited disorders of hemoglobin occur. (1) *Qualitative* changes in globin, diseases referred to as hemoglobinopathies, are exemplified by sickle cell anemia, in which both genes for the β chain are mutant. (2) *Quantitative* changes in the amount of normal α- or β-globin produced; these are called thalassemia syndromes, a catchall term for inherited disease in which globin is missing or produced in small amounts.

Sickle cell anemia is a qualitative globin defect.

A mutation in the gene for the β chain of globin leads to single amino acid substitution in the abnormal hemoglobin (Hb-S) that causes human sickle cell anemia, a serious genetic affection of the black race; 10% carry the sickle trait (their erythrocytes contain about half Hb-S), but only 0.2% develop anemia (>90% is Hb-S). This drastically reduces solubility of hemoglobin in its deoxygenated state, so that it precipitates into fibers, causing erythrocytes to become elongated and rigid and to wrinkle the cell surface, resulting in increased fragility and erythrophagocytosis.

Thalassemia: A quantitative globin defect

In thalassemia globins have a normal amino acid sequence but are reduced in amount. Genes for either α- or β-globin can be completely or partially deleted. They can have mutations that shut off globin protein synthesis or mutations that affect gene regulation. In β-thalassemia, it is the regulation of β-globin genes that is disturbed. The molecular defect is not in the gene's nucleotide sequence but in the intervening sequences of DNA that connect gene pieces.

ANEMIA DUE TO INSUFFICIENT ERYTHROCYTE PRODUCTION

Underproduction of erythrocytes can result from primary bone marrow failure or from diminished stimulation of marrow erythropoiesis. Put more simply, the mechanism of the deficiency may be a stem cell defect or a normal stem cell within an abnormal environment. Deficiency of the environment, usually a deficiency of *erythropoietin,* is not clearly established in animals. Erythropoietin is implicated in anemia of chronic renal disease, disseminated metastatic tumors, and hepatic failure. In most cases a deficiency of erythropoietin is implied. In rare cases, erythropoietin is synthesized in adequate amounts, but it is inactivated or does not reach the site of erythropoiesis in the bone marrow.

Bone marrow suppression

Normally, extremely large numbers of erythrocytes are formed continually; in some mammals as many as 3 million per second are released into circulating blood. Because of this high rate of cell division, bone marrow is highly susceptible to chemical agents that suppress metabolism. Erythropoietic cells are rapidly destroyed by radiation, immunosuppressive drugs, plant toxins (bracken fern), and infectious agents (feline leukemia, infectious feline panleukopenia, *Ehrlichia* spp.). With most of these agents the bone marrow undergoes atrophy and in severe cases becomes aplastic. The antibiotic chloramphenicol is a notorious bone marrow toxin that kills by producing aplastic anemia. In dead animals, the bone marrow is hypocellular and filled with plasma and fibroblasts.

Estrogens induce bone marrow toxicosis.

The initial response to estrogens (either natural or therapeutic) during myelotoxicosis is transient, increased granulocytopoiesis and neutrophilic leukocytosis. This is rapidly followed by decreased hematopoiesis, which leads to progressive leukopenia, thrombocytopenia, and nonregenerative anemia. Clinical disease may result from hemorrhage (due to platelet suppression), anemia, and bacterial infection associated with leukopenia.

Ferrets are highly sensitive to estrogen and may become anemic during prolonged estrus. Dogs are also sensitive and may develop anemia after clinical estrogen therapy and during increased endogenous estrogen production associated with ovarian granulosa cell tumors or Sertoli cell tumors of the testicle. Dr. Gary Kociba and co-workers, at Ohio State University, have reported anemia and bone marrow hypoplasia in male dogs with Sertoli cell tumors, hyperestrogenism, and feminization. Dogs develop pancytopenia and, because of reductions in circulating granulocytes and platelets, often have fever and infections.

Because of high rates of erythropoiesis, marrow is also susceptible to deficiencies of several essential dietary factors (e.g., iron, folic acid, vitamins B_{12} and B_6, and protein). The most important dietary deficiency that causes anemia is that of iron.

Iron-deficiency anemia

Deficiencies of iron result in small erythrocytes with decreased hemoglobin. Hypochromic red cells develop chiefly because of the lack of sufficient iron for formation of heme molecules; erythrocytes are released into the circulation before receiving their full levels of hemoglobin. Other minor mechanisms also operate in defective iron-deficiency erythrocytes. The surface membrane is overly susceptible to oxidative damage because of enzymic defects. Glutathione peroxidase activity is markedly diminished in iron-deficient cells (this enzyme normally acts on peroxides, preventing them from oxidizing sulfhydryl groups in the membrane).

Iron-deficiency anemia is seen as a dietary disorder in newborns, as part of chronic blood loss due to intestinal parasites, and as part of intestinal malabsorption diseases of adult animals. In some cases sufficient iron may be in the diet but it is made unavailable. For example, reduced intestinal absorption of iron occurs in mink kits fed raw marine fish; the cause is formation of insoluble crystalline ferric oxide hydroxides by trimethylamine oxide in fish.

In plasma, iron is complexed to the protein *transferrin*, which has the electrophoretic mobilization of a β_1-globulin and serves as an iron carrier. Plasma iron represents the balance between iron of hemoglobin breakdown and iron absorbed from the intestine minus iron removed by heme synthesis, cell metabolism, and storage.

Transient iron-deficiency anemia occurs in cats and dogs.

A mild, transient anemia develops in young kittens as a result of iron deficiencies associated with rapid growth and all-milk diets. Dr. Glade Weiser, now at Colorado State University, showed that kittens with low serum iron values at 2–4 weeks rapidly developed a microcytic subpopulation that was most prominent at 5 weeks of age. In dogs, iron-deficiency anemia is rare, being associated only with bloodsucking parasites and chronic external blood loss. Anemia is hypochromic, microcytic, and nonregenerative or "hypoproliferative."

Iron deficiency is common in baby pigs.

Piglets are born with low iron in their tissues. Their extraordinarily rapid rate of growth coupled with low iron levels in sow's milk require that they obtain large amounts of dietary iron. The plasma iron, which is normally 100–300 μg/100 ml may drop to 50 μg in anemic piglets. The iron-binding capacity of the plasma is increased (when iron is given therapeutically, it is rapidly complexed to transferrin and accepted by erythroblasts).

In affected pigs, the mucous membranes are pale, and systemic signs of anemia such as dyspnea and cardiac abnormalities occur. At necropsy, cardiac pallor, dilatation, and hypertrophy of ventricular walls are common.

The sequence of events is as follows: dietary iron deficiency, depletion of tissue iron stores, decreased saturation of transferrin, decreased delivery to erythroid cells, impaired hemoglobin synthesis, and anemia. Bone marrow is hypercellular. An estimate of iron deficiency can be made in marrow smears by finding hemosiderin granules stained with Prussian blue. The continued division of erythroblasts produces excessive numbers of small, pale erythrocytes with a shortened life span (i.e., hypochromic, microcytic anemia).

Models of iron-deficiency hypochromic anemia

Anemia in inbred strains of mice are used to study defects of iron absorption and transfer by the absorptive cells of the intestinal mucosa. Mice with microcytic anemia (*mk* mice) have an iron entry defect (iron never reaches the intestinal absorptive cells); mice with sex-linked anemia (*sla* mice) have a defect in exit of iron (large amounts of stainable iron are in the ileal mucosa but cannot be transferred to the lamina propria and from there into the circulation).

An erythropoietic stem cell defect occurs in gray collies with cyclic hematopoiesis. The most overt manifestation of the stem cell defect is the disappearance of neutrophils from the circulation every 10–12 days. Reticulocytes also undergo this curious cyclic depression, and there is a reduction in the formation of erythrocytes. The cycle reflects competition of differing hemic populations (granulocytes, platelets, and

erythroblasts) for the limited number of stem cells produced.

Iron metabolism is disturbed in inflammation.

Iron metabolism is altered in severe inflammatory disease. In dogs, plasma iron and iron-binding capacity are reduced. This is unusual because iron stores are actually increased in inflammation because of active phagocytic cells. Iron is in a less-labile form (as hemosiderin and ferritin) during the active inflammatory process (see inflammation, Chapter 18).

Lead toxicity anemia

Lead toxicity occurs by ingestion of flaking lead-based paints or ingestion of contaminated grasses near lead smelters. It leads to various gastrointestinal, neurologic, and osteologic disorders. Mild anemia occurs due to the suppression of hemoglobin production and the reduction of erythrocyte life span. In blood smears of poisoned animals, diagnosis is aided by the presence of dustlike particles in erythrocytes (referred to as *basophilic stippling*).

Defects are produced in mitochondrial pathways of uroporphyrinogen synthesis in lead toxicity. Lead inhibits ferrochelatase and levulinic acid dehydratase, involved in heme synthesis, and reduces the incorporation of iron into the porphyrin ring. Heme synthesis is suppressed, and there is an increase in protoporphyrin in erythrocytes.

Lead causes other cellular defects, although their role in lead toxicity anemia is not clear. Lead binds to mitochondrial membranes and suppresses both oxidative phosphorylation and the citric acid cycle. Lead also inhibits Na-K-ATPase in the surface membranes of erythrocytes and may enhance erythrocyte fragility.

POLYCYTHEMIA

Increased numbers of erythrocytes per cubic millimeter of blood are seen in dehydrated or hyperthermic animals. This *relative polycythemia,* also called hemoconcentration, is due to a diminution of the quantity of plasma in the blood. The erythrocyte count, hemoglobin, and hematocrit are elevated, but the total erythrocyte volume is normal. Hemoconcentration occurs because water is lost from the blood beyond the capacity of the interstitial fluids to replace it. It is seen in water deprivation, vomiting, diarrhea, and excessive water loss in fever. It is often a serious sign and should be treated with fluid therapy.

Absolute polycythemia exists whenever the erythrocyte volume is elevated above normal. Absolute erythrocytosis secondary to low oxygen content in the atmosphere is fairly common, occurring in mammals at high altitudes and in fish in warm waters. Absolute erythrocytosis may also accompany cardiac failure and diffuse pulmonary disease.

Familial primary polycythemia occurs as a simple autosomal recessive condition in Jersey cattle. Affected calves are weak, lethargic, and dyspneic and usually die by 6 months of age with hyperemia of the pulmonary capillary bed. Isolated cases of primary polycythemia have also been reported in dogs and cattle. Human familial polycythemia is a stem cell defect, probably of clonal origin.

ADDITIONAL READING

Auer, L., and Bell, K. Transfusion reactions in cats. Res. Vet. Sci. 35:145, 1983.

Feldman, B. F., et al. Anemia of inflammatory disease in the dog. *Am. J. Vet. Res.* 42:586, 1981.

Harvey, J. W., and Gaskin, J. M. Feline hemobartonellosis: Attempts to induce relapse of clinical disease in chronically infected cats. *J. Am. Anim. Hosp. Assoc.* 14:453, 1978.

Harvey, J. W., et al. Chronic iron deficiency anemia in dogs. *J. Am. Anim. Hosp. Assoc.* 18:946, 1982.

Leighton, F. A., et al. Heinz-body hemolytic anemia from the ingestion of crude oil: A primary toxic effect in marine birds. *Science* 220:871, 1983.

Prasse, K. W., et al. Pyruvate kinase deficiency anemia with terminal myelofibrosis and osteosclerosis in a beagle. *J. Am. Vet. Med. Assoc.* 166:1170, 1975.

Rebar, A. H., et al. Microangiopathic hemolytic anemia associated with radiation induced hemangiosarcomas. *Vet. Pathol.* 17:443, 1980.

Sherding, R. G., et al. Bone marrow hypoplasia in eight dogs with Sertoli cell tumor. *J. Am. Vet. Med. Assoc.* 178:497, 1981.

Smith, J. E. Erythrocyte membrane. *Vet. Pathol.* 24:471, 1987.

Smith, J. E., et al. Interaction of amphipathic drugs with erythrocytes from various species. *Am. J. Vet. Res.* 43:1041, 1982.

Stormont, C. J. Blood groups in animals. *J. Am. Vet. Med. Assoc.* 181:1120, 1982.

Weiser, M. G., and Kociba, G. J. Erythrocyte macrocytosis in feline leukemia virus associated anemia. *Vet. Pathol.* 20:687, 1983.

Weiss, D. J., et al. Studies of the pathogenesis of anemia of inflammation. *Am. J. Vet. Res.* 44:1864, 1983.

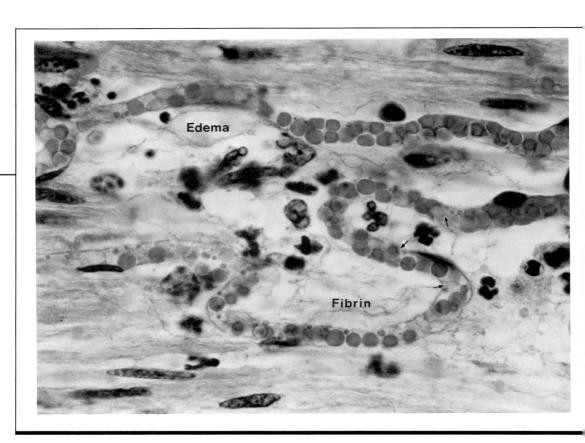

Degeneration and necrosis of endothelial cells with exudation of fluid (*edema*), fibrin, and leukocytes into the interstitium; thrombi within capillaries (*arrows*); equine viral arteritis.

INFLAMMATION AND HEALING

5

NFLAMMATION (L. *inflammare,* to set on fire) is a complex progression of vascular and tissue changes that develops in response to injury. The cardinal signs of redness, heat, swelling, and pain that were defined in Chapter 1 all result from the movement of plasma fluids and cells out of the vascular system into the tissues. The entire process is designed to dilute, destroy, and sequester the causal agent of injury and to repair the damaged tissue.

The first event in the inflammatory response is an *increase in permeability of endothelium of the capillary bed,* a change that may be subtle, as in allergic dermatitis resulting from flea bites, or massive, as is typical of trauma. The increase in vascular permeability leads directly to *exudation of leukocytes and plasma proteins* from blood vessel lumina into the tissue interstitium. As fluid accumulates in tissue spaces, toxins, microbial components, and tissue debris are complexed by specialized proteins, processed by phagocytic cells, and drained away into the lymphatic system. In essence, inflammation *extends the defense mechanisms existing in circulating blood into the tissues* and mobilizes the body to activate all its mechanisms of immunity to overcome injury.

During early inflammation, as all the mechanisms of local tissue protection are being activated, several important humoral signals are released from damaged tissue. These soluble signal molecules travel in the bloodstream to act at sites of *hematopoiesis* (bone marrow), *lymphopoiesis* (lymph nodes and spleen), and *plasma protein synthesis* (liver). As a result, leukocytes and stimulatory proteins (called "acute phase proteins") pour into the bloodstream, travel back to the inflammatory site, and enter the tissue to provide appropriate stimulation to keep the inflammatory process going.

Some of the acute phase proteins that rapidly appear in tissue fluids, lymph, and blood are strongly *vasoactive.* These peptides mediate inflammation not only by increasing permeability of capillaries but also by specifically directing the migration of circulating leukocytes, a process called *chemotaxis.*

Inflammation is not a neatly organized event but evolves like a three-ring circus with many interrelated acts occurring at the same time. The *inflammatory process incorporates several different biologic mechanisms:* edema is an integral component, phagocytosis is very active, and both coagulation factors and platelets are activated.

In late stages of inflammation, reconstructive processes are initiated that repair the tissue damage. *Vascular regrowth* (also called angiogenesis), *fibroplasia,* and *epithelial regeneration* flourish in the protein-rich tissue matrix established in early inflammation. Populations of leukocytes, which are often called "inflammatory cells," persist to clean up tissue debris and to provide specific mechanisms that remove microbial and foreign substances.

In the end, inflammation usually brings about recovery. In general, *immunity* is resistance to disease. In the higher animals, *inflammation is the primary process by which the mechanisms of immunity are implemented.* Phylogenetically, the inflammatory process becomes increasingly complex as one progresses from lower forms to the higher vertebrates. It consists largely of nonspecific fluid and cellular mechanisms in lower forms of animal life. In mammals, inflammation involves most of the more ancient mechanisms of immunity but also induces specific mechanisms such as production of antibodies and very selective types of lymphocytes.

Anatomical terminology of inflammation

Bile duct	cholangitis		Meninges	meningitis
Bladder	cystitis		Mouth	stomatitis
Blood vessel	vasculitis		Muscle (skeletal)	myositis
Bone	osteitis		Myocardium	myocarditis
Bone marrow	osteomyelitis			
Brain	encephalitis		Nerve	neuritis
Bursa	bursitis			
			Ovary	oophoritis
Cecum	typhlitis		Oviduct	salpingitis
Connective tissue	cellulitis			
Cornea	keratitis		Pancreas	pancreatitis
			Pericardium	pericarditis
Dura mater	pachymeningitis		Peritoneum	peritonitis
			Pleura	pleuritis
Ear	otitis		Prepuce	posthitis
Eustachian tube	eustachitis			
Eye	ophthalmitis		Renal glomerulus	glomerulitis
Eyelid	blepharitis		Renal pelvis	pyelitis
Fascia	fasciitis		Salivary gland	sialadenitis
Fat	steatitis		Sinus	sinusitis
			Skin	dermatitis
Gallbladder	cholecystitis		Spermatic cord	funiculitis
Gill	branchiitis		Spinal nerve root	radiculitis
Glans penis	balanitis		Spleen	splenitis
			Stomach	gastritis
Heart	carditis			
			Testicle	orchitis
Intestine	enteritis		Tongue	glossitis
Iris	iritis		Trachea	tracheitis
			Tympanum	tympanitis
Kidney	nephritis			
			Uterus	metritis
Lacrimal gland	dacryoadenitis			
Ligaments	desmitis		Vagina	vaginitis
Lip	cheilitis		Vas deferens	vasitis
Liver	hepatitis		Vein	phlebitis
Lung	pneumonitis		Vertebra	spondylitis
Lymph nodes	lymphadenitis		Vessel	vasculitis
Lymph vessel	lymphangitis			

The Inflammatory Process

18

INTRODUCTION

When an irritant passes an epithelial barrier such as skin, it gains access to mesenchymal tissues, which react in an attempt to destroy the irritant and to form an inflammatory barrier. In *acute inflammation,* tissues become distended with fluids and inflammatory cells because the vascular wall is altered. Plasma proteins such as albumin, fibrinogen, antibody, complement, and lysozyme pour into the tissues. This is followed immediately by exudation of phagocytic cells, chiefly neutrophils and monocytes. Although severe lesions can be life threatening when they occur in vital organs such as lung and brain, the inflammatory process is essentially curative. It is designed to dilute, inactivate, and remove irritants.

Variations in the inflammatory response

Inflammatory lesions as seen microscopically vary in intensity and in dominance of a particular component. Differences depend on the type of irritant and on the *animal species* involved. Nonvertebrate animals depend largely on phagocytosis and encapsulation as mechanisms for removal of irritants. Vertebrates, however, have developed the highly complex set of interdependent reactions that, considered together, are termed *acute inflammation.* Despite phylogenetic variables, inflammation is a remarkably uniform biological reaction against a wide variety of physical, chemical, and biological irritants. It is an evolutionary, adaptive response enhancing survival for those animals that possess vascular systems. Individuals of vertebrate species lacking the capacity to produce a vigorous inflammatory response do not survive.

The *age* of an animal influences the character of the reaction. The adult has a greater capacity to react than does the neonate, and the neonate greater than the fetus. Fetal inflammatory reactions, like those of lower animals, are largely histiocytic; pluripotential cells respond by becoming phagocytic. The inability of the fetus to respond relates to inert or retarded vascular responses. They have only immature, slowly reacting pregranulocytes in the circulation and low levels of complement and other chemoattractants in serum.

In the developing mammalian *fetus,* the maturation of the neutrophil population heralds the capacity to react with an inflammatory process. This occurs in the later phases of gestation and provides the fetus with a newly acquired capacity to resist infectious agents. In fetuses of most species, phagocytic capacity develops slightly before bactericidal activity. In the pig fetus, both mechanisms approach adult levels at or near 100 days of gestation, that is, at about three-fourths of the time spent in utero.

Historical views of inflammation

Celsus, a Roman philosopher and a contemporary of Christ, enunciated four cardinal signs that are observed grossly in acute inflammation: *redness, swelling, heat,* and *pain* (*rubor, tumor, calor,* and *dolor*). Rudolf Virchow in 1858 added a fifth: *loss of function.*

With the application of the light microscope to pathology in the middle 1800s, Julius Cohnheim, a German experimental pathologist, revealed the vascular alterations that are the basis of the inflammatory response. By examining mesentery from a loop of intestine pulled through an abdominal incision of a curarized frog, he observed the early changes in blood flow and vascular permeability. Cohnheim recognized that increased capillary permeability was due to direct injury to endothelium and that this explained the initiating reaction in inflammation; that is, hyperemia and the exuding fluid had given rise to redness and swelling.

Cohnheim saw that blood leukocytes migrated through the walls of injured capillaries and small venules to reside in tissue. Like other great pathologists of his day, he taught that the observation of these cells filled with bacteria indicated a highly favorable environment for bacterial growth and that leukocytes provided a means of dissemination. The significance of *intracellular degradation of microbes* was demonstrated by the Russian zoologist Elie Metchnikoff, who investigated the ingestion of particular matter by invertebrate animals. After introducing rose thorns into starfish larvae, he noted that roving cells in the blood localized around the thorns and appeared to ingest and devour them. He termed these cells *phagocytes* (more specifically, *macrophages*) and their process of engulfment *phagocytosis*. His subsequent studies revealed similar activity of "microphages" analogous to the granular leukocytes of vertebrates. These cells have evolved into populations of highly specialized cells (neutrophils, eosinophils, basophils). In the acute phases of inflammation, they migrate through the vascular wall at rates determined by their ameboid potential and their capacity to react to the chemotactic influences that develop in inflammation.

The cardinal signs of inflammation were further explained by Lewis's observations, in 1927, of the *triple response* of skin to a linear stroke produced by a marker (Fig. 18.1). A few seconds after injury, the stroke line was reddened. Slightly later a diffuse pink flare surrounded the red area, and in several minutes a wheal displaced the injury line. The interpretations of these reactions based on Lewis's experiment are (1) the initial redness is caused by the immediate release of vasoactive chemical mediators such as histamine and leukotrienes that cause capillary dilation and subsequent endothelial cell disunion, (2) the pale pink flare surrounding the injury is caused by arteriolar dilation due to an axon reflex arc, and (3) the wheal

forms from subsequent exudation of fluid and cells. The following sections will deal separately with these components of inflammation, how they develop, and advances in our understanding of them.

Pathogenesis

Acute inflammation usually develops along a common pathway (Table 18.1). However, inflammation is highly dynamic, with complex reactions developing simultaneously or at differing times according to the extent and type of injury. Heat produced at sites of inflammation exerts a pronounced effect on the entire process. Blood flow and phagocytic activity are enhanced by even small increases in temperature. Starling observed that if the foot of a dog was placed for 5 minutes in water at 60°C, lymph flow from the limb increased in quantity and content of protein. In inflamed tissues, this enormous increase in lymph flow prevents stagnation of interstitial fluids and allows debris to be drained away. In this process, microbial components can be dealt with by macrophages and lymphoid cells in regional lymph nodes, which are sites sufficiently distant from the inflammatory process that normal host defense mechanisms can be produced.

ENDOTHELIUM AND ITS ROLE IN INCREASED VASCULAR PERMEABILITY

Changes in the endothelial cell are the most crucial factors in the pathogenesis of inflammation. Whether endothelium is injured directly by trauma or toxins or is affected secondarily by hypoxia or by endogenous mediators such as histamine or leukotrienes, endothelial cell alterations determine the extent of the plasma protein–containing fluid that escapes to the extravascular spaces.

Blood flow

Blood flow to inflammatory lesions is increased. Within the inflammatory site, however, flow is slowed due to opening of the capillary bed and to dilatation of all blood vessels. Slowing and stasis of blood permits fluid and cellular exudation. Factors that influence the rate of

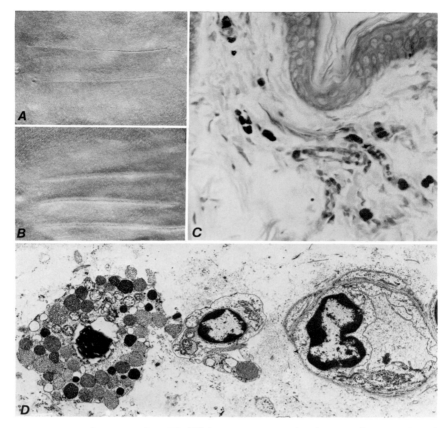

Fig. 18.1. A and B. Triple response: vascular changes with exudation of fluid, experimental injury, horse skin. A. Changes in skin immediately after scratching. B. Changes 4 minutes later. C. Perivascular mast cells, skin, cat. D. Ultrastructure of mast cell degranulation and edema in tissue spaces. Granular debris in interstitium represents exuded plasma proteins, myocarditis, cow with malignant catarrhal fever.

blood flow involve the arterioles, capillaries, and postcapillary venules.

Arteriolar dilatation is an early reflex.

Local tissue injury induces an immediate axon reflex arc, that is, one not traversing the spinal cord of the central nervous system (CNS). This arc is the main cause of arteriolar dilation, which underlies the pale red flare of the triple response. Following stimulation of sensory nerve endings at the site of injury, a nerve impulse passes centrally along the axon to its division and then peripherally to the arteriole supplying the injured area. Synaptic vesicles within the adrenergic synapse liberate adrenalin, which dilates the peripheral blood vessels. In Lewis's

experiments, sectioning of cutaneous nerves prior to producing skin injury abolished the flare of the triple response (but not the injury line or wheal). Furthermore, the flare was retarded in direct correlation with the presence of wallerian degeneration and death of the nerves sectioned.

Two other factors can also affect the inflammatory response by causing vasodilation upstream from the inflammation. First, impulses from the *central nervous system* can control arteriolar blood flow via vasodilator and vasoconstrictor nerves; however, all the essential elements of inflammation can occur without these central influences. Second, the passage of signal molecules between endothelial cells can cause a vasodilatory response that spreads peripherally from the site of injury (independent from the reflex arc).

Hemoconcentration inhibits blood flow.

Dilated blood vessels become filled with blood, and as the fluid content begins to exude

Table 18.1. Events in acute inflammation

1. *Capillaries and venules become abnormally permeable.*
   a. Tissue damage at the site of injury (trauma, hypoxia, or infection) releases products that promote inflammation. Endothelium becomes more permeable and releases soluble *procoagulant factors* and vasodilatory *prostaglandins.* Mast cells degranulate to release *histamine* (increases permeability of postcapillary venules), *heparin* (prevents coagulation and stimulates angiogenesis), *serotonin,* and *leukotrienes.*
   b. Endothelium peripheral to the site of injury becomes leaky (due to release of the above substances) and expands the inflammatory focus.
   c. Microbes release toxins and activate the complement system; *complement components* are released that attract leukocytes and cause mast cell degranulation, sustaining capillary permeability.

2. *Blood flow increases, then decreases.*
   a. Arterioles dilate due to nerve stimuli from an axonal reflex arc and the capillary bed expands.
   b. Stasis of flow is caused by filling of capillaries with blood, endothelial swelling, and exudation of fluids into the interstitium.
   c. Cells in flowing blood are redistributed: leukocytes marginate (move to the peripheral zone of flowing blood) and become sticky.

3. *Fluids and cells exude from capillary into prevascular spaces.*
   a. Plasma proteins exude into interstitium: tissues are expanded (wheal formation), antimicrobial proteins accumulate, and there is hemoconcentration. Thickened blood moves more slowly, further retarding blood flow.
   b. Neutrophils pass the vascular wall (increasing permeability further).

4. *Leukocytes degranulate in tissue spaces.*
   a. Neutrophils release *antimicrobial factors* (cationic proteins, hydrogen peroxide, hydrolytic enzymes, lysozyme), *proteases* that produce widespread tissue damage, and *kinins* (bradykinin) that cause additional vasodilation, vascular permeability, and nerve end stimulation (pain).
   b. Platelets release platelet activating factor, platelet factor 4, proteases, coagulation factors, and cationic proteins that sustain the increased vascular permeability.

5. *Microorganisms are killed and tissue is damaged.*
   a. Blood and lymph flow are suppressed. *Fibrinogen* polymerizes to form fibrin in tissue spaces, and *thrombi* develop in blood vessels. Lymphatic blockade occurs and leads to lymph stasis.
   b. Leukocytes are destroyed, with massive release of neutrophil granules and extensive tissue damage.
   c. Parenchymal cells of the host are damaged, with release of *pyrogens,* which act systemically to produce fever and muscle breakdown, and synthesis of the *acute phase proteins* (fibrinogen, complement, et al.) in liver, and *cytokines* that enhance inflammation.

into tissue, erythrocytes become increasingly concentrated. Sluggish movement of hemoconcentrated blood through tissues in an active state of metabolism results in an enhanced depletion of oxygen and glucose. Erythrocytes and leukocytes begin to show altered surface properties and to interact with endothelial surfaces.

Endothelial swelling retards blood flow.

Direct injury to endothelium causes acute cell swelling, and injured endothelial cells protrude into the vessel lumen. They markedly retard blood flow in larger capillaries and cause stasis in small vessels. The resulting hypoxia enhances endothelial injury, which produces its effects at the cell surface by causing changes in interendothelial cell junctions and in endothelial surface coats that control endothlelial-leukocyte interactions.

Endothelial junctions open to permit fluid exudation.

Classically, the earliest signs of endothelial damage had been depicted at the intercellular junction by the German pathologist, Julius Arnold, in 1875. Carbon particles, when injected intravenously, were found to outline intercellular junctions of endothelium where inflammatory lesions had been produced. Histologic examination revealed that when capillaries and venules were dilated, granular precipitates of albumin were present in perivascular spaces, and carbon was identified in the blood vessel wall.

A simple modification of Arnold's method is used to demonstrate local fluid exudation and to assay mediators of inflammation. The dye trypan blue, when injected intravenously, binds to albumin in plasma. Albumin-dye complexes do not pass the endothelial barrier except at sites where it has been damaged. When histamine is injected subcutaneously, followed by intravenous trypan blue, albumin beings to leak, allowing the site of histamine injection to become blue. It does so in relation to the extent of the histamine-induced endothelial injury, and the reaction can be quantified. This dye test is used to characterize toxins that directly damage endothelium.

When early inflammatory lesions are examined by electron microscopy, one sees subtle changes in the capillary endothelial cells (Fig. 18.1). Endothelial junctions are distorted. The massive amounts of fluid that exude do so through gaps and cavities between endothelial cells. Plasmalemmal vesicles, which normally transport fluid from one side of the endothelium to the other, are increased at luminal and basal surfaces, but these vesicles play only a minor role in inflammatory exudation.

Perivascular mast cells release factors causing increased permeability.

Tissue mast cells, which keep intimate company with capillaries and fibroblasts, act early in inflammation by liberating granules. Mast cell granules contain potent vasoactive factors such as histamine, serotonin, leukotrienes, and heparin. *Histamine* acts directly on endothelium of terminal capillaries and postcapillary venules to cause hyperemia and to increase vascular permeability (Fig. 18.2). It causes gaps between endothelial cells, partly by inducing endothelial cell contraction. *Heparin* is also released by mast cells, and its anticoagulant effect prevents the polymerization of fibrin from the exuding fibrinogen, thereby sustaining the exudative process.

The location of mast cells in lungs, brain, and intestine explains some of the clinical signs seen in these organs. By their action on the capillary bed, mast cells play important roles in

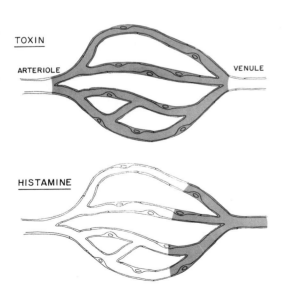

CAPILLARY PERMEABILITY – SITE OF EFFECT

TOXIN

ARTERIOLE   VENULE

HISTAMINE

Fig. 18.2. Sites of effect of histamine and toxin in capillary bed.

pulmonary edema, brain edema, and diarrhea. Species differences in mast cell numbers and location are important in variations in inflammatory reactions.

Endothelial cells peripheral to sites of injury are activated.

Activated endothelial cells surrounding the sites of injury enlarge and become sticky to circulating leukocytes. Metabolic changes within the endothelial cell cytoplasm occur that promote inflammation and coagulation. Prostanoids (prostaglandins and leukotrienes) are synthesized and have marked effects on enhancing the inflammatory process.

Endothelial cells are both a source of and target for the hormone *interleukin-1* (IL-1). This novel autocrine mechanism is responsible for much of the endothelial stickiness. IL-1 is secreted by monocytes and regulates several major events in acute inflammation, such as fever, neutrophilia, lymphocyte activation, and synthesis of acute phase proteins by hepatocytes. IL-1 causes endothelial cells, which normally have anticoagulant surfaces, to secrete procoagulant glycoproteins onto their luminal surfaces, thereby promoting coagulation.

Endothelial cells secrete other inflammation-enhancing products. Ramzi Cotran and colleagues at the Harvard Medical School have identified a protein synthesized by activated endothelial cells that is not found in normal endothelium. When skin sections of acute inflammation were stained with labeled antibodies against this protein, there was widespread staining of capillaries throughout the section.

Exudation of cells
Leukocytes attach to and penetrate endothelium.

In normally flowing blood, cells are concentrated in the central *axial zone* as opposed to the peripheral cell-free *plasmatic zone*. With slowing and stasis, leukocytes marginate, attach to the vessel wall, and begin to emigrate through it. They penetrate endothelial cell junctions, and pass through the endothelial cell basement membrane into the interstitium.

Migration of neutrophils is driven by chemoattractants produced in inflammatory tissue, many of which are complement fragments. Endothelial cell surfaces also play an active role in neutrophil migration by secreting proteins that function in adhesion. Monocytes also penetrate endothelial junctions but are not driven by the strong chemotactic forces that are so effective for neutrophils.

INFLAMMATORY EXUDATES

Serous Exudates

The initial exudate in the early phases of most inflammatory lesions is largely serous; that is, leakage has been confined to fluid and albumin. The large amount of albumin in the tissue appears histologically as homogenous eosinophilic granular material. In serous exudates, cells in tissue are spread apart by edema fluid, serving to dilute the irritant and to ease the migration of inflammatory cells that is soon to follow. Some of the most striking examples of serous inflammation occur in the respiratory tract, such as the severe, acute, serous rhinitis of upper respiratory viral infections (Fig. 18.3). These lesions rapidly form more complicated exudates but in early stages the "runny nose" syndrome results from serous exudation.

Blisters begin as serous exudates.

Blisters are caused in skin when excessive friction, burns, or chemical toxins damage sub-

epithelial capillaries. Epithelium reacts with a general loosening of cell attachments, due to intercellular fluid accumulation. Keratinocytes pull apart, remaining attached only at desmosomes (intercellular bridges). As fluid exudes into the epithelium, cell bridges break and serous, intraepidermal microvesicles form. These enlarge and coalesce, forming grossly visible blisters. As fibrinogen exudes into the serous exudate, it polymerizes to form fibrin and the lesion is called *serofibrinous*. Later, neutrophils will enter the vesicle to form pus, and the lesion is called *fibrinopurulent*. In the end, the blister breaks and fluid is absorbed, leaving fibrin and pus behind to form a scab.

Plasma proteins leak through endothelium at different rates.

Differing molecular weights of plasma proteins (albumin 69,000, globulin 150,000, and fibrinogen 340,000) are responsible for the type of exudation and thus reflect the degree of endothelial injury. Albumin, the smallest and fastest migrating protein on electrophoresis, is the first plasma protein to leak through the vessel wall. The globulin fractions of serum (α, β, and γ), which also leak early, contain a wide variety of specifically active substances that are highly important in defense, such as *antibodies* (also called *immunoglobulins*).

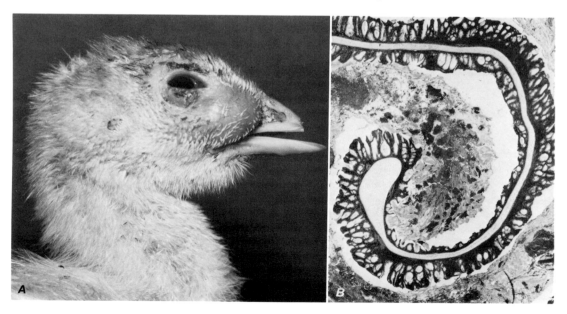

Fig. 18.3. Severe, diffuse, acute serocatarrhal sinusitis, mycoplasmosis. A. Turkey with markedly swollen sinuses. B. Histology of nasal turbinate surrounded by exudate.

Bacteria replicate in serous exudates.

When host defenses are compromized, pathogenic bacteria replicate in foci of serous fluid. If antibodies and "immune" lymphocytes are missing in these tissues, bacteria win the race for immunity or disease. These conflicts are especially important in the respiratory tract. Early inflammatory lesions contain exuding globulins, but if none of these have antibody activity, the host lacks the means for an immediate response.

Progressive tissue swelling leads to pain.

When severe injury allows free passage of plasma proteins, the equilibrium between hydrostatic pressure of the blood and osmotic pressure of the tissue fluid is altered. Extravascular protein abolishes the osmotic suck of the plasma proteins, and more fluid exudes. Increased hydrostatic pressure in dilated arterioles augments fluid loss. The tissue swells, giving rise to pain (two of the five cardinal signs of inflammation). Another source of pain is the action of some vasoactive substance on sensitized nerve endings.

Fibrinous Exudates

Severe injury to endothelium and basement membranes allows leakage of fibrinogen, which polymerizes perivascularly as fibrin (see blood coagulation, Chapter 16). Grossly, fibrinous exudates appear as pale tan, stringy, shaggy meshworks on tissue surfaces. Fibrin is bright pink in most histologic sections and can be identified presumptively with a phosphotungstic acid stain.

Fibrin prevents the spread of inflammation.

Meshes of fibrin around blood vessels impede the escape of plasma proteins. Fibrin also creates a network in tissue spaces that prevents spread of irritants, particularly bacteria (although some bacteria secrete factors that dissolve fibrin). Clotting in lymph vessels suppresses migration of bacteria-laden leukocytes. This effectively slows and often prevents the further spread via lymphatics of infectious agents and toxins (Fig. 18.4). The deposition of fibrin also provides the fabric around which healing occurs.

Fibrinous exudates may destroy tissue.

Fibrinous exudation may be so severe that it is a serious matter for the host. In some infections, a disastrous process occurs wherein the

clinician is obliged to treat not only the injury but the inflammatory process (Fig. 18.4). Pressure from tissue fluids, destructive enzymes from dead cells, and hypoxia enhance the primary injury. Degradation of basement membranes and endothelium may allow vascular injury far greater and longer-acting than the transient histamine-induced changes over which it is superimposed.

Mucous (catarrhal) exudates

Mucous hyperplasia of epithelial surfaces with liberation of large amounts of glycosaminoglycans and glycoproteins accompanies inflammation of respiratory and intestinal epithelium. The massive accumulation of goblet cells is released, and mucus floods damaged epithelial surfaces. It protects them and provides the tenacious material that, when expectorated, removes much of the debris and irritant. Catarrhal exudates contain not only the mucopolysaccharides of mucus but also many soluble defense factors secreted by leukocytes (antibodies) and epithelial cells (lysozyme).

Mucus stimulates cilia.

Mucus accumulates in inflammation on mucosal surfaces. In the upper respiratory tract, mucus is a stimulus to cilia. Increased ciliary movement propels bacteria, debris, and other materials forward. The irritant effect to sensory nerves induces the cough reflex, which is highly important in diluting and removing irritants and bacteria from the upper airways.

Mucous exudates are antibacterial.

Mucus contains many soluble antimicrobial substances. *Lysozyme,* formed by leukoctyes and epithelial cells, is secreted onto mucosal surfaces. It occurs in fluids of the respiratory and intestinal tracts and is markedly elevated in inflammation. Lysozyme functions as a mucolytic enzyme (at pH 3–6) on bacterial cell walls and is particularly effective on gram-positive bacteria. Gram-negative bacteria are not lysed because their cell walls contain lipids as well as mucopeptides.

Antibodies inhibit colonization of microorganisms, neutralize toxins, lyse viruses, and generally prevent penetration of antigenic proteins through mucosal surfaces. Secretory antibody (S-IgA) is the principal mediator of specific immunity (see immunity, Chapter 22).

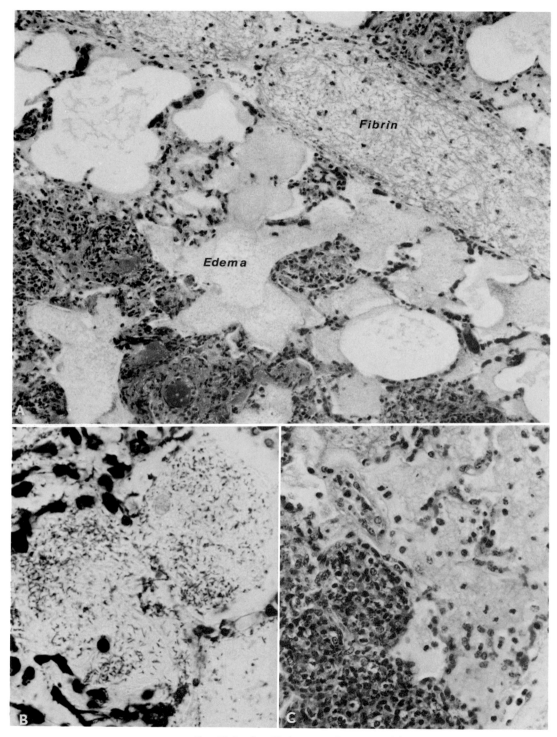

Fig. 18.4. Serofibrinous exudate, cow with pasteurellosis. A. Edema, fibrin, and vasculitis and monoctye infiltrates in alveoli and large amounts of fibrin strands in interlobular areas. B. Bacteria (*Pasteurella multocida*) in alveoli. There were 7 billion live organisms per gram of lung tissue. C. Fibrin in alveoli, recent lesion (*upper right*). Macrophages and monocytes displacing alveoli, earlier lesion (*lower left*).

Some bacteria produce IgA-destroying proteases.

On mucosal surfaces, IgA is exposed to various proteolytic enzymes of both host and microbial origin. Some species of bacteria have enhanced virulence because they produce an *IgA protease* that is capable of degrading S-IgA. Streptococci and *Haemophilis* spp. produce proteases that are active on serum IgA in vitro, but little is known about activity in vivo.

Purulent exudates

As neutrophilic leukocytes enter an inflammatory site, the transparent serous exudate becomes thickened, opaque, and cream-colored. Grossly, these lesions are called *purulent* (or *suppurative*). Microscopically, the exudate can properly be described as *neutrophilic*. In the case of severe, acute, neutrophilic meningoencephalitis caused by *Escherichia coli* (Fig. 18.5), enormous numbers of degranulate neutrophils accumulate in and distort tissue spaces.

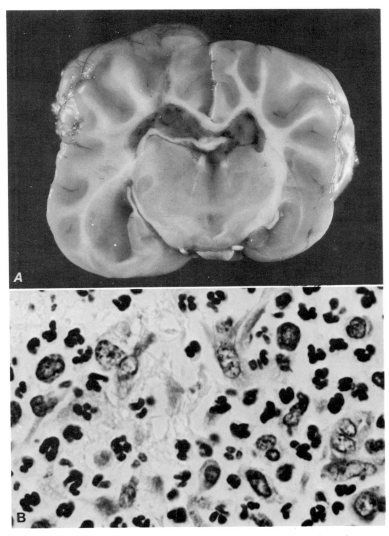

Fig. 18.5 Acute purulent encephalitis, *E. coli* and *Corynebacterium* spp. isolated from pus in meninges, young dog. A. Asymmetry of brain due to brain swelling. Surface of purulent tract extending deep into neuropil is seen in center left cortex; expansion of ventricles and purulent material in choroid plexus. B. Exudate of neutrophils and macrophages free in ventricle lumen.

Bacteria cause most purulent exudates.

In infected tissue spaces, bacterial products cause neutrophils to degranulate. Microscopically, neutrophils in pus lack the granules present in normal circulating neutrophils. They are usually dead and have all the characters of a necrotic cell. These cells should be examined closely because they often contain bacteria that can be classified by special stains and identified if the appropriate immunologic reagents are available.

With time, monocytes (which transform into macrophages) accumulate in inflammatory foci. Some bacteria survive within the macrophage after being engulfed; for example, bacteria that cause tuberculosis, listeriosis, and brucellosis are known for their capacity to grow within macrophages.

Abscesses develop in necrotic tissue.

An *abscess* is a local collection of pus formed by disintegration of tissue. Abscesses begin as microabscesses that coalesce to form large cavities (see Fig. 20.9). Abscesses rapidly become surrounded by a connective tissue barrier that represents a mechanism for sequestering bacteria and other microbes.

Scabs protect wounded surfaces.

Purulent lesions resolve as pus is removed by macrophages and fluids are drained away in lymphatics. Inspissated exudates remain over the surface to protect exposed subepithelial tissues. This is especially important in skin, which is exposed to bacteria and fungi (Fig. 18.6).

Bacteria in the bloodstream.

The number and quality of white blood cells obtained from circulating blood provides reliable and often striking evidence of disease, particularly on the nature and progress of infectious diseases. The most significant change occurs in populations of neutrophilic leukocytes (hereafter referred to as neutrophils). Analogous cells in lower vertebrates are termed heterophils, and in insects, amebocytes.

The precise function of these aggressively phagocytic cells varies, but in all species they exert potent phagocytic and bactericidal effects. Neutrophils also remove small amounts of tissue debris and fibrin polymers from the vascular system to maintain normal homeostasis. In systemic febrile diseases these functions are markedly increased.

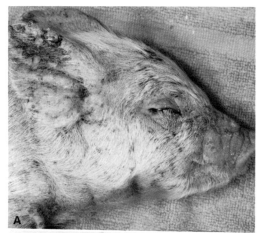
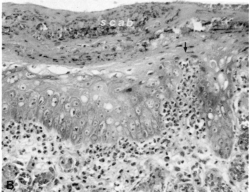

Fig. 18.6. A. Severe multifocal subacute purulent dermatitis caused by *Streptococcus epidermidis*, pig. B. Neutrophilic leukocytes have extended through the epidermis (*arrow*) into the surface scab. Note the vacuolation of keratinocytes.

Pathologic changes in neutrophils may be evaluated as to (1) number per cubic millimeter of blood; (2) structure, which involves the evaluation of the number and size of cytoplasmic granules by microscopy; and (3) chemotactic index, which is the capacity to attract, phagocytize, and digest determined quantities of bacteria and is a measure of granulocyte function. Other less utilized tests include those for degranulation and for the detection of specific enzymes and biochemical intermediates.

Leukocytosis: Increase in number of circulating leukocytes

Striking increases in white blood cells develop in inflammation and necrosis. The degree of leukocytosis is related not only to the inciting agent but to the capacity of the sites of production and storage of neutrophils in the spleen and bone marrow. By examining stained blood smears, the specific nature of the reaction can be determined (e.g., neutrophilic leukocytosis and monocytosis). Mild leukocytosis occurs during digestion and pregnancy, and this must be considered in evaluating inflammatory responses.

Leukopenia: Decrease in number of circulating leukocytes

Leukopenia is commonly seen in systemic viral diseases in which viruses replicate in and destroy leukocytes and organs that produce them. It also occurs as a result of the destruction of leukocytes in the terminal stages of overwhelming bacterial infections, during the sequestration of neutrophils in the pulmonary capillary bed in septic shock and anaphylaxis, and in any disease involving the depression of granulocytopoiesis. Mature leukocytes, like erythrocytes, originate from a pool of self-perpetuating bone marrow stem cells. Any factor that supresses the bone marrow tends to cause anemia and leukopenia.

CHRONIC INFLAMMATION

As the exudation of acute inflammation subsides in damaged tissue, processes concerned with repair begin. These involve (1) alterations in ground substances, (2) phagocytosis of necrotic cells and debris by invading monocytes and macrophages, (3) invasion by and reorganization of capillaries to facilitate blood-tissue interchange, and (4) fibroblast invasion with deposition of collagen, which provides a scaffold for future parenchymal regeneration. As the the inflammatory lesion begins to be dominated by these processes, it is termed *chronic*.

Ground substance

Wound fluids are mixtures of plasma proteins and ground substance. They provide the milieu in which tissue reconstruction takes place. Ground substance is the amorphous, mucoid, gel-like material that separates cells and fibers. It is composed of glycosaminoglycans (mucopolysaccharides) bound to protein. The long chain polymers that impart the gel consistency

to ground substance are broken by depolymerization in inflammation, and the gel becomes fluid. Some bacterial enzymes, such as clostridial hyaluronidase, hasten this process.

As acute inflammation progresses in mesenchymal tissue, there is rapid formation of hyaluronic acid. Ground substance becomes rich in glycosaminoglycans, and regeneration of connective tissue is initiated. Fibroblasts are the source of glycosaminoglycans and mast cells contribute some forms. Hyaluronic acids and hexosamine begin to disappear as fibroblasts produce collagen (Fig. 18.7).

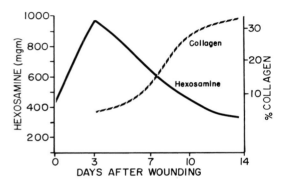

Fig. 18.7.   Rise and fall of mucopolysaccharides in experimental healing wound. (Data from Dunphy et al., *New Engl. J. Med.* 253:847, 1955)

Fibroblasts and collagen deposition

Fibroplasia begins early after injury. Existing fibrocytes are the source of fibroblasts in healing wounds, although the pluripotentiality of vascular endothelium and pericytes indicates that these cells may provide collagen-synthesizing cells.

In uninfected, uncomplicated skin wounds, fibroblasts multiply and collagen is laid down until the wound is completely bridged at about 5–7 days. In the subsequent 2–3 weeks, scar tissue is organized and the progressive process of *wound contraction* develops. By 4 weeks, when collagenization is largely completed, short, dense, elastic fibers begin to appear (Fig. 18.8). They consist of globules of elastin complexes with a hydrated glycosaminoglycan. The fibrillar-globular elastic fibers weave among the collagen fibrils, giving the newly formed connective tissue stretchability and elasticity. Large

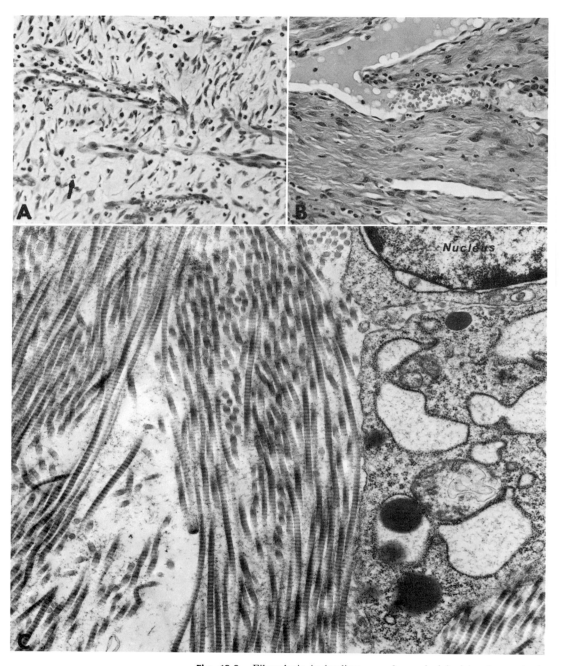

Fig. 18.8. Fibroplasia in healing wound, surgical incision in a cat. A. Endothelial cell invasion with extension of fibroblasts parallel to endothelial cell buds (1 week after incision). There are collagen deposits with few neutrophils (*arrow*). B. Advanced fibroplasia, connective tissue scar in healed wound (4 weeks after incision). C. Electron micrograph of collagen-producing fibroblast. Large groups of collagen *fibrils* (*center*) make up collagen *fiber*. The fibroblast (*right*) contains ribosomes and endoplasmic reticulum, with inspissated material within cisternae.

amounts of basement membrane material and reticulin are deposited in wounds and can be demonstrated by special stains.

Myofibroblasts cause wound contraction.

The process of contraction depends on specialized fibroblasts. After about 1 week of wound growth, peculiar modifications of fibroblast structure develop. These new cells, called *myofibroblasts,* have increased cytoplasmic microfilaments and surface attachment sites.

Systemic and local factors can inhibit healing.

Aging, protein deficiency, vitamin C deficiency, and several endocrine deficiencies are associated with inhibition of wound healing. Ascorbic acid deficiency markedly retards fibroplasia because this vitamin is required as a cofactor for proline hydroxylase.

Fibroplasia, extremely active in neonates, is delayed in aged animals, perpetuating the chronicity of the healing process. In aged animals, elastic fiber degeneration can be identified as splitting and granulation of the fibers (senile elastosis). The deposition of collagen and of matrix material is also restricted in cartilage and bone of aged animals, which seriously affects wound healing in these tissues.

Fibroplasia in wounds is inhibited by tissue debris and bacterial infection. Other, less important local factors include decreased temperature, irradiation, and foreign bodies such as talcum powder granules. Clinically, fibroplasia is enhanced by elevated temperature and by debridement, the removal of necrotic tissue.

Vascular hyperplasia and ingrowth

At the surviving vascular border of injured tissue, vascular sprouts appear. Endothelial cells throw out filopodia and migrate toward the stimulus. Curiously, they do not separate but remain fused as an advancing endothelial sheet. Factors that promote migration of vascular buds are released from platelets and neutrophils. Other stimulants to vascular growth include hypoxia, products from injured tissue, blood pressure differentials, and changes in the connective tissue stroma. Whatever the cause, vascular syncytia (cords of cells) form and rapidly differentiate and canalize. These vascular syncytia fuse and gradually establish a network of patent capillaries.

Endothelial cell mitosis and proliferation are due to direct injury and are most intense in areas lacking epithelium. When wounds become covered with epithelial surfaces, endothelial mitotic activity decreases. *Heparin* released from mast cells has a significant secondary role in stimulation of capillary endothelial proliferation.

Fibrin provides a scaffold for vascularization.

Fibrin is absorbed during vascular ingrowth. It persists beyond the disappearance of neutrophils and is not entirely removed until vascular invasion is accomplished. The newly formed endothelial cells are fibrinolytic. Unlike fibroblasts, they contain an activator of plasminogen. Removal of fibrin polymers is necessary as capillary buds migrate into the wound.

Like fibroplasia, vascularization is retarded in conditions of nutritional deficiency or other severe systemic disease. In scurvy, endothelial cells are abnormal and do not enter wounds at rates comparable to those in wounds of normal animals.

Collagen directs capillary growth.

Collagen does not lie as an inert bridging material but is constantly reformed to strengthen a wound. It plays in inductive role in new capillary formation, and when collagen synthesis in a wound is inhibited, capillary ingrowth is markedly delayed. Experimentally, when collagen is added to endothelial cells growing on the surface of a gel, cells reorganize into a network of branching and anastomosing capillary tubules.

Platelets and coagulation factors contribute to healing.

Platelet-derived growth factor is a mitogenic peptide secreted by platelets trapped at sites of inflammation. It stimulates proliferation of fibroblasts and smooth muscle cells and stimulates vascularization. Factor XIII not only catalyzes cross-linking of fibrin molecules but also promotes cross-linking of fibrin to the connective tissue matrix and to fibronectin on the surfaces of mesenchymal cells in the healing wound.

Macrophages

Macrophages are large, pale cells designed for phagocytosis and intracellular digestion. They constitute a second line of defense. They are not rapidly attracted by chemotactic substances that attract neutrophils and are less discriminating in the material they phagocytize. Whereas neutrophils degranulate and spew proteases and oxygen radicals into inflamed tissue, macrophages function more slowly to engulf particulate material. Uptake is slower and degradation is less complete. Digested debris accumulates in large membrane-bounded lysosomes called residual bodies, which may, by exocytosis, be shunted outside the cell.

In normal tissue, macrophages are continually involved in degradation of aged erythrocytes, cholesterol, fibrin polymers, pulmonary alveolar secretion, and other proteins. In necrobiosis, they clear and process dead cells and debris. In the atrophy of the involuting uterus following pregnancy, macrophages take up massive amounts of collagen, which is removed for the return of the uterus to normal size.

The unequaled ability of macrophages to process foreign proteins in a slow, limited manner (without enzymatically destroying protein) completely allows them to fulfill a vital role in processing and retaining antigens for specific lymphoid immune reactions.

Macrophages are activated by particulate material.

Activated (stimulated) macrophages are distinguished from nonactive forms by increased numbers of lysosomes, phagosomes, and mitochondria. They have increased amounts of hydrolases in their lysosomes, hypermobility of cell membranes, and markedly increased synthesis of lysozyme and cytokines. Activated macrophages secrete complement, interferon, plasminogen activators, and, probably most important, the multifunctional cytokine interleukin-1 (Table 18.2).

Macrophage blockade

The functional capacity of the macrophage system, or collectively the reticuloendothelial system, can be calculated from the clearance of carbon particles injected intravenously. The *phagocytic index* (PI) can be formulated where C_0 and C_t are the concentration of carbon in the blood at 0 time and at time t.

$$PI = \frac{\log C_0 - C_t}{t}$$

Blockade of the reticuloendothelial system can be transiently induced by overloading its macrophages with substances such as carbon. Macrophages are temporarily unable to phagocytize added particulate material. Paralysis of macrophages accompanies some severe infectious diseases. Substances such as the capsular material of anthrax bacilli inhibit cell membranes of macrophages, thus rendering them incapable of phagocytosis. Surfaces of fungi such as *Cryptococcus neoformans* also produce this direct inhibitory effect on macrophages.

Experimental blockade of the reticuloendothelial system increases an animal's susceptibility to infection, shock, and intravascular coagulation. Blockade is traditionally viewed as physical saturation of macrophages with particulate material. It also involves depletion of fibronectin and serum proteins (opsonins) that interact with particles to promote phagocytosis.

Granulomatous inflammation

Granulomatous inflammation is a special subtype of chronic inflammation. The granulomatous reaction is dominated by activated monocytes and macrophages, which infiltrate the inflammatory site in immense numbers. Tubercle bacilli, fungi, aberrant parasites, and inert particles such as asbestos and silica are notorious initiators of granulomatous lesions. All contain components that macrophage lysosomes cannot degrade. Macrophages become large and foamy because they accumulate both the causal agent and debris of degenerate tissue. These foamy cells, called "epithelioid cells," are the hallmark of granulomatous inflammation (Fig. 18.9).

Granulomatous lesions develop more slowly

Table 18.2. Products secreted by macrophages

For Host Defense	Cytokines	Enzymes
Lysozyme	Interleukin-1	Lysosomal enzymes
Complement components	Tumor necrosis factor-α	Collagenase
Interferon		Elastase
Microbicidal peptides		Plasminogen activator

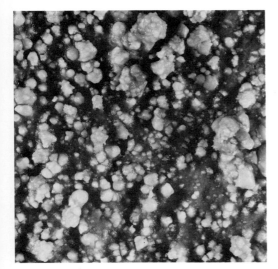

Fig. 18.9. Multifocal, granulomatous peritonitis, cow with tuberculosis.

than do purulent lesions. For example, the lesions of tuberculosis or histoplasmosis take weeks or months to cause disease whereas streptococci can cause acute inflammation lesions in 24 hours. Most microbes that cause granulomatous inflammation are not strongly chemoattractive to neutrophils. Monocytes are attracted to sites of infection and ingest but do not degrade or kill the etiologic agent. Additional blood monocytes migrate to the lesions, transform to macrophages, and rephagocytize the agent and its associated cell debris. New macrophages collect in progressively enlarging foci called *granulomas*. Although the bacterial substance may not be destroyed, the granuloma provides an effective means of localizing it and allowing other inflammatory and immunologic mechanisms to act for longer periods of time. A certain sign of chronicity, granulomas involve multiple episodes of necrosis, monocyte infiltration, and fibrosis.

Special stains such as the Gram stain for bacteria and the periodic acid–Schiff reaction for fungal capsules are used on granulomatous tissue lesions for etiologic diagnosis. Microcolonies of microorganisms are commonly present and are often surrounded by club-shaped bodies, especially in actinomycosis, actinobacillosis, and botryomycosis. These bodies are called "asteroid bodies" and the process of development the "Splendore-Hoeppli phenomenon." Electron microscopical studies of granulomatous tissue by

Drs. Gilka in Ottawa, Obihura in Japan, and Mandella in Italy have revealed granular material that probably represents products of an antigen-antibody reaction.

Immune reactions contribute to granulomas.

The induction phase of infectious granulomas is a macrophage response to insoluble material; the tissue reaction is purely inflammatory. For example, streptococcal cell wall polysaccharides induce granulomas with no immunologic basis; neither antibody nor cell-mediated immunoreactivity plays a role in evolution or resolution of the early lesions.

As infectious granulomas expand, however, they become increasingly complex. Although the dominant cell type remains the macrophage, many other cells invade. The pattern of immigrating cells is altered considerably by the agent involved and by the immunologic response it induces in the host. The lesion becomes, in a sense, an immunologically induced granuloma.

In some lesions, *plasmacytes* are common, indicating a role, even though ineffective, of these antibody-containing cells in attempting to overcome the organism involved. Antibodies may develop in the serum of the host, but these are of little significance either in recovery of the host or in resolution of the lesion.

The effect of cell-mediated immunity in producing and increasing the severity and duration of granulomatous lesions involves *small lymphocytes*. Lymphocyte mediators released in the reaction induce, in turn, the infiltration and activation of macrophages. This effect is clearly shown in an experimental model in which plastic beads linked to various proteins (called haptens) are injected intravenously into guinea pigs. In normal animals, the beads are trapped in the lung and induce only a mild inflammatory response. In guinea pigs previously immunized with the specific protein hapten, severe granulomas develop on recognition of the protein bound to the bead surface. This immunologically induced granuloma differs from its nonimmune counterpart only in intensity and lymphocyte content.

Giant cells are common cells in granulomas.

Fusion of monocytes and macrophages gives rise to huge, multinucleate cells called *giant cells*. Fusion occurs in regions of extensive

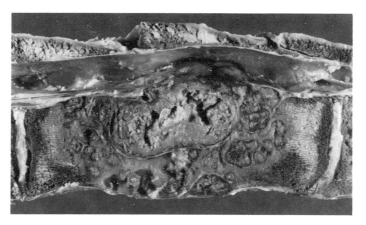
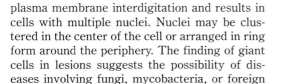
plasma membrane interdigitation and results in cells with multiple nuclei. Nuclei may be clustered in the center of the cell or arranged in ring form around the periphery. The finding of giant cells in lesions suggests the possibility of diseases involving fungi, mycobacteria, or foreign bodies and is a valuable aid in diagnosis (Fig. 18.10).

In most infectious diseases, giant cell formation occurs by *fusion of monocytes and macrophages.* The stimulus for fusion is believed to be cytokines released from lymphocytes that mi-

Tubercles begin as small aggregates of neutrophils and macrophages that sequester and ingest bacilli. If macrophages take in bacteria but do not kill them, they themselves are killed. Foci of necrotic cells become surrounded by a mantle of new macrophages. The lesion progressively expands due to the continuous entry of "immune" monocytes. These cells phagocytize dead macrophages and their viable bacteria and are, in turn, destroyed. At the periphery of the lesion, monocyte activity is most intense and large plump macrophages known as *epithelioid cells* are prominent. These cells contain markedly undulant and interwoven cell surfaces, and fusion of their plasma membranes leads to formation of the giant cells that characterize tuberculosis. The massive necrosis and cavitation in pulmonary tuberculosis in some mammals is due less to the virulence of the bacterium than to the hypersensitivity of macrophages in that particular host.

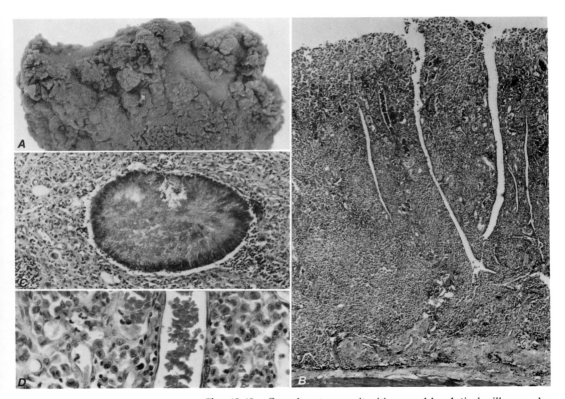

Fig. 18.10. Granulomatous peritonitis caused by *Actinobacillus* sp., dog. A. Diffuse granulomatous growth on surface of diaphragm. B. Fronds of granulation tissue project from muscle of diaphragm (*bottom*). C. "Sulfur granule," a large mass of bacteria and bacterial secretions among granulomatous tissue. D. Large macrophages in spaces between blood vessels.

grate into granulomas. That is, when stimulated by specific antigens, T lymphocytes produce a soluble protein that causes circulating monocytes to fuse and form giant cells.

Giant cells also form by *division of nuclei without cytoplasmic division*. This mechanism occurs in neoplasms and in congenital dysplasias; it rarely is involved in granulomatous inflammation. The fungal metabolite *cytochalasin* produced by some aspergilli affects cell division by altering microtubules of macrophages. It inhibits cytokinesis (cytoplasmic division) without affecting karyokinesis (nuclear division), and the giant cells found in granulomas of the lungs in aspergillosis may arise from this mechanism.

ADDITIONAL READING

Folkman, J. What is the role of endothelial cells in angiogenesis? *Lab. Invest.* 51:601, 1984.

Issekutz, A. C. Role of polymorphonuclear leukocytes in the vascular responses of acute inflammation. *Lab. Invest.* 50:605, 1984.

Kuehl, F. A., and Egan, R. W. Prostaglandins, arachidonic acid, and inflammation. *Science* 210:978, 1980.

Snyderman, R., and Goetzl, E. J. Molecular and cellular mechanisms of leukocyte chemotaxis. *Science* 213:830, 1981.

Unanue, E. R., et al. Regulation of immunity and inflammation by mediators from macrophages. *Am. J. Pathol.* 85:465, 1974.

Pathogenesis of
Acute Inflammation

CELLS OF THE
INFLAMMATORY EXUDATE

"Inflammatory cells" is a term used unrestrictively to lump together a large population of infiltrating leukoctyes in an inflammatory exudate. Pathologists use this term, especially when individual cells are difficult to identify. In this section we examine the basic biologic character of these cells—their structure, behavior, and pathologic appearance.

Neutrophils

Neutrophils are aggressively phagocytic cells that constitute a first line of defense against invading microorganisms and foreign materials. Distinctions of these cells are (1) rapid ameboid movement, particularly in contact with chemoattractants; (2) intense phagocytic activity; and (3) elaboration of granules bearing potent enzymes capable of extensive intracellular digestion. Neutrophils have the ability to degranulate and spew enzyme-laden granules into tissue at local sites of inflammation. Although highly mobile, they lack stability and cannot withstand the low pH and high temperature of severe inflammatory lesions.

Neutrophils have two major types of granules: azurophil (primary) granules and specific (secondary) granules (Fig. 19.1). *Azurophil* granules are small, primary lysosomes. In most mammals they contain lysosomal digestive hydrolases, mucosubstances, and peroxidase, most of which function at pH optima in the acid range. Azurophil granules have nearly all of the myeloperoxidase, one-third of the lysozyme, and some lactoferrin. The larger and more numerous *specific* granules contain alkaline phosphatase, cat-

ionic proteins, lactoferrin, and most of the leukocyte's lysozyme. Specific granules also contain proteolytic enzymes that act on collagen and elastin, and some lipases (which are lacking in most macrophages).

Neutrophil chemotaxis

The capacity to react to chemical attractants is an essential character of the neutrophil. Cinematographic studies of leukocytes in vitro reveal surprisingly rapid movement of neutrophils toward certain microbes. Under the influence of bacterial chemotactic factors in early inflammatory exudates, circulating neutrophils move more slowly through the capillary, peripheralize in the blood vessels, and stick to the endothelium.

Diapedesis: The process whereby
neutrophils emigrate through vascular walls

As neutrophils migrate across endothelium they enhance capillary permeability and hyperemia begun by histamine, probably via the release of prostaglandins and leukotrienes. As cells cross the endothelial barrier, there is direct movement through intact endothelium without its disruption, chiefly by way of intercellular junctions.

Neutrophils respond to many
chemoattractants.

Most chemoattractants are derivatives of normal plasma peptides. Substances that are cleaved from normal proteins in foci of injury and are (directly) strong chemoattractants for neutrophils include *complement fragments, fibrinopeptides, collagenolytic products,* and soluble *cytokines* released by antigen-stimulated lym-

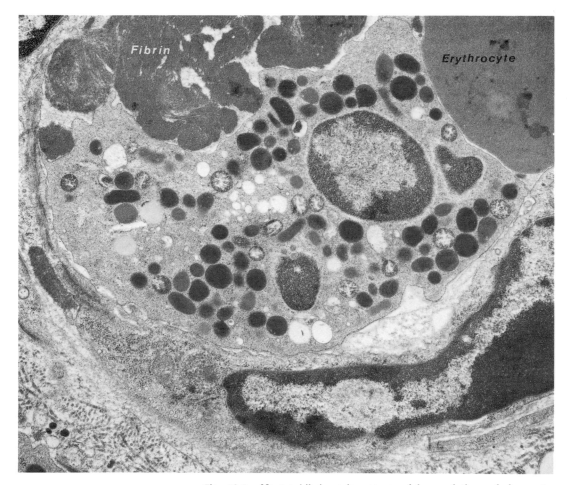

Fig. 19.1. Neutrophils in various stages of degranulation and phagocytosis of virions and fibrin, infectious bovine rhinotracheitis (see Fig. 4.1). Vacuoles, clefts, and lipid are seen in the neutrophils.

phocytes. *Platelet factor 4,* a potent heparin-binding protein released from α-granules when platelets adhere at sites of vascular injury, is also a strong neutrophil chemoattractant.

Pathogenic bacteria are chemotactic for neutrophils.

Most pathogenic bacteria will slowly attract neutrophils directly by releasing soluble products in infected tissue. Among the most potent of bacterial *chemotactic factors* are certain hydrophobic peptides released by bacteria. The peculiar feature that imparts chemotactic characteristics resides in the *N*-terminal amino groups of these peptides. Experimentally, the tetrapeptide *N*-formyl-methionyl-leucyl-phenyl-alanine (called *F-Met-Leu-Phe*) is synthesized and used to induce chemotaxis in vitro.

Complement fragments are strongly chemotactic.

Reactions that initiate the C cascade with the attendant liberation of *complement chemotactic fragments* C3 and C5 will attract neutrophils. Enzymes that act in this way (via complement fragments) include bacterial proteases, plasmin, trypsin, thrombin, and other tissue proteases. The complement system is especially potent for microbes. During infections, chemotaxis is markedly accelerated when complement adsorbs to microbial surfaces, a reaction most efficiently activated via the classic pathway by antibody. The complement system is so effective because it liberates chemotactic fragments directly into tissue fluids and because the mature neutrophil has specific surface receptors for the C4b-C3b complex (immune adherence receptors) that cause the migrating neutrophil to attach to the complement-coated microbe.

Opsonins: Substances that adsorb to bacterial surfaces.

In infection the processes of opsonization, release of complement chemotactic fragments, and phagocytosis are interrelated. When a bacterium is deposited in tissue, it becomes coated with various proteins that circulate and perco-late through tissue. Immunoglobulins (antibodies) and complement fragments are the most potent opsonins. They bind to specific receptors on neutrophil surfaces to initiate movement in the subsurface cytoskeleton of the cell and thus cause phagocytosis and degranulation.

Neutrophil enzymes also cause tissue damage.

Unfortunately, some enzymes in tissue (including elastase, collagenase, and cathepsin G) can actually retard neutrophil chemotaxis by splitting the chemotactic fragments C3 and C5 to render them inactive. These enzymes thus contribute to lowered opsonic activity and to pro-

---

FOCUS

Antibodies recognize surface proteins on bacteria.

Antibodies are Y-shaped globulin molecules synthesized to combine specifically with protein antigens that induce their production (see immunity, Chapter 22). Produced by protein synthesis in plasmacytes, antibody molecules circulate in blood and exude into foci of inflammation. They neutralize viruses, inactivate toxins, enhance (as opsonins) the phagocytosis of bacteria, and lyse bacterial cells. Antibody functions to recognize specific invading organisms and to attract complement, which actually does the work of lysis. In other words, the antibody molecule acts as a bridge between the invading microorganism and the complement proteins that cause lysis. Antibody binds tightly to proteins on the microbe surface and attracts complement, which in turn has a wide range of activities, one of which is to attract neutrophils.

Antibodies exude onto mucosal surfaces. During inflammation of the respiratory and intestinal tracts, the protein content of lung or gut fluids increases markedly. This is a nonspecific effect caused by increased vascular permeability, and in primary infections, the exuding proteins are albumin and globulins. If the animal has not previously experienced the disease, specific antibody activity is not seen in the initial outpouring of globulin. Later, specific antibody activity does develop and can be measured in the secretions (see Fig. 19.5).

In the 1890s it was shown that serum from guinea pigs immunized with *Vibrio cholera* lysed these bacteria specifically. Bordet demonstrated that lysis was due to two components in serum: one (proven later to be antibody) was heat-stable and present only in immune serum; the other was heat labile (destroyed by $1/2$ hour at 56°C) and present in both normal and immune serum. The term *complement* was adopted for the latter because it joins with specific antibody to produce lysis of bacteria.

longed inflammation. Streptococci and some other bacteria contain proteins on their surfaces that bind fibrinogen, and the protein-fibrinogen complex impedes access of complement components to the bacterium and thus suppresses chemotaxis and neutrophil attachment.

Neutrophil phagocytosis

As a prelude to phagocytosis, striking surface projections develop on the surface of the neutrophil and rapidly surround the target particle. Scanning electron micrographs show that these projections invaginate to form large "phagocytic cups" around particles at the cell surface. In *immune phagocytosis,* induced by antigen-antibody-complement coating of particles, there is an increased affinity of the cell surface for the target. Long tentacles form at a polar position in the neutrophil and provide increased surface area for the phagocytic process.

As the phagocytic vacuole forms, oxidases (previously on the cell surface) are "internalized" as the surface membrane folds in on itself. The enzymes immediately begin to catalyze the formation of superoxide anions and hydrogen peroxide. Lysosomes rapidly begin to fuse with phagosomes to form the complex vesicles called phagolysosomes. Phagolysosomes are large dense structures, and their content of dense debris and splintered bacteria reflect the high degree of degradation brought about by their potent hydrolytic enzymes.

Intracellular killing and digestion in neutrophils

Contact of neutrophils with stimuli that initiate phagocytosis results in activation of an oxygen-consuming metabolic pathway, which is dormant in the unstimulated cell. The manifestations of this pathway include increased oxygen uptake, glucose consumption by way of the hexose-monophosphate shunt, and production of oxygen-related toxic agents: superoxide anion O_2^-, hydroxyl radical $OH\cdot$, and singlet oxygen O_2. This group of events taken together are called the *respiratory burst,* and all occur as neutrophils are activated.

The respiratory burst

The respiratory burst is a consequence of activation of the enzyme NADPH oxidase that catalyzes the reduction of oxygen to superoxide anion:

$$2\ O_2 + NADH \rightarrow 2\ O_2^- + NADP^+ + H^+$$

NADPH oxidase is located within the lipid bilayers of membranes with part exposed to the cytoplasm, which utilizes NADPH (produced by the hexose-monophosphate shunt) as a substrate. Hydrogen peroxide released during the burst originates from the dismutation of the superoxide produced by the enzyme superoxide dismutase (SOD):

$$2\ O_2^- + 2\ H^+ -(SOD) \rightarrow 2\ O_2 + H_2O_2$$

Subsequent reaction between O_2 and H_2O_2 produces the bactericidal hydroxyl radical:

$$O_2^- + H_2O_2 \rightarrow OH\cdot + OH^- + O_2$$

Increase in the hexose-monophosphate shunt activity reflects an increase in NADPH turnover due to the nucleotide requirement for the O_2-forming reaction and, in part, to the activity of the glutathione peroxidase–glutathione reductase cycle, a metabolic pathway that functions to detoxify H_2O_2 diffusing back into the cytoplasm (Fig. 19.2).

The respiratory burst is a self-limiting phenomenon. It declines within 1 hour because of loss of activity of the O_2-forming enzyme. This limitation does not adversely affect bactericidal activity because bacterial killing requires only agents produced during the burst. Furthermore, damage inflicted by these toxic agents on tissues would be limited by termination of the burst after a short period.

Neutrophils kill phagocytized microorganisms by one or a combination of toxic systems, both oxygen-dependent and oxygen-independent. Among the former, myeloperoxidase-H_2O_2 is the most potent; but hydrogen peroxidase (by itself), superoxide, hydroxyl radicals, and singlet oxygen are also antibacterial. The oxygen-independent agents include lysozyme, lactoferrin, phospholipases, and the granule-associated cationic proteins. Chymotrypsinlike cationic proteins of the primary granules are most effective on gram-positive bacteria.

Superoxide dismutase degrades superoxide anion.

Superoxide anion (O_2^-), a free radical form of oxygen, is generated in the early autoxidative processes in the phagosome. Superoxide dismutase protects the cells from O_2^- toxicity but may

Fig. 19.2. Production of toxic oxygen radicals and their metabolism.

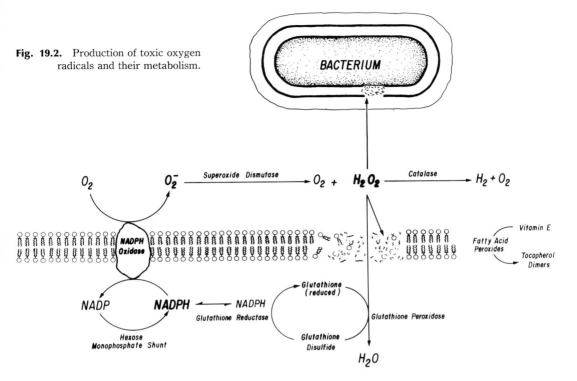

also inhibit bactericidal activity. Superoxide anion and H_2O_2 accumulate in the phagosome where they interact with bacteria and also generate other oxidants such as OH• and O_2. Within the vacuole they are not interfered with by superoxide dismutase or catalase, yet these enzymes protect the remainder of the cell from destruction.

Hydrogen peroxide is microbicidal.

Hydrogen peroxide kills most organisms in the absence of a catalyst but only in high concentrations. It is most effective in association with neutrophil peroxidase. Hydrogen peroxide formed by some microorganisms may contribute significantly to antimicrobial activity. For example, streptococci produce H_2O_2 (they lack catalase). Conversely, microbial *catalase* inhibits H_2O_2 function and may protect some bacteria. Catalase-rich strains of staphylococci are more virulent than are low-catalase strains.

Myeloperoxidase enhances hydrogen peroxide killing.

Myeloperoxidase (MPO), the name applied to the peroxidase of neutrophils, is in azurophile granules (it is responsible for the green color of pus). Like other peroxidases, MPO catalyzes the oxidation of substances by H_2O_2. MPO, H_2O_2, and an oxidizable cofactor such as halide combine to form a highly potent antimicrobial system. This MPO-mediated mechanism is effective against microbes at pH 4.5–5.0 and is inhibited by catalase.

MPO reacts with H_2O_2 to form an enzyme-substrate complex with strong oxidative capacity. The cofactor is converted from a weak to a strong antimicrobial agent. When iodide is the cofactor, iodination of bacteria occurs by direct halogenation of bacterial proteins and other groups in or on the bacterium.

Degranulation of neutrophils

During phagocytosis, neutrophils regurgitate lysosomal enzymes into the environment (they are released in massive amounts after cell death). Release of granules is particularly important when the neutrophil is in contact with very large particles, especially when these particles are coated with antibody. Neutrophil surface receptors specific for the Fc part of the immunoglobulin molecule can act as effector cells in killing antibody-coated microorganisms. In addition to killing bacteria by this mechanism, they also rapidly kill virus-infected cells that have become coated with antiviral antibodies; antibody-dependent cytotoxicity tests in cell cultures are indicators of neutrophil function.

Microorganisms and injured cells that become coated with antibodies and then activate the complement system are rapidly attacked by neutrophils. C5a is the major chemotactic component. C3b, the major opsonic component, combines with specific receptors embedded in the neutrophil surface to initiate movement required for both phagocytosis and granule release. When complement activation is limited and the target is very large, lysosomal enzymes and granules are released without altering neutrophil viability.

Neutrophil azurophil and specific granules are released at differing times during the degranulation process. Specific granules are immediately reactive after stimulus, while the lysosomal azurophil granules discharge more slowly. The rapid drop in pH that occurs in bacteria-containing phagosomes is reponsible for the sequential discharge of granules. The initial alkaline environment favors specific granule activity, while the later acid pH allows lysosomal enzymes to be more effective.

Tissue injury

Unfortunately, the microbe-killing activities of neutrophils are also directed against normal cells in inflammatory foci. *Oxygen radicals cause direct injury by forming hydrogen peroxide* (H_2O_2) and other oxygen metabolites such as OH•. For example, H_2O_2 and OH• are responsible for much of the neutrophil-induced endothelial injury in lungs.

Oxygen radicals can also induce tissue injury by generating additional chemotactic factors, by depolymerizing glycosaminoglycans in interstitium (especially hyaluronate), and by inactivating leukocyte protease inhibitors. Serum enzymes such as α_1-antiprotease normally suppress damage by neutrophil granule elastase and are inhibited by oxidation reaction of inflammation.

Neutrophil lysosomes also damage normal tissue. In tissue undergoing acute inflammation, neutrophils generate kinins, cleave complement, initiate clot formation, and synthesize and release peptides that cause fever. They activate mast cells and platelets to liberate histamine and directly attack endothelial cells and basement membranes to sustain increased capillary permeability.

Destruction of tissue is also initiated by at least two groups of substances in neutrophil lysosomes: *proteolytic enzymes* that degrade collagen, basement membranes, and elastin and *basic proteins* that increase capillary permeability. Four basic proteins that affect permeability have been obtained by purification of neutrophil granules followed by gel electrophoresis. One of these also induces mast cell degranulation and histamine release and is inhibited by antihistamine in vivo.

In chronic inflammation, the long-term effect of release of neutrophil enzymes may be irreversible tissue destruction. Prolonged elastase release from degenerating neutrophils will gradually destroy elastic fibers in the alveolar wall in chronic lung inflammation, a mechanism that underlies emphysema in man. The circulating enzyme α_1-antitrypsin suppresses the effects of neutrophil elastase; humans deficient in this enzyme are especially prone to emphysema.

Corticosteroids suppress tissue injury.

Therapy is occasionally needed to control the deleterious effects of inflamation. Corticosteroids stabilize lysosomal membranes and are potent inhibitors of neutrophil granule movement and intracellular digestion. They also inhibit chemotaxis.

Corticosteroids cause leukocytosis, possibly by suppressing production of glycocalyx material for the cell surface. By reducing the stickiness of the neutrophil, they prevent its ability to adhere to endothelium and to migrate into tissue.

Toxic neutrophils

In severe bacterial infections, neutrophilic leukocytosis is the usual hematologic finding. The increase in leukocytes is due both to *premature expulsion of neutrophils* from sites of formation and to *enhanced leukopoiesis*. Because demand often exceeds supply, these new cells are usually immature. The appearance of increasing numbers of immature neutrophils in the circulation is called a "shift to the left" (based on the Schilling index of neutrophil maturity) and indicates a relatively severe disease process. Very large neutrophils (over 22 μm in diameter) sometimes found in blood smears (especially in the cat and horse) are the result of inhibition of mitotic activity in precursor cells.

Toxic neutrophils appear in circulating blood during severe infection. These cells have cytoplasmic vacuoles and "toxic granules" (dense, azurophil granules). The chemotactic activity of toxic neutrophils is markedly reduced, and their bactericidal effect is less than that of normal neutrophils. Severely burned animals have toxic neutrophils with markedly diminished chemotactic responsiveness a few days after burning, and this promotes septicemia, a common consequence of severe burns. *Dohle bodies,* which are light blue amorphous regions in the cytoplasm, may also be present in toxic neutrophils.

Eosinophilic leukocytes

Eosinophils are large, ameboid, sluggishly phagocytic cells. Their unique granules hold the key to the specialized functions. Like neutrophil lysosomes, they function in phagocytosis to degrade substances. *Eosinophil basic protein* is especially toxic to parasite larvae (it can also cause host tissue damage). When released from eosinophils migrating into epithelium of the respiratory tract, eosinophil basic protein causes ciliostasis and degeneration of bronchial epithelium and may play a role in allergic respiratory disease.

Eosinophils respond to chemotactic factors.

Eosinophils respond to antigen-antibody complexes much like neutrophils. They are less responsive to most other chemotactic factors, however, including complement components. Eosinophilic chemotaxis occurs in various inflammatory lesions but is especially noted in parasitic infections of the intestine and in the nasopharynx during some allergic diseases.

The role of immune complexes in eosinophil chemotaxis is critical. They activate the complement system to produce factors that attract eosinophils. Chemotactic factors specific for eosinophils include histamine (mast cells are often associated with eosinophil exudates). Mast cell tumors usually have many eosinophils.

Blood eosinophilia

Elevation of eosinophils in circulating blood is common in parasitic infections. Eosinophilia has not been correlated with specific parasite components or with antibody levels. It has, however, been proposed as an immune phenomenon; that is, the ability of rats to respond to trichina infection with eosinophilia was associated with interaction of parasite and lymphocytes. Soluble factors that stimulate eosinophilopoiesis arise from the lymphocyte secretions.

Tissue eosinophilia

Most metazoan parasites produce marked tissue eosinophilia, especially in invasive and migratory phases of infection. Eosinophilic activity is generated both by release of chemoattractants by the parasite and by chemotactic activity of the host's inflammatory response.

Eosinophils kill parasites by several mechanisms.

Eosinophils kill by degranulating onto surfaces of parasites. This is done by depositing *eosinophilic basic protein* (contained in eosinophil granules) onto the parasite cuticle. Eosinophilic basic protein has a killing effect in the parasite.

In animals that have developed specific immunity, other mechanisms are superimposed on the activity of eosinophilic basic protein. Parasites become coated with antibody and complement, and this attracts eosinophils. In schistosomiasis, larvae that enter immune animals are damaged as they penetrate the skin because aggregates of eosinophils firmly adhere to the antibody-coated parasite. Eosinophils contain specific receptors of complement and immunoglobulins on their surfaces. After they attach to the antibody-complement complexes on the parasite surface, they secrete *peroxidases.* Focal lesions are produced in the parasitic tegument, causing it to separate from the body of the worm.

Damage also results from activation of the alternate complement pathway (eosinophils adhere to complement-coated parasites through their C3 receptors), but this is not an important mechanism for killing parasites. Recently, soluble factors (called "eosinophil cytotoxicity enhancing factor") that are released by monocytes and lymphocytes aid in some unknown way in killing parasites.

When large numbers of parasites are killed by chemotherapy, enormous amounts of eosinophilic basic protein that coat the dying parasite are released into the tissue lymph and bloodstream and may result in clinical signs. Syndromes of erythema, edema, and urticaria have been reported in animals treated with parasiticides (e.g., diethylcarbamazine). Called the "Mazzotti reaction," it occurs most strikingly in human onchocerciasis.

Eosinopenia leads to severe parasitism.

Inability to respond with eosinophilias leads to increased tissue localization of parasites. When animals cannot produce eosinophils experimentally, there is no effect on expulsion of *Trichinella spiralis* from the intestines, but the number of larvae invading muscles is almost doubled.

Basophilic leukocytes

Basophils are present in blood in such small numbers that increases, when noticed, are seldom meaningful. Under specific chemotactic influences, basophils migrate into tissue spaces. They localize in perivascular sites where their degranulation has a maximal effect on vascular permeability (Fig. 19.3). Although tissue *mast cells* play a greater role in acute inflammation, *basophils* migrating into tissue are more important in chronic inflammation.

Basophils are often a component of chronic lesions arising from immune reactions. They are attracted by lymphocyte cytokines. Basophils have surface receptors for complement fragment C3, which enhances phagocytosis and the ability of basophils (and mast cells) to adhere to parasites that have become coated with complement.

Basophils are involved in immediate and delayed hypersensitivity (see Chapter 23). Special cell-fixing antibodies attach to the basophil cell membrane and react on subsequent contact with antigen by inducing cell lysis and liberation of granules.

Monocytes enter inflammatory lesions simultaneously with neutrophils.

Substances chemotactic for neutrophils have no specific effect on monocytes so that these cells do not appear in large numbers in early stages of acute inflammation. Furthermore, monocytes are not as aggressively ameboid as neutrophils, their numbers in circulating blood are much lower, and their reproduction and release are stimulated at a much slower rate (Fig.

19.4). Once in tissue, monocytes avidly attach to microorganisms and either phagocytize them or, in the case of larger fungi, release soluble substances that are lethal for the microoganism.

Bone marrow is the source of monocytes.

Promonocytes originate in bone marrow. The sequence of promonocyte, monocyte, and histiocyte has been shown experimentally by the difference in isotope labeling of mononuclear phagocytes of bone marrow, blood, and peritoneal cavity. Monocytes are circulating, immature phagocytes. When activated they emigrate through the capillary wall into inflammatory lesions (Fig. 19.5) and promptly transform into macrophages. Early evidence of synthesis of new digestive enzymes can be detected in monocytes as they adhere to endothelium.

Monocytosis

Monocytosis is elevation of monocytes in circulating blood beyond the range considered normal. It is seen in recovery phases of bacterial infections and is characteristic of acute stages of certain diseases. Only under severe conditions do monocytes phagocytize while in the bloodstream to become circulating macrophages.

In some forms of severe intravascular hemolysis, monocytes become phagocytic, absorb erythrocytes, and degrade hemoglobin. Their role in erythrophagocytosis is related to the capacity of their plasma membrane to attach to immunoglobins and complement on erythrocyte surfaces.

Monocytes release cytokines that mediate inflammation.

Release of *interleukin-1* (IL-1), a polypeptide that induces many features of the acute phase response of inflammation, occurs as monocytes are activated. IL-1 acts as a hormone and circulates to affect distant organs. Its functions include (1) stimulating neutrophils to circulate and release granules by a direct effect both on the bone marrow and circulating neutrophils, (2) activating T and B lymphocytes, (3) stimulating fever and prostaglandin E_2 synthesis in the *hypothalamus,* (4) increasing synthesis of acute phase proteins in liver, and (5) increasing catabolism of skeletal muscle to provide amino acids for use by the liver.

In the late stages of inflammation, IL-1 acts as a growth factor for fibroblasts and other cells involved in repair. For example, in brain, it is a

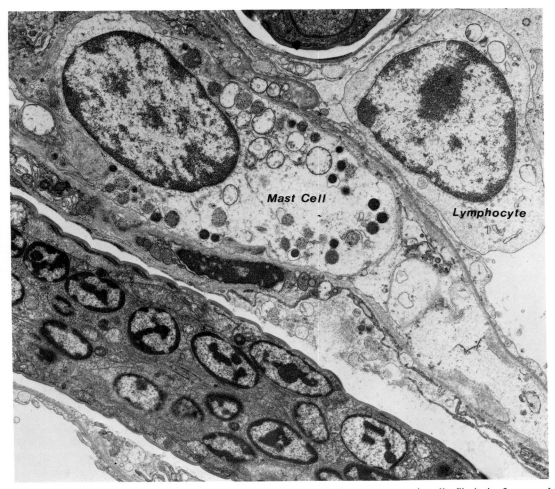

Fig.19.3. Mast cell in alveolar septum, canine dirofilariasis. Larvae of *Dirofilaria immitis* (*lower left*). The mast cell is partially degranulated.

potent mitogen for astroglia (it has no effect on oligodendroglia) and the brain content of IL-1 rises after injury.

Lymphocytes

In most mammals, lymphocytes make up 20–40% of the leukocytes in blood and over 90% of the cells in thoracic duct lymph. Lymphocytes are tiny round cells with a narrow rim of cytoplasm. Dense azurophil granules (5–15 per cell) and clear vacuoles are often present in the cytoplasm. Nuclear chromatin is densely packed, particularly at the periphery of the nucleus. The smallest lymphocytes are resting cells, and the reactions of ameboid movement, phagocytosis,

and chemotactic responses are weak or absent. Larger lymphocytes found in smears of normal blood usually represent transformed cells. They are blast cells with intensely basophilic cytoplasm. Increased numbers of these cells are found in recovery stages of pyogenic infections and some viral diseases and are, in fact, immature plasmacytes.

Lymphocytosis, the increase in numbers of lymphocytes in circulating blood, is seen in transient reponses to severe muscular exercise, fever, and other stress. Lymphocytosis of long duration is less common (it is usually a prelude to or actually is lymphatic leukemia).

Lymphopenia, a decrease in numbers of lymphocytes, occurs in viral diseases in which the

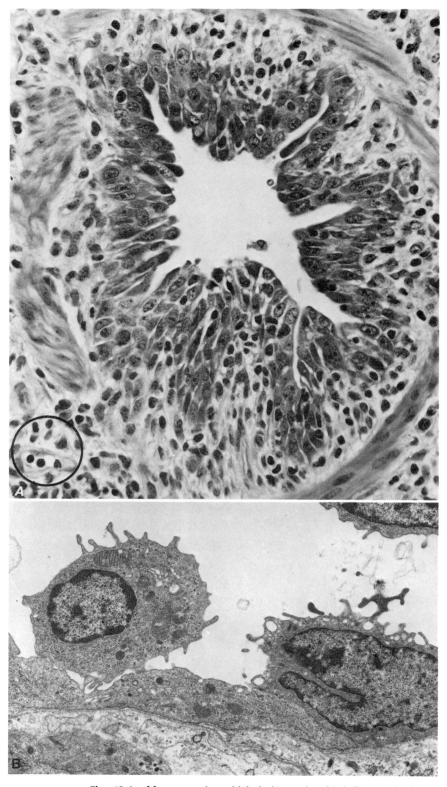

Fig. 19.4. Monocytes, bronchiole in lung, pig with influenza. A. Acute, monolymphocytic peribronchiolitis (*circle*) with hyperplasia of bronchiolar epithelium. B. Ultrastructure of circulating monocytes in process of emigration through capillary wall during inflammation. Note the long processes on cell surfaces and their interdigitation with processes on the endothelial cell.

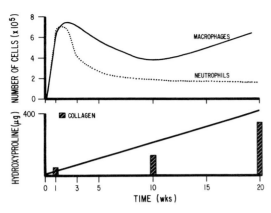

Fig. 19.5. Times of appearance of neutrophils and monocytes in lung exudates, experimental silicosis. (Data from Adamson and Bowden, *Am. J. Pathol.* 117:37, 1984)

virus attacks the lymphoid system (e.g., canine distemper, hog cholera, and bovine viral diarrhea) and during therapy with such lympholytic agents as cortisone, radiation, and immunosuppressive drugs.

Recirculation

Small lymphocytes originate by lymphopoiesis in the cortex of lymph nodes where they are shed into the lymphatic circulation and enter the bloodstream via the thoracic duct and then recirculate. By hematogenous distribution to the lymph nodes, they migrate through the extracellular spaces of the endothelium of *postcapillary venules* in the paracortical regions and reenter the lymphatic circulation.

In the 1960s, Gowans at Oxford cannulated the thoracic duct and periodically examined cells in lymph; enormous numbers of small lymphocytes entered the blood daily by this route. When lymph was continuously drained away in the cannula, the animals became depleted of small lymphocytes. The thoracic duct lymphocyte flow was restored in the animals by the intravenous injection of lymphocytes obtained from a closely related donor animal. By autoradiographic labeling, Gowans showed that donor lymphocytes entering the lymphatics of the lymph node migrated through the postcapillary venules with high endothelium.

Small lymphocytes have memory.

The small lymphocyte is the purveyor of immunologic memory; that is, a segment of the population is immunologically committed to antigens previously contacted. When triggered by that specific antigen, these small lymphocytes transform into large basophilic blast cells.

FOCUS

Influenza

Influenza occurs in birds and four species of mammals: swine, horses, sea lions, and humans. Influenza virus replicates in epithelial cells of the respiratory tract. By budding from cell surfaces, the plasma membrane of the host cell is modified and becomes the external coat of the virus. Spikes of neuraminidase and hemagglutinin project from the virion surface and are important in infecting epithelial cells elsewhere in the respiratory tract and in the transmission of influenza to other hosts.

In a typical severe infection, influenza viruses initiate an acute, intense, inflammatory response (rhinitis, tracheitis, and pneumonitis). Mucus is produced by epithelial cells. Plasma exudes into the airways from leaky capillaries to produce a *serous rhinitis.* The lesions eventually become *catarrhal,* and then *mucopurulent.* Cytokines, prostaglandins, and leukotrienes are released from participating inflammatory cells and cause many of the signs of disease such as fever, myalgia, and anorexia.

▶

►

Soon after the initial focus of infection begins in epithelium of the nasal turbinates, virus spreads to involve the entire upper respiratory tract. In the lungs, *alveolitis,* or inflammation of the septal walls, is the hallmark of acute influenza. In the 1960s, fluorescent antibody studies in the laboratory of Dr. Marvin Twiehaus, at the University of Nebraska, showed that viral antigens developed in cells lining the alveolar septal walls. Recently, Dr. Gian Winkler, now at the University of Zurich, has shown that virions of swine influenza can be detected budding from surfaces of pneumocytes as early as 5 hours after inoculation of baby piglets. Affected epithelial cells swell and develop cytoplasmic basophilia, but inclusion bodies are not present.

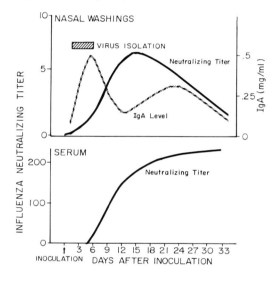

Levels of IgA and anti-influenza-neutralizing activity in nasal washings and serum. The first peak of IgA exudation is nonspecific and not associated with antibody activity. Later, IgA again rises, this time due to increased levels of specific antibody to influenza.

Virus can be isolated from nasal swabs taken from affected animals for several days after clinical signs appear. Disappearance of virus from the respiratory tract is associated with appearance of immune T cells and antibodies in the bloodstream. Recovery from influenza begins before antibody is detectable, however, and factors such as fever, interferon, and cell-mediated immune mechanisms play important roles in cessation of viral injury.

For example, small lymphocytes taken from animals immunized with tetanus toxoid transform to blast cells when placed in contact with tetanus antigen in the same culture.

KININ SYSTEMS IN INFLAMMATORY FLUIDS

Kinins are polypeptides in the bloodstream that arise from circulating plasma globulins. They are implicated as mediators of inflammation because of their presence at sites of tissue injury and their capacity to reproduce inflammatory lesions experimentally. Lysis of cells, particularly leukocytes, releases enzymes that generate kinins, which then sustain and enhance the early transitory capillary alterations begun by histamine.

Discovery of plasma kinins had origins in the old observation that urine, injected intravenously, lowered blood pressure. In the 1930s this hypotensive peptide was characterized and shown to be present in saliva, plasma, and other secretions. Since pancreas was a rich source, it was named kallikrein (Gr. *kalli,* beautiful, plus pan*kreas*). Later, it was shown that kallikreins act indirectly, as enzymes to split a plasma kininogen to form a kinin.

Bradykinin is the prototype kinin.

Bradykinin induces vascular leakage by opening gaps between endothelial cells in postcapillary venules. In sensitive tissues such as skin, it is 10 times more active than histamine. Bradykinin was discovered as an active factor released from an α_2-globulin by incubation with snake venom and was named for the slow or "brady" contractions it elicited from guinea pig ileum. Although it can be synthesized in the laboratory, studies on its function are difficult because of the short life span of kinin molecules and the instability of their precursors in the living animal.

Kinins mediate inflammation.

Kinins are potent mediators of vasodilation, pain, and increased capillary permeability, the major signs of acute inflammation. Action on arterioles and venules is mediated through contraction of smooth muscle. Smooth muscle contraction also causes bronchoconstriction.

Kinins are destroyed in passage through the lungs.

Kinins are degraded by inhibitors almost immediately as they are generated in serum. Inactivation has been attributed to a carboxypeptidase B in serum that removes the D-terminal arginine residue on the peptide molecule. Most kinins are inactivated by enzymes on the surface of the pulmonary capillary endothelial cells and thus do not survive passage through the lung.

Kallikreins activate plasma kininogen to kinin.

Kinins are released from a plasma α_2-globulin substrate by a plasma enzyme system called *kallikrein.* These kinin-generating enzymes are present in neutrophils, and these cells, when lysed, sustain the inflammatory reaction. Kallikreins are proteolytic enzymes of plasma that generate vasoactive *kinins* from globulin substrates. They are extracted by chemical precipitation of plasma protein, purified by chromatography, and identified by rat uterus bioassay (the recording of muscle contractions of the isolated rat uterus suspended in bath solutions).

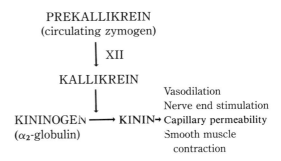

Prekallikrein also regulates coagulation.

Prekallikrein influences the rate of activation of factors XI and XII; that is, in the absence of prekallikrein, factor XII is activated more slowly. Kininogen brings prekallikrein and factor XI in close proximity to surface bound factor XII. Reciprocal activation occurs as prekallikrein is converted to kallikrein by factor XII. Factor XII is then cleaved by kallikrein into α and β fractions. The β fraction and kallikrein dissociate from the kininogen on the surface and enter the fluid phase to activate the kinin system.

Prekallikrein deficiency is a rare hereditary defect reported only in the dog. It is usually an incidental finding on hematologic workup. Although dogs have reduced kinin levels, prekallikrein deficiency remains clinically inapparent.

PROSTANOIDS: PROSTAGLANDINS AND LEUKOTRIENES

Arachidonic acid, produced during degradation of phospholipids in injured cell membranes, is the precursor for prostaglandins and leukotrienes. These molecules are important regulators of normal cell activity and participate in inflammation by directly causing smooth muscle contraction, vasodilation, and sensory nerve end stimulation.

Leukotrienes

Leukotrienes (LTs, named because they are produced by leukocytes and have three conjugated double bonds) are progressively altered enzymatically to produce molecules with different activities. The prototype, LTB_4, has potent chemotactic action on leukocytes. LTC_4, after enzymatic removal of one glutamic acid molecule, becomes LTD_4; LTD_4, after removal of glycine is LTE_4; and so on. LTE_4 increases permeability in postcapillary venules by causing contraction of endothelial cells. Several LTs are the active principles in *slow reacting substance of anaphylaxis,* a substance known for years to be released into fluids after injury and to cause potent smooth muscle contraction.

Prostaglandins

Prostaglandins (PGs) may exert enhancing or depressant effects on tissue, depending on changes in their molecular structure. Much of the effect is caused by enhancement of actions of bradykinin and histamine that pour into inflamed tissue. They also act to stimulate aggregation and degranulation of neutrophils. PGs of the E type are most prominent in mediating inflammation. Macrophages are important sources of PGE and, when activated, rapidly convert arachidonic acid to PGE. Both the production and effects of PGs depend on the enzyme content of tissue affected. Platelets make primarily thromboxane A_2, whereas smooth muscle forms prostacyclin (PGI_2).

Prostaglandins are increased in inflammatory fluids.

Efferent lymph draining inflammatory lesions has increased amounts of PGs within a few hours. PGs also appear in draining lymph nodes. They may facilitate antigen processing, as their amounts peak at the time when uptake and processing of microbial proteins is maximal.

Aspirin and indomethacin depress inflammation and pain by blocking PG synthesis. Their action is chiefly on cyclooxygenase, the first enzyme to act in the oxygenation sequence of arachidonic acid.

ACUTE PHASE PROTEINS

Clinical signs and lesions of early inflammation are associated with the appearance in tissue fluids of certain proteins that sustain the inflammatory process. The initial stimulus that incites inflammation causes these substances to enter the bloodstream rapidly. They are not normally present in plasma (or are present in very low amounts) but increase markedly immediately after injury. They are called *acute phase proteins* because their presence in blood is a diagnostic sign of tissue injury and inflammation (Table 19.1). Most are synthesized in the liver (the same hepatocyte has been shown to produce over four acute phase proteins).

Most acute phase proteins are actually glycoproteins. Because they initiate or enhance inflammation they are called "endogenous humoral mediators"; that is, they play an active role in some phase of the inflammatory process. Humoral mediators may act by increasing vascular permeability or by attracting leukocytes (chemotaxis).

Vasopermeability factors sustain the capillary permeability initiated by histamine and the leukotrienes; these factors work via their ability to open endothelial cell junctions by inducing contraction of actin-myosin filaments of endothelial cells (they also by cause contraction of smooth muscle of arterioles).

Chemotactic factors, distinct from vasopermeability factors, act mainly on neutrophils to cause them to migrate, aggregate, secrete lysosomal enzymes and increase their rate of glycolysis.

Table 19.1. Acute phase proteins in plasma

Acute Phase Protein	Relative Increase in Inflammation	Electrophoretic Migration	Function
Fibrinogen	50%	β	Coagulation; forms fibrin polymers
C3 (complement)	50%	β	Fulcrum for C cascade; leads to cell or bacterial lysis (membrane phase) and liberation of chemotactic fragments (fluid phase)
C-reactive protein	1000X	γ	Initiates C-dependent opsonization (facilitates phagocyosis)
Ceruloplasmin	50%	α_2	Copper transport
Protein SAA	1000X	α_2	? (forms amyloid fibrils)
Haptoglobulin	2–3X	α_2	Hemoglobin transport
α_1-antitrypsin[a]	2–3X	α_1	Inhibition of proteases in serum
α_1-acid glycoprotein[a]	2–3X	α_1	Blocks binding of microorganisms to cells

[a]Well-characterized only for man.

Fibrinogen

Fibrinogen is synthesized in the liver and circulates normally at uniform levels (see hemostasis, Chapter 16). During the acute phase of inflammation it is released by the hepatocytes and shows markedly increased levels in plasma. Much of this fibrinogen is used at the site of inflammation to form fibrin. The increase in fibrinogen in plasma also enhances erythrocyte aggregation, which is reflected in an increased *erythrocyte sedimentation rate* in the laboratory.

C-reactive protein

C-reactive protein (CRP) was the first acute phase protein to be described and was used (nonspecifically) in the 1930s to diagnose the presence and extent of inflammatory processes, especially those involving necrosis. CRP is a circulating protein that binds to phosphorylcholine molecules in surface membranes of macrophages, platelets, and some lymphocytes. This attachment causes complement to attach to the cell, which in turn facilitates attachment of bacteria; that is, it initiates the complement-dependent opsonization that leads to phagocytosis of microorganisms.

During acute inflammation, CRP can rise 1000 times within 48 hours. Changes in plasma levels of CRP are nonspecific and occur to the same extent in diverse diseases. Thus CRP measurement provides information similar to an increased erythrocyte sedimentation rate associated with fibrinogen elevations during acute disease. For example, CRP rises markedly within hours of surgery and subsides after a few days (in the absence of infection and severe inflammation or necrosis).

CRP reacts with only some types of bacteria. It was discovered because of its strong affinity for the C-polysaccharide fractions of capsules of *Streptococcus pneumoniae*. CRP-like proteins are found in most mammals, birds, and fish. Composed of five subunits, they have certain specificities and are known to have high affinity for some galactosyl polymers and to phosphocholine (the basis for its binding to pneumococcal capsules). Once bound to membranes, CRP then recruits *complement* much like antibody; that is, CRP is a surrogate for antibody in activating the classical pathway. It facilitates initiation of immune-related activities during early phases of inflammation, before specific antibody is produced.

Complement

Complement (C) is a self-assembling, extracellular system of proteins present in inactive form in plasma and body fluids. Activation occurs in a precise sequence (similar to the clotting cascade) on cell or microbial surface membranes (Fig. 19.6). Its consequences are *clumping of bacteria, enhancement of inflammation,* and *cell lysis.*

Lysis (of either cells or bacteria) occurs when

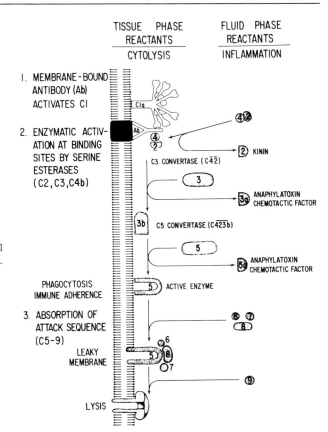

Fig. 19.6. Complement action on cell membranes.

the final products (C6–9) aggregate to form doughnut-shaped attack sequences that embed in the plasma membranes of the target cell to form pores (see Fig. 5.10). Inflammation is promoted by release of vasoactive and chemotactic C fragments cleaved during activation that enter surrounding fluids. Thus, C plays significant roles in inflammation in mediation of the chemotactic attraction of leukocytes, in killing of bacterial cells, and in activation of granule release mechanisms, (e.g., histamine from mast cells, procoagulants from platelets). It is essential for immunologic bacteriolysis, in which it functions as a nonspecific effector of specific antibody activities.

Complement activation occurs by two pathways. The alternate pathway is more primitive and less specific. The classic pathway is specific due to its initiation by antibodies. Both pathways lead to activation of a critical enzyme, *C3 convertase,* that activates a final common pathway generating the *membrane attack sequence* C5–9 (Fig. 19.7).

Classic pathway

Classic C activation begins when membrane-bound antibody molecules (or antigen-antibody complexes free in plasma) interact with circulating C1. The C1s subunit is exposed and mediates cleavage of C4. After attaching to the membrane surface, C4 binds C2 so that it may be cleaved to C2a by C1s. C4 then binds circulating C3 so that it is susceptible to cleavage by C2a. Thus C42 is the *C3 convertase* for the classic pathway. Activation of C1 leads to many C42 complexes capable of cleaving C3 and thus is an amplification step.

Alternate pathway

The alternate pathway includes five plasma proteins that interact to form C3 convertase without participation of circulating components

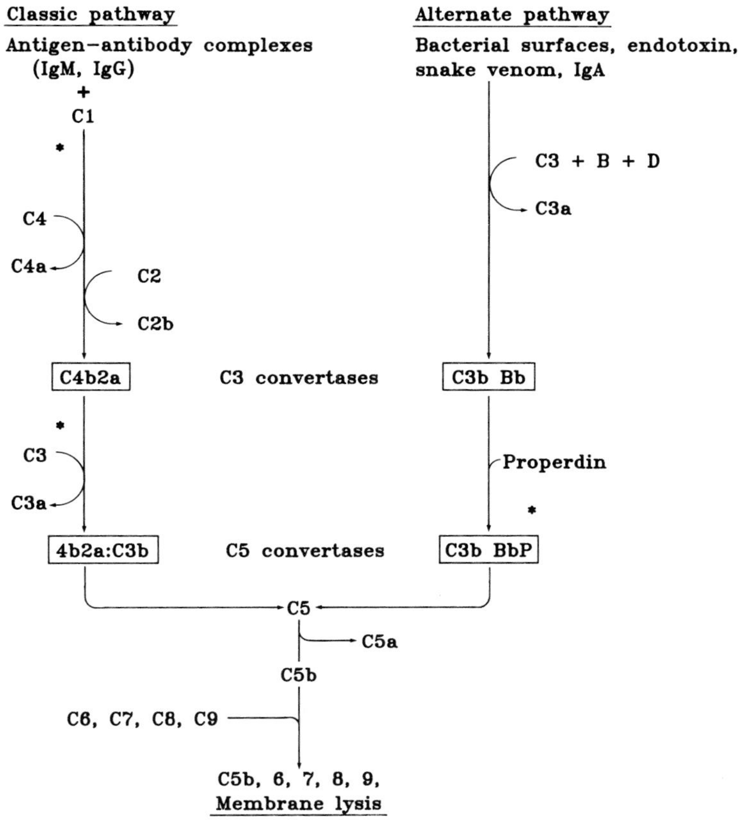

Classic pathway

Antigen–antibody complexes
(IgM, IgG)
+
C1

Alternate pathway

Bacterial surfaces, endotoxin,
snake venom, IgA

Fig. 19.7. Classic, alternate, and common pathways of complement (see text). Reactions occur as complement components in serum attach to components bound to cell membranes. Pathways are blocked by controlling proteins at certain sites (*asterisk*).

C1, 2, and 4. It is a mechanism to provide protection during early phases of microbial invasion before antibodies are produced. The alternate pathway is initiated when a plasma globulin (factor D, which circulates in active form) binds to particle surfaces, commonly the polysaccharide cell walls of bacteria and fungi. When D cleaves factor B the molecular rearrangements in B expose an enzyme site that interacts with C3 to form C3bB, the C3 convertase of the alternate pathway. Properdin, the first protein to be identified, stabilizes the C3bB molecule.

Common pathway

Factors C3–C9 circulate in unassembled but active form. C3 convertases (C42 or C3bB) attract and cleave circulating C3 into C3a and C3b. C3a is released into fluids to act as an *anaphylatoxin,* a substance that induces mast cell degranulation with release of histamine (thereby increasing vascular permeability). C3b,

depending on the type of cell or particle involved, may continue the C cascade or act as an *opsonin,* a substance that renders bacteria susceptible to phagocytosis (Table 19.2). To continue C activation, C3b binds C5 and cleaves it into an active enzyme on the membrane (C5b) and a fragment (C5a) that is both an anaphylatoxin and a potent chemotactive factor for neutrophils.

C5a aggregates the terminal components of C into an attack complex, which burrows into the membrane, allowing electrolytes and water to enter the cell. Affected bacteria then swell, and the plasma membrane may rupture.

Neutrophils have specific receptors for C3b on their surfaces.

Membrane-bound C3b is also the major opsonic protein (it can be assisted by C5b). It is a signal for adherence of neutrophils and monocytes to C-coated surfaces. The attachment of

Table 19.2.   Components of complement that mediate inflammation

Component	Functions
C3a and C5a	Mast cell histamine release → increased vasopermeability
C5a	Chemotaxis of neutrophils
Antigen-antibody-C3b complexes	Immune adherence to cells → lysosomal release
C3b	Platelet aggregation, monocyte chemotaxis, B lymphocyte transformation

bacteria coated by C3b with specific C3b receptors embedded in the neutrophil surface causes adherence and promotes subsequent phagocytosis. C3b receptor molecules are proteins embedded the plasma membranes of neutrophils (they also occur in monocytes and B lymphocytes), and their distribution has been studied using fluorescein-labeled antibodies.

C3a and C5a play significant roles in inflammation.

These two C fragments cause (1) histamine release from mast cells, (2) chemotaxis and degranulation of neutrophils, and (3) smooth muscle contraction (Table 19.1). The net effect is that neutrophils and other leukocytes are induced to migrate through highly permeable capillaries into a progressively expanding inflammatory focus. The complement system interacts with the kinin and fibrinolytic systems (Fig. 19.8).

C3a and C5a are rapidly inactivated.

Plasma carboxypeptidases rapidly inactivate anaphylatoxins (which are not effective in systemic reactions). These "anaphylatoxin inhibitors" act like pancreatic carboxypeptidase B, cleaving carboxy termini of basic amino acids. Activities of kinins and fibrinolytic peptides are also controlled by these enzymes.

Hypocomplementemia may suppress inflammatory responses.

Excessive consumption of C during some severe infections may result in hypocomplementemia. This occurs when antibodies react with antigens to use C. C3 is particularly important in opsonizing bacteria. The serum of human patients with hereditary C3 deficiency cannot sustain bacterial opsonization, and these patients are susceptible to repeated bacterial infection despite normal amounts of immunoglobulins. The role of C in inflammation is not completely understood; C depletion has little effect on the nonspecific inflammatory responses, yet in bac-

terial diseases C may launch all inflammatory reactions.

Lysozyme

Lysozyme (muramidase) is a small ubiquitous cationic enzyme that catalyzes the hydrolysis of linkages between N-acetyl-muramic acid and N-acetylglucosamine, moieties of peptidoglycans abundant in the cell walls of bacteria. It digests glycopeptide cell wall debris of bacteria killed by other mechanisms, and it seems that the antibacterial role of lysozyme is of less significance than that of substances that kill bacteria directly. Lysozyme is present in large amounts in various body fluids, notably milk, tears, saliva, and genital secretions. Fluids are examined for their content of lysozyme by adding them to wells in agar containing suspensions of mycobacteria (Fig. 19.9).

Lysozyme is found within granulocytes, monocytes, and macrophages, and serum lysozyme reflects its liberation from these cells. Lysozyme also is produced by epithelial cells of mucosae and ducts and glands of respiratory and intestinal tracts. It occurs in granular pneumocytes of the lung, in thymic corpuscles, and in intestinal Paneth cells. In vaginal mucus, the concentration of lysozyme is lowest at midgestation and highest in the early follicular and late luteal phases. By overlying frozen sections of cervix with bacterial substrates for lysozyme and determining the amount of lysis, it has been shown that lysozyme is within the secretory granules of cervical mucous cells and that its concentration varies in response to hormones.

Interferon

Interferons are cellular proteins induced and released following stimulation by microbes and some other foriegn substances. They were discovered as virus-inhibiting soluble factors released by cells infected with influenza virus (some viruses are potent inducers of interfer-

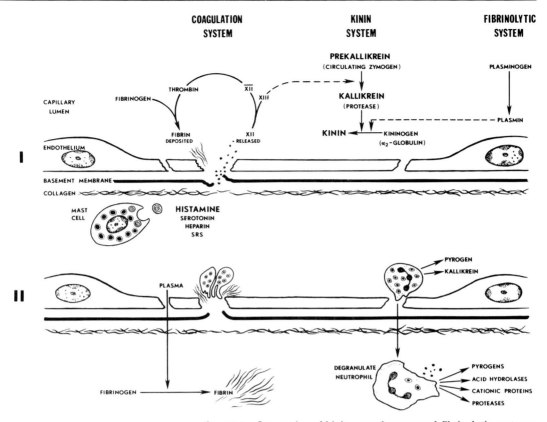

Fig. 19.8. Interaction of kinin, complement, and fibrinolytic systems.

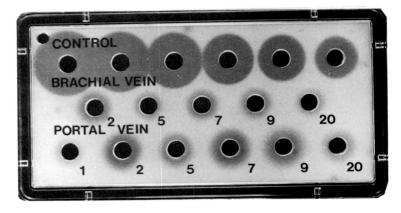

Fig. 19.9. Assay for lysozyme in serum. Dilutions of serum to be analyzed are placed in wells cut in a plate of agar containing a culture of mycobacteria. After incubation, the width of the zone where serum lysozyme has lysed the bacteria is measured. In this case, blood was taken from the jugular vein and from the portal vein in a case of severe bacterial enteritis from 1 to 20 h after infection. Lysozyme levels are higher and appear earlier in portal vein blood.

ons). Interferon does not inactivate viruses but blocks intracellular viral replication by inducing an antiviral protein in the cell that inhibits ribosomal production of proteins.

Interferon is nonspecific in action.

Although species specific, most interferons are nonspecific in their activity. This is in contrast to antibody, which is specific, extracellular in action, and produced by specific lymphoid cells distant from primary infection sites. Interferon is one of the first host defense mechanisms to appear in viral infection. It diffuses to surrounding cells and enters those cells that have receptors for interferon on their surfaces. The spreading virus thus meets an intracellular barrier to continued replication.

Interferon also occurs in the blood and body fluids.

Considerable amounts of interferon appear in the bloodstream. Interferonemia rapidly disappears because of loss via the renal glomerulus (Fig. 19.10). Interferonuria develops rapidly, and levels of interferon are often higher in urine than in blood. Salivary secretion also occurs and may be significant in oral infections.

Fibronectin

This glycoprotein is associated with fibroblast surfaces and basement membranes. Present in serum as a dimer, it is deposited in tissue as a multimer. Fibronectin occurs in normal canine plasma at about 240–340 μg/ml; it is decreased in plasma during the first phases of acute inflammation because it enters injured tissue sites

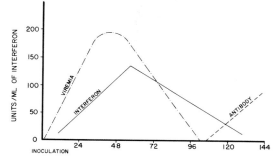

Fig. 19.10. Rise and fall of interferon in circulating blood relative to viremia and antibodies in an acute infection with an interferon-producing virus.

and because it is used to coat bacterial surfaces. It disappears especially rapidly during bacteremia. Plasma fibronectin (an α_2-glycoprotein) is an opsonin; that is, it enhances bacterial aggregation and promotes phagocytosis. It plays a very important role in stimulating Kupffer cells of the liver to remove circulating bacteria.

Fibronectin promotes healing.

Fibronectin accumulates in inflammatory lesions and plays a role in adhesion of cells during healing. Normally absent in dense connective tissue, it appears coincident with invading fibroblasts and disappears as collagen matures. Fibronectin functions as a matrix for organization of new collagen and promotes cell migration and adhesion.

Ceruloplasmin

This copper-containing α_2-glycoprotein also increases in inflammation. It has antioxidant activities and suppresses the damaging effects of oxygen radicals on cells, probably by its ferrooxidase activity. Fe^{++} can promote lipid peroxidation through reaction with oxygen radicals, and ceruloplasmin converts reduced iron (Fe^{++}) to oxidized iron (Fe^{+++}). Transferrin, the normal iron-binding protein of serum, may act similarly although it is reported that lactoferrin, which also binds iron, can potentiate tissue damage during neutrophil granule release by releasing its iron.

α_1-acid glycoprotein

Abundant in normal plasma, this acute phase protein rises abruptly in acute inflammation due to release by the liver. It closely resembles cell membrane sialoglycoprotein (it is 24% sialic acid) and may function as a nonspecific competitor for cell surfaces. In malaria it blocks the binding of *Plasmodium falciparum* to surfaces of human erythrocytes.

Iron-binding proteins in inflammation

The plasma concentration of ionic iron and iron transferrin (the normal iron-binding protein of plasma and lymph) declines in severe inflammation. This hyposideremia results from release of lactoferrin from neutrophil granules. *Lactoferrin* is an iron-free (but iron-binding) glycoprotein that removes iron from iron-transferrin complexes in inflammatory fluids. This occurs especially in an acidic environment, which causes transferrin to release iron and lactoferrin to accept it. Macrophages take up iron-lactoferrin complexes (receptors for lactoferrin have been identified on macrophage surfaces), which clears the complexes from the circulation.

In birds, the protein ovotransferrin is deposited in the egg and functions to bind iron in a similar way.

Stimulation of ferritin synthesis diverts iron.

Reduced serum iron and transferrin saturation are sustained in chronic inflammation by this second mechanism. Ferritin synthesis diverts labile iron into ferritin stores with reduced availability for release from tissue. This may result in iron-deficient erythropoiesis, low erythrocyte hemoglobin, and increased erythrocyte protoporphyrin concentration.

Hyposideremia withholds iron from bacteria.

Hyposideremia is a biologic mechanism of the host to withhold an essential nutrient from pathogenic bacteria. Iron concentration in plasma and tissue is less than that required for growth of some bacteria. Thus animals with plasma iron may be less susceptible to some bacterial infections. Conversely, animals with increased plasma labile iron (with hypoferritinemia and hypotransferrinemia) may have increased susceptibility to these same bacteria.

Enteric bacteria such as *Escherichia coli* produce iron chelators called *siderophores,* which remove iron from iron-binding protein. Called enterochelin (or enterobactin), they are synthesized only during iron-restricted growth and efficiently transport iron into the bacterial cell. Other organisms, such as *Neisseria gonorrhoeae,* remove iron from iron-binding proteins directly via a mechanism by which surface receptors on the bacteria combine with the iron-binding protein.

Experimentally, the number of bacterial cells (injected intraperitoneally) required to kill mice is lowered 3–5 log units by a concurrent injection of iron. The number of *Clostridium perfringens* growing in guinea pig muscle increases 6000-fold after iron injection; the number of *E. coli* in rat kidney increases 1000-fold. The injected iron saturates both transferrin and lactoferrin, causing increased fatalities by blocking the inhibitory effect of lactoferrin and providing increased iron for bacterial metabolism.

FEVER

During severe local inflammatory lesions or in generalized infections, neutrophils are lysed intravascularly. The release of protein components of their lysosomes is chiefly responsible for the signs of fever: increased body temperature, respiration, and heart rate.

The hypothalamus controls temperature.

Normal body temperature is maintained by hypothalamic regulation of the production and dissipation of heat. Stimuli originate from superficial thermoreceptors in skin and deep receptors near the hypothalamus that respond to temperature change. During fever, the hypothalamic "thermostat" is elevated by endogenous pyrogens of neutrophil origin. Monocytes and macrophages are also major cells of pyrogen release. They secrete the cytokine *interleukin-1,* which has many functions, one of which is to act as an endogenous pyrogen.

Animals become unresponsive to exogenous pyrogen.

Repeated injections of exogenous pyrogens experimentally induce a state of refractoriness termed *tolerance.* The animal no longer responds to further doses of pyrogen by increasing body temperature, because its own endogenous pyrogenic mechanism has become exhausted. Repeated injections of granulocytic pyrogen, however, continue to cause a full response, for they act directly on the hypothalamus. Thus animals made tolerant to exogenous substances by exhaustion remain fully responsive to endogenous pyrogen.

Fever is more than elevated body temperature.

In summary, the progression of events leading to fever involves leukocytes, plasma, the hypothalamus, and effector end organs that disseminate body heat (by cutaneous vasoconstriction, sweat production, and shivering). Antipyretic drugs can act by (1) interfering with synthesis or release of endogenous pyrogen by leukocytes and other cells, (2) inactivating circulating endogenous pyrogens, (3) interfering with the action of endogenous pyrogen in the brain, or (4) interfering with the effector pathways. Aspirin, the most common antipyretic substance, antagonizes the action of endogenous pyrogen within the hypothalamus.

ADDITIONAL READING

Baracos, V., et al. Stimulation of muscle protein degradation and prostaglandin E_2 release by leukocytic pyrogen (interleukin-1). *New Engl. J. Med.* 308:553, 1983.

Berggren, K. A., et al. Cytotoxic effects of *Pasteurella haemolytica* on bovine neutrophils. *Am. J. Vet. Res.* 42:1383, 1981.

Bertram, T. A. Neutrophilic leukocyte structure and function in domestic animals. *Adv. Vet. Sci.* 30:91, 1985.

Caspi, D., et al. C-reactive protein in dogs. *Am. J. Vet. Res.* 48:919, 1987.

Dinarello, C. A. Interleukin-1 and the pathogenesis of the acute phase response. *New Engl. J. Med.* 311:1413, 1984.

Kephart, G. M., et al. Deposition of eosinophil granule major basic protein onto microfilariae of *Onchocera volvulus* in the skin of patients treated with diethylcarbamazine. *Lab. Invest.* 50:51, 1984.

Matilla, T., et al. Depressed bacterial growth in whey during endotoxin induced mastitis. *Zentralbl. Veterinaermed.* [B] 32:85, 1985.

O'Flaherty, J. T. Lipid mediators of inflammation and allergy. *Lab. Invest.* 47:314, 1982.

Tvedten, H. W., et al. Mediators of lung injury in mice following systemic activation of complement. *Am. J. Pathol.* 119:92, 1985.

Weiss, S. J., et al. Long-lived oxidants generated by human neutrophils. *Science* 222:625, 1983.

Repair

REPAIR is a fundamental process of all living things. It begins soon after injury and utilizes both the fluids and cells that have exuded into the tissue during the acute phase of inflammation. Repair involves both fibrous reconstruction and hyperplastic regeneration. The enormous differences in repair processes among animals result from the regenerative capacity of the species involved, cleanliness or contamination of the site of injury, and the tissue in which repair is occurring.

REGENERATION

Regeneration is a remarkable characteristic of lower animals. Wounds heal rapidly, and lost parts may be replaced. Hydras and other coelenterates can be cut into small pieces, and each will develop into a completely new organism. Earthworms cut in half regenerate new heads and tails. Some of the lower vertebrate forms retain these remarkable capacities. When a newt's leg is amputated, the stump gives rise to pluripotential mesenchymal cells that differentiate to form a new leg including bone and muscle. Growth is not inherent in the stump, for if it is transplanted to the tail region it develops into a new tail. Frog tadpoles have similar powers of regeneration that are largely lost during metamorphosis.

In mammals, few functional gross regenerative changes occur. Epithelial and connective tissues regenerate extensively, but most tissues have a very limited ability to reduplicate. The process of repair in higher vertebrates is therefore chiefly the revascularization, fibroplasia, and reepithelization that occur in the late phases of the inflammatory response.

Epithelization

Growth of new epithelial cells over a reconstructed wound is a requirement for complete repair in skin and other surface tissues. In epidermis, basal cells of the surviving epithelium at the periphery of the wound begin to slide across the bare, fibrin-covered wound surface soon after injury. Migrant epithelial cells are pleomorphic and have blunt pseudopods that project, by ameboid movement, into fibrin strands. Epithelial cells also cover gaps in epidermis by growing up from skin appendages, such as hair follicles, providing these structures remain intact.

Peptide growth factors in body fluids promote healing. *Epidermal growth factor* in saliva appears to accelerate epithelization over skin injuries as animals lick their wounds.

Small wounds may be covered in 12 hours.

Mitosis begins in migrant epithelial cells, and new cells rapidly fill in the gaps in the new surface. New keratinocytes develop binding intercellular junctions with other epithelial cells and with the basement membrane to complete the repair process. Epithelial cell proliferation ceases when cells contact one another. *Contact inhibition* is the poorly understood phenomenon involving cell recognition and establishment of normal intercellular communication. Information causing epithelization to cease is somehow transferred from cell to cell (probably through specialized gap junctions), for cell proliferation does not cease if mechanical barriers are placed in the path of advancing cells.

New epithelial surfaces lack appendages, such as hair follicles and glands, and are usually poorly pigmented. Mammalian skin heals in a well-defined sequence but there are marked species differences in wound healing among lower vertebrates. Fish skin contains large numbers of extraordinarily large "alarm cells" interspersed among keratinocytes and contain an aqueous substance causing other fish to move away; alarm cells are not present in new epithelium over wounds.

Mucosal surfaces regenerate rapidly.

Mucosal epithelial surfaces regenerate more quickly than does epidermis. In small experimental wounds of the rat trachea, injured mucosa is covered by new epithelium in 48 hours; cilia and goblet cells appear in 14 days. Similar experimental wounding of the cat duodenum has shown equally rapid growth. Simple epithelium covers the clot-filled defect in a few days and subsequently remodels to form new villi and glands.

Granulation tissue is required for epithelization.

Massive wounds will heal progressively, providing a proper base of granulation tissue is present. In some patients surgical incisions are deliberately left unsutured to promote drainage and to avoid pockets of infection below the suture line. If infection is controlled, these wounds heal efficiently by granulation. When an *ulcer* erodes though the wall of an organ so that a base of granulation tissue cannot form, the epithelial margins of the wound do not grow together (Fig. 20.1). The stimulus provided by collagen is missing, and the wound edges will not coalesce.

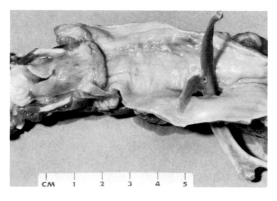

Fig. 20.1. Subacute focal fibrous esophagitis, aged dog. Ulceration and penetration of the esophagus by a foreign body (avian rib bone).

CONTAMINATION OF WOUNDS
Healing of a clean, incised wound: First intention

Surgical incisions are generally sharp and free from large numbers of bacteria and tissue debris. Because the vessels have been ligated and the wound edges approximated, they contain little free blood. Repair is rapid. Fibroblasts generally bridge the area in 12 hours. Capillary buds invade, allowing a framework of blood vessels to form and assisting fibroplasia and collagen deposition that impart tensil strength to the wound. Within 4 or 5 days, epithelium has grown over the wound, acute inflammation has ceased, and repair is sufficient to allow movement of the injured area (Fig. 20.2).

Healing of an open wound: Second intention

Lacerations of tissue that are not sutured must heal by new tissue formation at the base of the wound. They are usually filled with tissue debris, free erythrocytes, and dead bacteria. While bacteria usually do not persist, continual recontamination has the same effect, prolonging the phase of chronicity. The regularly spaced invasions of capillary buds in this tissue give it, when freed of exudate, a granular appearance, hence the term *granulation tissue.*

Organization: The regular and uniform bridging by connective tissue

As resolution of the wound occurs and resorption of exudates takes place, capillary ingrowth and fibroplasia dominate. Organization begins to form a scar, or *cicatrix.* As collagen production increases, the fibroblasts become less active. The scar appears white and glistening because of the dominance of collagen.

Collagen is constantly remodeled.

Collagen does not lie as an inert bridging material but exists in a dynamic state in which synthesis and removal is slowly occurring. With time, collagen fibers become progressively stronger by increased bonding among the fibrils. Collagenases, the enzymes that degrade collagen, occur in wounds several years old. Even though wounds may be completely healed, they may break down if the animal experiences a severe systemic disease that represses collagen synthesis for long periods.

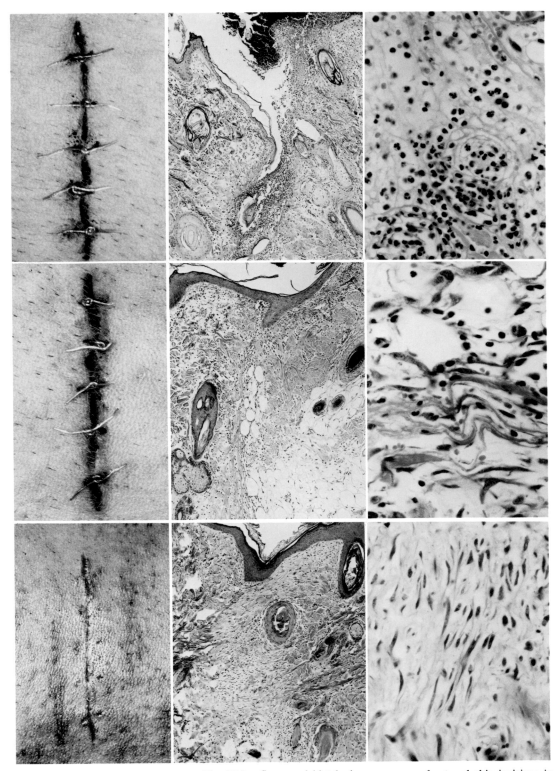

Fig. 20.2. Gross and histologic appearance of sutured skin incisions in abdominal skin, dog, at 2 (*top*), 5 (*center*), and 14 (*bottom*) days after incision.

Scabs retard epithelization.

Scabs form in wounds exposed to the air (Figs. 20.3 and 20.4). Although the dry exudate is a protective cover against pathogenic bacteria on the skin, it may also inhibit wound healing. The advancing epithelial cells do not attach to the scab and must grow beneath or circumvent the necrotic material. This is accomplished more quickly if the wound is kept moist and free of bacteria.

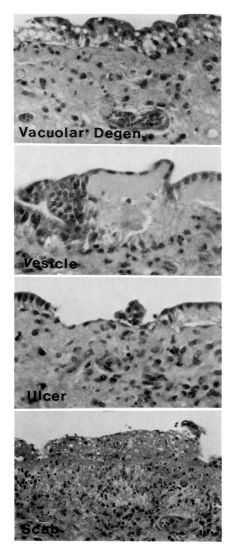

Fig. 20.3. Sequence of changes in bovine teat epithelium during staphylococcal mastitis. *Vacuolar degeneration* in epithelium, *microvesicles* formed by exuding plasma, *ulcer,* and *scab.*

Systemic disease inhibits healing.

Aging, protein deficiency, vitamin C deficiency, and several endocrine deficiencies are associated with inhibition of wound healing. Ascorbic acid deficiency markedly retards fibroplasia because this vitamin is required as a cofactor for proline hydroxylase. In the 1800s, seamen who developed scurvy noticed that scars several years old would break into open wounds.

Fibroplasia, extremely active in neonates, is delayed in the aged animal, perpetuating the chronicity of the healing process. In aged animals, elastic fiber degeneration can be identified as splitting and granulation of the fibers (*senile elastosis*). The deposition of collagen and of matrix material is also restricted in cartilage and bone of aged animals, which seriously affects wound healing in these tissues.

Wounds of starved animals heal slowly.

In starvation and protein depletion there is an impairment of collagen synthesis and granulation tissue formation. This seems to be most critical in proteins containing methionine and cystine. These sulfur-containing amino acids are important in the intermediate forms of collagen.

Cold inhibits wound healing.

Generally, wounds heal more slowly in cold weather, and experiments on poikilotherms have shown that the rate of wound healing is proportional to the temperature of the environment at which they are kept. A rise of 10°C results in a 2-fold increase in the speed of wound healing. In hibernating squirrels at 5°C, epithelization of granulation tissue is totally inhibited.

Many local factors inhibit wound healing.

Fibroplasia in wounds is inhibited by tissue debris and bacterial infection. Other, less important local factors include irradiation and foreign bodies such as talcum powder granules. Clinically, fibroplasia is enhanced by elevated temperature and by *debridement,* the removal of necrotic tissue.

Wound dehiscence

Dehiscence (the bursting open of a wound) is especially important in surgical incisions of the abdomen. Weakening of the sutured wound results from severe inflammation. Edema puts marked tension on sutures, which, if not properly placed, will fail to hold fascial planes and

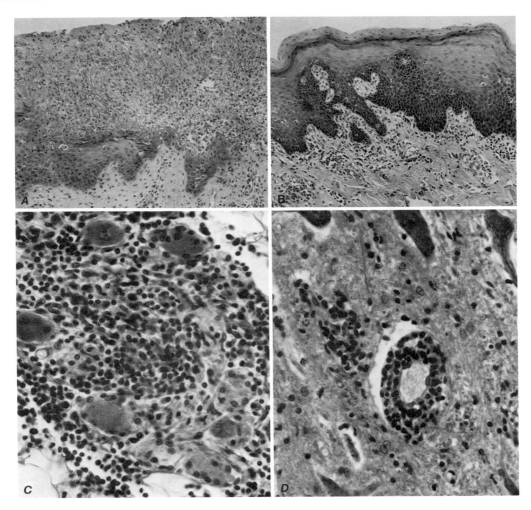

Fig. 20.4. Late-stage lesions, monkey with *Herpesvirus B*. A. Scab over lip ulcer, 7 days after appearance of first lip lesions. B. Healed epithelium with subepithelial lymphocytes, 12 days. C. Lymphocytic ganglionitis, trigeminal ganglion, 21 days. D. Lymphocytic perivasculitis, nucleus of trigeminal ganglion, brain.

peritoneum. *Movement* delays healing by persistent trauma; it also appears that exercise can delay healing through an effect on adrenal corticosteroid secretion. Vomiting, coughing, and any straining movement that puts pressure on the wound may precipitate dehiscence.

Mortality is high after wound dehiscence; this is largely due to bacterial infection, aided by contamination of the wound by soil and organic matter. *Peritonitis* (inflammation of the peritoneum) is often fatal and makes further attempts at wound suturing more difficult.

CONSEQUENCES OF CHRONIC INFLAMMATION AND ABNORMAL TISSUE HEALING

Hyperplasia

Stimulation of tissue growth that accompanies acute and chronic inflammation is stopped as tissue returns to normal. In some instances the irritant persists, causing tissue overgrowth that requires clinical attention.

Occasionally, in some species such as the horse, granulation tissue has a tendency to become excessive and may restrict function. This *keloid,* or "proud flesh," proliferates massively, often resembling tumor formation.

Epidermal hyperplasia is protective.

Hyperplasia of epithelium is a response to chronic irritation. In skin, this response is common in parasite infestations. Grossly, the skin becomes thickened, hairs disappear, and the expanded stratum corneum causes the epidermis to scale (Fig. 20.5). This barrier prevents a parasite and its toxins from interacting with tissue.

In viscera, hyperplasia of epithelium may lead to proliferative lesions that influence normal function. Hyperplasia of the epithelium of the terminal bronchioles in pneumonia can produce lesions that inhibit normal lung function. Several diseases of the intestine involve excessive proliferation of mucosal epithelium. Proliferative enteritis of pigs and of hamsters is associated with thickened intestinal walls made largely of reduplicated mucosal epithelium (Fig. 20.6).

Atrophy

Destruction of tissue during acute inflammation may lead to atrophy. A common response to enteric infection is atrophy of intestinal villi. Villi shrink from the normal, slender, elongate forms to short, stubby protuberances. The marked reduction of mucosal absorptive surface area results in malabsorption. *Villous atrophy* is due both to destruction of epithelium and to contraction of smooth muscle in the lamina propria of the villus, which pulls the villus toward the base of the gut wall. In transmissible gastroenteritis of piglets, the infecting virus has a tropism for epithelium of the upper villus; destruction causes the core of the villus to retract, resulting in shortened villi. In contrast, panleukopenia virus of cats, which replicates in crypt epithelium (killing off the progenitor cells that are destined to populate villous surfaces) also causes severe villous atrophy.

Chronic infection of the nasal cavity results in turbinate atrophy.

Atrophy of the bony and connective tissue components of the nasal turbinates is a conse-

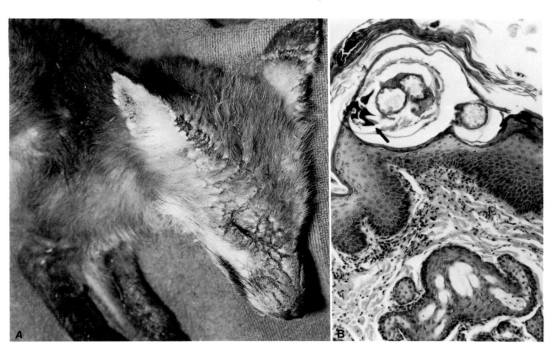

Fig. 20.5. Severe, diffuse, chronic dermatitis, fox with sarcoptic mange caused by *Sarcoptes scabei.* A. Extensive epidermal hyperplasia is responsible for thickening of skin. B. Parasite is present in cornified layers (note hooks, *arrow*).

Fig. 20.6. Chronic diffuse enteritis with dilatation of the intestinal lumen and thickening of the gut wall, hamster with proliferative ileitis.

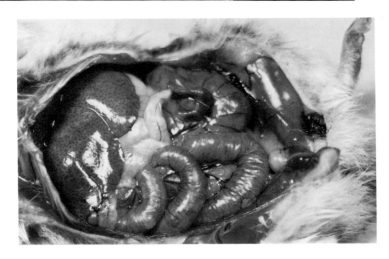

quence of chronic rhinitis. For example, gray collies with cylic hematopoiesis suffer recurring episodes of chronic mucopurulent rhinitis. After a few episodes the nasal turbinates have become smaller than those of normal dogs. *Atrophic rhinitis* is a major disease of swine (Fig. 20.7); tissue destruction is due to soluble toxins secreted by bacteria that colonize the turbinate surfaces (*Pasteurella multocida* and *Bordetella bronchiseptica* are the most often implicated).

REPAIR IN BONE

In the simple traumatic fracture of a long bone, the broken ends of the bone are disaligned and adjacent soft tissues are torn. Blood vessels are ruptured. *Hemorrhage* occurs throughout the fracture zone, and if blood seeps past the torn periosteum, it occurs in muscle. *Coagulation* of blood soon forms a clot that fills the spaces of the fracture. *Necrosis* occurs because of vascular damage; this develops in bone because the osteocyte, which depends on nutrients from canaliculi of the haversian system, is deprived of its precarious source of nutrition. Periosteum and marrow are better vascularized normally, so that necrosis is much less evident in these tissues. As trauma-induced *inflammation* develops, monocytes pass into the fracture area and transform into macrophages that play a major role in bone repair (Table 20.1).

Fracture is repaired by callus formation.

Within 48 hours after fracture, the blood clot is invaded by osteogenic cells of the deep layer of the periosteum, the endosteum, and the marrow. These cells proliferate at the margins of

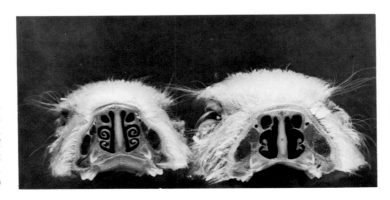

Fig. 20.7. Tissue destruction and atrophy, pig with atrophic rhinitis (normal nose, *left*). Purified toxin given intranasally produced rapid atrophy of nasal turbinates. (Photograph: Mark Dominick, *Am. J. Vet. Res.* 47:1532, 1986)

Table 20.1. Stages in fracture healing

1. Hematoma formation

2. Trauma-induced acute inflammation with edema and deposition of fibrin

3. Demolition: macrophages invade and remove fibrin, erythrocytes, debris

4. Granulation tissue formation: invasion of capillary buds and mesenchymal cells derived from periosteum and endosteum; pH low

5. Soft callus of woven bone and cartilage formation: mesenchymal osteoblasts differentiate to form bone or cartilage

6. Lamellar bone formation: woven bone removed by osteoblasts

7. Remodeling: continued osteoclast removal and osteoblast formation; external callus removed; internal callus hollowed to form bone marrow

the fracture and quickly invade the clot and adjacent necrotic areas (Fig. 20.8).

The *callus* is the tissue mass that connects fractured bone ends. Early, when the mass is granulation tissue, it is a "soft callus" and later, when formed of cartilage and bone, a "hard callus." If bone ends are inadequately immobilized, as is common in animals, the granulation tissue phase is prolonged and formation of hyaline cartilage is favored over bone formation in the callus.

Cartilage is formed early.

By 1 week proliferating cells have begun to differentiate into chondroblasts and cartilage is laid down. Matrix material released from the surface of chondroblasts is deposited in a halo surrounding the cell. In calcifying cartilage, tiny matrix vesicles are released that possess enzymes (alkaline phosphatase and enzymes for ATP-dependent calcium transport) that increase the local concentration of orthophosphate and lead to hydroxyapatite formation. At 7–10 days the pH in the callus increases, and this "alkaline tide" favors deposition of calcium salts.

The cartilage that forms has only a temporary existence and is eventually replaced by bone. The intercellular matrix calcifies, which causes the chondrocytes to die.

New bone is formed as cartilage disintegrates.

New trabeculae of bone are firmly cemented to old bone, even though the old bone ends may be dead. Osteocytes develop from pluripotential mesenchymal cells and fibroblasts and deposit

osteoid. As dead calcified cartilage disintegrates it is removed, and osteoblasts lay down osteoid that calcifies to form bone.

As the provisional bony callus is removed, osteoblasts lay down osteoid in a more orderly arrangement. The collagen molecules orient around blood vessels to form haversian systems.

Phagocytic cells are important in removal and rearrangement of the new bone. Osteoclasts, also phagocytic, are derived from bone marrow monocytes. The cancellous bone that is first laid down is gradually altered to form compact bone, and the callus continues to remodel itself. Eventually the original alignment of the bone is restored, and the thickened callus cannot be detected by palpation.

Osteomyelitis

Bacterial infection of the bone marrow commonly leads to progressive debilitating inflammatory disease and lameness. Osteomyelitis is often resistant to antibiotic therapy and persists until dead and infected bone chips are removed. Traumatized and dead pieces of bone become colonized with bacteria (so do orthopedic prostheses). "Polymicrobial" infections are common and usually involve symbiosis of aerobic and anaerobic bacteria, all held together in a matrix of bacterial polysaccharides. Adherence of most bacteria in microcolonies in tissues is through highly hydrated anionic exopolysaccharide polymers that bind to teichoic acid polymers (of gram-positive bacteria) or to lipopolysaccharides (of gram-negative bacteria).

HEALING IN THE JOINT CAPSULE

The joint capsule of synovial joints consists of an outer fibrous layer, continuous with the periosteum of the bone, and the synovial membrane or inner layer synovial membranes line the joint everywhere except over articular cartilage. Disease of the synovial joints is a cause of disability. *Arthritis,* inflammation of the joint, cripples both in its acute and chronic phases. Acute fibrinous arthritis is particularly important in swine, in which mycoplasmas, streptococci, and erysipelothrix bacilli are common causes of acute arthritis when they localize in the synovial membrane and joint cavity.

The extensive exudation in most acute forms of arthritis distort and efface the architecture of

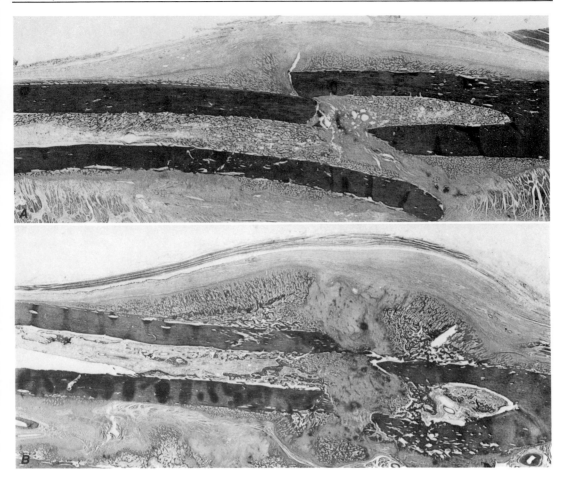

Fig. 20.8. Experimental bone fracture, dog. A. Ten days after fracture: swelling, increased vascularity, and residual hemorrhage. Callus (proliferating tissue) is formed by two sources: activated periosteum and activated endosteum. Resorption of old bone is limited. Trauma line contains a zone of debris (crushed tissue, extravasated blood, fibrin, bone fragments, and residual marrow). B. Large callus, 28 days after fracture. Callus is calcified, and there is layering of periosteal cells. Debris is inspissated and much has been removed. (Sections: American College of Veterinary Pathologists, Scientific Seminar, 1958)

the synovial membrane. Descriptions of early changes in membrane come from experimental studies. When staphylococci are injected into joints of rabbits, bacteria are phagocytized by synovial lining cells. Pyogenic arthritis is initiated by development of hyperemia and fluid exudation. Long filopodia develop on synovial cells, and they avidly take up bacteria. This is followed by rapid and intense neutrophil exudation.

Chronic arthritis involves fibrosis and synovial cell hyperplasia of the synovial membrane. These lesions tend to be self-sustaining; proliferative lesions into the synovial cavity provoke not only pain but a superimposed subtle inflammatory response. The chronic arthritis commonly seen in joints of aged animals begins as degenerative osteoarthropathy accompanied by fibrosing changes in the synovial membrane and synovial cell hyperplasia.

HEALING IN THE BRAIN

Inflammation of the brain, meninges, and spinal cord is called *encephalitis, meningitis,* and *myelitis,* respectively. The earliest events of inflammation (those that are involved in fluid accumulation) are critical in the brain because this organ cannot expand beyond the limits of the cranium. Even minimal swelling in the brain may cause neurologic signs. If swelling occurs in highly sensitive areas in the brain stem, death may occur.

Acute inflammation

Fluid accumulation within the brain substance, or neuropil, is separated classically into *brain swelling* (accumulation of fluid within glial cells) and *brain edema,* (accumulation of fluid in the extracellular spaces); in most cases, fluid is present at both sites. Astrocytes are most severely involved, and marked swelling of the

cell and its processes leads to secondary changes in adjacent myelin sheaths.

Purulent encephalitis is commonly caused by bacteria.

Exudation of inflammatory cells leads to serious consequences in the brain. Purulent encephalitis is nearly always due to bacterial infection. Neutrophils actively pass the capillary wall and accumulate in the neuropil. Bacteria most often arrive by way of the bloodstream, commonly during pyemia as metastatic emboli.

Purulent exudate in the neuropil tends to accumulate in microabscesses. If the animal survives, these abscesses become walled off by a capsule of connective tissue and lymphoid cells. Caseous necrotic material remains in the center of the abscess (Fig. 20.9).

Lymphocytic encephalitis is characteristic of viral infection.

Acute lymphoplasmacytic (also called "nonsuppurative" or "aseptic") encephalitis is usually

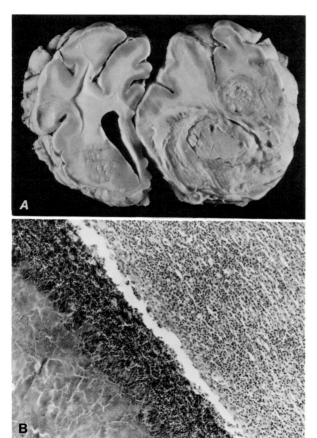

Fig. 20.9. Chronic focal purulent encephalitis with abscess formation in a cow. Abscesses consist of central areas of homogeneous necrotic debris (*bottom left*), margins of degenerate neutrophils, and capsules of inflammatory cells and connective tissue.

of viral origin. Most neurotropic viruses replicate in vascular structures prior to spreading to glia and neurons, but others arrive hematogenously or via nerve sheaths and affect neurons directly. The lymphoid response leads to accumulation of lymphocytes and often monocytes in pervascular spaces. Called *perivascular cuffing,* these inflammatory cell populations are often mixed; as disease progresses, plasmacytes appear. Plasmacytes can and do enter infected neurons although this process does not play a major role in recovery.

Repair

Healing in the brain occurs by proliferation of fibroblasts and glial cells along vascular networks. When the neuropil is punctured by a sterile instrument, the lesion heals by *astrocytic gliosis* and *fibrosis.* The lesion becomes filled with a fibrous core derived from the meninges and perivascular adventitia.

Astrocytes respond to injury.

The glial reaction to brain injury is rapid. Astrocytes are less vulnerable than are nerve cells and, if they are not destroyed during injury, react progressively to form a dendritic network around the wounded neuropil. Necrotic brain tissue initiates reactive astrocytosis. The *reactive astrocytes* (also called "fat astrocytes" or "gemistocytic astrocytes") are very large cells with homogeneous, acidophilic cytoplasm. They are stimulated by edema and ischemia and are most common in slowly progressing and diffusely sclerotic lesions. They develop at the margins of a lesion, and their cell processes extend into the affected area. Reactive astrocytes are phagocytic and may contain debris and microorganisms.

Oligodendrogliocytes are involved in demyelination.

Oligodendrogliocytes undergo acute swelling in injured areas. Their nuclei become pyknotic and the cytoplasm is vacuolated. These cells bear the same relation to myelin as do the Schwann cells of peripheral nerves, and they are most reactive in lesions characterized by extensive demyelination. The presence of several oligodendrogliocytes around a nerve cell body is referred to as *satellitosis.*

Microglia are phagocytic.

Microglia are migratory, actively phagocytic cells of the neuropil. They engulf lipids and degenerate portions of dendrites and necrotic neurons. In the process they accumulate large amounts of lipids and are referred to as *foam cells* (also "Gitter cells" or "lipid phagocytes"). *Neuronophagia,* the phagocytosis of nerve cells by microglia, should be distinguished from *satellitosis,* which is the residence of oligodendrogliocytes around neurons. In the process of reacting to injury in the brain, microglia undergo enlargement, hyperplasia, and autophagy. Nodules of hyperplastic microglia, called *glial nodules,* are characteristic of some rickettsial and viral encephalitides.

Monocytes also enter the neuropil.

Most of the macrophages found in inflammatory lesions in the brain in late stages of encephalitis originate from circulating monocytes. By labeling circulating monocytes with H^3-thymidine, it has been shown that these cells extravasate at sites of injury and transform into macrophages and that virtually all the macrophages at such sites bear the label in autoradiographs.

ADDITIONAL READING

Billingham, R. E., and Silvers, W. K. A note on the fate of skin autografts and homografts and on the healing of cutaneous wounds in hibernating squirrels. *Ann. Surgery* 152:975, 1960.

Page, R. C., et al. Pathogenesis of the chronic inflammatory lesion induced by group A streptococcal cell walls. *Lab. Invest.* 30:568, 1974.

Ross, R., et al. Wound healing and collagen formation. *J. Cell. Biol.* 44:645, 1970.

Rothschild, K. J., et al. Polypeptide transforming growth factors isolated from bovine sources and used for wound healing in vivo. *Science* 219:1329, 1983.

Schilling, J. A. Wound healing. *Physiol. Rev.* 48:374, 1968.

Squier, C. A., and Kremak, C. R. Myofibroblasts in healing palatal wounds of the beagle dog. *J. Anat.* 130:585, 1980.

Van Hattum, A. H., et al. A model for the study of epithelial migration in wound healing. *Virchows Arch.* [B] 30:221, 1979.

White, B. N., et al. Wound healing. *Proc. Soc. Exp. Biol. Med.* 101:353, 1959.

Sepsis and Septicemia

21

PRIMARY FOCI OF BACTERIAL INFECTION

The disease that results from pathogenic bacteria in the blood is called *septicemia.* The interaction of bacteria with leukocytes and endothelium causes fever and other manifestations of infection. More important, the circulation of pathogenic bacteria leads to dissemination of infection to important organs such as lung, kidney, and liver. This in turn induces a group of clinical signs that constitute septicemia (e.g., myalgia, respiratory difficulty, urinary abnormalities, and in severe cases, shock).

Although viruses, fungi, protozoa, and other microorganisms can enter the bloodstream and be disseminated to tissue, nearly all cases of septicemia involve bacteria. We will especially consider septicemia caused by gram-negative (e.g., *Escherichia coli*) and gram-positive (e.g., streptococci) bacteria, for they are the common etiologic agents that produce this condition.

Initiation of bacterial infection

Wounds that become infected with pathogenic bacteria often lead to the systemic spread of infection. Localized infections usually begin in wounds that penetrate epithelial barriers. Bacteria enter tissue along with tiny particles of dirt and inorganic debris. They replicate, release toxins, and cause local tissue destruction and inflammation. Microorganisms and their toxins escape local confinement, pass the regional lymph node barrier, and flow into lymphatics and from there to the bloodstream.

Traumatic wounds are common causes of septicemia.

Microorganisms seep into lymphatic vessels around contaminated wounds. A clinical finding in skin of dilated reddened lymphatics that radiate away from the wound and centrally toward the regional lymph node indicates that the patient is in trouble.

Traumatic wounds in animals are usually infected with several bacterial species, and in some cases these different populations have an interdependent relationship. In *synergy,* the presence of one bacterial species enhances the growth of another.

Anaerobic bacteria are the major residents of skin, teeth, and mucous membranes of normal animals. They seem to need to avoid oxygen as much as the host requires it. *Bacteroides* spp., which are commonly mixed with aerobic pathogens in abscesses, are a common cause of anaerobic septicemia in most animal species.

There are several factors other than bacteria that promote septicemia. Generalized inflammatory processes in skin or mucous membranes may predispose to the entry of bacteria into the lymphatics and bloodstream. Influenza virus will cause diffuse serous rhinitis with focal ulceration and facilitate passage of *Haemophilus* spp. and some other bacterial pathogens through the respiratory epithelial barrier into the bloodstream (Fig. 21.1). In some cases of influenza, the inflammatory lesion provides a growth factor in nasal tissue that enhances bacterial replication.

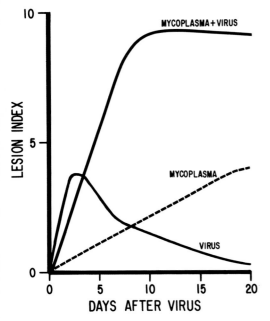

Fig. 21.1. Effects of viral infection on myco-plasmosis. (Data from Schoeb et at., *Vet. Pathol.* 22:272, 1985)

Infections that ascend from body orifices can cause septicemia.

Ascending infections are particularly important in the genitourinary tract. Localized in the bladder, bacteria may pass into the ureter to the kidney to cause nephritis and ultimately septicemia. Infection of the umbilical cord by *Escherichia coli* is a common cause of systemic infection and septicemia in neonates, particularly young calves.

Infection in visceral organs may lead to septicemia.

Bacterial infections that localize within various organs are common causes of disseminated infection and septicemia. Pyometra, mastitis, enteritis, and respiratory infections all may lead to septicemia. Large numbers of bacteria drain into and overload the phagocytic capacity of the lymphatics and thus are shed into the bloodstream. The bovine uterus, which is largely an anaerobic environment, normally harbors a variety of both aerobic and anaerobic bacteria. *Corynebacterium pyogenes* is the major bacterial pathogen, and recent studies suggest synergy between *C. pyogenes* and *Fusobacterium ne-*

crophorum (an anaerobe) in bovine metritis. Most infections occur at the time of ovulation, and clinical signs of pyometra occur some days after ovulation.

Covert infections may underlie septicemia.

Less obvious *covert infections* of body orifices can also cause sepsis: infected teeth, pustular tonsils, or reflux of bacteria from oviduct to abdominal cavity are all covert ways that sepsis can occur. In older animals, infected teeth are especially important in dissemination of bacteria into the bloodstream. Dental calculi are composed of masses of aggregated bacterial species (Fig 21.2) and are associated with gingivitis and dissemination of bacteria into the bloodstream.

Consequences of bacterial infection

If pathogenic bacteria are not destroyed at the site of infection, several different types of disease may follow: (1) localized infection with purulent inflammation and abscesses; (2) generalized infection, a spectrum from chronic disseminated abscessation and pyemia to peracute septicemia characterized by sudden death, the only meager gross evidence of inflammation being a watery putrid exudate in serous cavities and severe hyperemia; (3) toxemia from liberation of toxins that produce major lesions, despite localization and trapping of bacterial cells (e.g., clostridial myositis and tetanus); and (4) postinfectious immunologic disease in which syndromes of encephalitis, glomerulonephritis, or arthritis develop after the acute infection (caused by interaction of bacterial antigens with host antibodies or lymphocytes).

THE LYMPH NODE BARRIER

Microorganisms that survive local inflammatory processes at sites of infection migrate through lymphatics to regional lymph nodes. Arriving in afferent lymph vessels on the cortical surface of the node, they begin to percolate through the reticular cell–macrophage meshwork of the subcapsular sinuses.

Long dendritic tentacles on reticular cells avidly trap bacteria. As bacteria are phagocytized and destroyed, chemotactic factors and pyrogens are released that initiate the local acute inflammatory response and the systemic signs of bacterial infection.

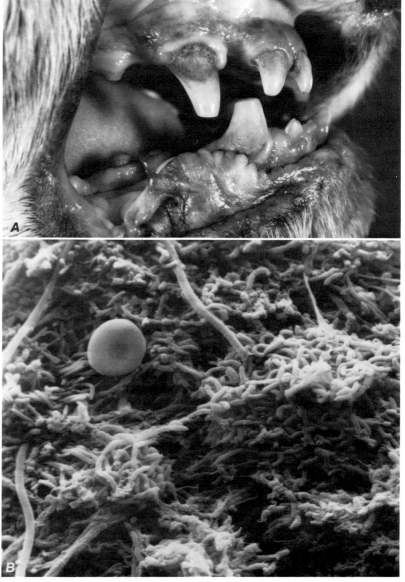

Fig. 21.2. Microbial plaque, tooth, dog. A. Supragingival calculi with fibrotic gingivae. B. Streptococci attached to large filamentous bacterium, probably *Actinomyces* sp. (scanning electron micrograph).

Microbial antigens are exposed to lymphoid cells.

The escape route for bacteria from the subcapsular sinuses is through the peritrabecular or intermediate sinuses. These sinuses surround the cortical parenchyma, which contains B lymphocytes in germinal centers and T lymphocytes in marginal zones. From the host's stand-point, it is essential to trap bacteria and degrade their antigens at these sites. As antigens are processed, they are passed along reticular cell dendrites and carried to germinal centers where they interact with B lymphocyte progenitors to stimulate production of antibody-forming plasmacytes.

Passing into the meshwork of the lymph node

medulla, bacteria are surrounded not only by macrophages but by columns of plasmacytes in the medullary cords. This is a plasmacyte-filled end of the funnel of reticular cell meshworks. In immune animals, it is in the medullary cords that bacterial migration is absolutely and finally prevented. Antibodies released by plasmacytes in the cords opsonize bacteria in the sinus lymph and present the bacterial clumps to activated macrophages.

Bacterial virulence

Bacteria produce disease by secreting soluble products that act as exotoxins, pyrogens, proteases, and chemotactic factors or by liberating structural components, such as endotoxin, a part of bacterial cell walls. As streptococci invade tissue, they liberate many different enzymes and toxic peptides. *Streptokinase* is a plasmin activator that initiates fibrinolytic dissolution of clots, and *hyaluronidase* depolymerizes connective tissue ground substance. These factors provide a tissue fluid medium that promotes replication of the streptococci, allowing their spread through the connective tissues. *Streptolysin* O is a prototype extracellular lysin (similar to those produced by clostridia) that binds to membrane cholesterol so that holes are formed in the plasma membrane and cytolysis occurs. Streptolysin O is capable of causing degranulation and lysis of leukocytes, and also causes suppression of chemotaxis. If phagocytized, a different protease, streptolysin S, may act intracellularly to kill leukocytes.

If the bactericidal processes within the lymph node sinuses are insufficient to kill virulent bacteria, multiplication of bacteria begins to dominate the balance between host defense and bacterial survival. Replication increases logarithmically within the milieu of exuding plasma proteins, degranulating neutrophils, and activated macrophages. Virulent bacteria are released into the efferent lymph to circulate via the thoracic duct into the bloodstream.

BACTEREMIA

Bacteremia is the presence of bacteria in the blood. It may occur silently or as the prelude to severe systemic disease. Bacteremia occurs far more often than does disease, however, for the highly responsive macrophages lining the si-

nuses of the liver and spleen effectively process circulating bacteria.

Removal of bacteria from the bloodstream

Bacterial clearance depends on the characteristics of the infecting organism. Avirulent bacteria are rapidly removed; virulent bacteria are not completely removed, and a portion of the population remains in low numbers until a secondary bacteremia occurs.

Bloodstream clearance varies with type of bacteria.

Although avirulent bacteria are rapidly removed from blood, the rate of clearance varies according to the species of bacteria; that is, staphylococci are removed much faster than *E. coli*. When 1×10^9 bacteria are infused into the jugular vein of pigs, *Staphylococcus aureus* is cleared rapidly with few lung lesions. Infusion of *E. coli* or *Pseudomonas aeruginosa* results in much slower clearance and leads to pulmonary hypertension (increased pulmonary vascular resistance), systemic hypotension, and inflammatory lung lesions.

The most virulent bacteria are not totally removed from the blood, but numbers remain low until a secondary bacteremia occurs that either leads to death or to activation of immune responses and recovery of the host (Fig. 21.3).

Bloodstream clearance varies with species.

Given proportionately equal numbers of bacteria according to weight, the rabbit clears *E. coli* in 5 minutes and the guinea pig in 25 minutes, while the mouse requires over 50 minutes.

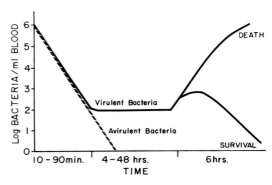

Fig. 21.3. Persistence of bacteremia in infection with bacteria of varying virulence.

These studies in rodents also translate into differences in larger animals.

Circulating bacteria are effectively removed during passage through the viscera. The liver and spleen are major organs for clearance in most animals. In liver, the Kupffer cells avidly trap bacteria slowly percolating through the sinusoids. In the spleen, blood flows through the tortuous channels of the reticular sheaths surrounding the terminal capillaries, and in this marginal zone the spleen effectively removes circulating bacteria.

In pigs, *lungs* are the major site of clearance and remove 60–80% of bacteria circulating in the venous system. In dogs, at the other extreme, only 10–20% of bacteria are removed from the lungs. Ruminants are between these extremes; the lungs in cattle and sheep will remove about 30% of circulating bacteria. The porcine lung is unusual due to a component of intravascular macrophages—macrophages that attach to the endothelium of the pulmonary capillaries, especially in neonatal piglets. Because the porcine lung so effectively traps bacteria, it is also more susceptible to pulmonary inflammatory disease.

Bacterial clearance varies with age.

An accurate method of measuring clearance of bacteria experimentally is to radioactively label bacterial cells, inject them intravenously, and follow the rate of disappearance of radioactivity in blood samples taken periodically. When *newborn* piglets (which lack antibodies and other opsonins) are injected with labeled salmonellae, clearance is slow. Bacteria are taken up chiefly in the spleen; small numbers of organisms are removed in the liver and lung. In adult pigs, which have activated macrophages, opsonins, and higher levels of complement, bacteria are more rapidly removed by the lungs and liver. Small numbers are also removed by the spleen, but only traces are found in other organs.

Host mechanisms
Macrophages acquire innate resistance to reinfection.

Listeria, brucellae, and the mycobacteria are virulent bacteria that replicate successfully within macrophages. During initial infection, macrophages develop a resistance that lasts for several weeks following infection (resistance is unrelated to specific antibacterial antibody). Subsequent infection with the same or similar organisms is followed by more rapid and efficient destruction of bacteria. For example, in cells from normal mice, inactivation of intracellular salmonellae does not begin for about 10 minutes and hardly more than 50% of the bacteria are killed. The killing of *Salmonella typhimurium* in cells of previously infected mice begins immediately after phagocytosis and proceeds rapidly until every intracellular organism has been killed.

Antibacterial antibody does not exert a profound effect on this type of reactivity. Animals infected with salmonellae are equally microbicidal for listeria. The augmented cells, once activated, are not specifically directed against the infectious agent that induced their activation.

Antibody identifies the bacterial cell.

Selective immunologic destruction of bacteria is mediated by antibody molecules in two ways: by opsonization (i.e., attaching to bacterial surfaces and enhancing their phagocytosis by macrophages and circulating granulocytes) and by affecting the complement system on the surface of the bacterial cells and inducing plasmolysis.

The simplest way to demonstrate *opsonization* is to mix two dilute suspensions of bacteria with leukocytes obtained from the buffy coat of centrifuged blood. To one sample, saline is added; to the other, specific antiserum. When smears are made after several minutes of incubation, it can be seen that neutrophils have engulfed large numbers of bacteria in the preparation containing antibodies. In the control, the neutrophils contain few if any bacteria. The *phagocytic index* is the number of bacteria ingested by 100 neutrophils. When this is determined on immune and normal (control) sera, an *opsonic index* can be calculated as a ratio between the phagocytic indices of the two sera. It is the measure of the "sensitizing power" of the serum of an infected animal for phagocytes.

Complement cooperates with antibody to produce bacteriolysis.

Invading organisms are identified by antibody and are then attacked by the components of the complement system. The antibody molecule, when it combines with antigens in the bacterium, serves to activate complement, which actually does the work of destroying the organism.

During lysis of the bacterial cell, complement components C5, C6, C7, C8, and C9 become enmeshed in the surface membrane of the bacterium. They aggregate to form a doughnut-shaped body with a central hole penetrating into the bacterium. This allows leakage of water and ions. Bacterial cells swell until the plasma membrane ruptures and the cytosol spills out.

Peptidoglycans on the cell walls of gram-positive cocci activate serum complement directly via the alternate pathway and provide "natural" immunity to some circulating staphylococci and streptococci.

SEPTICEMIA

Septicemia (from Gr. *septikos,* putrid, plus *haima,* blood) is the systemic disease associated with pathogenic microorganisms in the blood (i.e., septic bacteremia accompanied by fever, dyspnea, leukocytosis, hemorrhages, and severe systemic illness). Known generally as "blood poisoning," septicemia is always a serious clinical disease. Signs of intravascular coagulation and shock, which appear in late stages of septicemia, suggest a grave prognosis. Survival depends on therapy to shift the balance of bacterial virulence and host resistance. Animals with severe burns, diabetes mellitus, uremia, and acquired or congenital immunodeficiencies are especially susceptible to septicemia.

Bacteria can be isolated from venous blood in septicemia (Table 21.1). Organisms are present in high titers in peracute cases (e.g., anthrax in cattle, swine erysipelas, and colisepticemia in birds and the newborn of several species) (Fig. 21.4). Massive liberation of endotoxins, exotoxins, and bacterial peptide fragments rapidly lead to coma and death.

Septicemia associated with foci of infection in tissue is often less acute. Purulent metritis, mastitis, infected catheters, and abscesses of skin, teeth, and mucous membranes are associated with the sporadic release of pathogenic bacteria into the bloodstream, which are detected only intermittently. If the patient has been treated with antibiotics, it may not be possible to isolate any organism.

Table 21.1.   **Bacteria isolated from the blood in canine septicemia**

Bacterial Species	Dog
Streptococci	11
Staphylococci	34
Enterobacteriaceae	29
Anaerobes (clostridia and bacteroides)	9
Corynebacterium spp.	4
Actinobacillus spp.	. . .
Others	13

Note: Cultures of blood grew bacteria in 23% of 581 sick dogs.

Source: Data from Hirsch et al., *J. Am. Vet. Med. Assoc.* 184:175, 1984.

FOCUS

Anthrax

This classic disease of animals and man is caused by *Bacillus anthracis,* a gram-positive, spore-forming bacterium. Discovered by Robert Koch, *B. anthracis* was used by Metchnikof in his classic studies on phagocytosis. It infects most mammals and can cause a rapidly fatal septicemia. Goats, sheep, cattle, horses, pigs, and dogs are susceptible (in that order).

The bloodstream of septicemic animals swarms with chains of capsulated, square-ended bacilli. The host is killed by a combination of the lethal peptide toxins and massive amounts of antiphagocytic capsular material, which prevents opsonization and killing of *B. anthracis.* When the host animal dies, vegetative bacilli from the carcass are rapidly killed by putrefaction. However, bacilli contaminate the soil and form highly resistant spores that survive for decades.

▶

The absence of anthrax in an area for several years followed by an explosive outbreak with large death losses may lead to popular misconceptions regarding the origin of the disease. *B. anthracis* has been widely studied in the United States, Great Britain, and the Soviet Union in relation to biological warfare. In theory, airborne dissemination of spores could devastate livestock populations. Popular fears have been promoted in the press, adding to the generally popular fear of anthrax.

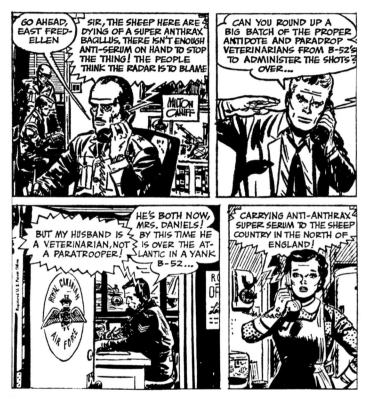

Reprinted with special permission of King Features Syndicate, Inc.

Grazing mammals ingest spores, which enter through mucous membranes, aided by local lesions. Cutaneous infection (common in man) is rare in animals. *Pulmonary anthrax,* a particularly lethal form, results from inhalation of spore-laden grasses and dust. Infection can also be transmitted by insects; this mode, however, has not been clearly established.

Infection in ruminant animals begins as lymphangiitis and lymphadenitis. Bacteria rapidly spread to the circulation. In ruminants dead of anthrax, blood is thick and dark and hemorrhages are common in mucous and serous membranes. Viscera are swollen and congested, particularly the spleen, which is so large and soft that it may rupture spontaneously. Histologically, splenic architecture is masked by the massive infusion of blood.

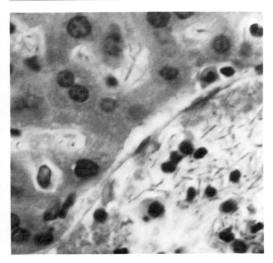

Fig. 21.4. Septicemia, anthrax bacilli in sinusoids of liver.

Pathologic changes

Liver, spleen, and lymph nodes are always hyperemic and swollen in septicemia, because these organs remove most of the bacteria. In spleen, virulent bacteria are trapped in splenic reticular sheaths and ingested by macrophages. In the peracute septicemias, bacteria may stick

to and be phagocytized by endothelial cells.

In contrast to the rapid clearance of avirulent bacteria, clearance of pathogens is retarded by bacterial virulence factors that suppress effective attachment to macrophages, phagocytosis, or killing. Although many virulent bacteria are destroyed, some remain to replicate and kill the host's phagocytes. Clinical and hematologic signs of septicemia arise from interaction of circulating bacteria with leukocytes and platelets during this secondary bacteremia (Table 21.2). Substances responsible for induction of fever and leukocytosis (and granulopoiesis) are bacterial peptides that differ from those of the bacterium associated with chemotaxis.

If skin is biopsied, bacteria can usually be found in endothelial cells in most cases of septicemia. Vascular lesions may be subtle but usually involve deposition of complement, plasma globulins, and fibrin. Drs. L.-Cl. Schulz, W. Drommer, and others at the Institute of Veterinary Pathology at the Hannovarian veterinary school have used swine erysipelas as a model of septicemia and tissue localization. *Erysipelothrix rhusiopathiae* circulates to cause severe cardiovascular lesions. Bacteria stick to and are phagocytized by endothelial cells. Subsequently, monocytes stick to endothelial surfaces and fibrin is deposited at such a rate that a systemic coagulopathy often results.

Table 21.2. Clinicopathologic signs in septicemia

Sign	Mechanism
Hyperemia	Vascular paralysis
Fever	Bacteria-neutrophil interaction with release of endogenous pyrogens that act on hypothalamus
Leukocytosis	Release of splenic and bone marrow neutrophils followed by "normal" leukocyte counts due to consumption in reactions with bacteria; toxic neutrophils in blood smear; leukocytopenia in terminal stages due to trapping in lung and other viscera
Thrombocytopenia	Marked in terminal stages due to trapping in thrombi
Coagulopathy	Coagulation factors depleted due to initiation of clotting mechanism; fibrin split products and fibrin monomers appear in late stages
Hypotension	Blood pressure diminished in terminal stages because of both venous pooling in viscera and decreased cardiac output
Anemia	Common but limited in amount and transient; caused both by complexing of endotoxins on erythrocytes and by trapping of cells in splenic cords
Hypoxemia	Terminal stages, from decreased cardiac output and increasing vasoconstriction
Hypoglycemia	Initial hyperglycemia followed by progressive decrease in blood glucose; associated with systemic metabolic deficiency in terminal septicemia
Hypertriglyceridemia	Impaired lipid disposal and activation of lipid clearing enzymes
Hypoinsulinemia	Impaired pancreatic islet perfusion and increased catecholamine output

Lungs

Death in septicemia is usually due to respiratory failure reinforced by terminal metabolic disease. The lungs are large, wet, and hyperemic, and hemorrhages are commonly present throughout the lung parenchyma. On cut surfaces, the frothy fluid is an index of pulmonary edema associated both with the shock state and with endotoxin-induced damage (in gram-negative bacterial sepsis). Histologically, the engorged capillaries of the pulmonary bed distend the alveolar walls (Fig. 21.5).

In early septicemia, lungs clear a significant portion of bacteria from the bloodstream. High lung clearance occurs in some animal species. Susceptibility to acute respiratory failure in septicemia occurs in those species whose lungs trap large numbers of pathogenic bacteria. For ex-

ample, lung injury is more apt to occur in septicemia of pigs than in that of dogs.

Pulmonary capillary endothelium is directly injured.

As septic shock progresses, expansion of the capillary bed is accompanied by slowing of blood flow, margination and accumulation of neutrophils at the periphery of the vessels, and polymerization of fibrin. Direct endothelial injury is caused by toxins from gram-positive bacteria. Anthrax toxin, experimentally injected intravenously, produces massive diffuse pulmonary edema and death within 2 hours. Microscopically, plasma rapidly exudes, forming blisters in the endothelium as it passes into the interstitial areas of the alveolar septae. This acute vascular injury is followed immediately by pulmonary capillary *microthrombosis*.

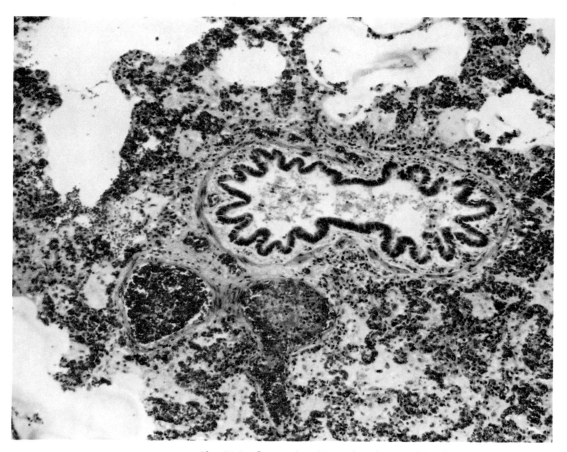

Fig. 21.5. Lung, pig with septicemia caused by *Salmonella cholera-suis*. There is severe hyperemia with fluid, macrophages, and extravasated blood in alveoli. Blood is also present in the bronchiole.

Microthrombosis, coupled with catecholamine-induced vasoconstriction, further retards blood flow and increases pressure in the pulmonary artery and right side of the heart. Although neutrophils engulf and become engorged with fibrin, they are not sufficiently effective and fibrin accumulates within the capillaries.

Dilated lymph vessels are blocked by fibrin.

Lymph vessels of the lung are expanded as edema fluids are drained from the lungs. They become filled with fibrin, which obstructs drainage. Fibrin is prominent in streptococcal and pasteurella septicemias, and fibrin membranes commonly line surfaces of alveolar septae.

The late effects of microthrombosis and disseminated intravascular coagulation can be helped by heparin therapy. If fluid can be rapidly removed by dilation of subpleural lymphatics, the killing effect of pulmonary edema is decreased.

Liver

Hyperemia of the liver is intense, and there may be centrolobular necrosis. Sinusoids are distended, and the reactivity of Kupffer cells varies from diffuse *reticuloendothelial hyperplasia* to *microabscess formation* (especially in the area of the central vein). Hepatocytes are often vacuolated, and because of the shift to anaerobic metabolism, glycogen is depleted.

In gram-negative sepsis (or experimental endotoxemia), liver sinusoids are expanded, with destruction of endothelium and accumulation of platelets and neutrophils. The liver removes bacterial endotoxins that are released into the portal circulation from the intestine. The endotoxins, which are fragments of cell walls of gram-negative bacteria, are removed by Kupffer cells. Liver necrosis can occur when large amounts of endotoxin pass into the portal vein.

Skeletal muscle

Sepsis is followed by rapid onset of muscle wasting, protein depletion, and urea excretion. Although some wasting is due to anorexia, most skeletal muscle breakdown results from protein degradation. Amino acids are released from limb muscles at rates 3–5 times normal and are used by the liver for gluconeogenesis, synthesis

of acute phase reactants, and other substances used in tissue healing.

Macrophage cytokines switch muscle metabolism.

A cytokine recently identified as *interleukin-1* is released from monocytes during septicemia and acts on skeletal muscle to stimulate protein degradation to form amino acids. In the muscle cell there are increased prostaglandin synthesis, lysosomal activation, and disappearance of muscle protein. Plasma from septic patients contains a proteolytic factor (probably a prostaglandin fragment) that causes muscle breakdown in vitro. *Myalgia* that accompanies systemic infection is probably due to protein degradation and amino acid depletion in the muscle cell.

Heart

Subendocardial hemorrhages, particularly of the ventricles, are characteristic of septicemia. Exudation also occurs in epicardium and endocardium. *Foci of necrosis* may develop in the myocardium, and bacterial colonization is apt to be seen around vascular walls at necropsy. Cardiac necrosis results from the combined effects of direct bacterial or endotoxic injury, excess circulating catecholamines, and the excess work load induced by increased pulmonary resistance.

Endocrine glands

Adrenal hyperemia is always intense, and hemorrhages are usually present in the cortex. Severe diffuse adrenal *cortical hemorrhage* is most common in the horse and is typical of severe human meningococcal infection (Waterhouse-Friderichsen syndrome). Lipids in cortical cells are depleted, and the cells change to an active metabolic state.

Adrenal cortical hormones protect in septicemia.

The normal pituitary-adrenal response is necessary for survival of the animal with septicemia. In an experiment with adrenalectomized mice maintained on graded doses of cortisol and inoculated with streptococci, survival was greatest in groups whose maintenance cortisol most closely resembled the normal. Mortality progressively increased toward the extremes of hypo- and hyperadrenocorticism.

In acute generalized infection the major corticosteroid hormones are stimulated early and become markedly elevated. Increases occur in the incubation or prodromal stages of disease, although high levels are seen only in the late stages of disease. In chronic disease, such as tuberculosis, adrenal cortical secretion is usually depressed. The fetal adrenal cortex undergoes hyperplasia during infection, and elevated levels of adrenocorticoids are considered a mechanism of abortion.

Severe, overwhelming, complicated infections are associated with increased levels of plasma corticoids. In swine erysipelas, plasma hydrocortisone levels are progressively elevated until death (Fig. 21.6). In survivors, they return to normal during the recovery phase.

Slow rates of corticoid clearance due to liver impairment or shock help to increase cortical steroid hormone levels. Hemorrhage and necrosis of the adrenal may occur in overwhelming infections in some species and are a manifestation of *disseminated intravascular coagulation* in the presence of shock.

Hyperactivity of the adrenal cortex also precipitates necrosis; a functional cortex is necessary in the development of hemorrhage following toxin injection. Lesions of septicemia are reduced by treatment with drugs that depress endogenous adrenal hyperactivity.

Hypoglycemia is a response to adrenal catecholamines.

Hypoglycemia is a direct consequence of increased plasma catecholamines, which increase the rate of glucose oxidation. A progressive de-

cline of blood glucose is indicative of impending death. Initially, amino acid production and utilization are increased, and up to 90% of newly produced amino acids are used for glucose synthesis.

Eventually, there is impaired gluconeogenesis from amino acids and a simultaneous rise of lactate with fall of glucose. When dogs are given live *E. coli* intravenously, they develop hypoglycemia, hypoinsulinemia, and hypertriglyceridemia. Endotoxins of gram-negative bacteria interfere with activation of lipid-clearing enzymes, leading to impaired lipid disposal.

Hypoinsulinemia accompanies hypoglycemia.

Depression of insulin is probably due both to catecholamine activity and to impaired pancreatic islet perfusion. The pathologic, diabeteslike glucose tolerance curves in late septicemia indicate that there is also a problem of glucose utilization. At any rate, abnormal blood glucose levels tend to impair phagocytic function in some unknown way and to augment the shock state due to suppression of reticuloendothelial clearance.

Thyroxin depletion

Increased cell uptake and metabolism of thyroxin (T_4) occurs in bacterial sepsis due to increased phagocytic activity. An early depletion of the T_4 pool is followed by rebound phenomena with increased plasma T_4, probably a host defense mechanism in which phagocytes use the iodine in T_4 for a peroxidase–hydrogen peroxide system for iodination and killing of bacteria.

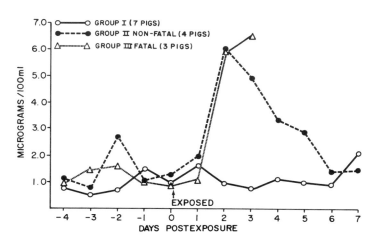

Fig. 21.6. Plasma hydrocortisone levels in pigs with erysipelas. Group I is a control group, II is survivors, and III is animals that died. (Data from Wood, *Cornell Vet.* 61:596, 1971)

Skin

Hyperemia in the septicemic animal, caused by blood-filled capillaries in the dermis, indicates the ominous sign of *vascular paralysis.* Hyperemic skin tends to be blanched in some areas, giving an overall appearance of blotchiness. This is especially apparent in white animals, such as pigs with erysipelas. The cold extremities seen in final stages are due to the combined effects of decreased cardiac output and arterial vasoconstriction and venous pooling.

Maculopapular rashes seen in some septicemias are due to widespread but focal vascular necrosis and thrombosis. They usually contain the causal bacteria. Cutaneous lesions resemble those of the endotoxin-induced Shwartzman reaction, but immunoglobulins and complement do not play major roles; it is probable that immunologic phenomena are involved in some of these skin lesions.

Kidney

Elevated blood urea nitrogen (BUN), an index of renal failure, occurs in terminal stages of septicemia as a manifestation of hypotension and severe cell swelling of renal tubular epithelium. Despite widespread evidence of disseminated intravascular coagulation in lungs, renal glomeruli are not usually greatly altered structurally in septicemia. Septic emboli and infarction may occur if the animal survives into a subacute process.

In gram-negative septicemia (e.g., salmonellosis), *bilateral renal cortical necrosis* accompanies severe endotoxemia. Septicemic salmonellosis in swine is frequently accompanied by lesions with hyalin ("fibrinoid") necrosis and degeneration in renal interlobular arteries. Dr. Kurt Nordstoga, at the National Veterinary Institute of Norway, has proposed that these lesions represent the generalized Shwartzman reaction; that is, they are a systemic effect of bacterial endotoxin and result from this progression: vasodilation → stasis → erythrocyte disintegration and fibrin deposition.

LOCAL MASSIVE NECROSIS

Large areas of necrosis sometimes develop that are not infected with bacteria or other microbes. Massive neoplasms that outgrow their blood supply, very large hematomas, and noninfectious infarcts are examples of necrotic tissue that undergo enzymatic dissolution and evoke neutrophilic leukocytosis, fever, and other manifestations of sepsis. These lesions are sepsis by definition, even though the bacterial component implied in the definition is not obvious.

ADDITIONAL READING

Dalldorf, F. G., et al. Transcellular permeability and thrombosis of capillaries in anthrax toxemia. *Lab. Invest.* 21:42, 1969.

Dehring, D. J., et al. Comparison of live bacteria infusions in a porcine model of acute respiratory failure. *J. Surg. Res.* 34:151, 1983.

Hirsh, D. C., et al. Blood culture of the canine patient. *J. Am. Vet. Med. Assoc.* 184:175, 1984.

Nordstoga, K., and Aasen, A. O. Hepatic changes in late canine endotoxin shock. *Acta Pathol. Microbiol. Scand.* [A] 87:335, 1979.

Olson, J. D., et al. Aspects of bacteriology and endocrinology of cows with pyometra and retained fetal membarnes. *Am. J. Vet. Res.* 45:2251, 1984.

Schulz, L-Cl., et al. Experimental erysipelas in different species as a model for systemic connective tissue disease. *Beitr. Pathol.* 154:1, 1975.

Thomson, G. W., et al. Endotoxin induced disseminated intravascular coagulation in cattle. *Can. J. Comp. Med. Vet. Sci.* 38:457, 1974.

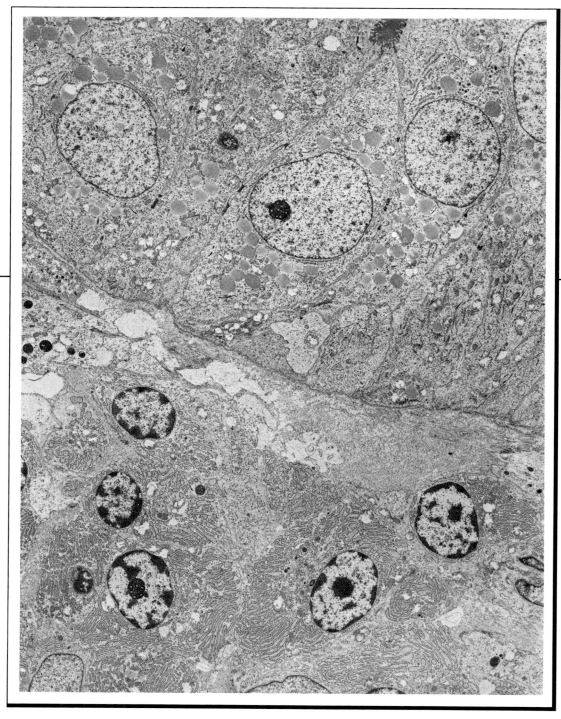

Plasmacytes below surface of uterine mucosa, dog with cystic endometrial hyperlasia. The nuclei have "cartwheel" forms, and the cytoplasm is filled with antibody-producing endoplasmic reticulum.

6 IMMUNITY

IN the broadest sense *immunity is resistance to disease.* An animal is considered immune when it is resistant to a known disease process. In common usage, however, immunity usually implies resistance to *infectious disease.* The word originated to describe immunity to some of the great animal and human plagues, many of which are still serious causes of death, especially in young animals. When born into an environment of reasonable temperature, given adequate food and water, and not exposed to predators, young animals are at greatest risk from infectious diseases. Various biologic mechanisms for resistance have evolved to deal with these pathogenic microbes. These same mechanisms also operate against toxic chemicals, tissue grafts, and neoplasms, but in none of these do the mechanisms of resistance and recovery play the important role that they do in infectious diseases.

All living animals must recognize and eliminate foreign material to survive in a hostile environment. Lower animals depend heavily on nonspecific mechanisms such as encystment, phagocytosis, and intercellular digestion. Mammals possess the most complex immunologic apparatus and, in general, have three major ways to resist pathogenic microorganisms:

1. *Chemical and physical barriers* in skin and mucous surfaces. These prevent microbial invasion of tissue. Chemical barriers include antimi-crobial proteins in mucus, lipids in cornified layers of skin, and hydrochloric acid in the gastric lumen. Movement of surface hairs and of respiratory cilia prevent stable contact of microbes with tissue surfaces. Each body orifice has a characteristic normal resident microflora, the secretions of which prevent overgrowth of pathogenic bacteria. For example, nonpathogenic bacteria that colonize skin, teeth, urogenital tract, and intestine reduce the growth rates of some pathogenic bacteria.

2. *Nonspecific internal mechanisms* involving cells and fluids. Phagocytosis and killing by granulocytic leukocytes, monocytes (and their progeny, macrophages), and at least one subpopulation of small lymphocytes are potent nonspecific systemic defense mechanisms. Serum and body fluids also contain enzymes and peptides that are strongly antimicrobial, that is, lysozyme and complement.

3. *Specific mechanisms involving lymphoid cells,* i.e., plasmacytes (that produce antibodies) and lymphocytes (that can kill organisms by direct contact).

Generally, the first two groups play important roles as a "first line of defense." In contrast, the highly specific lymphoid mechanisms of the third group are more important in recovery and in prevention of disease on second exposure to the same agent. The actions of these cells and

355

their products are commonly called "immune" mechanisms because they have two striking characteristics: they are *specific* (reacting antibodies and lymphocytes are specifically designed for a particular antigen) and they have *memory* (that is, they are able to be recalled on second exposure to a microorganism, and fur-

ther encounter produces a more rapid and stronger immunologic response).

In the following chapter we will examine ways in which these cells produce immunity and how they interact with one another and with the phagocytic cells (such as neutrophils and macrophages) to protect the host.

Mechanisms of Immunity 22

LYMPHOID CELLS AND THE IMMUNE RESPONSE

In the late 1800s pathologists began to recognize the importance of lymphoid cells in tissues of patients that had survived infectious diseases. During recovery stages, as phagocytic cells such as neutrophils and macrophages disappeared from inflammatory lesions, a residual population of plasmacytes and a few small and medium-sized lymphocytes remained behind. When infection persisted, the plasmacyte population was larger, and in persistent unresolved infections there were massive infiltrates of plasmacytes. *Tissue plasmacytosis* was especially common in persistent bacterial infections. For example, in chronic leptospirosis, causal spirochetes persisted within the lumen of renal tubules; this constant stimulus attracted large numbers of plasmacytes, which did not enter the renal tubule but lodged and remained in the peritubular interstitium.

Near the turn of the century, von Behring discovered antibodies. He observed that serum of animals that had recovered from experimental diphtheria contained a specific substance capable of neutralizing the toxin produced by *Corynebacterium diphtheriae,* the causal bacterium of the disease. It was called *antibody* because it appeared to be directed against the "foreign body" of the disease. Bacteria were rapidly being established as etiologic agents from many animal and human infections, and it was soon clear that the presence of antibodies in circulating blood of recovered patients correlated with immunity. Furthermore, the large number of plasmacytes

in infected tissue and in draining lymph nodes and spleen suggested that the source of antibodies was the plasmacyte. The actual presence of antibodies in the cytoplasm of plasmacytes was demonstrated using fluorescent antibody techniques in the 1950s.

Plasmacytes synthesize antibodies.

Plasmacytes are large plump cells that reside in vascular channels of lymph nodes and spleen, in tissue spaces at sites of infection. They have a characteristic "cartwheel" nucleus (large clumps of chromatin at the periphery with a large central nucleolus), and their cytoplasm is filled with the machinery of protein synthesis (Fig. 22.1). The globulins that plasmacytes produce are called immunoglobulins (Ig) because they have antibody activity (Ig and antibody are physical and functional descriptions of the same entity and are used interchangeably). Antibodies are stable and persist for long periods in serum and extracellular spaces as the major humoral mechanism of immunity.

Plasmacytes release antibody into tissue spaces by merocrine secretion.

As immunoglobulins are secreted, they are drained into lymph and transported to the bloodstream. Immunoglobulins persist in circulating blood until the infectious process is resolved, and on reinfection they appear more rapidly in blood. Although antibody production occurs at sites of infection, most antibodies are released in lymph nodes and spleen. In septicemia, during which bacteria circulate in the blood, small

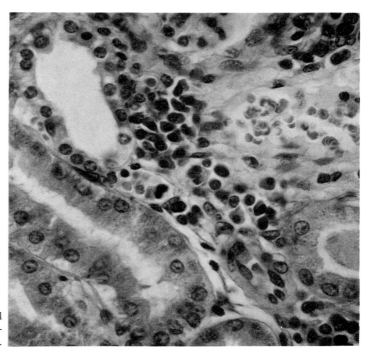

Fig. 22.1. Plasmacytes in interstitial spaces of kidney, dog with leptospirosis.

amounts of antibodies are released directly into the bloodstream by circulating plasmablasts.

Circulating antibody is especially efficient in preventing the spread of infection. It prevents both dissemination of microorganisms through the vascular system and bacterial colonization at sites distant from the primary infections. In some viral infections, plasmacyte precursors called plasmablasts migrate to infected cells, become attached to their plasma membranes, and secrete antibody directly into cells. Their membranes fuse, and antibody can be inserted directly into the cytoplasm of the infected cell.

Plasmacytes arise from bone marrow stem cells that differentiate to B cells.

The development of the plasmacyte involves the following progression: (1) *undifferentiated stem cells* are released from the bone marrow (Fig. 22.2); (2) residence of the stem cells in tonsils, Peyer's patches, and other intestinal lymphoid tissues allows the acquisition of special surface proteins that give stem cells the special characters of a plasmacyte precursor cell called the *B cell* (Table 22.1); (3) B cells are released from gut-associated lymphoid tissue to circulate and lodge in lymphoid tissue, particularly lymph nodes; (4) contact of the B cell with an antigen

drives the cell to develop into a *plasmablast*; (5) globulins (antibodies) are secreted by the plasmablast; and (6) antibody release ceases and globulins become inspissated in the cytoplasm, giving the cell the characteristic appearance of the plasmacyte. The plasmablast is actually the important secretor of antibodies while plasmacytes, even though identified in infected tissue sections, are end-stage cells that no longer actively release antibodies.

B cell characters are acquired in gut-associated lymphoid tissue.

Bone marrow stem cells acquire the capacity to transform into antibody-producing plasmacytes in lymphoid tissues at various sites, the most prominent of which are part of the alimentary canal. *Peyer's patches* of mammals are islands of lymphoid tissue in the submucosa of the small intestine that are closely associated with the gut epithelium and its microbial flora. Epithelium covering lymphoid follicles contains foci of specialized columnar lymphoepithelial *dome cells* (M cells) that bulge into the lumen of the gut. Distinct from absorptive cells, dome cells are covered with blunt microvilli that function in attachment and phagocytosis of microorganisms. Lymphocytes of Peyer's patches are

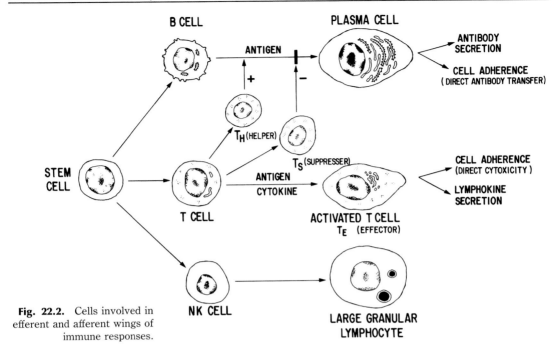

Fig. 22.2. Cells involved in efferent and afferent wings of immune responses.

both B and T cells, but it is here that B cells acquire their specialized characteristics.

Tonsils receive antigens from the oropharynx and transmit them via efferent lymphatics to cervical lymph nodes (there are no afferent lymphatics). Epithelial cells of the tonsillar crypts are phagocytic and play important roles in antigen processing and in transformation of stem cells to B cells. In birds, the *cloacal bursa* (bursa of Fabricius) is the dominant site of B cell differentiation. Removal of the bursa at hatching leaves the chick without the ability to form plasmacytes (provided radiation is used to kill lymphocytes seeded peripherally before hatching). Like the thymus, the bursa atrophies with age

and is no longer needed after the initial seeding of B lymphocytes that occurs after hatching.

Lymphocytes have both direct and indirect effects in immune reactions.

By the mid-1950s it was clear that, in some diseases, antibodies played very little role in recovery. In influenza, for example, the animal was cured before any meaningful antibody amounts were produced. Furthermore, treatment with passive antiserum did not alter the course of the disease, and patients with congenital failure of antibody production would pass

Table 22.1. Characteristics of small lymphocyte populations

Character	T Cell	B Cell	NK Cell
Produced in	Thymus	Peyer's patches, tonsils	Bone marrow
Function	Cell-mediated immunity	Antibody-mediated immunity	Nonspecific cytotoxicity
Cell type	Large blastic lymphocyte	Plasmacyte	Large granular lymphocyte
Surface properties	Thymic antigens[a]	Immunoglobulins, Fc receptors, C receptors	. . .

[a]Proteins that are embedded in the surfaces of mouse lymphocytes are identified as Thy L, L-1,2,3, etc.; those of other animals have different names.

through a clinical course of these diseases as though normal. Most important, the cellular aggregates in lesions of many of these infections contained not plasmablasts but collections of small lymphocytes (Fig. 22.3). The alveolar wall of the lungs in influenza, the perivascular spaces of the brain parenchyma in viral encephalitis, and the dermis below the epithelial lesions of poxviruses are all sites containing small lymphocytes.

The lymphocytes present in these tissues are associated with a different mechanism of immunity. Defense does not occur by circulating antibodies but by the *direct attack on the microbe* (or cells infected by the microbe) by the lymphocyte itself. Often called "cell-mediated immunity," these reactions are in contrast to the "humoral immunity" caused by antibodies. "Immune" lymphocytes are of prime importance in some kinds of graft rejection, hypersensitivity diseases, and viral infections. These *cytotoxic* lymphocytes kill infected or foreign cells by attaching and binding closely to the cell and then secreting toxic molecules that kill the "target" cell.

Recovery from influenza is largely due to a direct attack on influenza virus–infected cells by specialized lymphocytes that have been "sensitized" by previous contact with influenza antigens. These sensitized lymphocytes accumulate at sites in the terminal bronchiole where influenza virus replicates and act by directly killing the epithelial cells, which have influenza viral antigens on their surfaces.

Lymphocytes also have important effects in immunity by secreting *cytokines* that help or suppress the reactions of other cytotoxic lymphocytes. The contact of lymphocyte with microbe causes the cell to secrete a cytokine that causes other lymphocytes to proliferate and then to attack the microbe. Microorganisms that survive and replicate intracellularly are especially prominent in their capacity to induce T cell–mediated immunity, and this reactivity is the most significant reaction in recovery in tuberculosis, brucellosis, salmonellosis, and some of the fungal infections.

Small lymphocytes are functionally different populations of precursor cells.

Small lymphocytes that circulate in the bloodstream or that lodge in tissues represent several different populations of lymphoid cells, even though they cannot be distinguished structurally. Whereas plasmacytes in tissue are distinct cells with clearly defined functions, lymphocytes in tissue represent a diverse group,

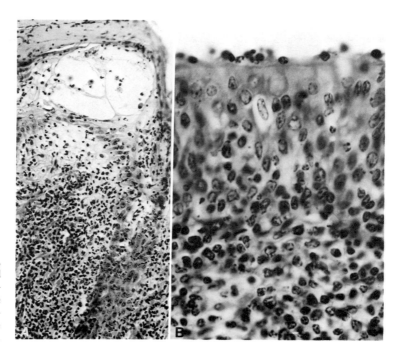

Fig. 22.3. Lymphocytes, skin, cow with malignant catarrhal fever. A. Lymphocytes throughout dermis and in a microvesicle in epidermis. B. Small lymphocytes below, within, and above epidermis.

most of which are specialized small lymphocytes called T cells; small lymphocytes in tissue sections may also be nonreactive or null lymphocytes, or even immature plasmablasts that have yet to acquire their distinctive cytoplasm. So confusing is this lack of correlation between appearance and function that pathologists often refer to these cells as mononuclear cells.

The specialized small lymphocytes originate from stem cells in bone marrow. They acquire their special characters by residence in the thymus. Their new functions are due to changes in cell surface proteins and glycoproteins that the T cells acquire. The thymus confers special reactivity on the bone marrow stem cells, which thereafter have the capacity to seed lymph nodes and to provide clones of lymphocytes with specific reactivity.

T cells, when activated by antigens, transform to *large lymphocytes* (they enlarge and develop abundant free ribosomes but, unlike plasmacytes, largely retain the characteristics of lymphocytes). Activated T cells secrete soluble cytokines, called *lymphokines,* which act in their immediate environment, but, unlike antibody, are rapidly destroyed and are not effective when circulating in the bloodstream.

The thymus is an organ for T lymphocyte differentiation.

The thymus is already a prominent lymphoid organ at birth, when the spleen and lymph nodes are poorly developed. It functions to trap bone marrow–derived lymphocytes, confer specialization on them, and induce them to replicate. Thymic, or T, lymphocytes can be differentiated from other small lymphocytes by the antigenic makeup of their cell membranes (although this is possible only in a few species, where purified antigenic reagents can be obtained). It is acquisition of thymic antigens that determines the role of these lymphocytes as cytotoxic, helper, or suppressor cells. T lymphocyte surface antigens are acquired as immature cells in the cortex. T cells are transformed to mature cells in the medulla and released into the bloodstream.

Thymic epithelial cells synthesize polypeptides that promote transformation of T cells. Extracts of thymus, when purified, show various proteins that stimulate lymphocytes. One of these is *thymosin,* which induces the differentiation of bone marrow precursor cells. Thymosin

has been used with some success clinically to treat human patients with congenital immunodeficiency disease.

T lymphocytes make up different functional subsets.

When examined for functional activity in the laboratory, T cells are found to be composed of several subpopulations. In addition to *cytotoxic lymphocytes* there are lymphocytes (T_S cells) that *suppress* or that *help* (T_H cells) the activity of other lymphocytes.

Small lymphocytes are responsible for immunologic memory.

The cellular residue that remains when inflammatory lesions heal consists of aggregates of small lymphocytes, the purveyors of immunologic memory. A segment of the small lymphocyte population is immunologically committed to antigens previously contacted. When triggered by that specific antigenic stimulus, these cells transform into large basophilic blast cells. For example, small lymphocytes taken from an animal immunized with tetanus toxoid will, when cultured, transform into blast cells when placed in contact with tetanus toxin.

Some lymphocytes do not have specific immunologic reactivity.

The term *null cell* has been applied to lymphocytes that are unreactive in laboratory tests to determine lymphocyte function; that is, they lack surface receptors or membrane proteins typical of T or B lymphocytes. Some null lymphocytes are said to have *natural killer* (NK) activity because they are effective without any previous exposure to antigens. These NK cells have been identified in tissue sections as *large granular lymphocytes* and are common in lymph nodes and visceral organs. In the laboratory, large granular lymphocytes cause lysis of virus-infected and malignant cells without previous exposure to provoking antigens and without involvement of antibodies or lymphokines.

Dr. Jerrold Ward, in an elegant study at the Frederick Cancer Research Facility, showed that large granular lymphocytes are common in acute inflammatory lesions in skin, lung, and intestine and suggested that they function as a first line of defense until specific reactions are induced by activated lymphocytes and plasmacytes. They are probably "prethymic T cells" and do what T lymphocytes do but do not require previous host contact with antigen from the agent producing the disease.

Development of specific immune responses: The "afferent phase"

Plasmacyte and lymphocyte immunologic responses are initiated when foreign proteins or glycoproteins called *antigens* interact with the surfaces of cells that are precursors to B and T cells. This interaction stimulates the blast cell to do two things: (1) synthesize new proteins that are released from the cell as soluble antibodies or cytokines and (2) cause the cell to produce other proteins that are inserted into the plasma membranes of the cell's surface, which then regulate the ways in which the transformed lymphocyte will react.

ANTIGENS AND ANTIGEN PROCESSING

An antigen is any substance capable of stimulating a specific immunologic response involving B and T lymphocytes. Proteins are good antigens if composed of over 20 amino acids. Polysaccharides are also highly antigenic, but most lipids are nonantigenic.

The structural part of the antigen molecule responsible for specific binding to antibody is called an *antigenic determinant* or *epitope.* Large protein antigens have multiple epitopes against which antibodies are directed. Antigenic determinants form a three-dimensional fit with the corresponding antibodies during the antigen-antibody reaction.

Haptens are substances that react specifically with corresponding antibodies but are unable to induce their formation unless they are complexed with a carrier protein. Antibodies produced in response to immunization with a protein to which a hapten has been artificially attached often show reactive specificity for epitopes identical in structure to the hapten.

In infectious diseases, most antigens that stimulate an effective immune response are glycoproteins present on the surfaces of viruses, bacteria, or other infectious agents. As integral components of the surfaces of microbes, glycoproteins are the antigens that first come into contact with the host's immune system. The specificity of an antigen-antibody reaction is determined by relatively small surface configurations of the epitopes on the antigen molecule.

Antigen processing and presentation

Macrophages process antigens by degrading them in lysosomes. They take up antigens by pinocytosis or phagocytosis and store them in tiny vacuoles or phagolysosomes. Here they are degraded. Once processed, the modified antigens can be delivered to either B or T cells to effect the immune response. T cells use macrophage processed antigens effectively.

Macrophage action is probably not required for every immune response. Macrophages may participate nonspecifically, simply as bystanders. It appears, however, that processing is necessary for and particularly effective with weak antigens; that is, partial degradation in the lysosome confers an adjuvant effect on the antigen.

Macrophages retain immunogenicity (ability to transmit information to lymphocytes) for long periods. Small amounts of antigen unassociated with lysosomes remain in the cell. Recent studies have given messenger RNA a role in transmitting information from macrophage to lymphocyte. The reaction of macrophage and antigen yields an immunogenic RNA that, when added experimentally to lymph node cells, elicits antibody.

Antibody helps macrophages trap antigen.

The trapping of antigens by macrophages in the immune animal is more efficient than in the nonimmune animal. On reexposure (i.e., in the presence of specific antibody) antigen is markedly taken up in specialized sites at the periphery of germinal centers in lymph nodes and spleen. In lymph nodes, immune complexes (antigen-antibody complexes) trapped in the subcapsular sinuses are rapidly transported by nonphagocytic cells to follicular regions along dendritic fibers.

Antigens are retained extracellularly by a large dendritic web of interlocking cell membranes of specialized reticular cells. They may be held there for several weeks, allowing exceptional access of the antigen molecule to the lymphoid tissues destined to produce antibody-forming cells. Some antigens persist for months or even years in lymphoid tissue of immune animals. They are retained in follicular dendritic cells and participate in maintenance of B lymphocyte memory.

Lymph nodes process antigens.

Antigens, which arrive in afferent lymph, percolate through the loose reticular cell networks of the subcapsular (cortical) sinus and into the networks of the medullary sinuses. As they pass through the cortical zones bearing germinal centers, they are trapped on the dendritic webs of *follicular dendritic cells.* These cells form a network of antigen-processing cells that have long dendrites that trap antigens and transport them to antigen-processing cells.

During the first immune response, vascular structures of the node expand in association with lymphoid proliferation and the medullary cords become filled with proliferating plasmablasts. In the presence of antibody the uptake of antigens becomes extremely efficient and plays a significant role in retention of antigens at sites of antibody production.

Germinal centers produce B lymphocytes.

Germinal centers are factories for large-scale production of plasmacyte precursors. They are seeded by B cells and develop through stages of production by expanding and contracting. *Primary centers* are small foci of dense lymphocytes in the cortical bed, *secondary centers* are large active nodules with pale centers and dense outer rims, and *tertiary centers* are large nodules composed of exhausted reticular cells. The active secondary germinal centers consist of a thinly populated center zone, a corona of dense small lymphocytes, and a mantle zone. Bone marrow stem cells populate the center zone, but differentiated B cells of gut origin are required for functioning mantle zones.

Paracortical areas are seeded by T lymphocytes.

Paracortical areas contain T lymphocytes and postcapillary venules with high endothelium, through which the small lymphocytes of the recirculating pool emigrate. These cells migrate through endothelial cell junctions. High endothelium is a special adaptation to allow excessive fluid loss; it is highly active in stimulated lymph nodes and is poorly developed in germfree animals.

In summary, lymph nodes are instruments for collecting, reacting with, and transmitting small lymphocytes. They receive large numbers of lymphocytes from blood and discharge them into lymph. In sheep, which have been extensively studied, at least 30 million lymphocytes per hour are discharged in efferent lymph. They enter the lymph nodes from blood, traverse the high endothelium of postcapillary venules, and enter sinuses. Lymphocytes may remain immobile in *desquamation zones,* extensions of medullary sinuses in paracortical areas. These zones, closely associated with postcapillary venules, are separated from the medullary sinuses by a sieve of bridging cells. Once free in the sinuses, cells move quickly down the sinuses, through the medulla, and out into the efferent lymph.

Macrophages present antigens to T$_H$ cells by a special mechanism.

The taking up of antigen and subsequent interaction with (and activation of) T$_H$ cells is called *antigen presentation.* T$_H$ cells will recognize processed antigen only if the macrophage presenting the antigen has the proper histocompatibility antigen on its surface. That is, T$_H$ cells recognize processed antigen only if associated with a histocompatibility antigen. Although several types of cells can present antigen, macrophages are the major "antigen-presenting" cells. Other cells that bear histocompatibility antigens (endothelial cells, B cells, and dendritic cells) lack the enormous phagocytic capacity of the macrophage. The important antigen-presenting cells are

Skin	Langerhans cells (phagocytic cells within the epidermis)
Lymph node	Follicular dendritic cells (interdigitating cells)
Gut	M cells (in Peyer's patches)
Bone marrow	Reticular cells (lining bone marrow sinusoids)
Liver	Kupffer cells (lining hepatic sinusoids)
Lung	Intravascular macrophages (inside alveolar capillaries)
Brain	Microglia

When foreign antigens first gain entrance past epithelial and inflammatory tissue barriers, they drain into regional lymph and circulate in the blood. In mammals, antigens must pass the elaborate biologic filters of the spleen. Located in the bloodstream the spleen is ideally suited to trap circulating antigens. Macrophages near reticular sheaths take up and transport antigens to germinal centers in white pulp. In these areas macrophages have a close association with plasmacyte precursors destined to produce antibodies. Antigens are first localized on cytoplasmic extensions of macrophages and are then taken into the cell and rapidly degraded.

Parts of the antibody molecule can act as an antigen.

Regions of a newly formed antibody molecule can act as an antigen to stimulate a new anti-antibody antibody. The unique antigen determinant on an antibody molecule is called an *idiotype.* The antibody produced in response to the idiotype is called an *anti-idiotype.* An idiotype network operates to shut off antibody production. As B and T cells and antibodies are produced during an immune response, say to an infection, the concentration of idiotypes rises to a point where anti-idiotypes are stimulated. Anti-idiotypes regulate the initial antibody response by binding to idiotypes on the surfaces of T cells that regulate other lymphocytes and by binding (and inactivating) antibody molecules.

Endogenous antigens: The histocompatibility antigens

Most of the proteins manufactured in an individual animal are identical to the same kind of protein in another individual. However, all cells in the body contain special proteins on their surfaces that differ among individuals and thus can act as antigen. One group of cell surface glycoproteins that is very important in immunology is called *histocompatibility antigens;* they function as guides by which lymphocytes of the immune system distinguish each other from all other types of cells, and also all cells of the body from noncells such as microbes. In other words, they function as receptors to lymphocytes.

Phylogenetic and ontogenetic differences

The greater the phylogenetic differences among species, the greater the differences in their antigenic makeup (called *antigenic disparity*). This is true of MHC and also other proteins; for example, serum albumins and hemoglobins of closely related species show more antigenic cross-reactivity than those in species further apart in the phylogenetic scheme. The antigenic panel of an individual becomes more complex with development (*ontogeny*). In the embryo, genetic information is not completely expressed so that many proteins found in the adult are missing.

There are two types of histocompatibility antigens.

The two different types of discrimination (T cell from T cell, and T cell from all other body cells) requires two different types of histocompatibility antigens. *Class I antigens* occur on cells and restrict access to other cell surface antigens to only lymphocytes bearing appropriate specific surface receptors; these are the major "transplantation antigens" that prevent tissue grafting between unrelated animals. *Class II antigens* occur on B cells and macrophages. They present foreign antigens to T_H and T_S lymphocytes. These are the antigens that regulate B cell antibody production. They are thus regulators of both the receptor and effector phases of T cell function.

Specific chromosomes code for histocompatibility antigens.

Genes that contain the codes to produce proteins that become histocompatibility antigens on the cell surface are clustered together on one chromosome. The gene cluster is called the *major histocompatibility complex* (MHC). In man and mice, specific chromosomes have been identified that contain these genes (in mice, the H-2 complex on chromosome 17; in man, the HLA complex on chromosome 6). For most other animals, the location of the gene complex has not been determined.

The amount of MHC antigens on cells can increase and decrease according to various stimuli. For example, the cytokine γ-interferon can act to selectively increase cell surface MHC antigens; for example, after treatment with interferon, MHC-bearing cells decrease in lymph nodes and spleen but increase in liver and other viscera.

T cells, unlike the antibody system, do not interact with antigen alone; the antigen must be presented on a cell surface adjacent to protein antigens of the MHC. T_C cells recognize an antigen in combination with class I MHC proteins (found on almost all cells); T_H cells bind to antigen associated with class II MHC proteins (only on macrophages and lymphocytes).

Major histocompatibility complex is used in transplantation testing.

Histocompatibility antigens function to restrict T lymphocytes. In the laboratory, they serve as antigens in tests that determine whether grafts between different animals are likely to be rejected. If tissue grafts are made between animals that differ at MHC gene loci, prompt immunologic rejection of the graft is apt to occur. Antibodies and cytotoxic T lymphocytes against the histocompatibility antigens will appear in the grafted animal.

In man, standard *lymphocyte microcytotoxicity tests* are used for MHC typing. Lymphocytes are isolated from blood and incubated with a battery of reagents (antisera containing antibodies against MHC proteins), and cytotoxicity is assessed microscopically.

Little of this information is available for larger animals. Prerequisites for work with animal histocompatibility antigens are inbred lines with significant variability for the system being assayed. A swine lymphocyte antigen (SLA) complex has been reported. It is divided into four closely linked gene loci with three loci controlling the class I antigen and the fourth controlling class II antigens. Differences among pig breeds can be correlated to preferred genetic characters such as resistance to disease.

MEDIATION OF IMMUNITY

The primary event in the immune response is the direct interaction of antigen and lymphocyte cell surface molecules. For B lymphocytes this occurs with immunoglobulin (Ig) molecules, which function as "receptors" on the cell surface (they are inserted into the plasma membrane early in B cell differentiation). When antigen combines with these surface globulins, the event triggers the lymphocyte into proliferation and differentiation to a plasmacyte precursor and to further synthesis of antibody, this time for export from the cell. B cells can be driven to proliferate and differentiate by interactions of soluble factors from lymphocytes, either cytokines (such as interleukin-1) or factors secreted by lymphocytes.

How far antigen-induced transformation of small lymphocytes will proceed is determined by the lineage of the lymphocyte involved. T cell responses are more complex. Most T cells do not recognize free antigen circulating in blood or lymph. Furthermore, they can respond to antigen on the surfaces of other cells only when the new antigen occurs in conjunction with an antigen of the host's own MHC proteins; that is, antigen receptors on the surface of a T cell must simultaneously recognize antigen *and* the MHC protein.

Antibody-mediated immunity

An *antibody* is a protein of the globulin type that is produced by plasmacytes upon antigenic stimulation and that has combining sites capable of reacting specifically with determinant groups on the antigen that has stimulated its production. The specificity of an antibody is determined by a relatively small part of the molecule constructed to combine with a particular determinant site on the antigen.

Antibody molecules are composed of two heavy and two light peptide chains joined by disulfide bridges (Fig. 22.4). Each chain is divided into *constant regions,* in which amino acid sequences are similar in all antibody classes, and *variable regions,* in which the sequence is different. The variable regions, which provide the specificity that characterizes the antibody, fold up in space to form a site that binds to the particular antigen against which the antibody was directed. Changes in its amino acid sequence change the affinity of the antibody for an antigen.

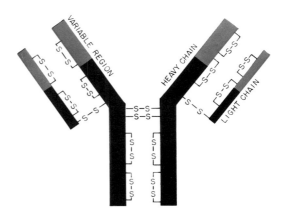

Fig. 22.4. Immunoglobulin (antibody) molecule.

There are two types of *light chains* in all vertebrate immunoglobulins, kappa and lambda. Light chains of every antibody molecule are of one type or the other. In any given species, the constant regions of each kappa or lambda light chain are identical with the constant regions of other chains of the same type. While in any one Ig molecule only one type of chain is present, normal serum has light chains of both types.

Antibody classes

Igs are separated into classes on the basis of molecular structure (Table 22.2). Each antibody molecule has one of five *heavy chain* types: gamma, mu, alpha, epsilon, or delta. The heavy chain type determines the class of the Ig (e.g., IgG, IgM, IgA, IgE, and IgD). In secreted antibodies of the IgM class, for example, all the heavy chains have the same mu constant region amino acid sequence and all the light chains have the same kappa or lambda constant region sequences. The variable regions differ from one antibody to the next and reflect their different antigen specificities.

Heavy chain constant regions determine the effector function of an antibody. If the gamma heavy chain is present, the resulting IgG antibody will circulate in the blood. If the epsilon chain is present, the antibody IgE binds to basophil and mast cell surfaces with high affinity to cause the liberation of histamine. If the heavy chain is the delta type, the IgD remains associated with the surface of the cell that produces it.

IgG

This is the dominant antibody molecule that circulates in the bloodstream and is protective in recovery phases of infectious diseases. In most species, IgG has been divided into subclasses such as IgG_1 and IgG_2, often with differing biologic activity (measured in terms of complement-fixation, induction of anaphylaxis, fixation to skin, or presence in body secretions). Bovine IgG_1, for instance, fixes complement and is the chief IgG in milk and saliva. It is the chief IgG in passive immunization of the calf.

IgM

IgM (macroglobulin), made up of five Ig units linked by disulfide bonds, theoretically has 10 identical binding sites for antigen. This gives IgM a peculiar effectiveness in activating complement to produce lysis of cell membranes, a thousand times more effective per molecule than IgG. Early primary immune responses are often IgM, and these are gradually replaced by IgG antibody (Fig. 22.5). For example, in the antibody response of bovine anaplasmosis, 19S IgM is produced 4–5 days prior to the appearance of IgG.

IgA is the dominant Ig in external secretions.

IgA ("secretory antibody") is the predominant Ig in saliva, tears, bile, and nasal and intestinal mucus in most species. Secretion of IgA is more than mere passive transfer, since its concentration in body fluids may be 20 times that in serum. Colostrum of dogs and horses contains IgA in much higher concentration than is present in sera.

IgA in these external secretions has a unique antigenicity conferred on the molecule by a non-Ig component called *secretory piece*. IgA is synthesized in plasma cells below mucous membranes, and the secretory piece is added in its transit through glandular epithelium. In the intestine of the pig, the secretory component has been localized in crypt epithelial cells and associated mucins by immunofluorescent stains; it is not present in submucosal plasmacytes that stain for IgA.

Dimeric IgA is secreted by plasmacytes into the intestinal mucosa. It is bound to the basal surfaces of intestinal absorptive cells by polymeric immunoglobulin receptors). The IgA-receptor complex is taken into the cytoplasm in a vesicle, transported to the luminal surface, and, by fusion of vesicle with luminal plasma mem-

Table 22.2. Characteristics of immunoglobulin classes

Class[a]	Heavy Chain	Sedimentation Constant	Molecular Weight	Electrophoretic Migration	Characteristic
IgG	γ	7S	150,000	γ	2 subclasses
IgM	μ	19S	890,000	β_2	Macroglobulin
IgA	α	10–12S	180,000	β_2	Secretory antibody
IgE	ϵ	8S	200,000	β	Reaginic antibody

[a]IgD, a fifth Ig class, occurs in man.

Fig. 22.5. Hypothetical primary and secondary antibody responses.

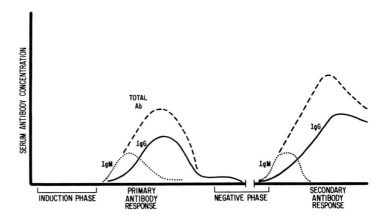

brane, exits into the gut lumen. At the cell surface the receptor is cleaved away from the IgA receptor complex by a protease (releasing IgA and approximately three-fourths of the receptor molecule attached to it). The receptor component remaining is the "secretory piece" of the IgA molecule.

For intestinal immunity, B lymphocytes acquire commitment to IgA production in Peyer's patches, migrate to mesenteric lymph nodes where they divide and differentiate to plasmablasts, and emigrate via the thoracic duct. In the bloodstream, they home to the lamina propria of the intestine, where they lodge and undergo terminal differentiation to IgA-bearing plasmacytes.

IgA produced by plasmacytes in intestine may also enter portal venous systems and pass through the liver. Secretory piece is added in hepatocytes (via transport vesicles on sinusoidal surfaces), and IgA then passes through the bile ductule to the gut lumen.

The presence of IgA is essential to the antimicrobial activity of the respiratory and intestinal tracts. It also dominates in salivary glands. In mammalian tears, the dominant Ig is IgA. Disease of the eye is characterized by large accumulations of plasma cells in the lacrimal glands, and most of these contain IgA. Extracellular IgA occurs between and within acinar cells and in the lumina of lacrimal acini.

IgE

IgE (reaginic antibody) has the peculiar ability to fix itself firmly to cells. Its Fc fragment binds with high affinity to surface receptors on basophils and mast cells; cross-linking of the Fc-IgE receptor complex induces these cells to re-

lease histamine and other vasoactive substances. IgE also binds to monocytes and eosinophils. Although these cells have fewer (or different) IgE receptors than do mast cells, they bind to eosinophils with lower affinity so that dissociation can occur before any meaningful cell response develops. IgE appears to play some role in phagocytosis and killing of IgE-coated parasites, although this mechanism has not been defined.

No certain protective function exists for IgE, and it is known only to produce disease. As a "homocytotropic" antibody, it sensitizes cells for hypersensitivity reactions such as anaphylaxis, asthma, and atopic dermatologic responses. In the dog, disease induced by antigens combining with IgE is manifested as dermatitis; rhinitis is more typical of other animals, especially man.

IgE disease was first demonstrated when Prausnitz injected serum from his allergic patient Kustner into his own forearm, inducing passive sensitization. When the allergen (fish) was applied later to the same site, it produced an erythematous wheal (the Prausnitz-Kustner reaction).

Antibodies in serum

The antibody-active proteins of serum were narrowed by Tiselius and Kabat in 1938 to the globulin fraction showing the least electrophoretic mobility, the γ-globulins. Electrophoretic migration is determined by the net charge of the protein; this separates the protein fractions of whole serum. Serum globulins may also be purified by inducing their precipitation in saturated solutions of ammonium sulfate. The precipitate is centrifuged and redissolved in distilled water, providing large amounts of crude antibody.

The net charge of serum globulins is also the basis of ion exchange chromatography. Ion exchange resins, such as diethylaminoethyl (DEAE) cellulose, absorb serum proteins according to their size and net charge. When serum is poured into a column of DEAE cellulose and the column is eluted successively with buffers of increasing molarity and decreasing pH, it yields successive γ-globulin peaks of increasing net charge.

Agar gel diffusion technique

Globulin will, when serum is placed in wells in agar, diffuse and precipitate with similarly diffusing antigen, thus forming observable lines. This technique distinguishes various globulins immunologically when serum is reacted with antisera produced in rabbits using the appropriate Ig as antigen. Immunoelectrophoresis combines this technique with electrophoresis: serum is applied to agar or cellulose acetate strips and induced to migrate in a charged field; antiserum is then applied and allowed to diffuse, and the resulting precipitate is stained for observation.

Biologic properties of antibodies

Functional activities of different antibody classes vary, and all classes participate in several types of antigen-antibody reactions. Adjectives such as agglutinating, neutralizing, and complement-fixing define this reactivity in vitro (Table 22.3). An individual Ig molecule may react in several tests.

Cytophilic antibodies bind to cells.

Antibodies attach to cells via binding sites on the antibody molecule that differ from those sites that react with antigen. Cytophilia is deter-

mined both by the antibody molecules and by the character of the cell membrane of the target cells. IgE has strong cytophilic affinity for mast cells and basophils. By binding, it confers immunologic reactivity on these cells; should they encounter the specific antigen again, they react by releasing their cytoplasmic granules. Subclasses of IgG in some species are also cytophilic for mast cells.

Immunologic tagging of antibody

Antibody molecules can be labeled with specific substances serving as indicators for the detection of antigens. The fluorescent antibody (FA) test is widely used in diagnostic microbiology. Globulins are precipitated from serum of immunized animals, and the antibody molecules are conjugated with fluorescein isothiocyanate. Smears, frozen sections of tissue, and infected cell cultures can be fixed, stained with the conjugate, and examined under ultraviolet light, inducing fluorescein (attached to the antigen) to fluoresce.

An indirect FA test uses an initial application of unlabeled but specific antibody that attaches to the antigen being sought. This is followed by fluorescein-labeled antiglobulin that binds to the unlabeled specific antibody. The advantage of this procedure is that one labeled antibody preparation can be used for the detection of many different antigens.

Development of the B lymphocyte line.

Antibody production is initiated in the plasmacyte nucleus when gene codes are transcribed for subsequent protein synthesis in the cytoplasm (Fig. 22.6). The paradox of a limited num-

---

Table 22.3. Definitions of antibodies

Antibodies	Characteristics
Autoantibodies	Those produced in a host that react with the host's own tissue
Cell-associated	Those in or on cells, either on antibody-synthesizing cells or cytophilic antibodies on other cells (*syn*: cytotropic antibodies)
Isoantibodies	Those produced in one individual that react specifically with an antigen present in another individual of the same species (*syn*: alloantibodies)
Natural	Those occurring naturally without deliberate antigenic stimulation
Opsonins	Those acting on particulate antigens to induce phagocytosis
Precipitating	Those reacting specifically with soluble antigens to form a precipitate (*syn*: precipitins)

ber of genes and an apparently limitless capacity to produce different antibodies is explained by *gene shuffling*. Instead of containing a set of complete linear genes for production of Ig chains, the antibody-producing B lymphocytes contain pieces of gene codes that are rearranged to form a coherent genetic message for production of a single protein chain. This rearrangement of DNA and its mRNA template during differentiation is called somatic recombination. The mRNA sequences are assembled by RNA splicing to form a continuous light or heavy chain mRNA.

Nonsensitized B lymphocytes

These cells produce Igs without directed antibody activity. Genes for the mu and delta heavy chains are transcribed and genes for the kappa or lambda light chains are formed. Later, the virgin B lymphocyte displays some of its newly formed Igs on its surface as receptors. These receptor Igs are IgD and a membrane-bound form of IgM. Early IgM differs from later forms of secreted IgM in that its synthesis ends in a short sequence of hydrophobic amino acids that anchor the μ chain to the hydrophobic lipids of the B-lymphocyte plasma membrane.

Clonal selection of B lymphocytes

The first contact of antigen with Ig receptors on the B lymphocyte surface initiates differentiation. By this ligand-receptor interaction the B lymphocyte is driven into development of the plasmacyte. IgM and IgD disappear from the cell surface, and either IgM, IgG, IgE, or IgA is secreted. Massive amounts of rough endoplasmic reticulum develop in the cytoplasm to produce the large amounts of antibody.

Heavy chain switching occurs as plasmablasts develop.

Within the developing plasmacyte, the order of appearance of Ig classes (in both phylogeny and ontogeny) follows a sequence of IgM, IgG, and IgA or IgE. Different Ig classes are produced against the same antigen. In most cases IgM is the first response, but its synthesis is followed and overtaken by IgG production. In Igs, the same variable region can associate with different heavy chain constant regions. This process, called *heavy chain class switching,* can occur by either DNA recombination or by differential RNA transcription and splicing.

Antibody synthesis

Fluorescent antibody studies of single synthesizing plasmacytes indicate that only one type of Ig is produced at one time. Light and heavy chains of the molecule are synthesized on separate ribosomes. The polypeptide backbone of the antibody molecule is synthesized in the rough endoplasmic reticulum and then transported to the Golgi apparatus where carbohydrate moieties are incorporated. Light chains appear to be formed on the endoplasmic reticulum membranes, while heavy chain production occurs in polyribosomes.

The route by which antigen enters an animal is important in the type of plasmacyte response.

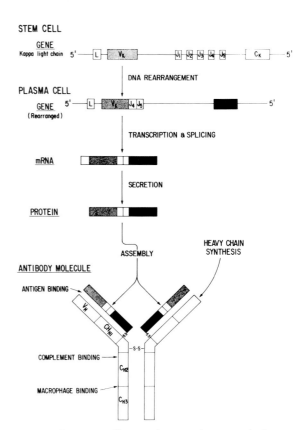

Fig. 22.6. Changes in gene that controls formation of components of antibody molecules. The gene for the kappa light chain is rearranged as the virgin stem cell differentiates into the plasma cell. The messenger RNA (mRNA) codes from the rearranged gene to instruct the plasma cell to form the appropriate kappa light chain, which is then assembled into the complete antibody molecule.

In animals immunized *subcutaneously,* large numbers of IgM-containing plasmacytes appear in peripheral lymphoid tissues, and this is followed by a progressive increase in IgG-containing cells. A few IgA-containing plasmacytes are found in the intestine. In *oral immunization,* however, IgA antibody-containing cells are abundant throughout the intestine. Plasmacytes in the gut are selectively committed to IgA synthesis.

Control of antibody synthesis

Segments of the variable region of the antibody molecule function as antigenic determinants called *idiotypes.* The specific amino acid sequence in the variable region of the antibody molecule acts as an antigenic determinant and is recognized by B cells to produce *anti-idiotype* antibodies. Idiotype and anti-idiotype interactions serve as positive and negative feedback controls that regulate the antibody response.

T LYMPHOCYTE–MEDIATED IMMUNITY

Small lymphocytes, when harvested from blood or lymphoid tissue, can be examined in the laboratory using tests for function. These tests show that individual T cells fall in three major categories: (1) *Helper T cells* (T_H cells), which enhance the actions of other T cells, (2) *suppressor T cells* (T_S cells), which inhibit the activities of other lymphocytes, and (3) *cytotoxic T cells* (T_C), which directly kill target cells that are infected or that contain antigens to which the T_C cell is sensitized (Table 22.4). T_C cells have much overlapping with T_S cells, and the distinctions between these groups is unclear in most animals.

The specificity of interaction of T cells with target cells results from the association of T_H and T_S cells with class II and class I major histo-compatibility complex (MHC) proteins respectively. Any target cell to which the T cell binds must have the appropriate MHC antigens on its surface.

T cells are identified by laboratory tests.

The various types of T cells are differentiated in vitro on the basis of life span, response to mitosis-inducing drugs, and reactivity of their cell surfaces with highly specific reagents. Commercial reagents (usually monoclonal antibodies to T cell surface proteins) are available that stain cells in smears or that will identify T lymphocytes as they flow through a flow cytometer. These tests are so expensive that the routine interpretation of blood smears or tissue sections leaves the pathologist in the dark as the specific function of lymphocytes.

Reagents are only available for human T cell antigens; in most animals, other, less specific techniques are used as presumptive evidence of T cell function, such as adherence or non-adherence to certain substances. In laboratory jargon, T_H cells are referred to as OK4+ and T_S as OK8+ cells because the OK reagents are widely used to determine subpopulations in human disease. This functional distinction is not absolute because some T4+ cells can cause suppression or cytotoxicity in the living animal.

A summary of differences between helper and suppressor lymphocytes includes:

Designation	T_H	T_S
Function	helper	suppressor
Surface glycoprotein	T4	T8
Class of MHC gene product that target cell must express	class II	class I

Surface receptor molecules determine T cell reactions.

T lymphocytes have proteins called *T cell receptors* embedded in their surfaces that function

Table 22.4.   Populations of T lymphocytes

T Cell Type	Subclass	Function
Cytotoxic	T_C	Kills cells with foreign antigens on their surfaces (virus infection, cancer cells); early defense mechanism, ahead of antibody responses; recognizes antigen only in combination with histocompatibility antigens
Helper	T_H	Enhances B cell function; secretes local-acting helper factor; requires interleukin-1 (IL-1) from macrophages for optimal responses
Suppressor	T_S	Regulates immune responses by suppressing B, T_H, or T_C cells; turns off effector cells after they have completed their function; produces γ-interferon after interacting with antigen

Note: T cells are identified by assays that detect specific proteins embedded in their plasma membranes. These "markers" are detected by reagents (monoclonal antibodies) that stain cells in smears.

to recognize microbes and other foreign proteins. Immunologic reactions are initiated by union of these receptors with specific antigen. The *recognition* event, in which surface receptors on the immune T lymphocyte interact with antigen, triggers *activation,* the conversion of the resting small T lymphocyte to a larger cell that produces cytokines.

Activated T Cells

Activated T cells function in many different ways. One subset (T_C for cytotoxic) kills cells directly by secreting toxic peptides as it attaches to target cells. Other T cell subsets influence *macrophages* and *natural killer cells* (the peripheral arm of the immune system) to function as effectors by secreting cytokines (such as interleukin-2) or by direct contact. In many T cell–mediated lesions, most of the effector cells in the lesion are monocytes and macrophages attracted by cytokines excreted by activated T lymphocytes (circulating antibodies may be present in these reactions, but they are not considered important in recovery of the animal).

Activated T_C lymphocytes can be killer cells.

Activated T_C lymphocytes attack and kill cells bearing appropriate antigens on their surfaces. For example, T_C cells against *Mycobacterium tuberculosis* will attach to macrophages infected with this bacterium. Sophisticated electron microscopic studies have shown tiny membranous bodies called *porins* that are released by the killer lymphocyte and punch holes into the membrane of the target cell.

A different mechanism, called "antibody-dependent cytotoxicity," appears to operate in cells coated with antibodies. T cells attack antibody-coated target cells by forming long surface projections that push deeply into infected cells to cause lysis. Binding of the T_C lymphocyte to the target cell membrane antigen induces secretion of cytoplasmic granules (by exocytosis) between the effector lymphocyte and its bound target. The granules contain lysosomal enzymes (unrelated to cell killing) and a membrane-active *granule cytolysin* or "lymphotoxin."

T_H cells and T_S cells modulate the response of B and T cells.

T_H cells are necessary for B, T_C, and T_S cells to function. They secrete cytokines called inter-

leukin-2 and γ-interferon that bolster natural killer cells and stimulate macrophages. For example, to respond to a viral antigen, B cells require a signal from the helper T_H cell in the form of cytokine or direct contact. The antigen-specific B cell then multiplies into a clone of antiviral plasmacytes. Plasmacyte function peaks before suppressor T cells begin to function. T_S cells inhibit both B and T_C cells and in effect turn off the immune response (T_S also turn off T_H cells).

B and T_H lymphocyte cooperation is required for effective immune responses.

To produce maximal antibody responses, cooperation between B and T lymphocytes is required. The specificity of the B lymphocyte is for the antigenic hapten, which, when it reacts with the B cell surface, slowly stimulates the cell to differentiate. To enhance this reaction, T lymphocytes recognize the same antigens (on a carrier part of the molecule distinct from the sites recognized by the B cell) and thereupon stimulate the B cell to differentiate to a plasmablast. The precise reaction occurs at the surface of the B cell when T_H cells "recognize" both specific antigen *and* histocompatibility antigens embedded in the B cell surface.

Macrophages are required because they concentrate or focus the antigen so that a critical number of B cell receptors are stimulated. They enhance B cell function by secreting a cytokine (interleukin-1) that cross-links with surface receptors on the B lymphocyte.

Soluble cytokines regulate T cell actions.

On contact with specific antigen, immune T lymphocytes release soluble cytokines (also called lymphokines), some of which are attractant to monocytes. By virtue of cytokine secretion, the T cell induces large numbers of nonspecific effector cells to participate in the cell-mediated reaction. Although cytokines develop concomitantly with infection, the cumbersome laboratory tests used for their assay are not used as uniform and valid criteria for routine diagnosis of disease.

Interleukin-1

Interleukin-1 (IL-1) is critical for initiation of T lymphocyte–mediated immunity (Table 22.5). Produced by macrophages, it binds specifically to receptor molecules on the surface of T lymphocytes that are committed to react against a

Table 22.5. **Cytokines that interact with lymphoid tissue**

Cytokine	Abbreviation	Produced by	Causes
Interleukin-1	IL-1	Macrophages, lymphocytes, monocytes, keratinocytes, et al.	T lymphocyte activation; many systemic effects
Interleukin-2	IL-2	T lymphocytes	T cell proliferation
Interferon (gamma)	γIF	Lymphocytes	Increases histocompatibility antigens on macrophage surfaces; enhances response to Ag
Thymosin		Thymic epithelial cells	T lymphocyte differentiation
Macrophage colony stimulating factor	M-CSF	All tissues	Promonocyte replication (macrophage production)

certain antigen. The T cells are thus stimulated to release another cytokine, interleukin 2, which in turn induces other T cells to proliferate.

Interleukin-2

Interleukin-2 or IL-2 (originally called T cell growth factor) is released by T lymphocytes during immune responses. Release is stimulated when antigen (in cooperation with major histocompatibility proteins) and IL-1 contact the T lymphocyte. Although all T lymphocyte subclasses can release IL-2, T_H lymphocytes are the major source of this cytokine. IL-2 binds to specific receptor glycoproteins on the surface of activated T lymphocytes and induces proliferation; that is, it promotes proliferation of *other* activated T lymphocytes that have IL-1 surface receptors (IL-2 receptors are absent on "resting" T cells). IL-2 markedly enhances the ability of NK lymphocytes to kill neoplastic cells and has been used clinically in man to suppress metastatic melanomas and renal carcinomas.

Cytokines act synergistically

IL-1 reinforces actions of other cytokines, such as tumor necrosis factors and interferons. These cytokines enter the bloodstream during infection and trauma to cause systemic effects such as metabolic changes, fever, and necrosis.

Genes for T cell receptor proteins undergo rearrangement.

Recently, the T cell receptor for antigen has been identified, and the *gene* for its production has been cloned (actually, the gene for the α-chain of the T cell receptor protein). This gene has sequences similar to the Ig heavy chain gene and undergoes rearrangement during T cell maturation analogous to Ig gene rearrangements.

DEVELOPMENT OF IMMUNOCOMPETENCE OF THE FETUS AND NEONATE

The placental barrier protects the fetus.

The mammalian fetus, having inherited antigens from its sire, is immunologically incompatible with its mother. Following implantation of the embryo, it becomes, in a sense, a homograft in utero. Rejection of the fetus and placenta by the mother is prevented by several mechanisms.

Fetal T cells inhibit the mother's immune response.

Suppressor, or T_S, cells develop in midpregnancy that inhibit T and B lymphocyte differentiation in the mother. They do this in the placenta by in two ways: by direct cell-to-cell contact or by secretion of soluble substances, thought by some to be prostaglandins. PGE_2 has been implicated in T_S suppression; PGE_2 receptors are absent on the fetal T_S cells so that they do not inhibit themselves.

Proteins produced by the fetus may have some role in suppressing the mother's immune response. α-fetoprotein, produced in the yolk sac of the embryo and liver of the fetus, is a major protein in serum during intrauterine development, decreases in late pregnancy and is gradually replaced in serum by albumin. Experimentally, α-fetoprotein suppresses mitogen-induced lymphocyte proliferation. It is elevated in serum of pregnant females.

Placental trophoblasts are immunologically unreactive.

Trophoblasts are the cells in direct contact with maternal tissues. Histocompatibility antigens (inherited from the sire) are irregularly distributed over the trophoblast surfaces. They are present on basolateral surfaces but diminished or absent on apical surfaces, which are exposed to maternal fluids. Furthermore, trophoblast apical surfaces are covered with a thick glycocalyx, a coat of glycosaminoglycans that helps to mask surface histocompatibility antigens.

Anatomical arrangements of the placenta inhibit lymphocyte interchange.

The lack of vascular interchange between dam and fetus varies among species. In some animals it does not permit large numbers of maternal immunocompetent cells to pass the placenta into the fetus. Even if antibodies are stimulated in the fetus, the placenta appears to act as a concentrating apparatus and acts as an immunologic filter.

Endocrine functions of the placenta suppress the female's immune response.

Adrenal corticosteroids from the fetus reinforce immunosuppression of the dam's lymphoid system. They probably play a greater role as parturition approaches and explain the drop in antibody production and T lymphocyte immune reactions that occur just before birth. Other hormones of minor importance that contribute to immunosuppression include hormones produced by the placenta: chorionic gonadotropin, progesterone, placental lactogen, and γ-globulins (pregnancy zone protein); these hormones have been shown to suppress immunity experimentally, but their role in vivo is not known.

Histocompatibility antigen differences affect the trophoblast.

In mice, disparity between maternal and fetal histocompatibility antigens favors greater invasiveness of the trophoblast and large size of the placenta. In humans, females who share many histocompatibility loci with their husbands have a higher rate of chronic idiopathic abortions. However, histocompatibility differences have not been identified as a cause of abortion in animals.

Is there an IgG blocking factor?

A factor that blocks IgG has been found in placental extracts and maternal serum. It inhibits cytokine production by maternal lymphocytes. Elevated levels of this factor are reported in human females with "idiopathic" abortions. The role of this factor in abortion in animals has not been established.

Antibody in the fetus

Because its environment is sheltered from antigens, the fetus usually does not make antibodies and is born immunologically virgin. Passive immunity in the developing animal is acquired from the dam. Transmission of Igs from dam to young may occur before birth, after birth via the colostrum, or (in most species) by a combination of these pathways (Table 22.6). While the maternal antibodies transmitted are usually protective, they may also inhibit fetal antibody production or cause disease.

If fetal antigens (which are not present in the mother's tissue) enter the maternal circulation, antibodies are formed against them by the dam. When these antibodies are returned to the fetus in the circulation, they may induce disease. The fetal immunogenic substances of most significance are the plasma globulins, erythrocytes, and platelets.

Fetal blood reaches the dam, even in species with tight epitheliochorial placentation, such as the horse and pig, by way of placental trauma and hemorrhage. Anemia may result from return of antierythrocytic antibodies to the fetus. In primates, where antibodies pass the hemoendothelial placental barrier prenatally, anemia

Table 22.6. Transfer of antibody in different species

Species	Route of Transfer	Dominat Ig	Time and Duration
Primate	Placenta	IgA	Prenatal (late gestation)
Horse	Intestine	IgG	36 hours after birth
Cow, sheep	Intestine	IgG	36 hours after birth
Pig	Intestine	IgG	36 hours after birth
Cat, dog	Intestine	IgG	Birth to 8 days (variable)
Rabbit	Yolk sac	IgA	Prenatal, from 15 days gestation
Rat	Placenta, gut	IgA	Before and 3 weeks after birth
Mouse	Yolk sac, gut	IgA	Variable
Chicken	Yolk sac	IgG	17 days incubation to 2 days posthatch

may occur in utero. In horses, mules, and pigs, in which antibodies are transmitted in colostrum, hemolytic anemia occurs following suckling.

Only IgG reaches the fetus.

These diseases would be far worse if all Igs passed the placental barrier. Fortunately, only IgG enters the fetus. Failure of IgA, IgM, and IgE to pass the placenta in significant amounts is important. The major blood group isoantibodies in primates are IgM. The reaginic antibodies associated with hypersensitivity are IgE. If these Igs reached the fetus, intrauterine disease would be an immense problem.

Avian embryos receive immunoglobulins from yolk.

In the chicken embryo, antibody transmission occurs through the yolk sac. Before the ovum is ovulated in the hen, antibodies (IgG) are selectively secreted by the ovarian follicular epithelium into the yolk. The close relation of oocyte and follicle in the hen's ovary permits this early globulin transmission. When the egg is hatched, the yolk contains all the antibodies destined for the chick. Beginning at 12–14 days of incubation of the egg, yolk sac epithelium begins to selectively transport immunoglobulin molecules. IgG in the yolk is specifically bound by IgG receptors on epithelial cells, taken into the epithelial cell, and passed into embryonic blood vessels underlying the epithelium. Igs are transported to the liver of the embryo via the vitelline veins. This process continues after hatching, since the yolk sac persists in the newly hatched chick.

Fetuses develop immune reactions.

Although the developing fetus is immunologically virgin, it becomes immunocompetent with the embryonic development of its lymphoid system. If stimulated antigenically, it will produce plasmacytes and Igs. Fetuses infected with pathogenic microorganisms have extensive plasmacytosis in affected tissues and develop high serum antibody titers. If a pregnant cow develops leptospirosis, the fetus becomes infected and reacts immunologically against the leptospires. Dr. H. D. Liggitt, at Colorado State, has shown that bovine fetuses develop immune responses 5–10 days after becoming infected with parvoviruses.

If proteins pass the placenta they can stimu-late the developing immune response of the fetus. Dr. Donald Cramer, a veterinary pathologist at the University of Pittsburgh School of Medicine, has used a rat model to show that antigens circulating in the female can cross the placenta to stimulate the immune system of the fetus. Antigens that passed into the fetus were deposited in the liver; by birth they were found in both liver and spleen and at 3 weeks of age they were largely in bone marrow.

Antibodies in the neonate
Mammary glands secrete globulins into colostrum.

Nearly all newborn mammals receive antibodies from the colostrum of the mother. The pregnant female develops antibodies against potential pathogens in her immediate environment and therefore can offer, in her milk, passive protection to her newborn. Passive immunity protects the neonatal animal until its own rapidly developing immunologic mechanisms are sufficiently mature for active protection. It protects the newborn in two ways: by inhibiting bacteria in the gut lumen and by passing into the bloodstream to protect the tissues.

IgA protects the gut lumen but is not absorbed.

IgA is the major Ig in colostrum of mammals that transmit immunity through the placenta. After ingestion by the newborn, IgA is not absorbed by the intestinal epithelium but acts locally to protect the gut wall against infection. This is an especially effective mechanism for enteric microbes. IgA-producing plasmablasts in gut-associated lymphoid tissues of the mother (responding to her gut microbial population) pass through the mesenteric lymph node and "home" to the mammary gland where they produce IgA against those same gut organisms. The IgA molecule is complexed with a *secretory piece* as it passes the mammary acinar epithelial cell, and it is secreted into the colostrum.

Mammary acinar cells concentrate IgG.

In species that transfer antibodies from mother to young via colostrum, IgG is absorbed after ingestion by the nursing neonate. In the mother, acinar cells of the mammary gland also function to transport maternal serum antibodies during colostrum formation. Circulating IgG is concentrated by these cells immediately after birth, but this ability is reduced sharply after initial colostral section.

Globulin is absorbed by the intestine.

Most colostrums contain trypsin inhibitors that facilitate the passage of globulins undegraded through the stomach and into the intestine. The maternal IgG in colostrum is specifically transported across the intestinal mucosa into the fetal circulation. Transfer is mediated by *Fc receptors* on the surfaces of intestinal epithelial cells. Other Ig classes as well as milk proteins are instead digested within the gut absorptive cells.

The capacity to absorb globulin is transitory.

In the intestine of most species, globulin absorption by the intestinal epithelial cells lasts only a few hours. The structure and function of the absorptive epithelium rapidly becomes tight and selective. If colostrum is not fed until 48 hours after birth, it is then too late for antibodies to be absorbed. They may act within the gut lumen but will be digested and destroyed, for only degraded proteins reach the circulation after 48 hours.

Absorption of colostral antibodies is reflected in the neonate's plasma.

The rapid transmission of globulins from sow to suckling pig is revealed in parallel changes in serum proteins of the piglets. Globulin levels, low at birth, increase rapidly after suckling. By 24 hours, the piglet has absorbed enough colostral Ig to give serum concentrations as high as or higher than those of the sow. If pigs are deprived of colostrum, Igs in their serum are usually too low to be detected. Following injection of antigen into the newborn pig, a true primary immune response results within 48 hours. The first molecules to appear are IgM, followed by synthesis of IgG.

IgG dominates in bovine colostrum.

IgG_1 is the dominant Ig in bovine colostrum; that is, IgA makes up a smaller proportion of colostral antibody in the cow than in most mammals. During colostrum secretion, the interstitial fluid of the bovine mammary gland stroma increases markedly. Immunofluorescent studies reveal globulins as well as albumin and other serum proteins in this fluid. Few plasmacytes are present in the gland, and it seems that most globulins arrive from the maternal circulation. Consistent with their function of transporting maternal serum proteins during colostrum formation, hypertrophic acinar cells are packed with large secretory vacuoles containing globulins.

Calves are agammaglobulinemic at birth.

IgG is optimally absorbed in the lower jejunum in the calf. Absorption occurs only for 24–36 hours after birth (with a substantial loss of antibody absorption even after 12 hours). Any delay in suckling can have a striking impact on the development of neonatal infections. Failure to absorb colostral Igs frequently leads to neonatal disease, especially colibacillosis. Calves with less than 10 mg IgG_1/ml are considered hypogammaglobulinemic. *Severe passive transfer failure* is diagnosed when serum Ig values fall below 5 mg IgG_1/ml.

Embryonic development of immunocompetence

The first hematopoietic cells of the avian and mammalian embryo are formed early in the yolk sac. Called *hemocytoblasts,* these stem cells migrate and seed other sites (yolk sac suspensions from 4-day chick embryos can repopulate both lymphoid and myeloid organs of irradiated 13-day embryos). After seeding begins, yolk sac hemopoiesis is gradually replaced by liver and spleen, and finally bone marrow hemopoiesis, which persists throughout life. The first evidence of lymphoid development is the appearance of the thymus.

In most species bone marrow is the source of undifferentiated stem cells. Mice irradiated to destroy immunocompetence recover and produce antibody and lymphocytes near normal levels if bone marrow sites are shielded during radiation. Mice not shielded can be repopulated by injection of normal syngeneic bone marrow cells. However, these cells correct the immunologic defect only in a mouse with an intact thymus. From this and other studies, we know that small lymphocytes of marrow origin are trapped in the thymus (and other organs) for further differentiation. Specialization at these sites confers on the lymphoid cell progeny of marrow lymphocytes their special ability to react immunologically.

ADDITIONAL READING

Edelson, R. L., and Fink, J. M. The immunologic function of skin. *Sci. Am.* 252 (6):46, 1985.

Fetcher, A., et al. Regional distribution and variation of γ-globulin absorption from the small intestine of the neonatal calf. *Am. J. Vet. Res.* 44:2149, 1983.

Henkart, P. A. Mechanisms of lymphocyte-mediated cytotoxicity. *Ann. Rev. Immunol.* 3:31, 1985.

Jacoby, D. R., et al. Immunologic populations of fetal-maternal balance. *Adv. Immunol.* 35:157, 1984.

Kennedy, R. C., et al. Anti-idiotypes and immunity. *Sci. Am.* 255(1):48, 1986.

Kim, Y. B., et al. Natural killing (NK) and antibody-dependent cellular cytotoxicity (ADCC) in specific pathogen-free (SPF) miniature swine and germ-free pigs. *J. Immunol.* 125:755, 1980.

Newby, T. J., et al. Immunological activities of milk. *Vet. Immunol. Immunopathol.* 3:67, 1982.

Pearson, R. C., et al. Times of appearance and disappearance of colostral IgG in the mare. *Am. J. Vet. Res.* 45:186, 1984.

Hypersensitivity Disease

THE production of antibody and sensitized lymphocytes against microbes and foreign proteins is usually associated with *immunity.* Clinical disease does not develop on reexposure to a specific pathogenic microorganism. The range in which an animal reacts to antigens, however, includes, at one extreme, *tolerance,* in which antigen inhibits antibody production, and, at the other extreme, *hypersensitivity* (allergy), which is an exaggerated reaction to antigen.

Hypersensitivity diseases arise from several different mechanisms, all of which involve an excessive reactivity to antibody or lymphocytes (Table 23.1). In some of the prototype diseases (e.g., insect envenomation anaphylaxis, autoimmune hemolytic anemia, and immune complex glomerulonephritis), the reaction is solely due to one mechanism. Most naturally occurring hypersensitivity diseases are mixtures of these mechanisms, and the reaction that dominates must be differentiated in each individual disease.

This chapter deals only with diseases that are solely due to mechanisms of hypersensitivity. There are many other clinical syndromes in which hypersensitivity reactions play a minor role. For example, the chronic phases of many infectious diseases are complicated by a hypersensitivity component that aggravates the clinical situation but does not significantly affect the outcome of the disease.

IMMUNE COMPLEX DISEASES

Immune complex diseases are due to the damage induced in tissues by antigen-antibody-complement complexes that produce an inflammatory response. They occur in two ways: (1) when antigen-antibody complexes form in the bloodstream and circulate to lodge in delicate vascular channels such as the renal glomerulus, choroid plexus, or vascular channels of synoviae and (2) when circulating antibody attaches to antigens in tissue sites, with production of a damaging inflammatory reaction directly in the tissue.

The size and character of the antibody are often more important than the nature of the antigen. Small complexes remain in circulation and are not trapped in blood vessels. Large com-

Table 23.1. Mechanisms of immunologic injury

Mechanism	Disease	Immune Reactant	Additional Requirements
Immune complex	Arthus reaction Glomerulonephritis Serum sickness	Antibody	Complement, WBCs
Cytolysis	Hemolytic anemia	IgM (less often IgG)	Complement
Anaphylaxis	Anaphylactic shock	IgE	
Delayed hypersensitivity	Graft rejection	Lymphocytes	
Granuloma	Tuberculosis		

plexes are insoluble and are quickly removed by the reticuloendothelial system. Medium-sized complexes remain in circulation, fix complement, and are trapped in small capillaries.

Circulating immune complexes
The prototype disease: Serum sickness

Serum sickness was a disease of animals and man in preantibiotic days when large amounts of horse serum were injected intramuscularly to produce passive immunity to infectious diseases. Lesions began when antibody formed and appeared in serum before the injected antigen had been removed. Antigen-antibody complexes developed in the bloodstream and were deposited in joints, kidney, and sites of serum injection.

In 1891, Kitasato (a co-worker of von Behring) first treated a human disease with antisera. He injected 1.5 ml of rabbit (antitetanus) serum into a 9-day-old infant suffering from tetanus. His success led to the widespread clinical use of massive amounts of immune serum. Shortly thereafter the first human case of serum sickness was reported; a German groom with tetanus given 261 ml of horse serum developed violent itching at the site of injection, diffuse urticaria, lymphadenopathy, and arthritis 11 days after receiving the antiserum.

Acute serum sickness can be reproduced by the intramuscular injection of large amounts of bovine serum albumin into rabbits. Antigen is eliminated in three patterns from the circulation (Fig. 23.1). Clinical and pathologic signs of dis-

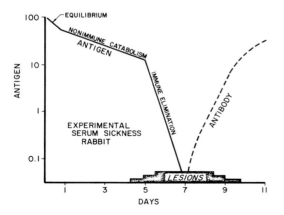

Fig. 23.1. Presence of antibody and antigen in circulating blood in experimental serum sickness, rabbit. Antigen was given at day 0.

ease first occur when antibody is formed, 5–6 days after injection of antigen. Necrotizing vascular lesions are widespread in kidney, heart, lung, and joints. In severe cases, polyserositis (effusions of serofibrinous exudates from pleura, pericardium, and peritoneum) is associated with immune deposits in lymph and blood vessels.

The renal glomerulus is the significant site of injury. Deposits of antigen, antibody, and complement below the capillary endothelium block the passage of glomerular filtrate. With immunofluorescent techniques applied to sections of kidney, the antigens, host immunoglobulin, and complement can be detected in the granular deposits along the capillary basement membrane. Regression of the lesion follows the disappearance of detectable circulating antigen-antibody complexes.

Complex disease: Anaphylactic shock

Serum sickness was common in animals used in serum laboratories in the 1890s. It was also known that some horses repeatedly immunized with tetanus or diphtheria antigens to produce antiserum suddenly collapsed and died when given a second or third injection. Theobald Smith, in his Boston laboratory for standardization of diphtheria antitoxin, noted shock, collapse, and death after repeated injections in guinea pigs. In 1894, Simon Flexner reported that dogs immunized to protein mixtures died abruptly after a second exposure to the protein. Human deaths, previously unreported, were brought to light after the notorious case of the daughter of the renowned pathologist Paul Langerhans (discoveror of pancreatic islets), who was taken to a clinic for preventative treatment for diphtheria and died within 5 minutes after receipt of antiserum.

These syndromes occur through complex mechanisms but are grouped together as *anaphylaxis,* a term coined in 1902 to describe the dichotomous response to immune serum; the immunizing or "prophylactic" response occurred when serum was given initially and the hypersensitizing or "anaphylactic" response occurred after repeated inoculation.

Early signs of anaphylaxis involve the lung; death is due to shock.

Anaphylaxis is an unusual or exaggerated allergic reaction. It is the most common after parenteral administration of drugs or vaccines but also can occur after inhalation or oral exposure. The signs of anaphylaxis are respiratory distress, a precipitous decrease in blood pressure, leukopenia, and decreased amounts of fibrinogen and complement in plasma (Fig. 23.2). All these clinical signs can occur, or any one of them may appear as an isolated manifestation. Horses are prone to die of respiratory problems and cardiovascular collapse during anaphylaxis and show tachypnea, harsh wheezing sounds, increased heart rate, weak thready pulse, cyanotic mucous membranes, and prolonged capillary refill times.

Different species show differing reactions in anaphylactic shock. In dogs and horses, the intestine may be an important "shock organ," especially if the antigenic challenge is prolonged. Increased peristalsis leads to diarrhea and hemorrhagic lesions in the intestine. Cattle, sheep, and swine may react similarly. In dogs, the liver is also an important shock organ. Severe congestion is followed by ischemic necrosis of hepatocytes, largely due to vasoconstriction causing

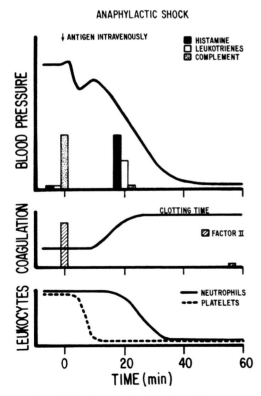

Fig. 23.2. Changes in blood and blood pressure during anaphylactic shock (aggregate anaphylaxis).

blood to pool in liver and intestine, which leads to hypotension and shock.

Anaphylaxis involves two mechanisms.

Anaphylactic shock, which is at the severe end of the clinical spectrum, is an immediate life-threatening reaction. It arises from two distinct mechanisms: deposition of immune complexes, which induces coagulation in the pulmonary capillary bed (*aggregate anaphylaxis*), and histamine/leukotriene-induced cardiopulmonary collapse (*cytotopic anaphylaxis*). Although a particular clinical case typically involves both mechanisms, one usually plays a dominant role. Which mechanism dominates depends on the type of antigen, how the antigen is delivered to the circulation, and the species of animal.

Aggregate anaphylaxis (immune complex anaphylaxis) occurs when large amounts of antigen are given intravenously. Antigens combine with IgG and the resulting antigen-antibody complexes bind complement. Complement causes the complexes to stick to endothelium and to attract leukocytes. In binding to complement, fragments of complement are released that induce blood coagulation and leukocyte degranulation. Aggregate anaphylaxis killed Flexner's dogs. The animals died because the pulmonary circulation was irreversibly blocked by clots of fibrin, platelets, and neutrophils trapped in the pulmonary vascular bed (Fig. 23.3).

Cytotropic anaphylaxis (IgE-mediated anaphylaxis) also occurs after rapid entry of antigens into the bloodstream, but collapse is sudden; blood levels of histamine are high, and disease can be reduced with antihistamines (before collapse) and epinephrine. Anaphylaxis is due to the immediate release of histamine, leukotrienes, and other vasoactive substances from mast cells and basophiles. These mediators cause vascular lesions (with increased vascular permeability) and activation of the coagulation system. Horses, man, and guinea pigs are prone to cytotropic anaphylaxis. In dogs, cytotropic anaphylaxis is the most common in atopic animals.

In situ deposition of immune complexes
Prototype disease: Arthus reaction

The classic Arthus reaction is produced in rabbits by two intradermal injections of the

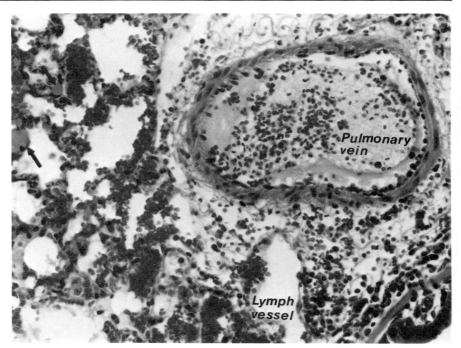

Fig. 23.3 Anaphylaxis, lung: dilatation of the pulmonary vein, capillaries of alveolar septae, and lymph vessel. Fibrin thrombi (*arrows*) block some capillaries. Erythrocytes in interstitial spaces (hemorrhage). Part of a bronchiole is at lower right corner.

same antigen at the same site at an interval of greater than 24 hours. Antibody produced locally after the sensitizing injection reacts with the antigen injected on the second, challenge dose. Antigen-antibody-complement complexes form directly within vascular walls and lead to acute vasculitis with hemorrhage, infiltration by neutrophilic leukocytes, and necrosis of the blood vessel wall (Fig. 23.4). Complement is strongly chemotactic for neutrophils, which rapidly degrade antigens. Unfortunately, lysis of neutrophils also occurs, and release of enzymes from neutrophil granules causes the disastrous tissue injury described above.

Arthus reactions are common, subtle components of parenteral immunization procedures. Antigens in the vaccine localize in the vascular wall, complex with antibody (produced during previous immunizations), and combine with complement. Most of these reactions are transient and subclinical. Although occasional bothersome dermal lesions occur after immunization, they are more likely to involve acute reactions induced by reaginic antibodies and histamine release.

Arthus-type reactions occur in the recovery stages of some infectious diseases, for example, the ocular lesions following acute infectious canine hepatitis (see Fig. 25.2). Partial resolution of the acute, primary, virus-induced iridocyclitis occurs, with viral antigens persisting in the anterior uvea. Antibody produced locally by plasmacytes in the iris and limbus reacts with cell-associated antigen, producing a hypersensitivity reaction that appears clinically as corneal opacity or "blue eye."

Focal edematous lesions of skin that appear as exacerbations of acute infectious disease may be due to the interaction of systemic antibody with persisting dermal antigens. A subacute dermatitis caused by *Sarcoptes scabiei* heals and disappears, and a generalized pruritis with erythematous skin lesions may appear several weeks after infection.

Complex disease: Allergic alveolitis

An immmunologic reaction, largely of the Arthus type, is induced on the alveolar wall of sensitized animals by large aerosols of extrinsic particulate antigens. Lesions in the lung include

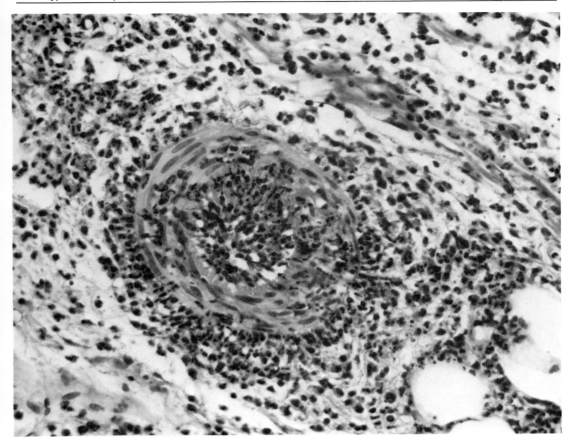

Fig. 23.4. Arthus reaction, skin, rabbit. Heterophils (rabbit neutrophils) have infiltrated and destroyed the wall of an artery.

infiltration of the alveolar wall with lymphocytes, macrophages, and plasmacytes. In severe cases, epithelioid granulomas that obliterate brionchioles occur, probably due to a complicating cell-mediated type of hypersensitivity.

The immunologic mechanism of a respiratory disease is proved by demonstrating (1) a latent period between exposure to antigen and onset of symptoms, (2) precipitating antibodies in serum, (3) an Arthus-type skin reactivity to suspect antigens, and (4) complement and immunoglobulins in lesions as shown by immunofluorescent staining of lung tissue.

Allergic alveolitis occurs in cattle and horses exposed to spores of *Micropolyspora faeni,* which are common in old, moist hay. *Thermoactinomyces* spp. are also responsible for pulmonary allergies in animals, especially *T. viridis,* one cause of "fog fever" of cattle. The large number

of allergic pneumonitides that occur in man are named according to the occupational hazard involved: for example, "farmer's lung" (due to *M. faeni*), "cheese washer's lung" (due to *Aspergillus clavatus* and *Penicillium casei*), "woodpulp worker's lung" (*Alternaria* spp.), "maple bark stripper's disease" (*Cryptostroma* spp.), and "paprika slicer's lung" (*Mucor* spp.). The lesions in these diseases are usually a chronic Arthus reaction, for there are multiple exposures of the lung to antigen. Lung biopsies reveal extensive fibrosis, vascular reactions, and perivenular lymphocyte accumulations. This suggests the participation of cellular hypersensitivity, which is often the case in these complex reactions.

Immunologic reactions of the respiratory system to organic dusts depend on the distribution pattern of antigens and on host reactivity. Atopic dogs and man give bronchial asthmatic reactions, which are mediated by nonprecipitating reaginic antibodies. Nonatopic individuals react to dust antigens predominantly with precipitating antibodies, which induce alveolitis typical of an Arthus-type reaction.

Glomerulonephritis involves circulating complexes or in situ deposition.

Immunologic injury to the renal glomerulus can result from the direct deposition of circulating immune complexes or from attachment of circulating antibodies to exogenous antigens trapped in the glomerular filtration barrier (Table 23.2). In the rare autoimmune glomerulonephritides, antibodies that cross-react with antigens that are components of the normal glomerular basement membrane will combine in situ with that material to produce glomerular disease.

All lesions of immune complex glomerulonephritis involve irregular granular hyalin deposits beneath the vascular endothelium (Fig. 23.5). Immunofluorescent staining can reveal the presence of antigens, complement, and immunoglobulins within these dense deposits. Affected glomeruli are hypercellular due to infiltration of inflammatory cells. Accumulations of monocytes (with some activation to macrophages) is the most common although neutrophils dominate in some types of immune complex reactions. The actual site of trapping in the glomerulus may be in the capillary endothelium, its basement membrane, or the slits of foot processes of the epithelium (Fig. 23.6). The normal renal filtration barrier restricts molecules greater than 4.5-nm diameter. Trapping in the glomerulus is influenced by the size of the immune complex (large complexes cause mesangiopathic glomerulonephritis while smaller complexes lead to membranous glomerulonephritis) and charge (highly cationic complexes are trapped most avidly). Systemic factors that influence trapping include (1) drugs (corticosteroid hormones and amine antagonists, (2) liver disease (failure of the liver to trap circulating immune complexes, especially IgA), and (3) thrombosis-enhancing factors. Furthermore, excess circulating antigen may cause release of complexes in glomeruli by conversions of large latticed deposits to smaller complexes.

Chronic infection is the major cause of immune-mediated glomerulonephritis.

Membranous glomerulonephritis is especially common in *bacterial sepsis,* especially chronic infections involving *Escherichia coli* (e.g., colisepticemia, coliform mastitis, and cystic endometritis of dogs). Local bacterial lesions have massive infiltration of plasma cells (see Fig. 22.1) and produce large amounts of immunoglobulins that in some unknown way become trapped in the renal glomerulus to cause basement membrane thickening and expansion of the glomerular mesangium.

Some *chronic viral infections* characteristically induce immune complex glomerulonephritis: bovine viral diarrhea, hog cholera, and equine infectious anemia. Malignant lymphoma in cats, mice, and man due to leukemia viruses induce renal glomerular deposits stainable for immunoglobulins and viral antigens (glycoproteins from the viral envelope).

Aleutian disease, a major problem of commercial mink ranching, is caused by a parvovirus that replicates in macrophages and persists in high titer in blood, spleen, and lymphoid tissues.

Table 23.2. Glomerulonephritis due to immunologic mechanisms

CIRCULATING ANTIGEN-ANTIBODY COMPLEXES (SOLUBLE IMMUNE COMPLEX DISEASE)	
Serum sickness	Multiple treatment with serum or proteins
Chronic sepsis	Coliform mastitis, bacterial septicemia
Viral disease	Aleutian disease of mink, feline and murine leukemia
Protozoal infection	Malaria (man)
Parasite infestation	Dirofilariases (dog)
PLANTED ANTIGENS (ANTIGENS TRAPPED IN KIDNEY BEFORE COMPLEXING WITH ANTIBODY)	
Viral infections	Hog cholera (swine fever), bovine viral diarrhea, measles (monkey)
Postbacterial disease	Poststreptococcal disease (man)
Parasite infestation	Dirofilariasis (dog)[a]
GLOMERULAR ANTIGENS (ANTIBODIES FORMED AGAINST COMPONENTS OF KIDNEY [RARE])	
Anti–basement membrane	Antiglomerular basement membrane lesions (horse), Goodpasture's syndrome (man), heterologous anti–GBM disease (experimental, rat)

[a]Soluble complexes and planted antigens both occur in dirofilarial nephropathy.

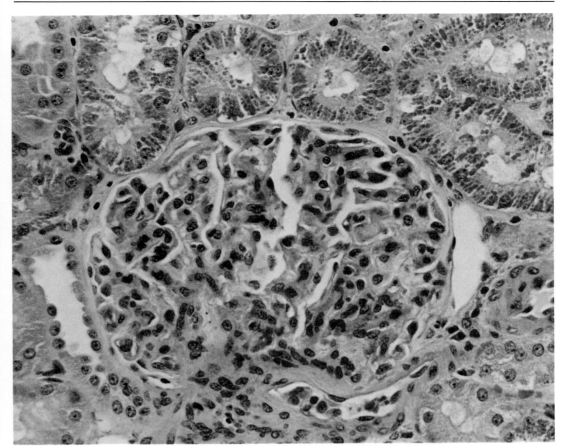

Fig. 23.5. Immune complex membranous glomerulopathy, dog with dirofilariasis. Capillaries in the glomerulus have markedly thickened basement membranes.

Viral replication is not associated with overt tissue lesions but induces an extreme immune response to viral antigens. Disease results from deposition of virus-antibody complexes and plasmacytes in tissues. Like many of the viral glomerulopathies, intravascular coagulation often contributes to the glomerular lesions.

CYTOTOXIC DISEASE

Cytotoxic diseases are initiated when circulating antibodies (either IgG or IgM) attach to antigens on cell surfaces. Cell lysis is caused when circulating complement attaches to the cell-bound antibodies. The attack sequence of complement components is responsible for the actual lysis of cells.

Complement-induced cytolysis

Clinical disease resulting from cytotoxic reactions involves blood cells. Although the most severe clinical reactions occur against erythrocytes (to cause anemia), cytotoxic diseases also develop from antibody-mediated, complement-induced attack on leukocytes (causing granulocytopenia) and platelets (causing thrombocytopenia). In all of these diseases, antibodies bound to the cell surface attract complement, the attack sequence of which causes 100-nm holes to appear in the plasma membrane. Lysis results from loss of potassium ions and entry of sodium and calcium ions and water into the cell.

Naturally occurring cytotoxic diseases are complex and may also involve cell-mediated mechanisms, that is, the direct action of sensitized lymphocytes on cell surface antigens.

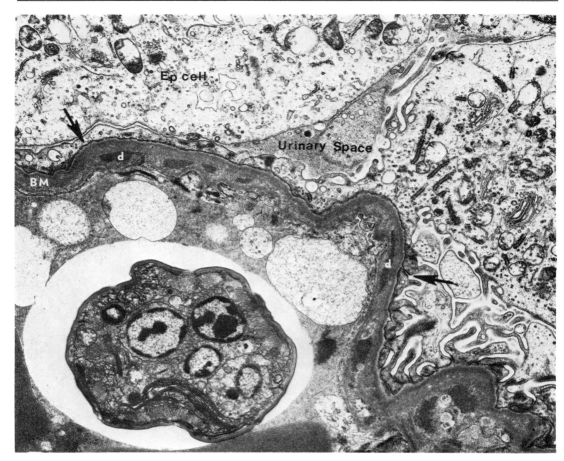

Fig. 23.6. Immune complex membranous glomerulopathy, ultrastructure of renal glomerulus. The basement membrane (*BM*) is thickened. There are fusion of foot processes (*arrows*) and dense aggregates (probably immune complexes) throughout the area of the membrane. A cross section of *Dirofilaria immitis* is at lower left.

Recent studies indicate that some lymphocytes (those with natural killer and T cytotoxicity activities) produce tiny membranous vesicles called *perforans* that are released on contact with target cells. Perforans attach to the cell surface of the target cells and induce holes similar to those produced by complement.

Transfusion reactions

Isoantibodies are formed against antigenic cell proteins (isoantigens), which differ among individuals of the same species. Generally, isoantibodies are important in relation to cellular antigens, such as those on erythrocyte surfaces. In normal baby pig sera, isoantibodies may de-

velop against globulins that have crossed the maternal-fetal barrier.

In 1900 Karl Landsteiner discovered the isoantigens A and B (and consequently the blood groups A, B, AB, and O) in human red blood cells. These form the strict limitations of human red blood cell transplantation. "Blood type" is based on differences in sugar moieties of glycoprotein isoantigens of the erythrocyte's plasma membrane: type A contains an enzyme that transfers acetylgalactosamine to the core protein, type B an enzyme that transfers galactose, and type O lacks both enzymes.

Similar antigenic differences exist in animals. While some of these are termed A, B, etc., they are unrelated serologically to human isoantigens or to each other. Isoantigens are not confined to red blood cells but are present on surfaces of endothelial and epithelial cells of the epidermis, thymic corpuscles, and intestines.

Transfusion reactions result when blood with erythrocyte *isoantigens* of one type is transfused to individuals with circulating *isoantibodies* against it, for example, blood with A isoantigen given to an individual with type B blood (and A isoantibodies). Clumping and lysis of the donor erythrocytes in the vascular system of the recipient result in embolization, pulmonary vascular blockade, and death. Because of the rapid dilution of donor antibodies, the opposite reaction of clumping of recipient erythrocytes by donor isoantibodies does not cause clinical disease.

Hemolytic disease of the newborn

Hemolytic disease occurs in newborn horses, mules, calves, and swine. The fetus, by virtue of inheritance from the sire, develops erythrocyte antigens not present in the mother. When these cells gain access to the mother's bloodstream, they induce antibody formation. If these antibodies are returned to the newborn via colostrum, severe hemolytic anemia is induced. Absorption of antibodies occurs via milk in horses and swine, but in man, transplacental transfer of antibody occurs, resulting in a similar disease called erythroblastosis fetalis. Thrombocytopenia caused by a similar mechanism has been reported in piglets and puppies with platelet deficiency and hemorrhages.

Hemolytic anemia caused by antibodies to erythrocytes can occur when the mother has been injected with blood or blood products, for example, antierythrocyte immunoglobulins appear in serum and colostrum of cows vaccinated against anaplasmosis with vaccines containing blood cells.

Hemolytic reactions to drugs

Hemolytic anemia during prolonged drug therapy, particularly penicillin, occurs in some animals. The most common mechanism involves the formation by the drug of a hapten on the erythrocyte surface that then binds antihapten antibodies to cause erythrocyte lysis. Other mechanisms have been reported in man (Table 23.3) but are not well documented in animals.

In cats, propylthiouracil is used for treatment for hyperthyroidism and may cause a hemolytic reaction. Clinical signs, which appear in 20–35

Table 23.3. Cytotoxic mechanisms in hemolytic reactions to drugs

Mechanism	Drug
Haptens on erythrocyte surface bind antihapten antibody	Penicillin
Immune complex of drug-antibody complex adheres to erythrocyte surface and attracts complement	Quinidine
Metabolic defect in RBC produces new surface antigens to which antibodies react	Methyl DOPA
Transfer of activated complement	Penicillin

days, include lethargy, weakness, anorexia, and bleeding. Severe anemia is accompanied by thrombocytopenia. The direct antiglobulin (Coombs') test is positive, and serum antinuclear antibody titers exceed 1:10. Cessation of treatment is accompanied by disappearance of anemia.

Anemia has been reported in an allergy to sulfadiazine in Doberman pinschers. The dominant sign was lymphocytic polyarthritis, and the dogs also had lymphadenopathy, myositis, and skin rashes.

Cytotoxic reactions contribute to other immune diseases.

Immune cytotoxicity plays a role in rare cases of human male sterility because antisperm antibodies are produced. In autoimmune thyroiditis and graft rejection, cytotoxic reactions play an early but limited role in tissue injury.

IgE-MEDIATED MAST CELL REACTIONS

IgE-mediated mast cell reactions occur when, after a second exposure to antigen, the antigen contacts antibodies bound to the surfaces of basophils and mast cells. On contact with antigen, sensitized basophils and mast cells release histamine and platelet-activating factor, which causes platelets to aggregate at the sites of reaction. Leukocytes release leukotrienes, which are more potent than histamine in producing vascular permeability and smooth muscle contraction (e.g., bronchoconstriction in the lungs) (Table 23.4).

IgE is involved in most reactions although cytotropic IgG may be involved in some species. Receptors on the surfaces of mast cells and basophils combine with the Fc part of the IgE molecule during the immune response. In subse-

Table 23.4.   **Skin test differentiation**

Type	Time	Mechanism
Immediate	15 min–1 hr	Anaphylaxis: histamine-induced vascular changes
	6–8 hr	Arthus reaction: antigen-antibody-complement complexes (via neutrophils)
Delayed	24–48 hr	Delayed hypersensitivity: mediated by T lymphocytes

quent exposure, antigen forms bridges between antibody molecules to trigger the release of inflammatory mediators.

Systemic reactions
Anaphylactic shock

Cytotropic anaphylaxis, discussed with immune complex hypersensitivity, results from the reaction of antigen with antibody fixed to mast cell plasma membranes. During the challenge incident, antigen enters the animal and attaches to the mast cell–fixed antibody. This causes uncoiling of mast cell granules, degeneration of the plasma membrane, and release of granules (see Fig. 19.3). Degranulation releases pharmacologically active agents (e.g., histamine, prostaglandins, and leukotrienes) that produce the clinical signs.

Rapid systemic distribution of antigen is one of the requirements of anaphylactic shock. As antigens combine with antibodies, there are precipitous decreases in blood pressure accompanied by smooth muscle contraction, capillary dilatation, and edema (Fig. 23.7). Accumulation of edema fluid is particularly severe in the upper respiratory tract (especially if that is the site of antigen entry), and affected animals may die from laryngeal obstruction and asphyxia.

If the animal survives for several hours, platelets and neutrophils are trapped in lungs and lead to intravascular coagulation. Lesions are similar to those of aggregate anaphylaxis from immune complexes, and immune complex reactions seem to complicate the late stages of IgE-induced anaphylaxis.

Local reactions
Postvaccination wheal-and-flare reactions

Vaccines prepared in cell cultures and chick embryos can induce wheal-and-flare lesions in the skin when used repeatedly. These "anaphylactoid" reactions involve several mechanisms, but mast cell degranulation and localized edema often dominate (see Chapter 25).

Insect envenomation also causes wheal-and-flare reactions.

Repeated bee stings and other insect venoms induce transitory postvaccinal-type reactions of edema and swelling. In dogs and cats, flea bites are seasonally recurring dermatitides with unusual dorsal body distribution and intense pruritis. Flea allergy is the most common small animal hypersensitivity skin disease. It probably results from a hypersensitivity reaction to insect saliva similar to that occurring in horses associated with repeated *Culicoides* spp. Cats with ear infections of *Otodectes cyanotis* have precipitins to mite antigens and develop wheal-and-flare reactions at sites of reinfection.

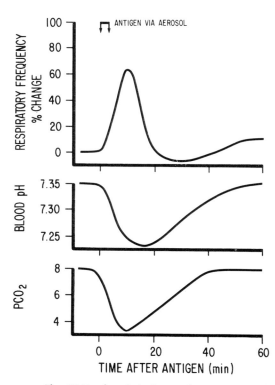

Fig. 23.7. Anaphylaxis: respiratory rate and changes in blood pH and oxygen.

In Australia, "Queensland itch" is an allergic dermatitis caused by hypersensitivity of horses to biting midges (*Culicoides robertsi*). Papules form and are followed by pruritis, alopecia, and crusting.

Atopic Reactions

The term *atopy* is used in allergic phenomena to imply a familial association. Reactions of this type are immediate and involve such shock organs as skin (urticaria), upper respiratory tract (rhinitis, or hay fever), and bronchioles (asthma). Antigens (reagins) can be demonstrated bound to affected tissues, particularly mast cells.

Skin tests are used to verify atopic reactions. The skin is clipped, cleaned, and disinfected and injected with 0.05 ml of a commercial antigen (e.g., "4-mold mix," "10-tree mix," "mixed feathers," and "house dust"). A saline control injection site must be included. Comparisons are made at 15- and 50-minute intervals after injection. Reactions are positive if the wheal is 3 mm greater or 2 times the control site.

Allergic inhalant dermatitis

Only in dogs has IgE-mediated atopic disease been adequately studied. Skin is the target organ and pruritis the primary sign; it is an "itch that rashes rather than a rash that itches." Like man, most atopic dogs are multisensitive and allergic to many allergens. Curiously, there is no significant difference in amounts of serum IgE between normal and atopic dogs.

The cause of allergic dermatitis in dogs is usually pollen allergy, most often ragweed pollen, and many pollens are unreactive in atopic dogs (e.g., nettle pollen). Clinical associations include age (most frequently 1–3 years), season (spring and summer) and intercurrent skin disease (flea infestation). In some areas nearly one-third of dogs admitted for dermatologic examination are atopic, and there is some breed predisposition. Of 29 atopic dogs in a California study, 38% were golden retrievers; 56% were born during pollen seasons, suggesting that sensitization during the first month of life is important. Viral infections appear to predispose to allergy in atopic dogs. Pups vaccinated for canine distemper before being given pollen extract had greater IgE antibodies in serum than did nonvaccinated pups.

Food allergy enteritis-dermatitis

Intestinal mucosal immune responses to food antigens may be due to atopic allergy. For example, atrophy of intestinal villi and lymphocytic infiltration into the lamina propria have been seen in calves and piglets fed soy proteins. Although atopic reaction may be responsible for malabsorption in neonates, cell-mediated immunopathic enteritis usually occurs in adults.

Milk allergy of human infants. In most humans IgE has a limited immunologic role. Although it helps to repel parasite invasions (elevated IgE is found in people in the tropics), elsewhere there is no "good" function of IgE and most humans synthesize very little of it. In atopic humans, IgE mediates hypersensitivity. In the absence of proper modulation by T cells, a clone of B lymphocytes is transformed by binding of antigen (allergen) that would not normally excite an immune response.

Human inhalant rhinitis

Allergic rhinitis in man is probably the most widespread allergic disease. Caused by pollen, pet hair, house dust, and mites (*Dermatophagoides* spp.) that live on human scales, they appear seasonally as seropurulent rhinitis.

CELL-MEDIATED HYPERSENSITIVITY DISEASE

Cell-mediated hypersensitivity diseases involve (1) *recognition* of antigen by T lymphocytes (T_{dh} subset), (2) secretion of *cytokines* by the activated T cell, and (3) *attraction of effector cells,* chiefly monocytes activated by the process and transformed into macrophages. Effector cells act to produce tissue injury by secreting lymphotoxins or by directly attacking target cells. One of the cytokines secreted by activated T cells is *transfer factor,* a dialyzable extract of lymphocytes that transfers this reaction from sensitized donors to negative recipients.

As a component of disease processes, cell-mediated hypersensitivity is very common, as the dominant component of a disease it is rare (one example is poison ivy), and as a sole component it probably never occurs, except as an experimental disease. In other words, cell-mediated hypersensitivity is usually complicated by exudative and necrotic processes that are induced by antibodies and that complicate the clinical signs and pathologic evidence of tissue injury.

Cell-mediated hypersensitivity in skin

Cell-mediated mechanisms are the most prominent in skin, largely because the sensitizing agent must diffuse through the skin barrier and can avoid stimulating antibody production, which would complicate the disease process. Drugs and toxins act as haptens in combining with protein in the skin epithelium. The conjugate is then carried to the regional lymph node, where it stimulates an immune response by lymphocytes. On the second exposure, the antigen is trapped in the epithelium by specialized macrophages. Skin contains specialized cells (epidermal Langerhans' cells) that are modified intraepidermal macrophages. They have Fc and immunoglobulin receptors and Ia antigens of the major histocompatibility complex on the surface. They play a key role in taking up and presenting antigens to lymphocytes during induction of delayed hypersensitivity in skin.

Contact hypersensitivities are common in animals and man.

Dermatitis caused by poison ivy, cosmetics, or drugs are the most frequent causes of human contact hypersensitivity. One of the most frequent contact hypersensitivities is "cement eczema" caused by allergy to hexavalent chromium salts present in cement. In animals, hypersensitivities to protein components in vaccines are probably the most common. Cell-mediated reactivity as a *component* of other syndromes is far more common and can be proved by testing on the skin using a dermal patch. A 1-cm filter paper soaked in dilute sensitizing antigen is placed on the skin, covered with tape, and examined after 12 hours. Swelling peaks at 24–48 hours and is taken as a positive sign of cell-mediated reactivity.

The tuberculin reaction is a diagnostic test.

Tuberculin (purified protein derivative, or PPD) is a relatively nonantigenic extract of soluble mycobacterial proteins. When injected intradermally into a tuberculous animal, it incites an inflammatory reaction characterized by increased vascular permeability to fluid and neutrophils and perivascular accumulation of lymphocytes and macrophages (Fig. 23.8). The character of the lesion is determined by the purity of the tuberculin and the severity of tuber-

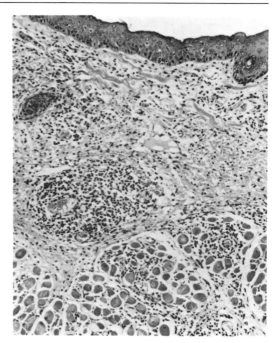

Fig. 23.8. Tuberculin reaction, eyelid, rhesus monkey. The dermis is expanded by edema fluid. Large aggregates of small lymphocytes occur in the dermis around venules.

culosis. Crude tuberculin is apt to provoke exudative reactions with many neutrophils.

Although a vigorous tuberculin reaction develops in the early stages of tuberculosis, *anergy* occurs in the terminal stages. Anergic animals do not respond to tuberculin, probably because of extensive dissemination of bacillary antigens throughout the host that depletes lymphoid tissue and renders host macrophages inoperable.

Hypersensitivities of this delayed type can be elicited in skin in most infectious diseases, but only in tuberculosis and some fungal diseases are they used clinically as diagnostic aids.

Graft rejection

If the technical aspects of skin grafting are correct (e.g., proper surgical alignment and absence of infection) skin transplants between *syngeneic* (genetically identical) animals vascularize and become accepted as host tissue. Grafts between *allogeneic* animals (not identical but of the same species) become necrotic and slough in 10–14 days. Rejection of grafted skin is preceded by infiltration of the dermis by small lymphocytes and monocytes, largely in a perivenous location. Vascular damage occurs and induces ischemia, which in turn causes death of the graft.

A second skin transfer and graft from the same donor will result in a more rapid rejection by the recipient. This rapid "second set" reaction is specific for the original donor skin and has other characteristics of a specific immune reaction; that is, rejection is inhibited by immunosuppressant drugs and can be transferred with lymphocytes but not with serum. In dogs given bone marrow grafts, two graft-versus-host syndromes occur. *Acute* rejections (median onset, 13 days; median survival, 29.5 days) are characterized by skin erythema, jaundice, diarrhea, and gram-negative bacterial infections. *Chronic* rejections (median onset, 124 days; median survival, 150 days) include skin ulceration, ascites, cirrhosis, gram-positive infections, and epidermal atrophy.

Histocompatibility antigens cause rejection.

The immunologic basis of rejection of grafted tissue is a direct expression of genetic differences between donor and recipient. Rejection occurs against *histocompatibility antigens*, which are proteins inserted in the membranes of the cell surface of the grafted cells. The nature of these histocompatibility antigens has been well defined in mice, somewhat less in humans and chickens, and hardly at all in other species. In all cases these antigens function to make immune reactions highly specific.

Lymphocytes directly attack graft tissue.

The majority of grafted organs in nonimmunosuppressed recipients are rejected with 4 weeks by mechanisms of cell-mediated immunity. Contact between sensitized lymphocytes and foreign cells destroys the latter. How the small lymphocytes mediate graft rejection is not precisely known. It is theorized that sensitized cell–antigen interaction releases a factor involving nonsensitized monocytes. The monocytes dominate in the graft, and release of lysosomal enzymes is responsible for tissue damage.

Kidneys are rejected by complex mechanisms.

Human organ transplantation has revealed complex mechanisms of tissue rejection. For example, kidney allografts may be rejected at three different time periods after grafting, each representing a different dominant mechanism. (1) Peracute rejection begins immediately and is mediated through activation of complement; platelets and neutrophils are prominent in the lesions and accumulate in glomerular and peritubular capillaries. (2) Acute rejection begins in a few days and is caused by the cellular immunologic processes decribed above; small lymphocytes accumulate around intertubular capillaries in the grafted kidney and destroy it. (3) Chronic rejection may occur after many months; it is related to vascular degeneration.

Graft-versus-host reaction

The graft-versus-host reaction is an immunologic response that occurs when lymphocytes are transplanted and proliferate to attack the recipient animal because they react against histocompatibility antigens of the host. The recipient of immunologically active lymphocytes is destroyed by the attack of these cells on its tissue.

There are three requirements for the reaction. (1) The recipient must be incapable of an efficient immune response to reject the graft, so neonatal animals are the best candidates. (2) Donor cells must be immunocompetent; adult lymphocytes are best, and the reaction is accelerated with cells from a preimmunized donor. Grafts such as epithelium cannot mount an immune response and so are incapable of initiating this reaction. (3) The donor and recipient must have different strong histocompatibility genes (Fig. 23.9).

Clinical signs of graft-versus-host reactions are growth failure (often called "runt disease"), diarrhea, and emaciation. At necropsy lymphoid depletion and hepatosplenomegaly are seen. Myocardium, intestinal mucosa, liver, and other

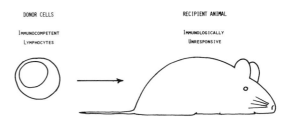

Fig. 23.9. Requirement for the graft-versus-host reaction.

organs contain accumulations of macrophages. In animals, graft-versus-host reactions are a complication of bone marrow grafting used in the treatment of immunodeficient or stem cell–deficient animals. In combined immunodeficiency of Arabian foals, injection of thymic cells has been followed by widespread infiltration of tissues with lymphocytes and death of the recipient.

ADDITIONAL READING

Atkinson, K., et al. Acute and chronic graft-versus-host disease in dogs given hemopoietic grafts from DLA-nonidentical littermates. *Am. J. Pathol.* 108:196, 1982.

Cummings, J. F., et al. Neuritis of the cauda equina, a chronic idiopathic polyradiculoneuritis in the horse. *Acta Neuropathol.* 46:17, 1979.

Davis, L. E. Hypersensitivity reactions induced by antimicrobial drugs. *J. Am. Vet. Med. Assoc.* 185:1131, 1984.

Giger, U., et al. Sulfadiazine-induced allergy in six Doberman pinschers. *J. Am. Vet. Med. Assoc.* 186:479, 1985.

Schwartzman, R. M. Immunologic studies of progeny of atopic dogs. *Am. J. Vet. Res.* 45:375, 1984.

Stormont, C. Neonatal isoerythrolysis in domestic animals. *Adv. Vet. Sci. Comp. Med.* 19:23, 1975.

Immunodeficiency Disease

24

THE immune system of normal animals deals effectively with a wide variety of microorganisms in the environment. Barriers in the skin, gut, and respiratory tract are bridged continuously with opportunistic bacteria that the host eliminates with remarkable efficiency. Normal animals breathe in dust bearing large numbers of fungal spores without ever suffering disease. These situations change markedly, however, when the immune system is crippled. No longer eliminated, these microorganisms of low virulence play an important role in causing disease.

The consequences of immunosuppression are infectious diseases that are rarely, if ever, seen in animals with normal structure and function in their lymphoid system. For example, horses with hereditary combined immunodeficiency often suffer acute respiratory disease due to an equine adenovirus or to the protozoan *Pneumocystis carinii,* two agents not known to affect foals that receive proper colostral antibodies and that have intact lymphoid systems. Fungi are notorious for causing disease in immunosuppressed animals, particularly those with cold stress (Fig. 24.1).

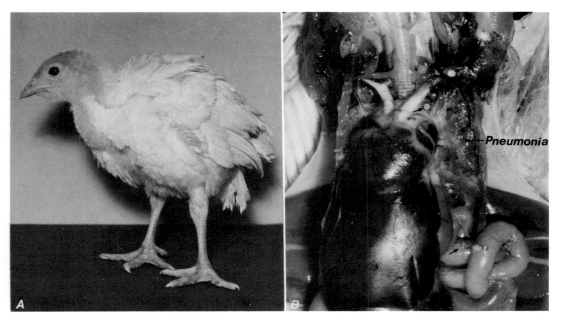

Fig. 24.1. Aspergillosis, turkey. A. Emaciation, lethargy, and anorexia. B. Purulent airsacculitis and colonies of fungi in the air sacs.

FAILURE OF BARRIER FUNCTIONS

Defects in epithelia of skin, mucocutaneous junctions, and gastrointestinal and genitourinary tracts may be associated with the suppressed capacity of animals to resist infectious disease. In most cases, epithelium is only a display tissue in which a defect in systemic mechanisms is manifest as a local epithelial disease. In rare instances, however, epithelial barriers themselves are defective and the host is prone to develop local infections.

Defects in normal bacterial flora

All body orifices and surface structures have a characteristic resident population of microorganisms. Secretions of this resident microflora play a role in preventing overgrowth of pathogenic bacteria. Nonpathogenic bacteria colonize skin, teeth, urogenital tract, and intestine and reduce growth rates of some pathogenic bacteria.

Disruption of normal microflora is particularly dangerous in the intestine, which is prone to bacterial overgrowth during therapy with antibiotics and corticosteroids. Dr. Ernest Sanford, at the Ontario Ministry of Agriculture, has reported overgrowth of Zygomycetes (mucormycosis) in the gastric mucosa of suckling pigs. There were large venous infarcts in the fundus, cardiac, and pyloric regions of the stomach, and fungal hyphae were in the lumens of thrombosed blood vessels. Disease occurred as an opportunistic infection, probably related to heavy doses of broad-spectrum antibiotics to pigs and their sows. Destruction of the normal bacterial microflora permitted overgrowth by fungi.

Defects in mucus and mucociliary movement

Mucus and fluids that cover the mucous membranes of the respiratory, gastrointestinal, and urinary epithelia are essential to maintenance of antimicrobial barriers. The antibacterial nature of these fluids includes the presence of proteins secreted from the epithelium, such as complement, secretory antibody (IgA), lysozyme, and several other proteins. The tenacious character of glycosaminoglycans of mucus also asserts an antibacterial effect.

Ciliary movement is essential for removal of bacteria.

Diseases of congenitally nonfunctional cilia, called the *immotile cilia syndrome,* have been found in dogs and man with prolonged retention (delayed clearance) of inhaled particulate material in the lungs. Canine patients with this syndrome have widespread evidence of abnormal cilia in the nasal cavity, ependyma, and spermatozoa. The disease is manifest as chronic sinusitis, bronchiectasis, and (in males) infertility. The basic defect is absence or abnormality of the dynein arms in ciliary axonemes. Cilia show slowed movements that are random rather than directed, as in normal cilia.

Lysozyme may be deficient in mucus, saliva, and tears.

Hereditary deficiency of lysozyme occurs in man, dogs, and rodents. Most are not associated with any severe predisposition to disease. Some strains of rabbits have leukocytes that are deficient in this antimicrobial protein, yet the rabbits show no marked susceptibility to bacterial infection.

DEFICIENCY OF NEUTROPHILS
Acquired neutrophil defects

Any depression of neutrophil function leads to an increased susceptibility to disease. Transient effects are common but are of such short duration that no significant clinical disease results. In other cases, an effect on neutrophils is produced, but the suppressive effects on specific lymphoid-induced immunity are even greater and this system dominates the clinical picture.

The importance of neutrophilic leukocytes in the inflammatory response and defense of the host can be seen when infectious diseases occur in animals that have insufficient numbers of cells to mount a neutrophilic response. Affected animals tend to have chronic, recurring infectious processes, and if the neutrophilic defect is marked, the animal will not survive.

Hormones affect neutrophil function.

The endocrine system has a subtle influence on neutrophils. For example, the hormones that appear during estrus in cattle have an inhibitory effect, which is sometimes translated into an increased incidence of mastitis. The bovine uterus is largely an anaerobic environment. However, a variety of both aerobic and anaerobic bacteria can be isolated from the normal uterus. *Corynebacterium pyogenes,* the major bacterial pathogen, often acts synergistically with the anaerobe *Fusobacterium necrophorum* to cause metritis (Table 24.1).

In dogs with diabetes mellitus, high blood glucose concentrations have a suppressive effect on neutrophil function, which makes diabetic patients susceptible to certain bacterial infections, particularly by staphylococci (Fig. 24.2).

Microbial factors suppress neutrophil function.

Microbial inhibition of neutrophils is a major factor in determining the virulence of bacteria and viruses. The polysaccharide components of the *capsules* and *cell walls* of anthrax bacilli, pneumococci, and some streptococci have a marked inhibitory effect on the phagocytic function of neutrophils. Some *exotoxins* secreted by bacteria are directly antiphagocytic. Streptolysins of streptococci inhibit neutrophil chemotaxis. Cryptococcal polysaccharides inhibit both neutrophils and macrophages; lesions caused by this fungus are notorious for their lack of cellular exudation. Intracellular bacteria such as *Brucella* spp., *Salmonella* spp., *Mycobacteria* spp., and *Listeria monocytogenes* all produce substances that allow their survival intracellularly. Most of these factors are effective for the macrophages within which these bacteria replicate, but the same factors also have an effect on circulating neutrophils. *Brucella abortus* causes a chronic, persistent infection of cattle in which components of its cell wall inhibit the myeloperoxidase–hydrogen peroxide–halide antibacterial system of bovine neutrophils. Dr. Tim Bertram, then at the National Animal Disease Center, showed that these nucleotidelike structures of the bacterial cell wall inhibit neutrophil degranulation, a defect that preferentially involves primary granules.

Viruses suppress neutrophils.

Systemic viral infections such as bovine viral diarrhea and canine distemper have a suppressive effect on neutrophil function, and although these effects promote secondary bacterial infections, these viruses have an even more disastrous effect on specific lymphoid immune mechanisms.

Chemical and physical suppression of granulocytopoiesis.

Chemical and radiologic suppression of granulocytopoiesis predisposes animals to infectious agents. *Corticosteroids* used therapeutically have a suppressant effect. Although most markedly affecting lymphocytes, they also inhibit neutrophil function. Studies of bovine neutrophils suggest that corticosteroids reduce neutrophil surface stickiness and attachment of neutrophils to endothelium, thus suppressing their margination and diapedesis during inflammation (even though bacterial killing remains unaffected).

Drugs termed *metabolic antagonists* have molecular structures so similar to the protein utilized in metabolism that they are incorporated into pathways in the cell. The molecular structure is sufficiently dissimilar, however, to cause blocks in the metabolic machinery of the cell, and rapidly proliferating hematopoietic stem cells are among the first to be depressed by such treatment (Fig. 24.3). Animals so treated (for immunosuppression or for anticancer therapy) are highly susceptible to fungi and bacteria.

Large doses of *radiation* cause depression of all white blood cells (panleukopenia). Although neutrophils are affected, there is no known selective inhibition of neutrophil function after low-dose irradiation.

Table 24.1. Bacteria in bovine pyometra

Bacteria	Normal Cows	Number isolates from uterine lumen	
		Cows with Retained Fetal Membranes	Cows with Pyometra
		(%)	
Corynebacterium pyogenes	40	58	66
Gram-negative anaerobes[a]	31	59	62
Coliform bacteria	1	11	25
Clostridia	26	46	46

[a]Source: Data from Olson et al., *J. Am. Vet. Med. Assoc.* 184:100, 1984.
[a]*Fusobacterium necrophorum* and *Bacteroides melanogenicus.*

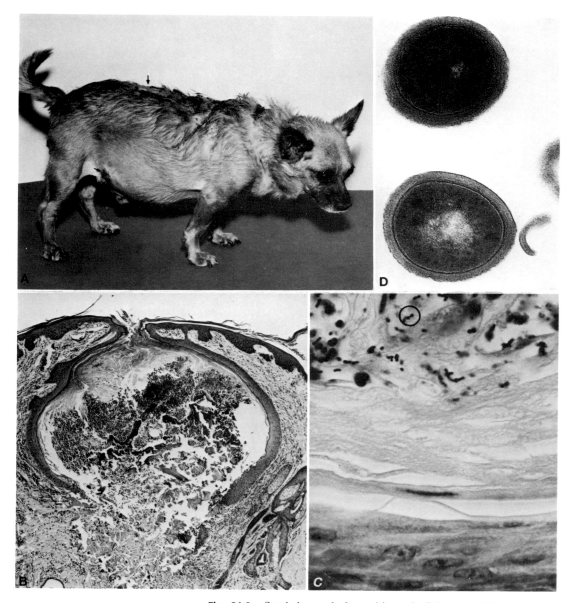

Fig. 24.2. Staphylococcal dermatitis and diabetes mellitus, dog. A. Severe serous dermatitis and folliculitis. B. Expansion of hair follicle by tissue debris and neutrophils. C. Enlargement of follicular epithelium in B show bacteria (*circle*) in cornified areas. D. Ultrastructure of staphylococci.

Congenital abnormalities of neutrophils

Some rare but intriguing genetic abnormalities in neutrophils exist. These "experiments in nature" readily illustrate the essential role of neutrophils in continual monitoring of the blood for microbes and tissue products. The three following models illustrate defects in neutrophil production, in neutrophil lyososome-phagosome fusion, and in bactericidal content of lysosomes.

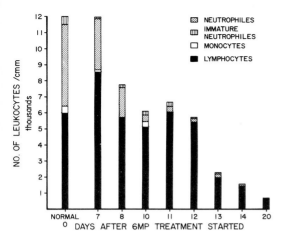

Fig. 24.3. Total and differential leukocyte counts of monkey receiving the antimetabolite 6-mercaptopurine.

Cyclic hematopoiesis (cyclic neutropenia)

This congenital disease occurs in collie pups that have a coat color mutation (the gray collie). The bone marrow defect involves cyclic depression of neutrophil maturation with consequential disappearance of mature neutrophils from the bloodstream every 11 days (Fig. 24.4). The disease occurs in human infants in cycles of 28 days. The nature of the defect involves insufficient stem cell production rather than control of hematopoiesis. Transplantation of marrow stem cells from normal to neutropenic dogs corrects the periodic depression of granulocytopoiesis. The transplanted cells mature normally in the defective recipient dogs.

The precise mechanism involved in cyclic neutropenia is unknown. Attempts to incriminate antineutrophil or elevated estrogen levels have been unsuccessful. Pathologic changes occur in neutrophils but indicate a secondary toxic degeneration as an effect of infection. Affected dogs develop periodic bacterial infections that coincide with phases of neutropenia (Fig. 24.5).

Chediak-Higashi syndrome

Another genetic neutrophil disease, the Chediak-Higashi syndrome, is characterized by anomalous giant granules in all granule-containing cells (including neutrophils), increased susceptibility to infections, and defective pigmentation. It occurs in mink, partially albino Hereford cattle, killer whales, inbred mice (beige strain), and man. Similar syndromes have been reported in bison, white mutant tigers, and Persian cats. The primary granules of neutrophils are defective, and although phagocytosis occurs normally, bactericidal activity is diminished.

Giant granules in neutrophils and other cells of Chediak-Higashi animals arise from abnormal fusion of primary granules during development. In *cattle,* the defect involves abnormal bacte-

---

FOCUS

Cyclic hematopoiesis

The *gray collie syndrome* is a lethal hereditary disease associated with abnormal hair pigmentation, cyclic depression of circulating neutrophils, and bilateral ocular scleral ectasia. Neutrophils disappear from the peripheral blood at intervals of 10.5 to 11.5 days, although intervals between neutropenic phases vary with the severity of disease. Episodes of fever, diarrhea, gingivitis, respiratory infection, lymphadenitis, and lameness (bone necrosis) follow neutropenic phases. Most untreated affected dogs die within a few days of birth, yet some survive only to succumb in early adulthood. The life span of those surviving puppyhood is markedly lengthened if they receive supportive clinical treatment; even so, they eventually develop lymphoid exhaustion, reticuloendothelial hyperplasia with monocytosis, anemia, and amyloidosis.

▶

> The wide spectrum of clinical signs and lesions in canine cyclic hematopoiesis is due largely to one basic defect, cyclic neutropenia. The basis for periodic cycling of blood cells is unknown, although in normal animals these changes occur in a very subtle manner.

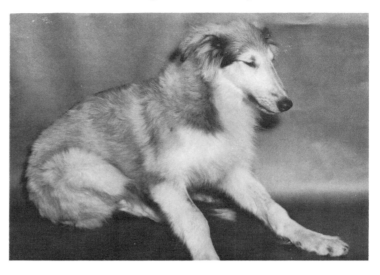

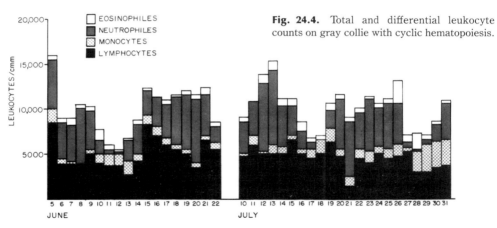

Fig. 24.4. Total and differential leukocyte counts on gray collie with cyclic hematopoiesis.

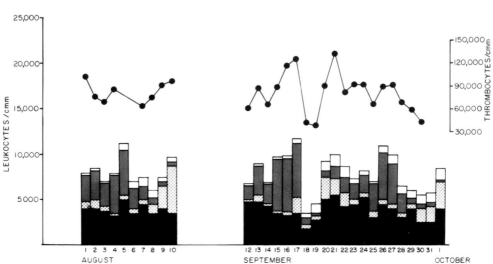

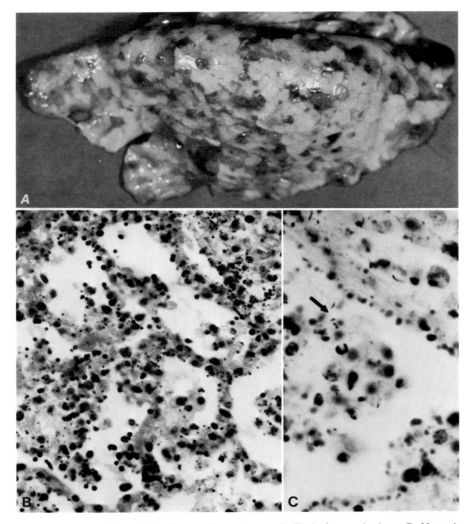

Fig. 24.5. Gray collie syndrome. A. Foci of necrosis, lung. B. Necrotic lung with tissue debris and mineral. C. Enlargement of necrotic stain especially stained for bacteria (*arrow*).

ricidal activity associated with the hexose-monophosphate shunt and delayed degranulation. The essential mechanism in *beige mice* is failure of neutrophil granules to migrate to phagosomes, causing delayed intracellular killing of bacteria. Neutrophils in some syndromes fail to show chemotaxis because of abnormal microtubule assembly and surface receptor functions.

Recurrent infections lead to early death. Affected animals also have defective pigmentation, thrombocytopenia, and lymphadenopathy. Giant cytoplasmic inclusions occur in many types of granule-forming cells including neurons, melanocytes, mast cells, and pulmonary granular pneumocytes. The Chediak-Higashi syndrome that characterizes the Aleutian mutant strain of mink is the basis for the remarkable susceptibility of these animals to the chronic, virus-induced plasmacytosis known as Aleutian disease.

Chronic granulomatous disease

A third neutrophil disease is found only in man. Affected children suffer severe recurrent infections caused by staphylococci and gram-negative rods, due to impaired bactericidal activity of their neutrophil lysosomes. Monocytes are similarly deficient. Despite vigorous neutrophil responses, normal degranulation, and adequate antibody formation, neutrophils are unable to kill bacteria. The major metabolic defect is an absence or inactivity of the membrane-associated enzyme that generates O_2^-. Leukocytes do not exhibit a respiratory burst and cannot kill bacteria that lack catalase and do not produce H_2O. Streptococci and other bacteria that excrete H_2O_2 into the extracellular environment are killed by the patient's leukocytes; bacterial H_2O_2 is utilized by the bactericidal system of the neutrophil lysosome. Bacteria, such as staphylococci, that produce catalase and do not excrete H_2O_2 are not killed and proliferate to cause disease.

Other hereditary defects

The *Pelger-Huet anomaly* is incomplete segmentation of nuclei of neutrophils and eosinophils, resulting in round or oval nuclei and large cytoplasmic granules. Neutrophils have impaired ability to migrate. This anomaly occurs in dogs, rabbits, and man. Studies in foxhounds (which do not show clinical disease) have revealed a serum factor that affects B lymphocytes.

Myeloperoxidase deficiency occurs in man, but patients do not suffer recurrent bacterial infections; leukocytes from some patients even produce an increase in oxygen radicals, probably to compensate for lack of myeloperoxidase.

In the *hyperglobulin E recurrent infection syndrome* of man, neutrophils are normal in size and number and phagocytize and kill normally but have a chemotaxis defect, probably due to a protein secreted by monocytes.

A hereditary defect in neutrophil glucose oxidation via the hexose-monophosphate shunt leads to a syndrome of recurring bacterial infections in dogs.

DEFICIENCIES OF COMPLEMENT

Acquired hypocomplementemia

Hypocomplementemia results from an excessive consumption of complement during most systemic microbial infections, that is, in any immunologic reaction in which antibodies react with antigen to use complement. The component C3 is particularly important in antibacterial reactions. In most bacterial infections, the host responds to produce complement, rapidly returning its levels in the bloodstream to normal.

Hereditary complement defects

Hereditary deficiencies of individual components of complement have been reported: the C3 deficiency of Brittany spaniels, C4 deficiency of guinea pigs, C5 deficiency of mice, C6 deficiency of rabbits, and C1-inactivator deficiency of man. In most of these abnormalities there is little or no increased susceptibility to disease, probably because the deficiency is compensated for by other antimicrobial systems.

The *C4 deficiency* of guinea pigs is inherited as an autosomal codominant trait. Plasma of heterozygous deficients have approximately 40% normal C4, and none is in the plasma of homozygotes. Deficient animals, which show little increase in susceptibility to infections, were discovered when they made antibodies to C4 when injected with normal guinea pig serum.

Several hereditary complement deficiencies occur in man, but most result only in minor changes in susceptibility to infection. Serum of human patients with hereditary *C3 deficiency* cannot sustain bacterial opsonization, and these patients have repeated bacterial infections despite normal levels of immunoglobulins. *Deficiency of C1 inactivator* (a major inhibitor of kallikrein, factor XII, and plasmin) results in angioneurotic edema; fluid from blisters produced in these patients contains large amounts of kallikrein.

DEFECTS IN SPECIFIC LYMPHOID-INDUCED IMMUNE MECHANISMS

The specific immune systems fail to respond to infectious agents and other antigens when the central or peripheral lymphoid organs are markedly abnormal. These structures may be absent congenitally or may have been damaged by infectious disease, toxins, or drug therapy (Table 24.2). The end result is that the host animal becomes unusually susceptible to infectious processes that would be of little consequence in the normal animal.

Table 24.2. Immunodeficiency syndromes

Primary
Humoral: agammaglobulinemia (Bruton type [man])
Cellular: thymic aplasia (Di George syndrome [man]); nu/nu mouse)
Combined: agammaglobulinemia (Swiss type [man])
Specific Ig deficiency: IgA deficiency (man)
Partial deficiency: Wiskott-Aldrich syndrome (man)

Secondary
Postviral immune deficiency: hog cholera, panleukopenia (cat), bovine viral diarrhea, measles, etc.
Neoplasm-associated: plasmacytoma, thymoma, lymphosarcoma
Aging
Malnutrition
Drug-induced

Congenital immunologic defects

Defective development of the organs responsible for immunologic reactivity may result in varying immunodeficiency diseases. These natural diseases illustrate the complexity of host defense mechanisms. *Thymic hypoplasia* leads to defective cell-mediated immunity with normal antibody production. There is absence of thymic tissue and hypoplasia of regions in peripheral lymphoid tissues (spleen and lymph nodes) normally populated in the neonate by T lymphocytes. In *agammaglobulinemia,* antibody production is depressed but cell-mediated immunity is normal. The most common and most severe defects in animals are *combined immunodeficiencies* in which both B and T cell populations are defective. Antibody production and cell-mediated immunity are both depressed.

Combined immunodeficiency of horses

A fatal, genetic, combined B and T lymphocyte immunodeficiency occurs in Arabian foals. The clinical diagnosis is based on lymphopenia (less than 1000/mm^3), hypoplasia of the thymus, absence of germinal centers and lymphoid sheaths in the spleen, and absence of one or more serum Ig class. IgM is invariably absent, and IgA is missing in about 50% of the affected foals. Skin graft rejection is prolonged. Laboratory tests for T lymphocytes show markedly diminished function of T cells.

Foals with combined immunodeficiency are highly susceptible to respiratory disease and usually die with some form of pneumonia. High mortality occurs from adenoviral infections and *Pneumocystis carinii* lesions. Neither of these diseases is of clinical importance in normal horses.

Combined immunodeficiency in Arabian horses appears to be an autosomal recessive trait. Affected foals do not live to breeding age; their sires and dams are not afflicted.

Thymic aplasia of mice

Nude mice (nu/nu) are a hairless, growth-retarded strain affected with thymic dysgenesis (not agenesis). The thymic rudiment does not contain lymphocytes of Hassall's corpuscles but consists of cysts whose walls are lined with squamous or glandular epithelium. As a result of this defect, nude mice are deficient in the inductive capacity of normal thymic epithelium. They have bone marrow precursor T cells but lack T lymphocytes. They are totally deficient in cell-mediated reactivity and will accept skin grafts not only from allogenic mice but from other animal species. Circulating lymphocytes of nude mice all contain surface immunoglobulins, indicating that they are B cells. Serum globulin levels are relatively unchanged, although IgA may be low and antibody formation slightly retarded.

Other congenital immune defects

Several immunodeficiency syndromes occur in cattle. A lethal syndrome caused by an autosomal recessive mode of inheritance occurs in black Danish calves, which have hair loss, parakeratosis, and marked hypoplasia of the thymus with depletion of peripheral lymphoid tissues. Antibody production is depressed but probably secondary to the thymic defect. Selective deficiency of IgG2 has also been reported in cattle, with increased susceptibility to infection.

Dysgammaglobulinemia associated with a defect in secretion of plasmacytes has been reported. Airedale terriers have a defect in *IgA production* that contributes to systemic infections and diskospondylitis. German shepherd dogs are susceptible to bacterial overgrowth in the proximal small intestine, allegedly due to low levels of IgA produced in gut-associated lymphoid tissue.

Acquired immunologic defects
Chemical immunosuppression

Immunosuppression can be induced therapeutically by many different mechanisms (Table

24.3). These methods are used clinically to prolong the survival of grafts, to suppress immunologic components of acute inflammation, and to kill neoplastic cells. Many immunosuppressive agents have nonselective effects. Cortisone has profound effects on both humoral and cell-mediated immune systems (Fig. 24.6). Some agents, however, cause selective destruction of either cellular or humoral mechanisms. For example, antilymphocyte serum preferentially affects cell-mediated immunoreactivity, and there is evidence that radiomimetic drugs have a greater effect on the T cell population than on B cells.

Table 24.3.   Methods of immunosuppression

Surgical	Bursectomy; removal of gut-associated lymphoid tissue Thymectomy Thoracic duct cannulation
Biological	Antilymphocyte globulin (ALG) Adrenal corticosteroids Viruses (lympholytic)
Chemical	Folic acid antagonists (methotrexate) Purine analogs (6mp, 5fu) Nitrogen mustards
Physical	Radiation Burns

Alkylating agents produce profound suppressive effects on immune responses by the toxicity to lymphocytes. They alkylate nucleic acids by forming cross-links with nucleoside bases, thereby interfering with DNA biosynthesis. Mercaptopurine, like most purine analogs, in-hibits multiple enzymes involved in purine synthesis and may suppress a number of cellular functions. Methotrexate functions as a powerful inhibitor of dihydrofolate reductase and thereby depresses DNA synthesis by suppressing thymidylate formation.

Failure of passive transfer of immunoglobulins from mother to offspring

Failure of transfer of colostral immunoglobulins is the leading cause of acquired immunosuppression in neonatal animals (see Chapter 22). Calves are agammaglobulinemic at birth and absorb IgG from milk only for 24–36 hours after birth. Any delay in suckling has a marked effect on enhancement of bacterial infection. Calves with less than 10 mg IgG_1/ml are considered hypogammaglobulinemic; values below 5 mg IgG_1/ml are evidence of passive transfer failure.

Animals with failure of Ig transfer are often treated with antibiotics and corticosteroid during the neonatal period. This extends the immune defect by permitting fungal overgrowth and by suppressing host defense mechanisms. Foals with passive transfer failure are prone to develop bacterial septicemia, and if treated with antibiotics, may develop systemic and oral fungal infections such as candidiasis.

Starvation causes immunosuppression.

Atrophy of lymphoid tissue is common in cachexia and starvation, especially in young animals. Thymic atrophy (or hypoplasia) is most prominent, and the thymus has long been considered a "barometer of nutrition." Thymic regression occurs in pituitary deficiencies, but the

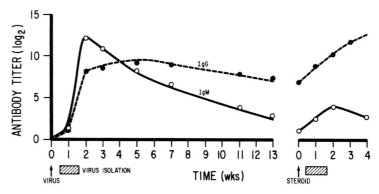

Fig. 24.6. Corticosteroid-induced disease: viral isolation and serum antibodies in calf with given infectious bovine rhinotracheitis. Cortisone treatment causes exacerbation of viral secretion. (Data from Potgieter et al., *Am. J. Vet. Res.* 46:893, 1985)

connection of growth hormone with thymic size is not known.

Viral immunosuppression

Many of the viruses that cause systemic disease are known to produce transient immunosuppression by virtue of replication in the lymphoid and reticuloendothelial systems. Bovine viral diarrhea, canine distemper, feline panleukopenia, hog cholera (swine fever), and Newcastle disease are some of the more important diseases in which immunosuppression plays a role in viral persistence (Figs. 24.7–24.10). The host's immune system usually loses the race with a particularly virulent strain of virus during the incubation period. Immunosuppression is caused by direct destruction of lymphoid cells and by several alterations in cell signal molecules that are secondary to lymphocyte cytolysis

(e.g., prostaglandin release, phospholipase activation, interferon production, and activation of acute phase proteins of inflammation). A variety of chronic diseases follows acute infection by these viruses because of lymphoid destruction and immunosuppression.

Lymphocytic choriomeningitis virus of mice causes a classic disease model of viral immunosuppression. The virus suppresses both antibody production and cell-mediated reactivity. Selective destruction of T lymphocytes and necrosis of the thymus and thymic-dependent areas of lymph nodes and spleen are responsible for the term "viral thymectomy."

Leukemia viruses silently cause immunosuppression.

Most leukemia viruses produce a phase of immunosuppression soon after infection. No overt

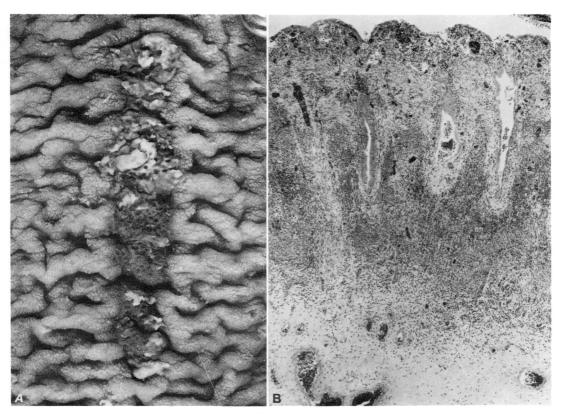

Fig. 24.7. Destruction of lymphoid tissue, submucosal lymphoid tissue, jejunum, bovine viral diarrhea. A. Exudate and necrotic debris on surface of lymphoid patch. B. Histology: epithelium contains areas of degeneration and hyperplasia. There are fusion of villi and marked depletion of lymphoid tissues.

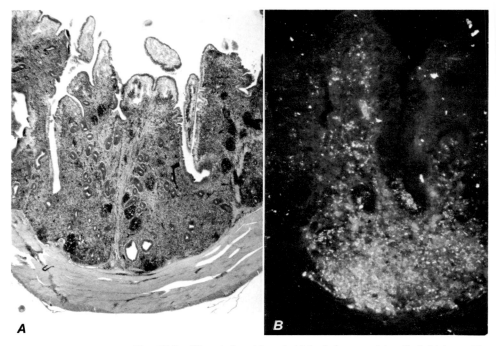

Fig. 24.8. Virus-induced lymphoid depletion, cecal tonsil of chicken with Newcastle disease. A. Severe inflammation, lymphoid destruction, and hyperemia. B. Fluorescent antibody stain, viral antigen throughout the lymphoid areas.

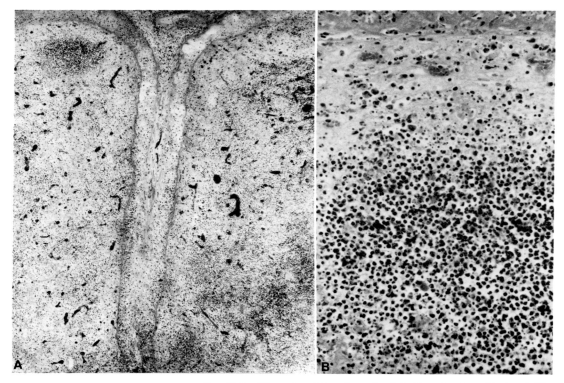

Fig. 24.9. Necrosis of lymph node, infectious bovine rhinotracheitis, steer. A. Total obliteration of lymphoid cells, cortex. Spaces of the subcapsular sinus penetrate into the medulla. B. Enlargement of A: necrotic lymphocytes.

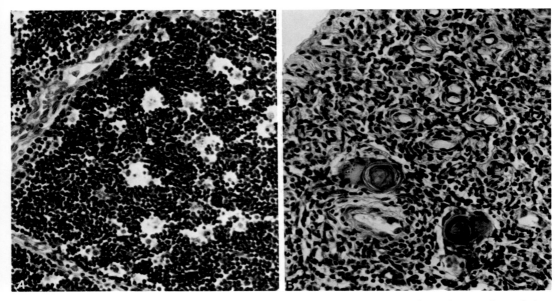

Fig. 24.10. Virus-induced lymphoid depletion, thymus, hog cholera (swine fever). A. Early phase of thymic infection: "drop-out" as lymphocytes are destroyed. B. Thymus, late stages of chronic infection: lymphoid tissues depleted and thymic cortical and medullary reticulum collapsed around thymic corpuscles.

clinical disease results, but affected animals develop infections and serious diseases from agents to which that species of animal is not normally susceptible. In cats, a major result of infection with feline leukemia virus (FeLV) is loss of normal immune function. More FeLV-infected cats die from consequences of immunosuppression than from leukemia. Young kittens infected with feline leukemia virus often develop hemobartonellosis and other opportunistic infections.

The immunosuppression caused by leukemia viruses is part of a widespread effect on host bone marrow. *Anemia* also occurs in early stages of infection, and although often not clinically important, it is clearly shown by hematocrit determinations at various intervals. Lymphoid leukosis virus of chickens, which replicates first in the cloacal bursa (a central lymphoid organ for antibody production), will induce an immunosuppressive phase.

Simian acquired immunodeficiency syndrome

Acquired immunodeficiency syndrome (AIDS) is a progressive wasting disease in which opportunistic microorganisms kill a host severely im-

munodepressed by a retrovirus. Several suspect viruses have been isolated, and some produce AIDS as quickly as 2–4 weeks after inoculation. Monkeys given the causal retrovirus develop swollen lymph nodes characterized by marked follicular hyperplasia and reduced paracortical areas (which contain mostly T_S lymphocytes). Pathogens isolated from tissue lesions include cytomegaloviruses, papovavirus SV40, *Cryptosporidium* spp., *Candida albicans,* and various septicemia-causing bacteria.

Adrenal corticoids cause lymphoid depletion and immunosuppression.

The adrenal cortex plays a protective role against infection; a normal pituitary-adrenal response is necessary for survival of an animal with severe bacterial infection and septicemia. In an experiment with adrenalectomized mice maintained on graded doses of cortisone and inoculated with pneumococci, survival was greatest in groups whose maintenance cortisol most closely resembled the normal. Mortality was progressively increased toward the extreme of hypo- and hyperadrenocorticism.

Chronic treatment with corticosteroids renders an animal increasingly susceptible to bac-

FOCUS

Acquired immune deficiency syndrome

This new progressive, fatal disorder was first recognized in man in 1981 by the Centers for Disease Control in Atlanta. Victims were largely male homosexuals (others were heroin users and hemophiliacs), and all died after a course of lymphadenopathy, fever, diarrhea, and weight loss. Terminal disease was associated with various rare forms of neoplasia and with infections considered to be "opportunistic." AIDS was soon shown to be associated with an immunosuppressive retrovirus called human immunosuppressive virus (HIV). The virus is highly cell associated. The persistent inflammatory lesions of the genitourinary tract of male homosexuals and the inflammatory cells in their semen probably play a major role in the ease of transmission in this group of humans. Virus spreads from person to person through wounds in the rectal mucosa.

AIDS virus destroys the immune system of the host, particularly the subset of T lymphocytes known as T_H, or "helper," cells (identified by specific cytochemical reagents as "T4" cells). T_H cells are missing from circulating blood and from lymphoid tissues. Swollen lymph nodes of AIDS patients contain many more T_S (or T8) cells than normal, and these cells invade the germinal centers (normally reserved for B lymphocytes). B lymphocytes of AIDS patients are present but do not function normally. B cells continuously secrete large amounts of nonspecific immunoglobulins because they never receive the T cell signal that normally would shut down this synthesis.

T_H cells are most susceptible to AIDS virus infection when they have been stimulated. Thus patients with chronic parasitic or viral infections are the most susceptible (homosexual males commonly are infected with hepatitis B virus, cytomegalovirus, and Epstein-Barr virus). Once T_H cells are infected, the immune response cascades downward into severe deficiency. There is a reduction in levels of the T_H cell cytokine interleukin-2 (IL-2), thus reducing the proliferation of mature T cell populations. Further reductions of IL-2 and γ-interferon depress activity of macrophages and natural killer lymphocytes.

Feline leukemia virus–infected cats resemble AIDS patients. Infected cats often die not from leukemia but from opportunistic infections such as panleukopenia or hemobartonellosis. Part of the FeLV protein envelope, p15E, has been shown to inhibit the feline T cell response. Kittens given purified p15E were more prone to develop sarcomas after subsequently being given feline sarcoma virus. A similar suppressor factor called gp41 has been identified from the AIDS virus. Recently, a replication-defective variant of FeLV that rapidly induces fatal immunosuppression has been molecularly cloned directly from infected tissue of cats. Do mutant viruses act in cat AIDS?

▶

▶

In human AIDS, not only are T_H cells reduced in number but those that remain are incapable of recognizing antigens, the first step in the immune response (e.g., T cells from AIDS patients do not respond to antigens such as tetanus toxoid). The virus in some unknown way suppresses the receptor for antigen on the surface of T_H cells so that the cell can no longer distinguish the antigen. A related phenomenon may protect the AIDS-infected cell from recognition by the host's immune system, by reducing the number of class I MHC proteins the cells express on their surfaces. Such an effect would enable the virus to elude any residual T cell function of the host.

The genome of AIDS virus contains a sequence called *tat* that encodes a regulatory protein that increases transcription of the virus itself. Perhaps the *tat* regulatory protein regulates transcription of viral genes. It might *inhibit* genes that should stimulate replication of T_H cells or *activate* genes that turn off division of host T_H cells.

terial and fungal infection. Glucocorticoids particularly cause lysis of lymphocytes and depletion of cells in central and peripheral lymphoid organs. A retrospective study of 16 cases of equine nocardiosis in California (1965–1983) showed that only 2 horses had local lesions associated with wound infection, 14 horses had disseminated infection, and all were immunosuppressed. Eight were Arabian foals with combined immunodeficiency, 3 had ACTH-secreting pituitary tumors with secondary hyperadrenocorticism, and 3 had systemic disease also known to be associated with immunosuppression.

Can mental stress cause immunosuppression?

Mental anxiety in man can reduce immune responses and may play a role in animals. In a study of medical students after final exams, T_H cells were reduced, and there was diminished natural killer cell activity. These results can be correlated with activation of herpes simplex and development of "cold sores." Pituitary secretion of ACTH and adrenal corticosteroid release are surely involved in this phenomenon. Recently, autonomic innervation of lymphoid organs has been demonstrated. In thymus, nerves follow blood vessels into the tissue and branch out into groups of lymphocytes into areas known to have T cell populations (B cell areas did not have nerve endings).

Gammopathy

Gammopathy is any Ig abnormality. Most are neoplastic diseases and are associated with increased plasma Igs. The Ig arises from neoplastic B lymphocytes or plasmacytes. Plasmacytomas (also called myelomas) are tumors of malignant plasmacytes and are characterized by massive production of light chains of the antibody molecules and defective assembly with the heavy chain components (light chains accumulate in the bloodstream and, because of their low molecular weight, spill over into the urine as "Bence Jones proteins").

If only one specific Ig is produced, the gammopathy is called *monoclonal* (e.g., IgA monoclonal gammopathy). Monoclonal components may also be IgG, IgM, or an Ig subunit such as kappa or lambda chains. If different Igs are present in plasma the disease is *polyclonal*, having arisen from more than one clone of Ig-producing cells.

Clinical signs in these gammopathies result from the remarkable elevations in plasma globulins. The *hyperviscosity syndrome* of dogs, characterized by weakness, congestive heart failure, distended retinal veins, and bleeding tendencies, is due to greatly thickened plasma with excess Igs.

AUTOIMMUNE DISEASE

In autoimmune (allergic) disease, the animal's own tissue acts as an endogenous antigen to incite production of antibodies or sensitized lymphocytes. The state of tolerance is broken; that is, an autoimmune disease results from breakdown of the tolerant state with production of autoantibodies and lymphocytes following circulation of autoantigenic material.

Both autoantibodies and immune complexes are ubiquitous in normal mammalian serum. They preserve immunologic hemostasis. A special class of autoantibodies (anti-idiotype antibodies) self-regulate the immune system.They are antibodies to antigens that are part of the combining site of the normal IgG molecule.

Rheumatoid factors, a group of human antibodies directed against γ-globulin, are among the most common autoantibodies of man. They are present in very low amounts in normal individuals and in higher concentrations in patients with immunologic disease, especially those with rheumatoid arthritis and lupus erythematosus.

Autoimmune hemolytic anemia of dogs

This disease is characterized by severe hemolytic anemia and thrombocytopenia. The anemia is usually regenerative; thus high reticulocyte counts are common, and increased erythroid activity is demonstrable in bone marrow smears. Erythrocytes have antibodies attached to their surface membranes that induce hemolysis or promote removal by macrophages in the spleen.

The spleen becomes filled with degenerate and dead erythrocytes.

Clinical tests corroborating the diagnosis of autoimmune hemolytic anemia include a positive direct antiglobulin (Coombs') test (Fig. 24.11) and low hemoglobin with spherocytosis of erythrocytes. The positive Coombs' test indicates that the dog has antibody or complement on erythrocyte surfaces (but it does not establish that antibody is specifically directed toward the erythrocyte), and false positive results may occur in drug toxicity and parasitemia.

Thrombocytopenia usually accompanies autoimmune anemia.

In 1963, Dr. Robert Lewis, now at Cornell University, reported 19 cases of autoimmune hemolytic anemia in dogs; 14 dogs had thrombocytopenia and 6 of these had purpura. Glomerulonephritis with "wire-loop" lesions (thick basement membrane encircling capillaries of the glomerulus) were seen in some cases. These phenomena must be differentiated from idiopathic thrombocytopenia (where only antiplatelet antibodies are present) and lupus erythematosus.

Autoimmune anemia may be acute or chronic.

The pathogenesis of this disease is complex due to the variation in types of antibodies involved. Affected dogs may have the following categories of autoagglutinins: (1) saline-reacting antibody, which causes erythrocyte clumping visible on drawing blood into saline solution (disease in these dogs is usually sudden with a poor prognosis); (2) in vivo hemolysin, which causes

Fig. 24.11. Coombs' test for detection of autoantibodies bound to surface erythrocytes.

COOMBS' TEST

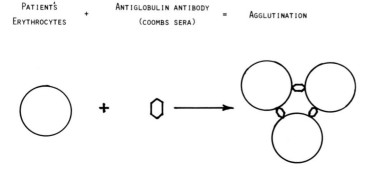

PATIENT'S ERYTHROCYTES   +   ANTIGLOBULIN ANTIBODY (COOMBS SERA)   =   AGGLUTINATION

massive intravascular erythrocyte destruction accompanied by sudden onset of icterus; (3) incomplete antibody, in which erythrocytes are coated but not lysed and are removed by the spleen (onset tends to be gradual); and (4) cold hemagglutinin, in which the autoantibody is not fully active at body temperature (hemoglobinuria may occur, and skin lesions develop caused by ischemia from intravascular agglutination). Coombs' tests are negative at 37°C but positive at 4°C.

Cold hemagglutinin disease occurs in dogs and horses.

Cold hemagglutinin disease, also called "cryopathic autoimmune hemolytic anemia," is a subtle syndrome. IgM-class autoantibodies are present in large amounts in serum. Anemia is much less evident than in "warm" anemia except when animals are exposed to cold. Skin lesions arise from capillary stasis because of erythrocyte agglutination and lysis. In dogs, they involve the nose, ears, and extremities.

Autoimmune thyroiditis

Naturally occurring lymphocytic thyroiditis with signs of thyroxin deficiency occurs in dogs, rats, chickens, and man. Thyroiditis may be caused either by autoantibodies or by lymphocyte-mediated mechanisms. Most of these have antithyroid antibodies in serum, but the precise mechanism of pathogenesis is not clear. Circulating antibodies to thyroid hormone are present in about 50% of hypothyroid dogs and circulating antigen-antibody complexes in about 20%.

Thyroiditis in chickens is B cell mediated.

Thyroiditis in a strain of white Leghorn chickens is used as a model of B lymphocyte–mediated thyroiditis. Adults have excess body fat, small skeletons, silky feathers, poor laying record, and sensitivity to low environmental temperature, all changes associated with hypothyroidism. Plasmacytes and even germinal centers develop in the thyroid and circulating autoantibodies to thyroglobulin are present in serum.

Two forms of thyroiditis exist in man.

In Graves' disease, antibodies form against *receptors for thyroid stimulating hormone* (TSH) that are normally present in thyroid epithelium. These antibodies bind to the TSH receptors and stimulate thyroid hormone production. The thyroid gland is infiltrated by activated T lymphocytes, and unlike normal thyroid epithelium, the epithelial follicular cells produce an excess of histocompatibility antigens on their surfaces. In the rarer Hashimoto's disease, there are *antithyroglobin antibodies* in serum and chronic lymphocytic thyroiditis.

Lupus erythematosus

Lupus erythematosus (LE) is a rare disease of dogs and man characterized by arthritis, anemia, lymphadenopathy, and nephritis. Widespread vascular lesions are induced by circulating antigen-antibody complexes. Thus the clinical and pathologic manifestations resemble those of serum sickness more than those of autoimmune "organ" diseases such as thyroiditis.

In general, flare-ups of disease correlate with drops in complement levels, and antigen-antibody-complement complexes can be demonstrated directly in vascular and renal lesions. Deposition of immune complexes in the renal glomeruli produce the critical signs of disease, but complexes also occur in other vascular organs such as choroid plexus, myocardium, skin, and gonads.

Autoantibodies develop to a wide variety of host proteins.

Autoantibodies to chromatin (DNA-protein complexes) produce dense, extracellular "hematoxylin bodies" (remnants of nuclear debris) in tissue. Other autoantibodies react with erythrocyte surfaces to cause mild hemolytic anemia. Anti-DNA antibodies are the basis of the LE test, in which suspect serum is added to leukocyte suspensions. Nuclei of susceptible cells undergo dissolution with release of nuclear chromatin, which is then phagocytized by other leukocytes. These appear as LE cells, large cells with hematoxylin-staining inclusions.

Canine lupus erythematosus

This complex disorder leads to progressive hemolytic anemia, thrombocytopenic purpura, proteinuria, and polyarthritis. Renal failure, due to irregular, spotty, chronic membranous glomerulonephritis with accumulations of plasmacytes, is a frequent cause of death. Lymphoid follicles develop in medullary areas of the thyme.

Anemia occurs as acute, severe hemolytic

crises, during which there is a strong, direct, positive antiglobulin (Coombs') test. Eluates from affected erythrocytes sensitize normal canine erythrocytes to an indirect antiglobulin test (confirming that autoantibodies are responsible for the hemolysis). Serologic abnormalities include autoantibodies against IgG, nucleoprotein, DNA, RNA, thyroglobulin, and erythrocyte membrane antigens.

Thrombocytopenia purpura, which occurs due to platelet destruction, is manifest as hematuria, epistaxis, and petechiae or ecchymoses in the skin and mucous membranes. Autoantibodies to platelets have been demonstrated. Circulating antigen-antibody complexes (unrelated to platelets) may also exert a cytotoxic effect.

Immune complex conjuctivitis

Bilateral conjunctivitis and recurrent vaginitis have been reported in poodles, associated with immune complex deposition. Severe keratitis and corneal ulceration often develops. In the human form (Sjogren's syndrome), plasmacytic aggregates develop in conjunctivae and lacrimal glands and there are autoantibodies against nictitating membrane epithelium (a tear-forming organ). Parenchymal destruction of salivary and lacrimal glands by invading lymphocytes leads to decreased secretion and fibrosis.

Immune complex orchitis

Immune complexes develop in the testes after vasectomy, which confines sperm to the epididymis and proximal vas deferens where they degenerate and are engulfed by macrophages. During this process, sperm antigens leak into the circulation and, in some animals, stimulate formation of autoantibodies. Experimental production of autoimmune orchitis is characterized by decreased size of epithelial cells, increased thickness of basement membranes, and deposition of dense deposits of immune complexes.

A naturally occurring infertility in black mink males is associated with autoimmune orchitis. Affected mink have antisperm antibodies in serum, aspermatogenesis, and monocytic orchitis.

Idiopathic polyneuritis (Guillain-Barre syndrome)

Idiopathic polyneuritis, a postinfectious paralytic disease of man, is usually transient and follows upper respiratory infections such as influenza. An autoimmune mechanism is involved in the segmental demyelinating lesions in the spinal nerve roots and peripheral nerves that cause the clinical signs.

Idiopathic polyneuritis of dogs ("coonhound paralysis") is a similar condition. Progressive paralysis begins 7–14 days after the dog has been bitten or scratched by a raccoon. Affected dogs are afebrile and alert, and signs of disease vary from weakness to flaccid symmetric quadriplegia. The ventral nerve roots of the spinal cord and some peripheral nerves have lesions of segmental demyelination and perivenular lymphoid infiltrates.

Experimental allergic neuritis of dogs (produced by injecting ground nerve tissue) has similar lesions. Neutrophil infiltration, both perivascular and in foci, occur early, followed by nerve degeneration and demyelination, especially in lumbar and sacral spinal roots.

Neuritis of the cauda equina, a disease of equine spinal nerves, resembles the Guillain-Barre syndrome. The clinical signs of paralysis of the tail and urinary and intestinal sphincters are due to disintegration of myelin and infiltration of monocytes and macrophages of the sacral intradural rootlets.

Myasthenia gravis

Progressive muscular weakness and low tolerance to exercise, the clinical signs of myasthenia gravis, result from autoantibodies that bind to and block acetylcholine receptors at motor endplates. Affected endplates become short with wide, attenuated secondary synaptic clefts (the terminal axon remains normal). In late stages, lymphoid cells invade synaptic clefts, diminishing the total area of the postsynaptic membrane and the release of acetylcholine.

Dogs affected with myasthenia gravis suffer from severe muscle weakness that responds to anticholinesterase therapy. Alterations have been demonstrated in the pre- and postsynaptic elements of the junctional regions of the motor endplate by electron microscopy. A *congenital form* of myasthenia gravis in Jack Russell and smooth fox terriers has reduced acetylcholine receptors in muscle without any demonstrable autoantibodies to receptors in serum.

Pemphigus

Pemphigus is a group of diseases of dogs and humans characterized by bullous lesions of the skin and mucous membranes. In canine pemphigus, which arises as an autoimmune disease of oral mucous membranes, bullae develop due to loss of coherence of epithelial cells and development of acantholysis. Autoantibodies in serum are directed against glycoproteins of epithelial cells.

Pemphigus variants

Pemphigus foliaceous is a variant of pemphigus in which bullae occur on the face and ears. Bullae form under the stratum corneum rather than just above the basal layer. They progress to scabs and alopecia. Footpad lesions develop in most dogs. Bearded collies, akitas, schipperkes, and Newfoundlands have an increased risk for pemphigus foliaceous.

Autoimmune *pemphigoid* is a similar disease, but autoantibodies are directed against the epithelial basement membranes and to antigens in the glycocalyx of keratinocytes.

Eosinophilic granuloma complex of cats

The eosinophilic granuloma complex of cats may be an autoimmune lesion. Dr. Howard Gelberg, in a retrospective study of sera of 19 cats with this complex, showed that 68% of cats with this complex had circulating antibodies to components of normal cat epithelium. These autoantibodies may be secondary, however; that is, the granuloma may release altered self-antigens to which the cat's immune system responds.

IMMUNE TOLERANCE

Immune tolerance (immunologic unresponsiveness) is a state in animals, resulting from previous exposure to antigen, in which the body ignores the antigen by not responding to it. There are two types: *central unresponsiveness,* in which there is a deletion of lymphoid cells competent to respond to a specific antigen, and *peripheral inhibition,* in which competent cells are present but are suppressed by T_S lymphocytes,

antigen, or antigen-antibody complexes.

The first natural example of immune tolerance was discovered in cattle. Red blood cell chimerism occurred in nonidentical bovine twins with vascular anastomoses and mixing of placental circulations. Such dizygotic twins can also accept skin grafts from one another and are chimeric as to circulating leukocytes. Similar red blood cell chimerism occurs in lambs.

To explain the lack of antibody formation to "self" proteins, Burnett theorized that when immunocompetent cells encounter antigens in fetal life, they are deflected forever from antibody production against that antigen. Medawar's experiments on skin grafting confirmed that if a pure-line mouse was inoculated as a fetus with cells from a donor mouse of a different allogeneic strain, it would subsequently accept a skin graft from the same donor mouse, while skin from a second unrelated donor was rejected. Medawar called this *acquired tolerance.* By injection of syngeneic immune ("sensitized") lymphoid cells into the tolerant graft-bearing mice, rapid rejection of the graft occurred. Tolerance was promptly ended by the activity of the lymphocytes on the graft.

All tolerance is multifactorial; that is, several factors contribute to the unresponsive state. In central *tolerance in the neonate,* deletion of immunocompetent cells by the continued presence of antigen is the primary mechanism. The presence of the antigen is required in the thymus, where stem cells differentiate to immunocompetent cells. Here the newly differentiated, thymus-dependent lymphocytes are sensitive to antigen, which arrests their maturation. The *blockade theory* of tolerance suggests that antigen saturates the Ig receptors on lymphocyte surfaces and provides an "off" signal that persists as long as antigen persists. Active tolerance is never permanent and is only prolonged when antigen or T_S lymphocytes persist for unusually long periods.

Although tolerance may be induced by making either T or B cells unresponsive, it is most often the T cell that is tolerant in natural disease. Macrophages are also crucial in tolerance when they fail to "fix" tolerogenic antigens and to properly present antigen to the lymphocyte. Antigens that diffuse fully are more apt to induce tolerance than are those that concentrate on macrophages; the latter are more immunogenic. Some believe that exposure to antigen in the absence of the cytokine interleukin-2 is a paralyzing event for T cells, causing them to be unreactive to the same antigen in the future (clonal anergy).

ADDITIONAL READING

Biberstein, E. L., et al. *Nocardia asteroides* infection in horses. *J. Am. Vet. Med. Assoc.* 186:273, 1985.

Colten, H. R. Molecular basis of complement deficiency syndromes. *Lab. Invest.* 52:468, 1985.

Gelberg, H. B., et al. Antiepithelial autoantibodies associated with the feline eosinophilic granuloma complex. *Am. J. Vet. Res.* 46:263, 1985.

Gosselin, S. J., et al. Autoimmune lymphocytic thyroiditis in dogs. *Vet. Immunol. Immunopathol.* 3:185, 1982.

Greene, C. W., et al. Cold hemagglutinin disease in a dog. *J. Am. Vet. Med. Assoc.* 170:505, 1977.

Guillemin, R., et al. *Neural Modulation of Immunity.* New York: Raven, 1985.

Halliwell, R. E. W. Autoimmune disease in the dog. *Adv. Vet. Sci. Comp. Med.* 22:221, 1978.

Hirsch, V. M., et al. Hereditary anomaly of neutrophil granulation in Birman cats. *Am. J. Vet. Res.* 45:2170, 1984.

Holmberg, C. A., et al. Immunologic abnormality in a group of *Macaca arctoides* with high mortality due to atypical mycobacterial and other disease processes. *Am. J. Vet. Res.* 46:1192, 1985.

Hurvitz, A. I. Canine pemphigus vulgaris. *Am. J. Pathol.* 98:861, 1980.

Ihrke, P. J., et al. Pemphigus foliaceus in dogs. *J. Am. Vet. Med. Assoc.* 186:59, 1985.

King, N. W. Simian models of acquired immunodeficiency syndrome (AIDS): A review. *Vet. Pathol.* 23:345, 1986.

Quimby, F. W., et al. A disorder of dogs resembling Sjogren's syndrome. *Clin. Immunol. Immunopathol.* 12:471, 1979.

Roth, J. A., and Kaeberle, M. L. Suppression of neutrophil and lymphocyte function induced by a vaccinal strain of bovine viral diarrhea virus with and without the administration of ACTH. *Am. J. Vet. Res.* 44:2366, 1983.

Winkelstine, J. A., et al. Genetically determined deficiency of the third component of complement in the dog. *Science* 212:1169, 1981.

Immunization and Adverse Reactions

VACCINES may be composed of live or killed microorganisms or of immunogenic fragments of disrupted microorganisms. Killed vaccines are produced by chemically inactivating the infectivity of virulent microbes while permitting retention of immunogenicity. Most live vaccines are attenuated mutant microorganisms that are relatively avirulent. The live microorganism multiplies in the recipient, eliciting an immune response, but causes little or no disease beyond a mild febrile reaction. Because of the biologic variability in both vaccine and host, adverse reactions to immunization occur and can be both costly to the owner and painful to the animal. These reactions arise from defective vaccines, inappropriate use of vaccines, and suppressed immune systems in the vaccinated animal (Table 25.1).

Clinically important vaccination reactions may be local or systemic. Local reactions are due to inflammation provoked by some nonantigenic component of the vaccine, usually an adjuvant. Systemic reactions occur in almost every immunization procedure. Characterized by mild fever and myalgia, these reactions are usually transient and of little consequence. On rare occasions, they are life-threatening.

REACTIONS TO NONMICROBIAL COMPONENTS OF VACCINES

Adjuvants

Adjuvants, according to the World Health Organization, are "materials that are added to vaccines with the intent of potentiating the immune response so that a greater amount of antibody is produced, a lesser quantity of antigen is required, and fewer doses need to be given." Some

Table 25.1. Adverse reactions to vaccine

Inappropriate use	
Wrong vaccine	Rabies vaccine in hamster
	Pseudorabies vaccine in sheep
	Canine distemper vaccine in wild canidae
Wrong route	Intraarterial or intravenous injection with any vaccine
Wrong time	Neonates with passive colostral immunity
	Pregnant females
Contaminated vaccines	
Hidden viruses	Hepatitis virus in yellow fever vaccine
	Scrapie virus in louping ill vaccine
	BVD virus in bovine coronavirus vaccines
	Bacteriophages in bacterial vaccines
Virulent vaccines	
Viruses	Newcastle disease virus
	Equine herpesvirus-1
	Rabies virus
Immunosuppressive viruses	Canine distemper
	Canine parvovirus
	Infectious bursal disease of chickens
Immunosuppressed host	
Cause unknown	Progressive vaccinia
	Rabies
	Canine distemper
Carriers in vaccines	
Carrier/adjuvant	Adjuvant granuloma
Tissue components	Postvaccinal encephalomyelitis (nerve tissue)
	Cell culture or egg proteins
Preservative	Mercurials (thimersol), formaldehyde

411

adjuvants incite considerable tissue injury; for example, adjuvants used with vaccines against *Clostridium perfringens* are highly irritating and frequently produce abscesses.

Aluminum phosphate and aluminum hydroxide gel (to which antigen is adsorbed) are commonly used. Oily adjuvants of the Freund type are used experimentally to produce remarkable immune responses but are not acceptable clinically due to severe granulomatous local reactions. Muramyl dipeptide, an active component of mycobacteria, is a synthetic adjuvant that can be conjugated to some antigens to produce an exaggerated immune response.

Carriers are proteins that are coupled to small molecules (haptens) to increase immunogenicity. They are important in increased cell-mediated immune responses, especially those involving helper T cells. An immune response to one of the proteins of foot-and-mouth disease virus is markedly augmented by its conjugation to the carrier keyhole-limpet hemocyanin. In testing this system, however, it must be clearly established that hypersensitivity to the protein does not occur.

Tissue components

As antibody titers to microbial antigens rise in an animal after vaccination, there may be a concomitant rise in antibodies to nonmicrobial components in the vaccine, especially in vaccines that are crude or not properly purified. These antibodies can lead to serious hypersensitivity reactions, either anaphylaxis or delayed hypersensitivity (in which lymphocytes in the vaccinated animal become sensitized and induce cell-mediated skin lesions).

Egg allergy

Use of chicken embryos to produce vaccines was once widespread, and anaphylactic reactions to egg proteins were common, especially in humans that had become sensitized to chicken egg protein. This was never a major problem for animal vaccinations and now is even less relevant due to preparations of more purified vaccines.

Nerve tissue: Postvaccinal encephalitis

The centenary of Pasteur's first successful rabies immunization in man was in 1985. These early vaccines, which were composed of nervous tissue, produced a variety of local and sys-

temic reactions. Although severe local cutaneous reactions and systemic anaphylaxis were major problems, the serious cause of mortality was postvaccinal encephalomyelitis. The patients died of an immune-mediated reaction against their own nerve tissue. It was not until 1928 that it was suggested that nervous tissue in the vaccine was responsible.

Canine postvaccinal allergic encephalomyelitis is a rare complication of repeated immunization using rabies virus grown in brain tissue. Clinical signs of paralysis and disorientation are a result of lymphocyte cuffing and demyelination in the white matter of the brain and spinal cord (Fig. 25.1).

Experimental allergic encephalomyelitis, produced by injecting a laboratory animal with brain tissue extracts, is a widely studied model of immunologic central nervous system disease. The encephalitogenic antigen is a protein in myelin. The lesions are mediated by T lymphocytes and are foci of demyelination surrounded by perivascular lymphocytic infiltrates. Antibodies are present in these animals but do not play a primary role in the disease.

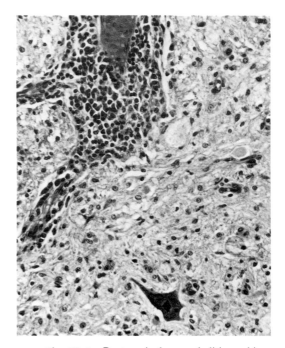

Fig. 25.1. Postvaccinal encephalitis, rabies, dog. Large collections of lymphoid cells occur around veins and venules.

Cell culture proteins: Foot-and-mouth vaccine reaction

Repeated use of a live foot-and-mouth disease virus vaccine grown in baby hamster kidney (BHK) cell cultures was responsible for a severe disease in Bavarian cattle in the 1960s. Eczema and proliferative and nodular dermal lesions with ulceration developed on the udder, perineal skin, and coronary band. Abortion was allegedly part of the syndrome. The reaction was traced to antibodies against proteins of normal BHK cells. Similar lesions have been implicated with *bluetongue virus* infections of sheep.

Reactions to preservatives
Formalin in vaccines

Formaldehyde is used as an inactivating agent in many veterinary vaccines, particularly clostridial vaccines. Excess formaldehyde may or may not be neutralized (with metabisulfite) after manufacture, but in either case, residual free formaldehyde remains in the product. Clinical signs of local burning occur in animals injected with vaccines containing over 1800 μg/ml formaldehyde. Although these vaccinations cause severe pain and discomfort, they are not known to result in serious disease.

Toxoids (vaccines prepared by detoxification of a toxin) often contain formaldehyde but in dilutions that are no problem. For example, tetanus toxoid is produced by purifying toxin, inactivating it with formalin, and adding an adjuvant to increase the immune response.

HYPERSENSITIVITY REACTIONS TO MICROBIAL ANTIGENS
Bacterial vaccines
Pasteurellosis

Pneumonic pasteurellosis is a major cause of mortality in feedlot cattle in North America. Use of certain killed bacterins in cattle against the causal bacteria *Pasteurella multocida* and *P. hemorrhagica* has been associated with severe respiratory disease after vaccination. When exposed to field viruses naturally, vaccinated animals often have more severe respiratory disease than do animals that have not received the vaccine. The suspicion that these bacterins induced more severe disease in vaccinated animals has been confirmed experimentally. Results of these studies were not always clear, and it is not

known what vaccine components are involved and how they act to make disease more severe. *P. multocida* produces a "cytotoxic factor" when it replicates in the presence of specific IgG, and this fact may underlie the more severe lung lesions in vaccinated calves.

Paratuberculosis

The chronic enteric disease paratuberculosis occurs when *Mycobacterium bovis* localizes and replicates in the intestinal wall in cattle and goats. Adult cattle infected with *M. paratuberculosis* have been given vaccines composed of large numbers of killed bacteria in oil adjuvants. Shortly after vaccination, animals develop severe, progressive diarrhea. Disease is due to a hypersensitivity reaction in the gut against the newly administered bacterial antigens.

Viral vaccines
Parenteral vaccination, respiratory challenge

Severe pneumonitis has been reported in animals vaccinated with a respiratory virus (and with high antibody titers) during later natural exposure to the same respiratory virus. The model for this disease is a formalin-inactivated vaccine against human respiratory syncytial virus used in the l960s in children. Given parenterally, it induced good neutralizing antibody responses. On encountering a naturally occurring respiratory syncytial virus during later epidemics, however, the immunized children suffered more severe disease than did nonimmunized controls. No clear example of this has been reported in animals, but the potential exists for neonates immunized parenterally that later receive a natural challenge by the aerosol route.

CONTAMINATED VACCINES

Reliable manufacturers of vaccines maintain quality control programs to detect and eliminate contaminating microbes. In addition, vaccine safety is monitored by governmental agencies. The United States Department of Agriculture conducts assays on random samples of all commercially produced biologically active vaccines. In Canada, similar monitoring of vaccines is done. Despite these efforts, contaminated vaccines are sometimes produced, often with infectious agents not considered in planning for vaccine production.

Hidden viruses

Louping ill vaccine (with scrapie agent)

In the 1950s a vaccine against louping ill in sheep was prepared from nervous tissue. Having proved effective against this arthropod-borne disease, it was cleared for use in sheep in Great Britain. Several months later, sheep began dying with a chronic central nervous system disease that later was shown to be due to scrapie agents present in the nervous tissue from which the louping ill vaccine had been prepared.

Coronavirus vaccine (with bovine viral diarrhea virus)

Vaccines against bovine coronaviruses began to be marketed in the 1960s for use against neonatal diarrhea in calves. Although they were seemingly effective, it was soon shown that some of the vaccines contained bovine viral diarrhea virus that caused a syndrome in calves characterized by mild enteritis and generalized weakness. Although tests for bovine viral diarrhea virus are applied today, this virus remains a serious problem for products containing bovine tissue or serum.

Yellow fever vaccine (with hepatitis virus)

Massive amounts of yellow fever vaccine were ordered for use in American soldiers during early World War II. The vaccine was prepared in chicken embryos using nonvirulent (strain 17) yellow fever virus that had proven highly effective and without side effects in animals and human volunteers. Immediately after vaccinations were begun, large numbers of soldiers developed hepatitis and icterus. The fear was that yellow fever virus had returned to virulence, but virologic studies showed that a human hepatitis virus had been inadvertently passed in the vaccine.

Poliovirus vaccine (with simian virus 40)

During the massive polio vaccinations of the 1950s, the formalin-killed Salk vaccine was widely given to children in North America. Unbeknownst to physicians, this vaccine contained a monkey virus (SV40) proved to be oncogenic in hamsters. Although vaccinated children developed antibody responses to this virus, no adverse effects were documented.

These reactions are especially important in human vaccination, since some vaccines are produced on monkey kidney cell cultures. Over 75 simian viruses have been identified. *Herpesvirus simiae* (B virus) is lethal for man and presents a clear hazard. Recently adenovirus-SV40 hybrids have been discovered in adenovirus vaccines grown in monkey kidney cells, and these recombinant viruses may be an important consideration for future vaccines.

Marek's disease vaccine (with reticuloendotheliosis virus)

In 1974, flocks of chickens given Marek's disease vaccine developed a syndrome of stunted growth, anemia, abnormal feathers, and leg paralysis. Reticuloendotheliosis virus was isolated from affected chickens and later from the vaccines.

Bacteria in vaccines

Vaccines may become contaminated with bacteria, especially when stored for long periods. Abscesses at injection sites that were caused by *Corynebacterium ovis* are an occasional problem both because of local injury and because of damage of the pelt.

Bacteriophages in vaccines

Bacterial viruses are frequent contaminants of bovine sera prepared commercially and are indicators of previous bacterial contamination. No known disease is associated with bacteriophages, but when they occur in biologically active products they may destroy that product's effectiveness. For example, phages specific for *Brucella abortus* have contaminated vials of the vaccine strain 19, making it useless for field use.

VIRULENT VACCINES

One of the most common problems in vaccine production is failure of attenuation of the microbial antigen. This is especially true with viral vaccines, which tend to be modified live viruses that must replicate in the host to produce immunity. In certain conditions, viruses of low virulence may produce disease.

Virulent viruses that directly cause disease

Infectious canine hepatitis

Vaccines against infectious canine hepatitis have in the past contained live canine adenovirus-1 strains, which replicate systemically when administered to dogs. The most common sequela occurs when vaccine virus replicates in the cornea to produce edema and corneal opacity, or "blue eye" (Fig. 25.2). Viral antigens persisting elsewhere in the eye produce hypersensitivity reactions in the iris and limbus. Canine adenovirus-1 also causes subclinical infections of the kidney. Replication in renal tubules with shedding of vaccine virus in the urine may cause nonvaccinated dogs to become infected. Current immunization programs use a related canine adenovirus-2 against infectious canine hepatitis.

Postvaccinal thrombocytopenia occurs in dogs given a modified live viral canine distemper–hepatitis vaccine, although it is not associated with clinical bleeding. When vaccination is done in conjunction with other stress, such as surgery, bleeding episodes are a risk.

Newcastle disease vaccine

Strains of Newcastle disease virus are used for vaccine production that replicate in mucosa of the upper respiratory tract and destroy epithelium. In most immunization protocols, a first vaccine is a relatively avirulent (mesogenic) strain, followed by a strain of low virulence (lentogenic strain). The mesogenic strains replicate throughout the upper respiratory tract; although

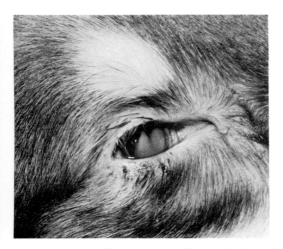

Fig. 25.2. Corneal edema ("blue eye"), infectious canine hepatitis; sequel to vaccination.

no overt disease results, the infection, while providing strong immunity to Newcastle disease, may predispose to bacterial infections when severe reactions occur.

Bovine viral diarrhea vaccine

Both cytopathic and noncytopathic bovine viral diarrhea (BVD) viruses have been isolated from spleens of cattle with fatal postvaccinal *mucosal disease*. Clinical signs of diarrhea, lameness, and seromucous oronasal discharges occurred 10–20 days after vaccination with BVD vaccines. These syndromes closely resembled the natural form of chronic BVD known as mucosal disease, except that skin, foot, and eye lesions were more prominent. Lesions include (1) necrosis and ulceration of tongue, gum, palate, and upper gastrointestinal tract; (2) seborrheic dermatitis (especially axillary, sternal, and inguinal areas); (3) serous lymphadenitis; and (4) necrosis and ulceration of interdigital spaces (pododermatitis).

Current evidence indicates that BVD vaccine viruses may be especially dangerous when given to calves persistently infected with noncytopathic strains of BVD virus. That is, calves with BVD viremia but no antibodies when given the vaccine develop antigen-antibody reactions and severe lesions of mucosal disease.

Equine herpes encephalitis

Equine rhinopneumonitis (caused by equine herpesvirus-1, or EH-1) is a common upper respiratory tract disease and cause of abortion and neurologic disease. Vaccines used in pregnant females in the 1970s were associated with abortion storms. EH-1 virus causes vascular necrosis and lymphoid infiltrates in the endometrium. Blood vessel changes tend to be confined to the endometrium in mares infected late in gestation but are widespread in those mares infected during early pregnancy. It has been suggested that EH-1 viral strains that cause abortion are different (and should be called equine herpesvirus-4).

Neurologic syndromes are associated with enzootics of respiratory disease and abortion due to EH-1. Vasculitis in the brain and spinal cord is severe, and arterioles are often necrotic.

IMMUNOSUPPRESSED HOST ANIMALS

Generalized infections

The vaccination reactions in immunosuppressed animals are closely related to those in the previous section. When disease develops the microbe is obviously too virulent, but this may occur because of some transient, unrecognized immunosuppressive event in the animal.

Progressive vaccinia

Vaccinia virus is a laboratory strain with origins in cowpox virus that was used for 200 years as a vaccine for smallpox. It is also used against monkeypox in several species of nonhuman primates. In normal monkeys the vaccine is scarified into the skin and gives rise in a few days to a series of changes: erythema, macule, papule, vesicle, and pustule. The pustule in the scarified dermis heals within a week or so.

In immunosuppressed monkeys, as in man, *progressive vaccinia* produces death and chronic tissue damage. Viral growth begins to produce satellite lesions around the original site of scarification (Fig. 25.3), and these progress to produce massive necrosis and often death. In very young animals *generalized vaccinia* (the systemic spread of virus) may occur with foci of necrosis in spleen, liver, and other viscera.

Progressive fowlpox

Chickens and turkeys are vaccinated against fowlpox and turkeypox by scarifying these viruses into the featherless skin on the wing (the "wing-web" procedure). Just as in progressive

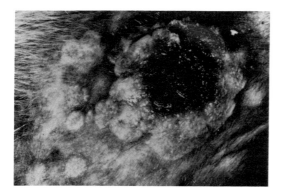

Fig. 25.3. Progressive vaccinia, lesion that developed after vaccination of monkey with vaccinia virus to protect against monkeypox.

vaccinia, progressive fowlpox can also spread in immunodeficient birds to produce massive vaccine reactions.

Rabies in immunodeficient dogs and cats

Live, attenuated rabies vaccines are used to provide preexposure prophylaxis in dogs and cats and less often in cattle. Although vaccine reactions do occur in these animals, they are rare. Under appropriate conditions of immunosuppression, disease can be produced by vaccine strains of virus. In cats given the high egg-passage vaccine, a syndrome of posterior paralysis has been reported. Paralysis began in one hindlimb and rapidly spread to the other and then to the forelimbs. Later signs of cranial nerve paralysis occurred. In the brain, inflammatory lesions resembling those of natural rabies were seen although, typical of vaccine-induced rabies, Negri bodies were not seen in the cytoplasm of affected neurons. Immunofluorescent tests showed that viral antigens were present in brain tissue; the rabies virus was isolated and shown to be a specific vaccine strain.

In dogs, the same pattern of ascending paralysis has been seen, usually occurring 12–14 days after vaccination with chick embryo origin, the low egg-passage Flury strain of rabies virus. More serious problems may arise when these vaccines are used in wild foxes, raccoons, and laboratory animals.

Canine distemper

Dogs treated with immunosuppressive drugs may die of vaccine virus–induced encephalomyelitis. Canine distemper may occur 2 or so weeks after vaccination and is characterized by diarrhea, then respiratory signs, and then central nervous system signs: myoclonus, trembling, decreased muscle coordination, and convulsions. These signs are due to necrosis of spinal cord funiculi and dorsal horns of gray matter. Eosinophilic nuclear inclusions occur in glia that stain with immunofluorescent stains. Interstitial pneumonitis is characteristic.

Canine parvovirus vaccine may be immunosuppressive in dogs.

Some parvovirus vaccines cause lymphopenia 5–7 days after vaccination, a manifestation of transient immunosuppression that can increase susceptibility to other infectious agents, including canine distemper vaccine viruses. Vaccination of dogs with mixed vaccines of canine distemper 5 days before inoculation of parvovirus enhanced the severity of canine parvovirus enteritis; vaccinated dogs became clinically ill, while unvaccinated dogs did not. Lymphopenia occurs after canine distemper vaccination, and parvoviruses may replicate during the rebound stage when lymphocyte proliferation is stimulated.

INAPPROPRIATE USE OF VACCINES

The wrong vaccine

Disaster can result from the administration of a vaccine to an animal species for which it is not designed. These accidents are human error, giving a good vaccine to the wrong animal. They are analogous to dietary deficiencies caused by mistakes made during diet formulation although proper standards are known.

Rabies vaccine

Most vaccine strains of rabies virus will replicate in (and produce rabies in) small rodents such as hamsters. They should not be used in these species as vaccines. In one case, a teacher, concerned that a classroom pet hamster might develop rabies, brought it to a clinic to be immunized. Unaware of this danger, the veterinarian administered the vaccine. The hamster subsequently developed signs of rabies, and the exposed students were required to receive prophylactic immunization.

Pseudorabies vaccine

Lethal pseudorabies has occurred when lambs have been given a vaccine designed for pigs. In some cases the vaccine was administered in error, but in most cases pseudorabies occurred in lambs vaccinated for some sheep disease using unwashed syringes that had previously been used to vaccinate swine with an attenuated pseudorabies vaccine. When such an unwashed syringe is used, about the first 20 lambs injected will develop pseudorabies.

Canine distemper

Vaccine-induced canine distemper commonly occurs when wild animals, particularly those confined to zoos, are given vaccines designed for dogs. Members of the order Carnivora are susceptible to canine distemper and those in the families Canidae, Procyonidae (raccoons, kinkajous, lesser pandas), Mustelidae, and Hyaenidae have been reported to develop canine distemper after vaccination. Ferrets and foxes are highly susceptible, the gray fox more than the red fox.

The origin of tissue in canine distemper vaccine is important. When three modified live vaccines were tested in foxes (dog cell line, dog tissue culture, and chicken tissue culture) and the foxes challenged with virulent virus, all those given dog tissue culture vaccine died while there was no disease in vaccinates receiving chicken tissue.

The wrong route
Intravascular injection

Inadvertent injection of an artery or vein during subcutaneous or intramuscular injection allows rapid dissemination of antigen. In a previously immunized animal that has developed circulating antibodies against antigens present in the vaccine being administered, this will cause anaphylaxis (see hypersensitivity disease, Chapter 23).

The wrong time
The animal is too young.

Death of newborn animals to infectious disease is a major problem that can be prevented by vaccinating animals as soon as possible after birth. If an animal has acquired passive immunity by receiving antibodies from its mother through colostrum, however, these antibodies can interfere with the maximum response of the vaccine.

The animal is pregnant.

Some vaccines that are safe in young animals can cause abortion when given to pregnant females. This is a danger with modified live viral vaccines, particularly with herpesviruses. Losses can be disastrous when large breeding herds are vaccinated during gestation.

Early modified live viral vaccines against *infectious bovine rhinotracheitis* (IBR) were effective in preventing disease with few side effects. In the early 1960s practitioners began seeing abortions in cattle after vaccination. These abortions occurred "without warning," especially in cows 5–6 months pregnant. Foci of ulceration and necrosis were present in the dead fetuses, and herpes inclusion bodies were found in liver, spleen, and adrenal. Dr. Peter Kennedy, at the University of California at Davis, showed that vaccinal strains of IBR virus inoculated intramuscularly frequently induced abortions secondary to virus infecting and spreading in the fetus.

Infectious bovine rhinotracheitis can persist in the genital tract some months after infection and is also a cause of loss of the conceptus and death of the early embryo, events that usually go undetected and are seen only as failure to conceive. Dr. Janice Miller, at the National Animal Disease Center, has found ovarian lesions in newly pregnant cattle when viruses obtained from commercial vaccines were inoculated intravenously into heifers on the day after breeding. The animals had severe corpora luteal necrosis and an abnormally low concentration of progesterone in plasma.

Congenital cavitary anomalies of the brain appeared in the late 1960s after vaccination of pregnant ewes with *bluetongue virus* vaccines. Porencephaly and hydranencephaly, in which cerebral hemispheres are reduced to membranous, fluid-filled sacs (the head of normal size, in contrast to hydrocephalus), were common lesions (Fig. 25.4). Experimental studies showed that lambs infected at 50–58 days of gestation developed severe bluetongue virus–induced necrotizing encephalopathy while those lambs that received virus later in gestation were less severely affected (see teratology, Chapter 30).

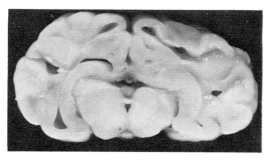

Fig. 25.4. Porous lesions involving primarily subcortical white matter in cerebrum of 120-day fetal lamb inoculated with bluetongue virus vaccine at 77 days of gestation. (Photograph: Bennie Osburn, *Lab. Invest.* 25:197, 1971, used by permission)

LONG-TERM SEQUELAE
Guillain-Barre syndrome

Recently, a high incidence of Guillain-Barre syndrome occurred following use of the "swine" influenza vaccination program in the United States. Approximately one case per 100,000 vaccinees occurred. This syndrome has also been reported to follow rabies vaccinations and may be a second type of sequela to these vaccinations.

Oncogenesis

To ensure that viruses to be used in vaccines do not induce tumors, the candidate viruses must be tested in rodents. Hamsters are extraordinarily susceptible to oncogenic viruses and are used as a sensitive test animal. Some canine adenovirus-1 strains used in commercial vaccine production have been known to produce tumors in rodents. Infectious canine hepatitis vaccines, however, have been used clinically in dogs for over 20 years and no tumor has ever been attributed to the vaccine virus.

Repeated and excessive hyperimmunization is reported to result in an increased incidence of *plasma cell myeloma* in man. That chronic antigen stimulation may lead to neoplasia of antibody-forming cells is interesting, but this finding has not been confirmed in man and not reported in animals.

Carcinomas at vaccination sites

In very rare instances neoplastic lesions have been reported at sites where vaccines were administered. Cutaneous squamous cell carcinomas develop at sites of papilloma vaccine injection. They have been reported in scars of poxvirus vaccination of primates, and suspicious cases of muscle tumors have been reported at sites where vaccines were given intramuscularly. These conditions are so rare that they have little clinical bearing on the use of vaccines.

ADDITIONAL READING

Bregman, C. L., et. al. Cutaneous neoplasms in dogs associated with canine oral papillomavirus vaccine. *Vet. Pathol.* 24:477, 1987.

Esh, J. B., et al. Vaccine-induced rabies in four cats. *J. Am. Vet. Med. Assoc.* 180:1336, 1982.

Jones, B.-E. Platelet aggregation in dogs after live-virus vaccination. *Acta Vet. Scand.* 25:504, 1984.

Kennedy, P. C., and Richards, W. P. C. The pathology of abortion caused by the virus of infectious bovine rhinotracheitis. *Vet. Pathol.* 1:7, 1964.

Krakowka, S., et al. Canine parvovirus infection potentiates canine distemper encephalitis attributable to modified live-virus vaccine. *J. Am. Vet. Med. Assoc.* 180:137, 1982.

McFeely, R. A., et al. Abortion in a dairy herd vaccinated for infectious bovine rhinotracheitis. *J. Am. Vet. Med. Assoc.* 153:657, 1968.

Martin, S. W., et al. Factors associated with mortality in feedlot cattle. *Can. J. Comp. Med.* 44:1, 1980.

Mayr, A., et al. Untersuchungen uber Art, Umfang und Ursachen von Impfschaden nach der Maul- und Klauenseuche-Schutzimpfung in Bayern in den Jahren 1967/68. *Zentralbl. Veterinaermed.* [B] 16:488, 1969.

Pedersen, N. C., et al. Rabies vaccine virus infection in three dogs. *J. Am. Vet. Med. Assoc.* 172:1092, 1978.

Peter, C. P., et al. Characteristics of a condition following vaccination with bovine virus diarrhea vaccine. *J. Am. Vet. Med. Assoc.* 150:46, 1967.

Van Alstine, W. G., et al. Vaccine-induced pseudorabies in lambs. *J. Am. Vet. Med. Assoc.* 185:409, 1984.

Van Der Maaten, M. J., et al. Ovarian lesions induced in heifers by intravenous inoculation of modified-live infectious bovine rhinotracheitis virus on the day after breeding. *Am. J. Vet. Res.* 46:1996, 1985.

Wilcock, B. P., and Yager, J. A. Food cutaneous vasculitis and alopecia at sites of rabies vaccination in dogs. *J. Am. Vet. Med. Assoc.* 188:1174, 1986.

Wilkie, B. N. Response of calves to lung challenge exposure with *Pasteurella hemolytica* after parenteral or pulmonary immunization. *Am. J. Vet. Res.* 41:1773, 1980.

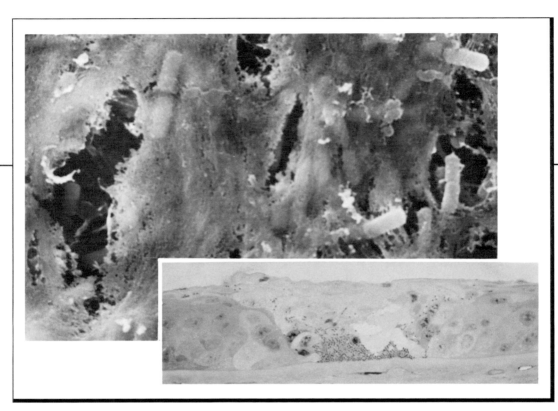

Moraxella bovis invading the surface of the cornea. Bacteria attach to, enter, and destroy corneal epithelial cells. Pits are formed on the corneal surface and newly formed bacteria dissect the cornea between epithelial cells. (Photograph: Douglas Rogers, *Vet. Pathol.* 24:200, 1987)

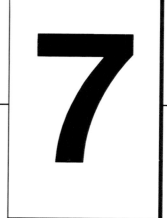

CAUSES
OF DISEASE

A N understanding of pathogenisis is founded on *etiology,* the study of disease causes. An *etiologic diagnosis* provides the precise cause of a disease. A simple classification of *external* etiologic agents is a division into physical, chemical, and microbiologic types (see Table 1.1). Some of these agents directly and consistently cause a pathologic reaction and a predictable series of consequences. Cyanide stops mitochondrial function and will kill and animal regardless of nutritional and immune status. Rabies virus, once established as an infection, replicates in neurons and invariably produces neuronal degeneration, inflammation of the brain, and death. The only determinants of disease for these dangerous agents are the total dose received by the host and the portal of entry.

It is rarely sufficient, however, to explain disease in terms of single causes and unremitting, step-by-step progress. With most agents, production of disease is not uniform. The tubercle bacillus causes tuberculosis, yet only a small fraction of infected animals develop the disease. Feline leukemia virus infects large numbers of kittens but will induce lymphosarcoma or leukemia in only a few. In these diseases, pathogenesis involves a balance of agent viability and host defense. The genetic, nutritional, immunologic, and environmental characters of the host animal determine, in large part, the development and extent of disease. Thus the pathologist must seek multiple factors as "causes" of disease, searching for patterns of lesions and groups of lesions that combine to produce the clinical manifestations of disease.

The relation of cause and effect may be masked by antemortem disappearance of the causal factor. Physical causes of disease such as heat and cold are often determined only by the pattern of tissue injury they produce. Drugs may be catabolized after lesions arise in the liver but before death occurs. Microbial agents may be destroyed by host defenses between the times of infection and death. Clinical treatment commonly obliterates the cause. Bacteria may be killed by antibiotics and cannot be cultured from even severe inflammatory foci in treated animals. In rare infections, antibiotic treatment may even promote death; in anthrax, for example, treatment kills the circulating bacteria but the host may die from the ensuing massive liberation of bacterial toxins.

One misleading aspect of pathologic tissue evaluation results from *multiple causation.* In the liver, one drug may inhibit detoxifying enzymes that predispose to hepatotoxicity by another drug; for example, a single large dose of ethanol produces a markedly enhanced susceptibility to barbiturate anesthetics. Two or more infectious agents may be involved in tissue injury. Viruses may induce respiratory disease of little importance, yet in so doing predispose the lung to

421

severe secondary bacterial infection, such as when influenza becomes complicated with bacterial pneumonia.

In the intestine, intracellular microbes (e.g., viruses, coccidia, treponemes) may destroy epithelium, permitting bacteria to colonize the gut wall. Bovine viral diarrhea virus replicates within intestinal epithelium to produce foci of destruction that support bacterial growth. Viruses that suppress the host's immune system are especially dangerous because they lead to disseminated bacterial or fungal infections.

Lymphoid tissue destruction produced in canine distemper permits growth of the protozoan *Toxoplasma gondii*. Bovine viral diarrhea virus also produces a smoldering chronic infection that destroys lymphoid tissues and permits widespread infection by several bacterial pathogens. When two or more of these processes are combined, they must be differentiated and the dominant causal factor of the lesion determined. Isolation of a microorganism from a tissue does not necessarily mean that it has caused the lesion in question.

26

Physical Causes of Disease

TRAUMA
Mechanical injury

Traumatic lesions arise from any force or energy that is applied to the body. In large animals, trauma is especially common during confinement and shipping. *Contusions* (bruises) arise from blood vessel rupture with disintegration of extravasated blood. *Abrasions* are circumscribed areas where epithelium has been removed; they may or may not penetrate to the dermis. The displacement of epithelium in an abrasion may indicate the direction of the force applied. On mucous membranes, *erosion* is used to indicate partial loss of surface epithelium.

Incised wounds or cuts are produced by sharp-edged instruments and are longer than they are deep. *Stab* wounds are deeper than long. *Lacerations,* or torn wounds, involve severance of tissue by excessive stretching and are common over bony prominences and on the skull; they occur with dull instruments that macerate and tear tissue with much blood loss.

Compression injuries result from the force of slowly applied pressure. These injuries are common during parturition or in the neonatal period, especially in swine (Fig. 26.1). In *blast injuries,* explosive forces are transmitted (in air or water) to body surfaces. In air blast injury a force of compression waves is exerted unidirectionally against surfaces, followed by a wave of diminished pressure. This can rupture muscles and viscera to cause extensive hemorrhage. Gas emboli may arise and lead to infarction of lung and other viscera. In water blasts, pressure is applied more uniformly to body surfaces, usually propelling the animal to the surface. In fish, rupture of the swim bladder is often lethal.

Factors that determine severity of wounding by mechanical trauma include amount of force, rate of application of that force, surface area involved, and the type of tissue that is wounded. Viscera are more friable than are skin and muscle. Abnormal tissues are usually more susceptible to mechanical injury than are normal tissues; that is, wounding to fatty livers and congested spleens will be more severe.

Bullet wounding

As it produces an entry wound in the skin, a spinning bullet indents, stretches, and scrapes out epidermis. Research done in the 1940s on dogs and goats showed that bullets hitting the skin at right angles produce uniform margins of abrasion; those that hit at less than 90° produce asymmetric margins in which the widest margin indicates the direction from which the bullet came. In exit wounds, bullets are traveling at slower speeds and are frequently deformed, so they tend to produce irregular, lacerated wounds with everted edges. Contamination of bullet wounds with bacteria occurs directly from bullet surfaces and indirectly by suction induced by violent cavity formation and collapse of tissue.

The wounding capacity of bullets can be determined by weight (W) and velocity (V) (e.g., force = $WV^2/2g$, where g is the acceleration of gravity). The kinetic energy of a bullet increases arithmetically in relation to weight and geometrically in relation to velocity. When two bullets weigh the same but one travels twice as fast as the other, the energy is 4 times as great in the fast bullet. A bullet fired from a rifle (2000–3000 ft/second) has a muzzle veolicty 3–4 times greater than that from a pistol (500–1000 ft/sec-

423

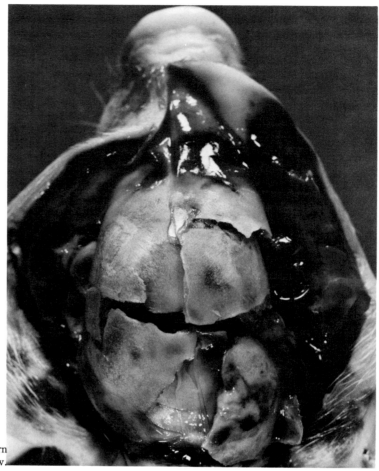

Fig. 26.1.   Fracture, skull, newborn
piglet crushed by sow.

ond), and such high-velocity bullets have kinetic
energies 9–16 times greater than at low velocity.
Rotation of the bullet also enhances its energy
and thus the injury production of flying metal.

ELECTRICAL INJURY

Injury depends on the kind (direct or alternating), amount (amperage), and electromotive
force (voltage) of an electrical current. The
path, duration, and area of current flow are also
important. A 60-cycle alternating current (common in domestic use) as small as 100 milliam-
peres is sufficient to cause ventricular fibrillation in a dog if it passes through the heart.

Electricity causes injury both directly (e.g.,
electric flow through cardiac conduction sys-

tems and respiratory centers of the brainstem)
and indirectly (e.g., heat produced in tissue and
fractures on falling during tetany). Death from
low-voltage current is usually due to ventricular
fibrillation. High-voltage currents induce tetanic
spasm of respiratory muscles and directly inhibit respiratory centers in the brain; high
voltage also produces severe flash burns that
are serious if the animal survives.

Lightning

The diagnosis of death due to lightning is
based on history (range animals found dead after a severe thunderstorm), absence of any other
disease, and presence of subtle lesions in the
dead animal. Characteristic skin damage and
singed haircoat are produced in about half the

FOCUS

Traumatic reticuloperitonitis and pericarditis

Cattle, which are notoriously unselective in eating habits, are prone to swallow metallic foreign bodies during grazing. Nails, wires, and other sharp objects commonly penetrate the wall of the reticulum and cause traumatic reticuloperitonitis. This event is promoted by contraction of the reticulum and is especially common during the increased abdominal pressure of late pregnancy. Sharp foreign bodies often advance to perforate the diaphragm and pericardium to incite pericarditis.

The pathway of the foreign body through the tissues is accompanied by contamination of ingesta, detritus, and bacteria. *Corynebacterium pyogenes, Fusobacterium necrophorum,* and various putrefactive bacteria are common in these wounds. As the pericardium is penetrated, a local fibrinopurulent peritonitis, pleuritis, and pericarditis develops. The pericardial space is filled with fibrin, bacteria, and foul-smelling fluid. Adhesions form between the visceral layer of pericardium and the endocardium over the heart surface. If the cow survives, the fibrinous adhesions may resolve somewhat, but it is doubtful if severe cases can return to normal.

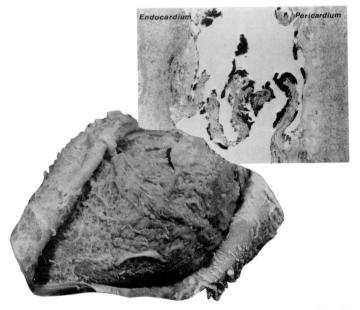

Subacute diffuse fibrinous pericarditis and endocarditis, cow with colibacillary septicemia caused by *Escherichia coli.* Inset: histology; open area is pericardial space between endocardium and pericardium (which are both thickened by inflammatory exudates and fibrosis). The dark material on vegetative growths is fibrin.

cases of lightning death in cattle. The carcass is often cyanotic, and postmortem bloat may be severe. Congestion is common in the viscera, and tiny hemorrhages are typically present in lungs, endocardium, and superficial lymph nodes. Lightning can kill without leaving any of these signs of injury, however, and the diagnosis of lightning as a cause of death has important legal considerations. In pregnant cattle, lightning may kill the fetus but not the cow. Post-lightning sequelae in surviving cattle include ocular degeneration and myoglobinuria, often with renal tubular necrosis.

Ground fault voltage

"Stray voltage" is used to describe electricity on metals and other conducting materials, especially on feeders and waterers on dairy farms. When cows are exposed to voltage that exceeds 1 volt alternating current, an increase in abnormal behavior occurs: poor milk production, reduced feed or water intake, and abnormal behavior at milking time. Water consumption is reduced when waterers are charged with as little as 3.7 volts, so dehydration may become a factor. An increase in clinical mastitis also has been seen in affected farms. In a recent survey in Michigan, 32 of 59 dairy farms had sources of stray voltage.

Affected piglets show excitability and abnormal behavior such as tailbiting.

TEMPERATURE
Thermal burns

The clinical significance of thermal burns depends on the proportion of the body surface involved and the depth of the burn. Burns may be "partial thickness" (first- and second-degree) or "full thickness" (third-degree). Only hyperemia and injury to the superficial layers of epidermis are involved in first-degree burns (e.g., sunburn of hairless, white-skinned animals). In second-degree burns, the epidermis is destroyed although hair follicles remain and provide a nidus for the epithelization of healing. In third-degree burns the dermis is also destroyed.

The effects of burns are *local tissue destruction* and, in severe burning, *fluid loss.* Increased vascular permeability with extensive fluid loss may lead to shock and death. These effects arise from blistering, serous exudation, and surface evaporation from large, denuded wounds. Late complications of severe thermal burns include (1) *laryngeal* and *pulmonary edema* from inhalation of smoke or toxic gases, (2) *renal failure* that accompanies shock-induced necrosis of kidney tubules, and (3) *sepsis* associated with secondary bacterial infections.

Immediately after burning, the wound is sterile for about 20 hours. Thereafter, bacterial contamination is progressive, and by 72 hours there may be millions of bacteria per gram of burned tissue. Bacteria invade the deep layers of skin to reach inflammatory zones that demarcate healthy tissue. Although staphylococci and streptococci are major problems, *Pseudomonas aeruginosa* has a predilection for skin where it invades vascular tissues and produces septicemia.

Thermal injury to skin results in transient neutropenia, sequestration of neutrophils in lung capillaries, and activation of the *complement system* in serum (C5-related chemotactic activity). Oxygen-derived free radicals released by activated neutrophils play a crucial role in lung injury in severe burns. Immunosuppression occurs in severe burns and is probably related to impaired phagocytosis by neutrophils.

Sunburn

Sunburn of the skin occurs in hairless, white-skinned animals. Dogs raised in temperate zones are apt to develop sunburn of the tongue due to prolonged pantings when transferred to hot, tropical climates. Fish held in shallow waters in uncovered concrete ponds (especially at high altitude) develop focal necrosis of the skin with blistering and ulceration. The cellular response of skin to prolonged sunlight exposure is keratinocyte swelling within basal epidermis. Called "sunburn cells," these dense, glassy, homogenous cells with pyknotic nuclei are a prelude to necrosis.

Hyperthermia

Hyperthermia due to high environmental temperature is, in mammals, accompanied by increases in blood pH, hemoglobin concentration, and erythrocyte counts. All of these are consequences of water loss. In *heatstroke,* there may be degenerative changes in the myocardium, renal tubules, and brain that lead to permanent damage. Heatstroke frequently occurs in small pets confined in a hot environment without water. The early signs of hyperpnea (abnormal increase in rate and depth of respiration), tachycardia (rapid heart action), and vomiting may be related to brain injury. Several days after heatstroke, there often is evidence of renal failure caused by degeneration and necrosis of renal tubules.

Mitochondria are major sites of heat production.

In most cells, about 25% of free energy released from oxidation of glucose is conserved as ATP; 75% appears as heat. Combustion in mitochondria is controlled by the ADP:ATP ratio and is dependent on adequate availability of substrates, oxygen, and calcium. Extracellular control is exerted by neuroendocrine systems that act directly on cells to modify thermogenesis. Catecholamines have a rapid effect that ceases when the hormone is removed; thyroxin produces a slow, longer-lasting action.

Vascular exchange networks cool blood for the brain.

Countercurrent heat-exchange networks occur in the brain of carnivores and artiodactyls (cattle and other even-numbered-hoofed mammals) but are lacking in horses, primates, rodents, and lagomorphs. On a hot day a whippet can keep a rabbit running until the rabbit dies of heat exhaustion. Running raises the temperature of both animals, and both are cooled by airflow over oronasal mucosae. The dog's brain, however, has a cooling system lacking in the rabbit; a network of blood vessels branching from the carotid artery to supply the brain (the carotid rete mirabile) passes through a venous sinus drawing cooled blood directly from the nasal cavity. The warm arterial blood loses heat to the cooler venous blood.

In all warm-blooded (homeothermic) vertebrates, body temperature is virtually independent of environmental temperature. Although control of body temperature by cellular mechanisms and metabolic energy is a selective advantage, homeothermy is not without its price. Even under the least-demanding circumstances, birds and mammals devote over 90% of the heat produced by metabolism to maintenance and regulation of body temperature. The energy cost of homeothermy increases markedly as environmental temperature decreases.

Environmental temperature is critical for poikilothermic (cold-blooded) animals because it directly determines body temperature. The rates of most chemical reactions double with each increase of 10°C. This is a particularly valuable influence on defense mechanisms, such as phagocytosis. In most vertebrates the complex reactions of inflammation are plainly enhanced by the increases in body temperature known as fever.

Hypothermia

Severe cold injury produces freeze-induced necrosis of tissue, especially of extremities. The more common cold injury in animals, however, relates to their requirement for increased caloric intake in cold temperatures. Range cattle can withstand very cold temperatures if the food supply is adequate, but their susceptibility to cold increases markedly if they are poorly nourished.

In fish, heat loss is not due to surface heat lost in cold water but to the process of respiration. The low oxygen (2.5% of that in air) and high capacity for heat absorption of water render homeothermy extremely difficult in aquatic animals. The low oxygen in blood allows for little accumulation of metabolic heat, and this small accumulation is lost immediately in passage through the gills. Large, rapidly swimming fish (and all aquatic mammals) require the adaptive advantage of elevated body temperature to enhance muscle power. In these animals another rete mirabile, a network of arteries and veins below the backbone, provides a countercurrent thermal barrier against heat loss. It short-circuits heat flow from muscle to gill and shunts accumulated heat back to the dark swimming muscles.

Hibernation is a precisely regulated lowering of the central thermostat in the hypothalamus designed to conserve energy. Regulated by the effects of day-length cycles on the pineal, hibernation is mediated by a protein called thermogenen and stimulation of heat production in brown fat cells in which mitochondrial oxidative phosphorylation and respiration are uncoupled.

Freezing

Frozen tissue undergoes necrosis because water crystallizes, leaving high salt concentrations in the cytoplasmic matrix. Freeze damage is enhanced by injury to blood vessels. As frozen tissue thaws, vasodilation, increased vascular permeability, and thrombosis occur and complicate parenchymal cell damage. There may also be significant damage to peripheral nerves. The necrotic tissue is swollen, blotchy, and discolored.

Glycerol prevents freeze injury to cells. It is added to semen in artificial insemination establishments to prevent freeze injury to sperm.

RADIATION INJURY

Radiation occurs in two forms: electromagnetic waves (X rays and gamma rays), and energetic charged particles (alpha and beta particles, protons, neutrons, pi-mesons, and heavy ions). Their effects on cells are similar, but there is great variation in the deposition of energy within tissue. Charged particles lose energy by multiple collisions with electrons in tissue, and energy deposition is relatively constant in the course of penetration (which is limited). Neutral particles (X rays and gamma rays) lose energy in infrequent random collisions, leading to exponential reduction of energy deposition in progressively deeper levels of tissue; penetration is much more significant.

Although the effects of radiation are dependent on dose, rate of delivery, and tissue absorption, the dose is the most critical. The unit of energy deposition of radiation at a given point in tissue is the *rad* (r), which is the deposition of 100 ergs of energy per gram of irradiated material (the emission of energy by the X-ray machine or therapy unit is defined as the *roentgen* [R], the liberation of 1 electrostatic unit of positive ions from 1 cc of air). Even with equal amounts of energy absorption, different radiations produce different biologic effects, called the *relative biologic efficiency* (RBE). In lethal effects on mice, the RBE for neutrons (compared with X rays) is about 10; that is, if 500 rad of X rays causes death, then 50 rad of neutrons produces the same effect. An alternate way to express this is to use the *rem* (Roentgen equivalent man) which is rads × RBE. A chest X ray in man gives about 20 or 30 millirem, and 400 rem is considered lethal for half the people exposed. Radioactive isotope activity is measured as *curies,* or Ci: 1 Ci of radioactive isotope suffers 3.7 × 10^10 disintegrations per second. One-half the atoms will disintegrate during one half-life of the isotope.

Radiation-induced cell damage

Radiation energy affects tissue by ionizing cell atoms and molecules with which it collides. Disruption of linkages and bonds of DNA is the most serious event although enzymes, membrane proteins, and other macromolecules are disrupted. Chemical changes may be direct; that is, the absorbed energy in the molecule itself results in ionization or excitation, which produces a chemical change. Alternately, a chemical change may occur due to action of free radicals or ions produced indirectly. For example, radiation causes ionization of cell water leading to formation of hydroxy and peroxide radicals that secondarily interact with crucial enzymes or other molecules.

Radiation-injured cells develop cell swelling, usually with vacuolation of endoplasmic reticulum, swelling of mitochondria, and nuclear swelling. Chromosomal damage, which can be identified by special techniques, include many kinds of injury (e.g., breakage, deletion, and translocation). Clearly, more subtle damage is also present, and this effect is probably more important in the long-term effects of radiation. Radiation injury to vascular and connective tissue is also prominent, and erythema is one of the early tissue changes seen in the radiated animal. In heavily radiated tissue, blood vessels may rupture or develop thrombosis.

Tissues vary in radiation sensitivity.

Radiation sensitivity is in direct proportion to a tissue's mitotic activity and inversely proportional to its degree of differentiation. Germinal cells of the ovary are the most sensitive, followed by sperm, lymphocytes, erythropoietic and myeloid cells of bone marrow, and intestinal epithelium. Neurons and muscle cells are relatively insensitive to radiation. Radiation injury is diminished in the absence of oxygen, and hypoxia is a protective factor in radiation. This is especially important in radiation therapy for cancer since the centers of tumor nodules are often hypoxic.

Animal species vary in sensitivity.

Various species show differences in sensitivity to radiation. Generally the higher the animal species is phylogenetically, the more sensitive it is to radiation. The dose that is lethal for 50% of a group of animals (LD_{50}) is 100,000r for amebae, 700r for frogs, 400–650r for mice and man, 315r for dogs, and 275r for pigs. These differences are partly due to variation in activity of cell replication. Frogs can be given a dose of radiation that will kill in 6 weeks. If irradiated frogs are kept at 5°C, they remain alive for several months, but on being warmed, will die within 6 weeks like the control animals kept at normal temperature.

Radiation damage is delayed.

The initial tissue damage in radiation is instantaneous, but the clinical effects may not be apparent for days. If a single dose of radiation is

---

FOCUS

Failure to conduct necropsies: The Utah radiation incident

During May 1953 two atomic bomb blasts at a test site in Nevada rained fallout on herds of sheep grazing nearby. The U.S. Atomic Energy Commission had tested "Nancy" and "Harry," two high-yield bombs. As clouds of dust and radiation rolled down Utah valleys, ranchers reported radiation burns on sheep grazing downwind of detonation sites. Wool sloughed off in clumps. Within a short period 2000 ewes and 2200 lambs died, roughly one-eighth of the ewes and one-fourth of the lambs.

Complaints were made, and a team of veterinarians was dispatched to collect tissues and bone samples from surviving sheep for radiologic analysis at the radiation lab in Oak Ridge. Later, sheep were experimentally exposed to intense radiation at Los Alamos in an attempt to duplicate the lesion. Scientists at a Hanford, Washington, lab who studied effects of radioiodine on ewes suggested that the "sheep did not die from irradiation because doses were too low; they did not die from doses to thyroid because that is a slower cause of death." However, two veterinarians concluded that the lesions on surviving sheep were similar or identical to those produced at Los Alamos and that "radiation was at least a contributing factor to the loss of these animals."

The sheep probably died from effects of contaminated grass in their stomachs. Sheep exposed to only 4 rads of external gamma radiation might have gotten a dose of 1500–1600 rads in the gastrointestinal tracts, and fetal lambs may have received a thyroid dose of 20,000–40,000 rads (*Science* 218:545, 1982).

Thirty years after this incident, previously classified documents were released that stimulated lawsuits against the government in relation to human leukemia. Utah ranchers initiated a lawsuit, also alleging suppression of information after atomic testing. The courts found that the U.S. government had suppressed scientific data and pressured veterinarians to revise their conclusion. Motivated by a desire to prevent general alarm, the Atomic Energy Commission had extensively investigated these events but had not revealed potentially compromising field observations and critical data from laboratory experiments.

given to the skin of a rabbit, erythema does not appear until about the 10th day, necrosis not until the 2nd week, and death weeks later.

Total body radiation

Acute radiation sickness from large doses of radiation given by a point source arises from killing of cells in the bloodstream, bone marrow, and intestine (Table 26.1). Anorexia and vomiting develop within 2 hours of radiation and may arise from brain injury. These signs decline, but at 24–48 hours they recur, accompanied by severe diarrhea due largely to necrosis of gastrointestinal epithelium and to dehydration, hemoconcentration, and shock (Fig. 26.2).

Table 26.1. Clinical signs and pathology of acute radiation injury

Signs	Pathology
Vomiting	Early (neurologic) and late (intestinal destruction) onset
Leukopenia	Immediate onset, especially lymphopenia
Thrombocytopenia	Bone marrow destruction
Hemorrhage	Effects prominent in heart, intestine, and urogenital tract
Bone marrow atrophy	Diminished production of blood cells
Anemia	Predisposal to cardiovascular injury
Epithelial necrosis	Intestine with diarrhea, tarry stools, ulceration
Edema	Loss of serum proteins
Lymphoid tissue necrosis	Widespread infections and necrosis in many body systems

Note: Late effects of radiation include sterility, cataracts, premature aging, and fetal malformations.

In the 1960s radioactive fallout from military bomb tests resulted in massive liberation of neutrons and gamma radiation. Effects of this type of radiation are complicated by cloud movement and deposition of radioactive particles on plants. Acute radiation sickness in exposed animals results not so much from external radiation but from internal radiation from ingestion of contaminated plants.

In the last decade a suprising source of radiation has occurred from the illegal dismantling of old radiographic equipment. In 1983 junkyard workers in Mexico opened a radiation therapy device (containing gamma sources) that spilled out several thousand metal pellets, each mm in

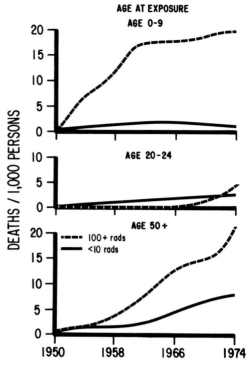

Fig. 26.2. Incidence of radiation-associated leukemia in humans among exposures to atomic radiation in Japan (Data from Beebe, *Am. Sci.* 70:35, 1982)

diameter and containing 70 microcuries of cobalt-60. Steel foundries melted the radioactive pellets along with scrap metal, and this was made into steel rods, table legs, and other items, which emitted 600–700 milliroentgens/hour. One worker received 10,000 rem and developed wounds on his hands. Four others received 300–450 rem in doses to the whole body, and at least 200 people received doses ranging from 1 to 50 rem.

Radiation during gestation has long-term effects.

Drs. Glenn Miller and Stephen Benjamin, at the Radiation Biology Laboratory at Colorado State University, studied thymic involution in pregnant beagles irradiated at 30, 40, and 45 days of gestation. Dogs were examined at 5 and 10 days after irradiation. Results were that the earlier in gestation the irradiation occurred, the greater the thymic destruction (injury to the medulla was greater than that in the cortex).

ADDITIONAL READING

Buckley, I. K. Tissue injury by high frequency electric current. *Austr. J. Exp. Biol.* 38:195, 1960.

Gleiser, C. A. The pathology of total body radiation in dogs which died following exposure to a lethal dose. *Am. J. Vet. Res.* 15:329, 1954.

Stoner, H. B., et al. Trauma and its metabolic problems. *Br. Med. Bull.* 41:201, 1985.

Till, G. O., et al. Lipid peroxidation and acute lung injury after thermal trauma to skin. *Am. J. Pathol.* 119:376, 1985.

27

Chemical Causes of Disease

NEARLY every chemical substance can be toxic. Even water and sodium chloride, which are required for life, will be toxic if given in massive amounts. In this chapter the major categories of toxins that cause natural disease are introduced and the mechanisms of action of a prototype toxin are discussed. The most lethal toxins are those that produce damage in the liver, kidney, heart, brain, or bone marrow. Even though some toxins produce highly specific injury to a particular organelle (e.g., cyanide kills by suppressing mitochondria), most toxins have widespread effects in the animal and produce injury by complex mechanisms.

In most cells, acute toxic injury leads to immediate cell swelling. Depending on dose, blood flow, and cell enzyme patterns, injured cells may recover or progress to more severe changes such as lysis, coagulation necrosis, vacuolar degeneration, or fatty degeneration. Toxins are quite selective in the tissue, cell, or even organelle that they destroy. Differences in cell tropism are due to the chemical nature of the toxin and to where it acts in the metabolic energy of the cell. Proximal convoluted tubules of kidneys, terminal bronchiolar epithelium in lungs, and Purkinje cells of the brain are all sites of predilection for toxic injury. The *liver* is a major organ of detoxification chiefly because most toxins enter from the gastrointestinal tract. Toxic damage usually occurs in centrolobular hepatocytes, which have large amounts of detoxifying enzymes but have the least oxygen supply due to the position in the hepatic sinusoid.

Poisons, like all chemicals, are metabolized in the hepatocyte by various oxidation, reduction, hydrolytic, and conjugation reactions designed to convert fat-soluble compounds to hydrophilic ones, which are more easily removed by the kidney and excreted in urine. Within hepatocytes, protective mechanisms against toxicity include (1) oxidizing enzymes of the smooth endoplasmic reticulum, (2) the catalase-H_2O_2 system of peroxisomes, (3) the sulfhydryl buffer or glutathione oxidation-reduction cycle, and (4) other specific enzymes in the cytosol. *Reduced glutathione* is a potent antioxidant; it has a free sulfhydryl group and serves as a sulfhydryl buffer to prevent the toxic effects of many drugs. The cycle of oxidation and reduction of glutathione is a major antioxidative reaction in hepatocytes.

BIOLOGIC TOXINS

Animals, microorganisms, and plants contain or secrete toxic substances that are protective or in some other way promote their survival in nature. In general, toxins become increasingly complex as one proceeds up the phylogenetic scale. For example, the toxin of the bacterium *Escherichia coli* is exquisitely precise, producing diarrhea by turning on production of adenyl cyclase in the intestinal absorptive cell to enhance secretion of fluid into the intestine. In contrast, snake venoms contain as many as 50 different peptides differing widely in biologic action. In rare cases, animals and plants cooperate to produce toxicity. The monarch butterfly feeds on and selectively absorbs toxic glycosides from the milkweed flower. Accumulating in high concentration in the wings, these toxins produce severe emesis when the butterfly is eaten by birds or other predators.

Arthropod toxins and venoms

Spider toxins

Spiders are uniformly venomous, but most attack only other arthropods, using venom to paralyze their prey. Venom of the black widow spider causes paralysis of the mammalian nervous system by affecting release of neurotransmitters. The result is severe inflammation at the site of the bite and ascending motor paralysis with destruction of peripheral nerve endings. Envenomation into blood vessels may lead to cardiovascular collapse and respiratory paralysis. The brown recluse spider produces a hemolytic and necrotizing venom that incites a chronic ulcerating wound, which is accompanied in early stages by the systemic effects of fever, nausea, and vomiting.

Hymenopterous toxins

Each year in the United States nearly twice as many humans die from hymenopterous insect bites (from bees, wasps, hornets, and yellow jackets) as from snake bites. Deaths are due to systemic anaphylactic shock, in which respiratory distress is followed by vascular collapse. Bee venom contains histamine, two enzymes (phospholipase A_2 and hyaluronidase), and several toxic peptides. The latter include mellitin (which is hemolyzing), apamin (which is neurotoxic), and a mast cell–degranulating peptide. Mellitin, 50% of the dry weight of bee venom, is the main toxin. It acts on plasma membranes of vascular endothelial cells to stimulate endogenous phospholipases, which in turn stimulate formation of cyclic GMP. These reactions, in the end, increase capillary permeability and incite other events of necrosis and inflammation. Venoms of wasps are often more potent locally and produce tissue necrosis with severe edema and inflammation. Venom of the oriental hornet causes local muscle necrosis.

Blister beetle toxicity

Blister beetles, when ingested in hay, produce necrotic lesions in the alimentary canal. This is a recurring problem in horses in the southwestern United States. Drs. Roger Panciera and Trentin Schoeb, at Oklahoma State University, reported hemorrhage and necrosis with ulceration in the gastrointestinal tract and urinary bladder in equine blister beetle toxicity. Focal necrosis of the myocardium and swelling of renal tubule cells contributed to the lethal effect of the toxin. Cantharidin ("Spanish fly") is the toxic principle responsible for the tissue necrosis.

Snake venoms

Snake venoms are mixtures of up to 30 different peptides, most of which are toxic, either directly or via activity as enzymes (Table 27.1). All snake venoms contain (1) phospholipase A_2, which has a direct lytic action on membranes of erythrocytes, platelets, and other cells; (2) hyaluronidase ("spreading factor"), which cleaves internal glycoside bonds of acidic mucopolysaccharides to facilitate diffusion of toxin into tissue; (3) phosphodiesterase; and (4) peptidases. Superimposed on these enzymes are different toxins in individual venoms that act specifically on nerve tissue, coagulation systems, and other organs.

Myonecrosis

Rattlesnakes and other pit vipers have fangs that reach deeply into muscle. They produce

Table 27.1. Toxins in crude snake venom

Venom	Crotalidae[a]	Viperidae[b]	Elapidae[c]	Hydrophidae[d]
Phospholipase A_2	+	+	+	+
Phosphodiesterase	+	+	+	+
Hyaluronidase	+	+	+	+
Peptidase	+	+	+	+
Kininogenase[e]	+			
Neurotoxin (presynaptic)				+
Neurotoxin (postsynaptic)			+	
Defibrinating peptide	+[f]			
Antithromboplastin			+[f]	

[a]Rattlesnake, moccasin, copperhead.
[b]Russell's viper, African puff adder, Gaboon viper.
[c]Cobra, coral snake, krait, tiger snake.
[d]Sea snake.
[e]Bradykinin, discovered in 1949 by Silva, who mixed euglobulin with *Bothrops* venom, producing a rapid drop in blood pressure.
[f]Some species.

large puncture marks that rapidly develop severe edema and erythema. In man, bites occur on extremities. In animals, in which curiosity leads to probing the snake, bites are apt to occur on the nose. These bites lead to swelling of facial and pharyngeal tissues and to respiratory distress. Hemolytic anemia (with hemoglobinuria) and kidney damage reflect the necrotizing toxins in venom. When much venom is involved, cardiac irregularities, fall in blood pressure, and shock may occur.

Neurotoxicity

Neurotoxins are the most potent constituents of snake venoms. They kill by blocking neuromuscular transmission at motor endplates of skeletal muscle, by blockade of the cardiac conduction system, and by producing central effects that suppress both respiratory and cardiac action. The most prominent of these is motor endplate dysfunction and paralysis of the respiratory muscles of the diaphragm and rib cage. Mechanistically, neurotoxin action on neuromuscular transmission is either (1) presynaptic, via inhibition of acetylcholine release; (2) synaptic, by cholinesterase acting within the synaptic cleft; or (3) postsynaptic, by binding to acetylcholine receptors to prevent the depolarizing action of acetylcholine.

Cobra and krait have postsynaptic toxins that bind tightly and irreversibly to acetylcholine receptors and act as antagonists, like curare. Injection of cobra venom in mammals produces a flaccid muscle paralysis, and death occurs by respiratory failure. Neurotoxic peptides bind specifically to nicotinic acetylcholine receptors, producing a nondepolarizing block.

In addition to postjunctional neurotoxins, cobra venoms contain large amounts of similar peptides that act directly on cell membranes. They are called "cardiotoxins" or "membrane toxins" because they cause depolarization and contracture of cardiac (and skeletal) myocytes. In large concentrations, cardiotoxins also cause degeneration and lysis of neurons and erythrocytes although these cells are not targets in vivo.

Fish and amphibian toxins

All toads contain skin glands that secrete repulsive chemicals. The more poisonous amphibians are the Colorado River toad (*Bufo alvarius*), the marine toad (*Bufo marinus*), and the poison-

dart frogs of central America (*Dendrobates* spp.). These species secrete complex venoms all containing a toxin that mimics the action of cardiac glycosides, which poison the electrolyte pumps of heart muscle. Batrachotoxin, the steroidal alkaloid of the poison-dart frog, irreversibly blocks sodium channels in neurons and leads to membrane depolarization. The *Bufo* species have parotid glands behind the eyes that secrete *bufotoxin*, a conjugation of bufagen, a digitalislike toxin, and bufotenine, which produces marked pressor action resembling oxytocin. Most poisonings occur in dogs and cats that attack and bite the bufo toads. Young kittens and puppies are especially susceptible and exhibit salivation, cardiac irregularities, ventricular fibrillation, and pulmonary edema.

Tetrodotoxin is concentrated in liver, ovaries, intestine, and skin of many species of puffer fish, which are prized as food in the Orient. It binds to sodium channels on nerve axons and suppresses conduction of nerve impulses. Generalized paralysis occurs, followed by convulsions and death. Tetrodotoxin is also produced by the California newt, the Australian blue-ringed octopus, and other amphibians, but poisoning from these species is rare.

Saxitoxin acts in the same way as tetrodotoxin. This molecule is produced by a genus of plankton, *Gonyaulax* spp., which under favorable conditions multiplies so rapidly that it reaches a density of many millions per liter and creates a "red tide," turning the ocean surface rusty brown by day and luminescent by night. Shellfish that feed in red tide waters concentrate the toxin in their tissues and are thus poisonous to man.

MICROBIAL TOXINS
Bacterial toxins

Microbial toxins include some of the most potent toxic substances known (Fig. 27.1). Toxins produced by bacteria fall into two major categories: (1) *structural components* of the bacterium, which are released after bacterial destruction, and (2) *soluble peptides,* which are released by the living bacterium (there is overlap in this dichotomy, since some structural toxins are shed by living bacteria and dead bacteria contain some soluble toxins).

The dominant structural toxins are *endotoxins,* which are lipopolysaccharides present in the cell wall of gram-negative bacteria. They produce profound effects on the blood-vascular system and are important in septicemia, in which they cause "endotoxic" shock.

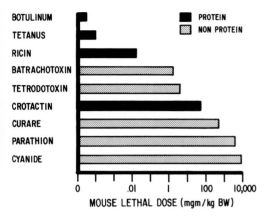

Fig. 27.1. Comparative toxicity of protein and nonprotein toxins.

Soluble exotoxins act by one of two general mechanisms.

Exotoxins may be potent lysins that *damage cellular membranes* (clostridial phospholipases, hemolysins, and other lysins), or they may act by entering the cell to *suppress metabolism.* In the first group, the toxins destroy phospholipids in the lipid bilayer of the cell surface. Small holes are produced in the membrane, the cell gains unwanted electrolytes and water, and cell swelling progresses to cell lysis. The highly lethal alpha toxin produced by clostridia in black-leg of cattle and gas gangrene of man, for example, is a lecithinase that destroys membrane lecithins. The enterotoxins of staphylococci, shigellae, and some of the other clostridia damage intestinal absorptive cells in the same way.

Soluble exotoxins that suppress metabolism are, like some hormones, large glycoprotein molecules with a two-unit construction: the A chain produces cell injury and the B chain binds to the cell surface. After the B chain binds to receptor molecules on the surface, the exotoxin molecule enters the cell by receptor-mediated endocytosis (into coated vesicles). The subsequent cleavage of the molecule allows fragment A to exert its toxic effect. Most exotoxins act by ADP ribosylation; that is, the toxin catalyzes cleavage of endogenous NAD with covalent attachment of the adenosine diphosphoribose moiety to a cell substrate. In some cases this process inactivates a critical component of protein synthesis (e.g., *Pseudomonas* toxin), while in others it increases cell activity (e.g., the toxins of cholera, pertussis, and *E. coli*).

Exotoxins of clostridia are extremely potent.

The minimum lethal dose for mice of botulinum toxin is 0.00012 mg/kg when given subcutaneously. Botulism toxin blocks irreversibly and with high specificity the release of acetylcholine from nerve termini at the motor endplates (Table 27.2). *Clostridium tetani* produces two toxins at sites of tissue infection: a *hemolysin* and a *neurotoxin,* tetanospasmin. The neurotoxin binds selectively to ganglioside receptors embedded in membranes at peripheral nerve endings.

Fungal toxins (mycotoxins)
Aflatoxins are hepatotoxins.

Mycotoxins include a diverse group of fungal peptides (Table 27.3). Aflatoxins, the best-known mycotoxins, are a group of hepatotoxic metabolites produced by some strains of *Aspergillus flavus.* They are synthesized by fungi growing in the feed, and they poison when these feeds are ingested by the animal. Aflatoxins were first isolated from peanut meal that had been associated with ill-defined intoxications of trout, turkeys, pigs, and cattle. Most animals are susceptible, and liver lesions depend on dose and chronicity of exposure. Ducklings, dogs, and swine are among the most susceptible animals.

The primary effect of aflatoxin is on the liver, where it causes hepatocyte necrosis, fibrosis, and bile duct proliferation (Fig. 27.2). Drs. Paul Newberne, at Massachusetts Institute of Technology, and William Carlton and George Szczech, at Purdue, have defined the hepatic lesions of aflatoxicosis. Hepatocytes around the central vein are most susceptible to the toxin, and the lesion is called *centrolobular necrosis.* Within the hepatocyte, aflatoxin is directly toxic to a DNA-dependent RNA polymerase in the nucleolus and the end result is a blockade of protein synthesis in the hepatocyte. In *chronic toxicity,* aflatoxin causes liver tumors. The natural occurrence of aflatoxin-induced neoplasia is difficult to prove, but in feeding experiments

FOCUS

Tetanus

From *The Veterinarian,* Volume 2:

MARCH 30, 1819, I was requested to attend a chestnut colt, four years old, that had been taken up to be broken, the property of Mr. Bamford Bradely, near Bilstone, Staffordshire. I was immediately convinced that it was Tetanus, from the following symptoms: Jaw completely closed, saliva flowing from the mouth; rigidity of the principle muscles of the body, pulse slow and irregular, and tail elevated.

Severe spasms of striated muscle spread progressively from muscle to muscle from a site of wound infection with *Clostridium tetani.* The bacterial toxin suppresses, as does strychnine, all synaptic inhibition. The cause of death is usually asphyxia following paralysis of respiratory muscles. The toxin causes disruption of spinal inhibitory pathways; the resulting unopposed stimulation of motor nerves is the primary cause of unremitting rigidity of skeletal muscle. Muscle rigidity leads to locomotor disturbances, stiffness of limbs, ears, and tail, and curious facial expressions.

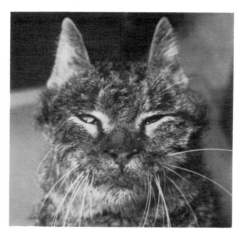

Cl. tetani produces several toxins. The most important is the neurotoxin *tetanospasmin* (generally referred to as "tetanus toxin"), which is highly toxic for horses and man. Tetanospasmin binds selectively to ganglioside receptors at peripheral nerve endings, is taken into the nerve, and passes via retrograde transport to nerve cell bodies in the spinal cord where it diffuses back to exert its action presynaptically. Its major effect is to suppress neuroinhibitory Renshaw cells. Within these neurons toxin localizes on membranes of endoplasmic reticulum and suppresses the production of neurosecretory substances.

▶

Tetanus toxin also produces central effects in the brain, for example, reflex motor convulsion. In rare cases, these effects may dominate in a syndrome of "cephalic tetanus." Toxin may also bind to cells of the sympathetic nervous system in later stages of disease, producing hypertension, tachycardia, and peripheral vasoconstriction.

A second toxin, *tetanolysin,* is a hemolysin that destroys cells by acting on plasma membranes. Experimentally, it causes hematologic alterations and cardiovascular alterations, and some of the signs seen in terminal tetanus are due to this toxin, for example, pulmonary edema and azotemia. There is a direct lytic effect on skeletal muscles late in the disease, and this effect may be due to tetanolysin, possibly by inhibiting ion flux in sarcoplasmic reticulum.

Table 27.2.   Clostridial toxins

Species	Type	Disease	Animal	Toxin
Cl. botulinum	A, B	Botulism	Man	One toxin produced by each single type; all toxins are similar in action; blocks release of acetylcholine by peripheral nerve
			Bird (limberneck)	
	Cα	Botulism	Chicken, wild duck	
	Cβ	Forage poisoning	Cow (Australia)	
	D	Lamziekte	Cow (South Africa)	
	E, F	Botulism	Man	
Cl. tetani	1 type[a]	Tetanus	Mammals	Tetanospasmin (neurotoxin), tetanolysin (hemolysin)
Cl. novyi[b]	A	Cellulitis/myositis	Man (gas gangrene)	α (lethal, necrotizing)
				γ (phospholipase C)
				ϵ (lipase)
				δ
	B	Infectious necrotic hepatitis	Sheep (black disease)	α
				β (phospholipase C)
	C	Nonpathogenic		
	D[c]	Bacillary hemoglobinuria	Cow	β
Cl. septicum	6 types	Cellulitis/myositis	Man (gas gangrene)	α (lethal, necrotizing)
			Cow (pseudoblackleg)	β (DNAase), hyaluronidase
			Sheep	
Cl. chauvoei	1 type[a]	Blackleg	Cow, sheep	Uncharacterized
Cl. perfringens[d]	A	Cellulitis/myositis	Man (gas gangrene) Other mammals (wound infections)	α (phospholipase C)
		Enterotoxemia	Lamb, calf, man	α, enterotoxin
	B	Enteritis/enterotoxemia	Lamb, calf, foal	β, ϵ, α
	C	Enteritis with necrosis and hemorrhage	Sheep, foal, pig, calf, man	β, ϵ, α
	D	Enterotoxemia	Sheep (pulpy kidney disease)	ϵ, α
	E	Enterotoxemia	Sheep	ι, α

[a]Based on toxin production, isolates differ in growth characteristics.
[b]*Cl. oedematiens.*
[c]*Cl. hemolyticum.*
[d]*Cl. welchii.*

Table 27.3.   Diseases caused by fungal toxins

Mycotoxin	Produced by	Animal	Pathologic Lesions
Aflatoxin	*Aspergillus flavus* *A. parasiticus*	Cow Pig Chicken Horse Fish	Acute hepatic necrosis, widespread hemorrhage

Subacute or chronic hepatic necrosis with cirrhosis Hepatoma |
Citrinin	*Penicillium citrinin* *P. viridicatum*	Pig Cow	Renal tubular degeneration
Ergot toxins, ergot-amine, etc.	*Claviceps purpurea*	Cow Sheep Pig Chicken Man	Vascular necrosis and gangrene of limbs Nervous signs, staggers, convulsions
Fusariotoxins T-2 toxin	*Fusarium* spp.	Pig Cow Chicken	Dermal necrosis, gastroenteritis, abortion
Zearalenone		Pig	Estrogenic stimulation of female genitalia
Vomitoxin		Pig	Emesis, enteritis
Diacetoxyscirpenol		Pig	Gastroenteric necrosis, hemorrhage
?		Horse	Leukoencephalomalacia
Ochratoxin	*A. ochraceous* *P. viridicatum*	Pig Chicken Turkey	Renal tubular necrosis
Penitrem	*P.* spp.	Dog Cow Sheep	Ataxia, convulsions
Rubratoxin	*P. rubrum* *P. purpurogenum*	Pig Cow	Hepatic necrosis, coagulopathy
Sporodesmin	*Pithomyces chartarum*	Sheep	Hepatic necrosis, photosensitivity (facial eczema)
Stachybotryotoxin	*Stachybotrys atra*	Horse	Gastroenteritis, dermal necrosis, bone marrow hypoplasia

where aflatoxins are given in small amounts over a long period, hepatomas have been induced in trout and hepatocarcinomas in rats.

Abnormal coagulation and bleeding occur in acute aflatoxicosis. Drs. Dale Baker and Robert Green, at Texas A&M University, have shown that this is primarily due to suppressed synthesis of coagulation factors by the damaged liver. In severe toxicity, peptides released from the necrotic liver can also cause consumption of coagulation factors and intravenous coagulation directly.

An accurate diagnosis of aflatoxicosis requires the demonstration of toxins in feed and urine of intoxicated animals. Four major toxins (B_1, B_2, G_1, and G_2) are differentiated by their chromatographic mobility and fluorescence under ultra-violet light. B_1 is the most toxic. The oral 7-day LD_{50} for aflatoxins in ducklings is (in μg): B_1, 18.2; B_2, 84.8; G_1, 39.2; and G_2, 172.5.

Sporodesmin causes liver failure and photosensitivity disease.

Sporodesmin, produced by the fungus *Pithomyces chartarum* (a saprophyte on pasture grass), causes *facial eczema,* a photosensitivity of sheep and cattle. It is a hepatotoxin that causes degeneration of hepatocytes and bile canaliculi, occlusion of bile ductules, periductal edema, and hepatitis. Photosensitivity results from failure of the damaged liver to remove *phylloerythrin* from the blood. Phylloerythrin circulates and absorbs energy from the sun as it passes through skin; the release of energy causes necrosis.

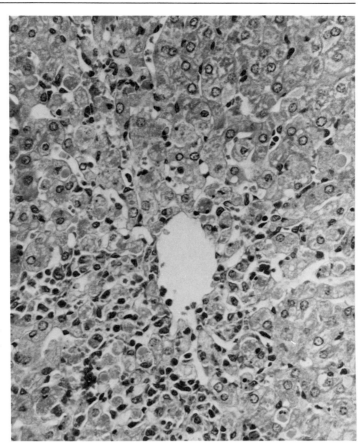

Fig. 27.2. Aflatoxicosis, liver. Necrosis of hepatocytes around central vein, with infiltration of monocytes.

Penitrem

Penitrem A, a product of *Penicillium* spp., produces acute neurologic disease: muscle tremor, seizures, ataxia, and death. It occurs in dogs fed moldy cheese and in large animals that eat moldy roughage. Penitrem suppresses *glycine*, the neurotransmitter of some inhibitory neurons. Signs resemble those of *strychnine* toxicity, for strychnine is also a glycine antagonist. Treatment with substances that raise glycine content of the brain (e.g., mephenesin and nalorphine) abolish penitrem-induced tremors. No cellular lesion has been documented for penitrem.

Ergot

Ergotism is a classic disease of cattle, horses, and other animals. In medieval Europe, human epidemics of gangrenous necrosis of the limbs resulted from ingestion of ergot-contaminated flour. Ergotism is caused by alkaloids of *Claviceps purpurea,* which turns cereal grains black and misshapen. Toxic compounds of the fungus include *ergotamine,* a vasoconstrictor, and *ergometrine,* a smooth muscle contractor. Other lysergic acid derivatives are also produced. Gangrene is produced by *chronic vasoconstriction, ischemia,* and *capillary endothelial degeneration* in the extremities. In horses and carnivores, nervous signs and convulsion may be the dominant signs.

A second syndrome of gangrene of the extremities called *fescue foot* occurs in cattle that ingest tall fescue grass (*Festuca arundinacea*) infected by another fungus, *Sphacelia typhina.* Infected tall fescue, when eaten in small amounts, also produces a wasting disease in cattle called "summer syndrome."

Fusarium toxins

Fusarium spp. produce two types of toxins that cause disease: estrogenic metabolites and trichothecene toxins. Formed in temperate climates or even in cold weather, they produce a wide variety of clinical syndromes. *Zearalenone,* produced in moldy corn, causes precocious sexual development with vulvar enlargement and mammary development in swine. Affected sows have ovarian abnormalities and proliferation of uterine glands. Offspring are born weak, and there is reduced litter size.

Equine leukoencephalomalacia is produced by feed contaminated with *Fusarium moniliforme,* although a specific toxin has not been isolated. In the brain there are areas of liquefactive necrosis of the subcortical white matter of the cerebrum, sometimes with cavitation.

Acute interstitial pneumonitis has been reported in cattle eating sweet potatoes damaged by the mold *Fusarium solani.* The disease can be reproduced with a furan (4-ipomeanol) isolated from the moldy potatoes. Studies in rodents by Dr. A. R. Doster, at the University of Nebraska, suggest that Clara cells in the terminal bronchioles contain enzymes that convert this furan to a reactive toxin. More recent studies by Dr. S. K. Durham and colleagues, at Cornell University, indicate that pulmonary endothelium, especially capillaries and small veins, play an important role. Endothelial cells metabolize the exogenous furans to highly reactive metabolites by the cytochrome P-450 mixed function oxidase system of pneumocytes, leading to lung injury.

Mushroom toxins

There are many toxic mushrooms, including some common ones, and a few of these are lethal. Most poisonous mushrooms are not lethal but produce signs soon after ingestion, that is, within 1–2 hours. Some contain *muscarine,* which causes blurred vision, sweating, increased peristalsis, and reduced blood pressure. The liberty cap (*Psilocybe semilanceata*) has been deliberately eaten for its hallucinogenic effects. Indoles of this fungus (e.g., psilocybin and psilocin) alter the concentration of indoles, including serotonin, in the brain and thereby interfere with transmission of stimuli regulating perception.

Mushrooms of the genus *Amanita* are the most deadly.

Most human deaths are due to a single species of this genus, *Amanita phalloides.* In contrast to most mushroom poisonings, signs do not appear for many hours after ingestion. A full day may pass before abdominal pain, diarrhea, and violent emesis occur. If medically treated, patients recover from the gastroenteritis but succumb later to lethal nephropathy. The two major groups of toxins from *A. phalloides* are the *amanitins,* consisting of at least five amatoxins (all cyclopeptides or ring-shaped amino acids) and the *phalloidins.* In renal tubular epithelium of poisoned animals, the major cellular change begins with disintegration of the nucleolus and nuclei of renal tubular cells. Damage is from α-amanitin, which attacks an RNA polymerase that directs synthesis of mRNA. Suppression of this enzyme stops protein synthesis and kills the cell.

PLANT TOXINS

Of about 700 species of plants known to be toxic to animals, action of the toxic principle is known for less than half (Table 27.4). The chemical classification followed below contains some overlapping. Solanine, the toxic principle of the nightshades (*Solanum* spp.), is a glycoside (because of its sugar residue, solanose) but is considered an alkaloid because on hydrolysis it yields the toxic alkaloid moiety solanidine.

Alkaloids

These bitter, soluble, organic acid-alkaloid salts are common in several plants, and over 5000 have been partially characterized. Unfortunately, they are often named according to the generic name of the plant from which they were extracted. The alkaloid content varies little with growing season or climate. It is distributed throughout the plant, so that any part may be dangerous to livestock.

Pyrrolizidine alkaloids

Species of *Senecio, Crotalaria,* and *Heliotropium* contain pyrrolizidine alkaloids that are toxic. Toxins are most often associated with chronic liver disease in grazing livestock. Signs of wasting, weakness, and icterus occur up to 2 months after ingestion of plants. Lesions consist of an initial necrosis of hepatocytes, followed by *cytomegaly* of remaining hepatocytes and progressive *cirrhosis,* that is, perisinusoidal fibrosis, proliferation of bile ductules, and regeneration

Table 27.4. Plant poisons

Group	Toxin	Genera (prototype)
	ALKALOIDS	
Pyridine	Coniine	*Conium* (hemlocks)
Pyrrolizidine		*Crotalaria*
		Senecio
		Heliotropium
Tropane	Atropinelike	*Atrupa* (belladonna)
Steroids		
Solanum type	Solanine	*Solanum* (nightshades)
Veratrum type	Veratramine	*Veratrum* (false hellebore)
		Zigadenus (death camas)
		Amianthium (staggergrass)
Polycyclic	Delphinine	*Delphinium* (larkspur)
diterpenes		*Aconitum* (monkshood)
Quinolizidine		*Lupinus* (lupines)
	AMINES	
β-aminopropionitrile		*Lathyrus* (sweet pea)
	GLYCOSIDES	
Cardiac	Digitalis	*Digitalis* (foxglove)
	Ouabain	*Strophanthus*
	Squill	*Urginea* (sea onion)
	Convallatoxin	*Convallaria* (lily of the valley)
	Oleandrin	*Nerium* (oleander)
Coumarin	Coumarinlike	*Melilotus* (sweet clover)
Cyanogenic	Amygdalin	Several fruit seeds
	Amygdalinlike	*Prunus* (chokecherry)
Goitrogenic	Thiooxazolidone	*Brassica* (cabbage)
Saponin	Hederagenin	*Hedera* (English ivy)
	Saponine	*Saponaria* (cow cockle)
	MISCELLANEOUS	
Oxalates	Oxalate	*Halogeton*
Tannins	Oak tannin	*Quercus* (oak)
Minerals	Nitrates	
	Selenim	
Resins		

of surviving hepatocytes. These alkaloids act as alkylating agents on DNA, producing cytomegaly by preventing mitosis while permitting cytoplasmic ribosomal synthesis to continue.

Crotalaria metabolites produce endothelial damage in the lung that leads to increased thickening of the media of muscular arteries in the lungs and to pulmonary hypertension. Right ventricular hypertrophy followed by heart failure occurs in some species. Heart lesions include focal cytolysis of myocytes, cell swelling, and fibrosis.

Swainsonine

An indolizidine alkaloid in locoweeds (*Astragalus* and *Oxytropis* spp.) and Darling peas (*Swainsona* sp.), swainsonine produces an oligosaccharide storage disease caused by its specific inhibition of α-mannosidase in lysosomes. Lysosomes accumulate, making affected cells large, pale, and foamy. Neurons, myocardium, and renal tubules are most severely affected. Poisoned animals become nervous and may fall backward, walk into objects, or leap over imagined objects. Ingestion is habit forming and grazing animals seek out the toxic plants. Cattle grazing at high altitudes are likely to die from congestive heart failure, which develops when the effects of high altitude are superimposed on the cardiac lesions.

Coniine

Poison hemlock (*Conium maculatum*) contains at least five alkaloids. Coniine dominates in the fruits and is responsible for the rapidly developing signs of ataxia, reduced cardiac function, dilatation of pupils, and coma in acute toxicity.

Some gastrointestinal irritation occurs, and vomiting is common. Pigs are most commonly affected and develop ataxia and trembling. Skeletal malformations occur in newborn piglets if sows are poisoned between 43 and 61 days of gestation. Arthrogryposis, lumbar-thoracic scoliosis, and twisted limbs result from the teratogenic alkaloid γ-coniceine.

Glycosides

Glycosides are more widespread in the plant kingdom than are alkaloids. They are a combination of an aglycone (or "genin") with one to four sugar molecules. Toxic activity resides in the aglycone, and sugars may modify solublility.

FOCUS

Foxglove as drug and toxin

Digitalis, the potent cardiac stimulant that is used clinically to strengthen the heartbeat, is also a potent toxin. It was discovered by physicians after investigating reports of the use of foxglove tea in human patients with congestive heart failure. William Withering's 1785 publication, "An Account of the Foxglove and Some of Its Medical Uses," gives signs of human digitalis toxicity: "vomiting, purging, giddiness, confused vision, objects appearing green or yellow; increased secretion of urine with frequent motions to part with it; slow pulse, even as low as 35 in a minute, cold sweats, convulsions, syncope, death." Digitalis toxicity leads to abnormalities of cardiac rhythm and atrioventricular (A-V) conduction, even to A-V block. These are due both to the direct effects of digitalis on the A-V node and Purkinje fibers and to vagal effects. Fibrillation is enhanced by the elevation in plasma potassium ions (K^+) that occurs in severe intoxication. Vomiting and diarrhea are due more to excitation of medullary chemoreceptors of the brain than to gastric or colonic irritation.

Digitalis and other cardiac glycosides work by altering the ionic content of muscle cells in the heart. Laboratory experiments on the mechanism of action have used *ouabain* to study how sodium (Na^+) and calcium (Ca^{++}) work by suppressing the ion pump Na-K-ATPase, which is embedded in the plasma membrane of the cardiac myocyte. Binding prevents the extrusion of Na^+ and intake of K^+ by the pump. There is a gradual increase in intracellular Na^+ and small decrease in K^+. Because myofibers can exchange Na^+ for Ca^{++}, the net result is an increased level of intracellular Ca^{++}, which then facilitates the contraction of myofilaments.

Cardiac glycosides

The glycosides *digitalis, digitoxin, ouabain,* and *squill* have in common a powerful action on myocardium: they increase the contractility of cardiac muscle (in a dose-dependent manner) by binding to and inhibiting the sodium pump in the membranes of myocytes. These drugs are also potent toxins and lead to severe electrolyte disturbances and injury of the myocardium when given in excessive doses.

Oleander (*Nerium oleander*), a common shrub, contains a highly toxic cardiac glycoside. Dogs and humans have been killed merely by putting a stem of oleander in the mouth. Cardiovascular collapse occurs immediately. Oleander toxins produce myocardial degeneration and other widespread changes in the heart muscle.

Cyanogenic glycosides

Members of the family Rosaceae commonly contain glycosides that yield free cyanide on hydrolysis. The high content of hydrocyanic acid (HCN) in wilted and frozen leaves is due to the hydrolytic effects of plant enzymes activated in the dying leaf. Toxicity of HCN occurs after ingestion and absorption. Once they are in the bloodstream, there is little difference between toxic and lethal levels of cyanide. HCN has a high affinity for iron and reacts with the trivalent iron of mitochondrial cytochrome oxidase, the terminal respiratory catalyst linking oxygen with metabolic respiration. Cell anoxia is immediate. The progression of staggering, prostration, coma, and death may all occur within 15 minutes. Since utilization of oxygen is blocked, venous blood is oxygenated and almost as bright red as arterial blood.

Goitrogenic glycosides

Plant thiocyanates and thiooxazolide mimic the effects of thiouracil and thiourea in preventing the accumulation of inorganic iodide in thyroid follicular epithelium. These glycosides occur in several species of *Brassica,* including cabbage, kale, and rape. Poisoning is associated with signs of hypothyroidism, and affected thyroids are hyperplastic. This toxicity is common in sheep. Pregnant ewes may be asymptomatic, yet their newborn lambs will be unthrifty and have large hyperplastic thyroid glands.

Other glycosides

Hepatoxicity of swine is associated with ingestion of *cocklebur* sprouts (*Xanthium* spp.).

Signs of ataxia, convulsions, and death are due to brain edema and neuronal degeneration. Hepatoxicity is prominent, and there is centrolobular necrosis, hepatic edema, and serofibrinous ascites. The glycoside carboxyatractyloside uncouples mitochondrial oxidative phosphorylation, producing hepatocyte degeneration and an associated hypoglycemia.

Saponins are large molecules that form colloidal solutions that produce froth when shaken with water. These common plant glycosides are rarely toxins. Most saponin-bearing plants are unpalatable, ingested only when grazing is restricted. They produce gastroenteritis and are absorbed through the injured intestine. A saponin in broomweed (*Gutierrezia microcephala*) produces toxic liver and kidneys in ruminants in the high plains areas of Texas and is a significant cause of abortion. Anemia and hematuria are often consequences of saponin toxicity.

Several plants produce *calcinogenic vitamin D analogues* that cause hypercalcemia, parathyroid hyperplasia, hyperostosis, and soft-tissue mineralization. Chronic poisoning leads to progressive debilitation and is peculiar to certain geographic areas (e.g., Manchester wasting disease in Jamaica, enteque seco in South America, and Naalehu disease in Hawaii). The hyperostosis caused by *Solanum malacoxylon* has been characterized by Dr. Jurgen Dobereiner, in Brazil. Dr. Bob Norrdin, at Colorado State, showed that toxicity was due to a water-soluble glycoside of 1,25-dihydroxycholecalciferol that stimulates bone formation on trabecular surfaces.

Thiaminases

Bracken fern produces a thiaminase that depletes thiamine reserves in monogastric animals. In grazing horses it causes a neurologic syndrome with encephalomalacia. Thiamine is a component of thiamine pyrophosphate, the prosthetic group of three important enzymes in the nervous system. Cattle, protected from this toxin because of production of large amounts of thiamine in the rumen, succumb to a second toxin in bracken fern that causes bone marrow destruction, thrombocytopenia, and widespread hemorrhages. In ruminants, thiamine-deficiency encephalomalacia occurs in poisoning by the anticoccidiostat drug *amprolium* and, under rare conditions, by overgrowth of thiaminase-producing rumen bacilli.

Fluorescent pigments and photosensitivity disease

Several plants synthesize fluorescent pigments, which are ingested by grazing animals and, when absorbed from the intestine, enter the bloodstream (Table 27.5). Although nontoxic, they localize in skin, where in hairless, nonpigmented areas, they are exposed to sunlight. Action of ultraviolet (UV) light produces fluorescence, the transformation of UV waves to longer wavelength. Energy released in the process damages capillaries and venules to cause endothelial degeneration, hyperemia, and edema. Ears, nose, and teats are particularly vulnerable and may develop raw ulcers and gangrenous necrosis.

The antinematode drug *phenothiazine* is directly toxic, primarily causing hemolytic anemia with hemoglobinuria and icterus. It also produces photosensitivity keratitis by fluorescence injury. During catabolism in the liver, the intermediate phenothiazine sulfoxide escapes into the circulation to enter the aqueous humor of the eye. It is also excreted in tears and, when exposed to sunlight, fluoresces to cause corneal edema and ulceration.

Table 27.5. Photosensitivity disease types

	EXOGENOUS[a]
Fagopyrism	Pigments from buckwheat, *Fagopyrum esculentum*
Hypericism	Pigments from St.-John's-wort, *Hypericum perforatum*
Phenothiazine	Sulfoxides in tears and aqueous humor (keratitis)
	HEPATOTOXIC[b]
Plant toxins	Mexican fireweed, *Kochia scoparia* Lechugilla Ngaio tree leaves Kleingrass
Mycotoxins	*Pithomyces chartarum* (mycotoxin production)
	CONGENITAL[c]
Congenital erythropoietic porphyria	Uroporphyrinogen cosynthetase defect (cow, cat, pig, squirrel)
Congenital protoporphyria	Ferrochetalase defect (cow)
Syndromes of defective bile excretion	Southdown sheep Corriedale sheep (Dubin-Johnson syndrome of man)

[a]Fluorescent pigments ingested, absorbed, enter bloodstream.
[b]Liver necrosis or bile ductule obstruction that blocks biliary secretion of phylloerythrin, a catabolite of chlorophyll.
[c]A defect in porphyrin metabolism.

Photosensitivity dermatitis is also produced when *phylloerythrin,* the fluorescent catabolite of chlorophyl, accumulates in tissue after liver damage. The sequence of grazing on lush pasture, ingestion of phyto- or mycotoxins, and exposure to sunlight is the most common. The liver lesion responsible for biliary stasis and failure to excrete phylloerythrin is usually pericholangitis with fibrosis; in rare instances, photosensitivity dermatitis can result from viral or congenital liver disease.

DRUG TOXICITY

Antibiotics

Antibiotics produce disease in two ways: by direct toxic injury and by disruption of normal bacterial flora of the gut (Table 27.6). Given to animals in excess dosages, they are always toxic. Most are nephrotoxic although many produce a wide variety of tissue damage. Anthracycline antibiotics are widely used as antineoplastic drugs. They intercalate into DNA and kill tumor cells by suppressing transcription of genes and subsequent protein synthesis. Adriamycin, the prototype drug, produces lysis of cardiac muscle, and poisoned patients die in heart failure.

Neomycin and lincomycin damage the intestine.

Neomycin toxicity is associated with malabsorption diarrhea. Lesions in the intestine are fragmentation of microvilli on enterocytes. *Lincomycin* given orally is toxic to horses, rabbits, and most rodents and causes severe diarrhea, dehydration, and even death. Lesions of hemorrhage and necrosis in the cecum and colon of horses are due to suppression of gram-positive aerobic bacteria and certain gram-negative anaerobes. Subsequent overgrowth of nonsensitive coliform bacteria and clostridia leads to damage to the gut wall.

Oxytetracycline is nephrotoxic in ruminant animals.

Oxytetracycline toxicity is common in cattle and sheep treated with multiple large doses. Typically, a herd is treated for a respiratory disease first by the owner and then by the veterinarian who is unaware of the previous treatment. Acute swelling and diffuse necrosis of the kidneys is obvious at necropsy (Fig. 27.3). The

Table 27.6.   Drugs that are toxic to animals

Tissue	Toxin	Animals Very Susceptible
Hepatotoxins	Acetominophen	Cat
	Halothane	Pig
	Furazolidone	Turkey
	Reserpine	Horse
Nephrotoxins	Oxytetracycline	Ruminant species
	Gentamicin	Birds, horses, dogs
	Sulfonamides	Ruminants
	Aminonucleoside	. . .
	Anthracycline antibiotics	. . .
Neurotoxins	Phenobarbital	. . .
	Isoniazid	. . .
	Succinyl choline	. . .
	Theobromine (in chocolate)	Dog
Intestinal toxins	Phenylbutazone	Horse
	Indomethacine	Dog
	Aspirin	Cat, dog
	Ibuprofen	Dog
	Cyclophosphamide	Small animals
	Lincomysin	
Myotoxins	Monensin (heart)	Horse
	Chloroquine	Primates
	Anthracycline antibiotics[a]	. . .
Hematopoietic toxin	Cyclosporine	. . .

[a]Adriamycin, daunomycin.

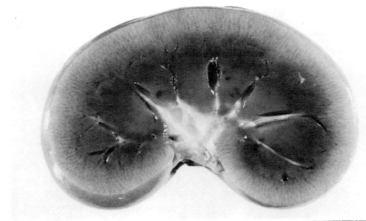

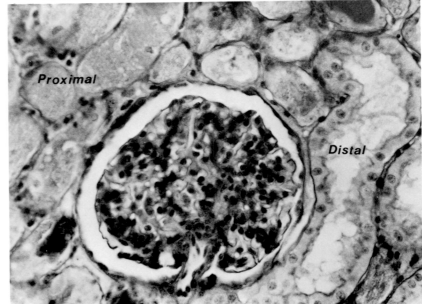

Fig. 27.3. Oxytetracycline toxicity, goat. Kidney is pale, swollen, and mottled (*above*). Proximal convoluted tubules are necrotic; distal tubules and glomerulus are less affected (*below*).

Proximal

Distal

proximal convoluted tubules are most severely affected; the distal convoluted tubules are usually spared.

Gentamicin

Gentamicin is nephrotoxic in mammals. It is also used to treat bacterial infections in newly hatched chicks and in wild birds; in these species it is nephrotoxic, but it also produces damage to the ear and neuromuscular junctions. Gentamicine has a narrow range between therapeutic and toxic levels.

Dr. William Spangler, working at the University of California in Davis, sequentially biopsied the kidneys of dogs poisoned with gentamicin. Proximal convoluted tubule cells became swollen, lost surface microvilli, and developed cytoplasmic granules. The granules proved to be large lysosomes filled with cellular debris, an attempt at repair of the cell. By 12 days the epithelium was denuded, renal function was depressed, and dogs developed uremia.

Sulfonamides

Sulfonamides are used against bacterial infections. At high doses they cause acute nephrotoxicity (sulfonamides also cause a more delayed type of injury by immunologic mechanisms; see

immunologic disease, Chapter 23). Acute injury is most common in calves, especially febrile animals that are dehydrated. At necropsy, kidneys are enlarged, congested, and pale; linear deposits of sulfonamide crystals are usually present in the medulla, and crystals may also be in the pelvis and urinary bladder. Histologically, the proximal convoluted tubules undergo acute cell swelling and necrosis. Other parts of the nephron are less affected. A mild but diffuse edema and fibrosis develop in the interstitial areas in the medulla and are most prominent at the corticomedullary junction.

Sulfonamide crystals are apt to be washed away in tissue processing. They must be differentiated from oxalate crystals in ethylene glycol (antifreeze) toxicity and in sheep poisoned by oxalate-containing plants (see Fig. 27.4).

Anti-inflammatory drugs
Acetaminophen

Acetaminophen is a widely used analgesic. Safe at therapeutic levels it causes fatal hepatic necrosis in large doses, especially in cats and man. Consistent dose-dependent liver lesions can be reproduced experimentally. Within the hepatocyte, acetaminophen is catabolized to

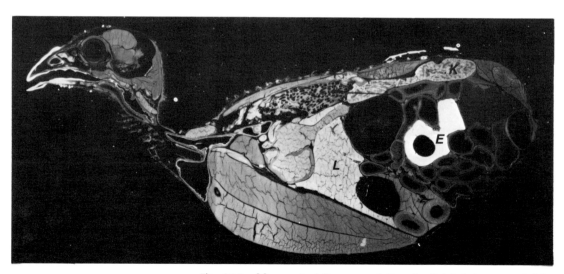

Fig. 27.4. Mercury toxicity: accumulation of radiolabeled mercury (*white areas*) 4 days after experimental inoculation, whole section of quail. There are heavy concentrations in beak, egg albumin (*E*), liver (*L*), and kidney (*K*). (Photograph: Jorgen Bäckstrom, *Acta Pharmacol. Toxicol.* 27 [Suppl. 3]:1, 1969, used by permission)

highly reactive intermediates within the smooth endoplasmic reticulum. Acute toxicity is due to biotransformation within this organelle and to depletion of *glutathione.*

Chronic acetaminophen toxicity and that of phenacetin (which is converted to acetaminophen in the liver) leads to hemolytic anemia, methemoglobinuria, and icterus. In cats, signs also include facial edema and cyanosis. Erythrocyte destruction in chronic toxicity is also related to glutathione depletion, since reduced glutathione maintains hemoglobin cysteine residues in the reduced state and keeps hemoglobin in the ferrous state.

Ionophores

Ionophores are drugs that act as ion channels in cell membranes. They become inserted into the cell surface and carry ions across the plasma membrane. Most of these diverse compounds have a common central ring of liganding oxygen atoms that forms a critical cavity to fit a particular ion.

Monensin

Monensin is the prototype sodium ionophore. It is used both as a coccidiostat (it inserts into coccidial surface membranes causing ionic imbalances that cause the coccidia to swell and burst) and to enhance rumen production of protein in ruminant food-producing animals. Monensin is particularly toxic for the horse but also poisons most other species. It causes necrosis of both skeletal and cardiac muscle, and poisoned animals die in acute heart failure. Dr. John Van Vleet, at Purdue, has worked extensively with this drug and suggests that in swine it selectively affects type I fibers.

Trace elements

Selenium

Selenium is the most toxic of all trace elements. Toxicity occurs in one of two ways: (1) when animals are fed grain grown on soils of high selenium content or (2) from errors in ration formulation. In addition, selenium drained from soils with heavy deposits into swamps may cause disease in fish and migrating waterfowl.

Grazing of ruminants on heavy selenium soils has caused a chronic debilitating disease called "blind staggers" or "alkali disease." *Chronic disease* in cattle includes emaciation and congestion, edema, and hemorrhages in viscera; cows commonly die of heart failure due to myocardial necrosis.

Plants that require and selectively accumulate selenium from soils include *Astragalus* (poison vetch), *Aster xylorrhiza* (woody aster), and *Oonopsis* sp. (golden weed). Clinical disease may be acute, subacute, or chronic. Species variation is common. Elemental selenium is relatively nontoxic, but the three oxidation states, selenate ($+6$), selenite ($+4$), and selenide (-2), produce disease.

Porcine selenium toxicity involves nervous tissue damage.

In the early 1980s Drs. Terry Wilson, at Pennsylvania State University, and L. H. Harrison, at the University of Georgia, reported focal, bilateral, symmetrical, poliomalacia in pigs with high tissue selenium. Gross lesions of cavitation were present in the ventral horns of all segments of the spinal cord. Microscopically, the foci of necrosis were replaced by endothelium and glial cells, and the malacic area was infiltrated with eosinophils. Necrosis also occurred in the coronary bands of the feet, and this caused sloughing of the hooves.

ENVIRONMENTAL POLLUTANTS
Metals

Metals interact biologically as soluble salts that dissociate in an aqueous environment to facilitate their transport into tissue. Gastrointestinal absorption is most common, and absorption is greater when ingestion occurs during a period of fasting. Intestinal absorption is affected by diet. For example, high levels of phosphate reduce uptake of lead because highly insoluble lead phosphate is formed. Pulmonary absorption is poor with insoluble compounds because they are cleared rapidly in the upper airways.

Metals existing as alkyl compounds in which metallic ions are firmly bonded to carbon pass readily across lipid membrane and unaltered into the circulation. Thus organometallic compounds such as methyl mercury and tetraethyl lead are highly toxic. The clinical significant lesions of heavy metal toxicity often occur in the brain (Fig. 27.4).

FOCUS

Mercury toxicity

The disappearance of seed-eating birds and their avian predators was observed by ornithologists in the 1950s. Large amounts of mercury were discovered in dead and intoxicated birds, and mercurials such as methyl mercury that are used for commercial seed disinfection were implicated. Studies of birds from museum collections showed increasing mercury in feathers from about 1890 onward. Methyl mercury is readily absorbed by and stable within the bird. It accumulates in most organs, with preference for kidney, liver, and oviduct. There is an intense concentration in egg albumin (females excrete mercury faster than males). Embryonal development is affected, and there is poor hatchability of the egg.

There are three toxic forms of mercury: *elemental mercury* (Hg) is an inhaled metal distributed to the alveolus and causes chronic toxicity; *inorganic mercury* (Hg^{++}, as in $HgCl_2$) can be highly soluble and thus highly toxic when ingested; and *organic mercury* (methyl, ethyl mercury, and the alkyl mercury diuretics) forms slats with acids and reacts with cell ligands such as sulfhydryl groups to complex with and pass through membranes. Organic mercury in the environment makes this form the most important animal metallic toxin.

The aquatic environment is contaminated by industrial and agricultural uses of mercurials. Freshwater fish become contaminated, and if large amounts of mercury are present, will develop gill disease and die. Dr. P. Daoust, working at the University of Saskatchewan, exposed rainbow trout to lethal amounts of inorganic mercury and demonstrated necrosis of epithelium and fusion of lamellae of affected gills. Fish gills function not only in respiration but in osmoregulation, acid-base balance, and excretion of nitrogenous wastes, which are functions of the kidney in higher animals. Mercury in fish enters the food chain and is responsible for toxicity in birds and man. In Minimata, Japan, a large number of people suffered severe acute neurologic disease from eating fish contaminated with effluents from a paper mill.

In large animals mercury poisoning is associated with ingestion of feeds contaminated with organic mercurial fungicides. In rare cases, inorganic mercurials poison when licked from blister ointments. Acute toxicity is associated with gastroenteritis and ulceration of alimentary mucosa and chronic toxicity with progressive renal disease, colitis, and stomatitis. Horses are more resistant than cattle or sheep and require 8–10 g for clinical signs to appear.

In the early 1970s Drs. Leander Tryphonas and N. O. Nielsen, then working at the University of Saskatchewan, documented the pathologic lesions in swine chronically poisoned by alkyl mercury. Neuronal necrosis was followed by secondary gliosis and capillary endothelial proliferation. Pigs that recovered had cerebral atrophy and dilated cerebral ventricals due to loss of brain mass. The pathogenesis of mercury neurotoxicity in mammals involves altered blood-brain-barriers, suppression of synaptic transmission, and degeneration of neurons.

Lead

Lead toxicity occurs after animals ingest flaking lead-based paints or contaminated grasses near lead smelters. Disease involves nervous, gastrointestinal, and hematologic signs. Weakness, periodic convulsions, and anemia appear early and progress to paralysis and death.

In cattle, lead poisoning is an acute disease, but in most other species it is subacute or chronic. Calves are especially affected and progress from muscle tremor, staggering, and falling to convulsions and opisthotonus and may die within 24 hours. Brain swelling contributes to clinical signs but is difficult to define histologically. Absorbed lead is immediately deposited in the liver and kidneys, and, in chronic toxicity, in bones. In the kidney and liver, lead-protein complexes form in nuclei of hepatocytes and renal tubular cells. Because these nuclear inclusions stain with the acid-fast stain, they are diagnostic for lead toxicity. Lead is slowly excreted in bile, urine, and milk.

Lead produces its most marked effects in the *brain.* In the nervous system lesions are primarily vascular. There is *necrosis of endothelial cells* in capillaries and arterioles, and damaged blood vessels are surrounded by *edema* and *hemorrhage.* The neuropil in affected areas is vacuolated (*status spongiosis*), and there is demyelination and necrosis. Necrotic brain tissue develops in layers, a pattern called *laminar necrosis.* In the early 1970s Drs. Ralph Christian and Leander Tryphonas studied brain lesions in both natural and experimental lead toxicity and showed that foci of vacuolation and demyelination were common in the cerebral cortex and in chronic toxicity the cerebral gyri were blunted and atrophic. Dr. Bernie Zook found similar lesions in 32 dogs poisoned with lead.

Anemia in lead toxicity is due both to suppression of hemoglobin production and to reduction of erythrocyte life span. In stem cells, mitochondria are affected in two ways: defects in uroporphyrinogen synthesis and suppression of oxidative phosphorylation and citric acid cycles. Other lesions in lead toxicity include hyperplasia of bone marrow, spotty necrosis of skeletal muscle, peripheral neuropathy, and persistence of thick cartilage in trabeculae of the long bones.

Arsenic

Phenylarsonic acid derivatives used for control of porcine enteric diseases are toxic. Arsanilic acid (*p*-aminophenylarsonic acid) and 3-ni-

tro (3-nitro-4-hydroxyphenylarsonic acid) are the most common toxic compounds. In 1973, Dr. Arlo Ledet reported the lesions of arsinilic acid. Dr. Seamus Kennedy, at the Veterinary Research Labs in Stormont, Northern Ireland, reported neuropathology of experimental 3-nitro toxicity. Clinically, pigs showed paresis and clonic convulsive episodes that were caused by demyelination and axonal degeneration in white matter of the spinal cord. There was preferential involvement of the cuneate and gracile fasciculi and peripheral regions of the ventral and lateral funiculi.

Fluoride

Ingestion of fluoride-contaminated feed has caused fluoride toxicosis in dairy cattle. Brown mottling of enamel of teeth is accompanied by swollen odontoblastic layers and abnormal dentine. In long bones, disruption of growth plates, decrease in trabeculae in primary spongiosa, and paucity of osteoclasts lining the remaining trabeculae are typical. Fluoride replaces hydroxyl ions in calcium hydroxyapatite, leading to fluoroapatite formation. Fetuses are affected since deciduous teeth are all formed in utero in cattle.

Aromatic halogenated hydrocarbons

Hexachlorophene was used as an antibacterial agent in soaps and deodorants in the 1970s and, since it persists in the environment, was detected in surface waters as high as 48 ppb. Hexachlorophene concentrates in myelin, and it causes encephalopathy and neuropathy in both man and animals.

Dioxin

Dioxin refers to the basic structure of a family of chemicals: a pair of oxygen atoms joins two benzene rings, and substitution of chlorine for hydrogen on the rings produces the chlorinated dioxins; for example, 2,3,7,8-tetrachlorodibenzo-*p*-dioxin (TCDD) is a toxic byproduct in the synthesis of 2,4,5-T.

An accident in West Virginia in 1949 exposed over 200 workers to TCDD. Of 122 who developed dermatitis, 121 were followed medically for 30 years. Total deaths in the groups did not differ significantly from that expected in the population at large, and there were no excess deaths due to cancer. Although some studies have claimed correlations between human abortions and sarcomas and TCDD exposure, most responsible investigators agree that there is no known connection. In 1976 an industrial accident in Italy released a chemical cloud of dioxins and other compounds over a wide area; despite evacuation, there was considerable acute disease in plants, animals, and man.

Highly toxic to animals, TCDD accumulates in soil from many sources and its long-term effects are not clearly understood. In man, acute effects include dermatitis, myalgia, and psychiatric disturbances. No case of human death has been associated with TCDD, and there is no unequivocal evidence of chronic sequelae.

Laboratory rodents vary in sensitivity to dioxins (Table 27.7). The oral LD_{50} for the guinea pig is 0.6 mg/kg body weight while that for the hamster is 2000 times greater. At very high doses over long times, dioxins are carcinogenic in rats and mice. However, a study by Dr. Robert Kociba, at Dow Chemical Co., showed that rats tolerated a daily dose of 1 mg/kg/day for 2 years without showing toxic effects.

Table 27.7.   Toxicity of dioxin (TCDD) to various species

Species	LD_{50} (μg/kg body weight)
Guinea pig	0.6 (male), 2.1 (female)
Rabbit	11.5
Monkey (female)	>70
Rat	22 (male), 45–500 (female)
Mouse	>150
Dog	30–300 (male)
Frog	1000
Hamster	1157

Pentachlorophenol (PCP), a widely used pesticide and defoliant, can be routinely detected in human and animal tissues as a result of contaminated foods. In the 1950s it was associated with the death of millions of chickens in the southeastern United States. Toxicity was traced to components in animal fat used in feed. The fat had been derived from hides preserved with PCP; the toxicity was not due to PCP, however, but to dioxin isomers in the technical grade of PCP used on the hides. Reproduction of dioxin-contaminated PCP disease in cattle induced progressive anemia, thymic atrophy, and villous hyperplasia of urinary bladder epithelium.

Acid water

Depression of pH in lakes causes widespread loss of animal life. Studies in Norway show that even Crustacea are vulnerable to acidification (although Diptera are not).

Acid precipitation effects have been simulated by addition of sulfuric acid to small lakes in Canada during an 8-year period. The natural balance of animal life was gradually destroyed. The first irreversible disturbances to simple organisms occur before marked changes in pH are apparent; phytoplankton remain relatively constant, but new species appear and numbers of organisms small enough to be eaten by zooplankton decline, adversely affecting zooplankton and their predators. Algae overgrow spawning grounds of lake trout, the normal prey of fish (such as shrimp) die, and trout lose weight and die. Lower verbrates die from hydrogen ion toxicity and from the secondary effects of parasitism by opportunistic microorganisms.

Inhalation toxicity

Lungs receive constant insults of dust, microorganisms, and toxic gases. The oxygen-exchanging membranes of the alveolar wall are protected from much of this by the mucociliary system of the bronchioles. The ciliated columnar epithelium of the respiratory tract is designed to purify air from the polluted environments for presentation to the respiratory lobule. Warmed and humidified by passage through the upper respiratory tract, the air is cleansed in the bronchioles by the continuous secretion of mucus, which traps and inactivates foreign substances.

Terminal bronchioles are especially equipped to deal with inhaled toxins. Their Clara cells are loaded with enzymes that catabolize inhaled pollutants. These are cytochrome P-450-dependent monooxygenases, bound to smooth endoplasmic reticulum, which catabolize toxic drugs, pesticides, and carcinogens.

Ozone

The current U.S. National Ambient Air Quality Standard for ozone is 0.12 ppm, a level commonly exceeded in metropolitan areas during summer. Alveoli in the proximal acinus are the primary sites of ozone injury. Drs. Boorman, Schwartz, and Dungworth reported slight increases in air-blood barrier thickness in rats after 90 days of exposure to 0.2 ppm.

Sulfur dioxide

SO_2 is a significant air pollutant in industrial areas that causes loss of cilia on short-term experimental exposure at 100 ppm (the concentration in severe London smog is 1.35 ppm). Cilia are also susceptible to low levels of ozone and nitrogen dioxide. Studies by Drs. Stephens, Schwartz, and Eustis have shown that exposure to these gases causes bronchiolar cilia to become blunted and broken.

Hydrogen sulfide (H_2S)

H_2S gas is produced in large amounts in farm slurries and pit silos. Farm workers in these areas may be unknowingly overcome by heavy concentrations of gas in enclosed spaces. Typically, one worker succumbs, another descends to help and is also affected, and so on. H_2S, like HCN, inhibits mitochondrial cytochrome oxidase, and death occurs suddenly without overt lesions of disease.

PESTICIDES AND HERBICIDES
Organophosphorous insecticides

TEPP (tetraethyl pyrophosphate), tabun, and sarin were secretly developed in Germany during World War II as possible nerve gas warfare agents. Although useful as insecticides, they were highly toxic to mammals and hydrolyzed in presence of moisture. Further research led to the synthesis of parathion in 1944. Extensively used in agriculture, parathion has been the pesticide most frequently involved in human fatalities in the past 30 years. It is now being replaced by other, less toxic organophosphorous compounds (Table 27.8).

Parathion is an *acetylcholinesterase inhibitor.* It prevents inactivation of acetylcholine at neural synapses, leading to excessive stimulation of

Table 27.8. Common agricultural poisons

Group	Compound	Mechanism of Action
		INSECTICIDES
Organophosphates	Parathion Malathion Dichlorvos Diazinon	Inhibits acetylcholinesterase; signs resemble stimulation of cholinergic nerves
Organochlorines	DDT, methoxychlor, aldrin, dieldrin, chlordane, endrin, heptachlor, toxaphene	Alters transport of Na^+ and K^+ across plasma membrane of nerve axons (prevents K^+ efflux); signs are tremor, convulsions, and paresthesia; multiple effects on lower vertebrates
	Lindane Mirex, kepone	Causes blood dyscrasia (chronic) and neural disease (acute)
Botanical insecticides	Pyrethrum Nicotine Rotenone	
		HERBICIDES
Chlorophenoxy compounds	2,4-D; 2,4,5-T	Mycotoxicity
Dinitrophenols	Dinitrophenol Dinitroorthocresol	Suppresses mitochondrial oxidative phosphorylation
Bipyridyl compounds	Paraquat	Causes lung injury during exhalation (subacute) and myocardiopathy (acute)
		RODENTICIDES
Warfarin		Inhibits coagulation
Red squill		Cardiotonic glycoside
Sodium fluoroacetate		Inhibits citric acid cycle
ANTU		Combines with -SH groups, alters carbohydrate metabolism; causes pulmonary edema and hemorrhage
Strychnine		Lowers threshold of spinal reflexes by blocking inhibitory pathways; causes tetanic convulsions
Reserpine		Depletes catecholamines

cholinergic nerves. The immediate cause of death from this and other organophosphorous insecticides is asphyxia resulting from respiratory failure. Effects contributing to disease and death arise from three major nerve sites: (1) motor nerves to skeletal muscle (*nicotinic* signs resulting from accumulation of acetylcholine at myoneural junctions are muscle weakness, twitching, and fasciculation), (2) postganglionic parasympathetic nerve fibers (*muscarinic* signs, which occur in cardiac and smooth muscle and exocrine glands, include bronchoconstriction, increased bronchial secretion and salivation, sweating, urination, diarrhea and defecation, and constriction of pupils), and (3) certain central nervous system synapses (accumulation of acetylcholine in brain is associated with restlessness, drowsiness, and other behavioral abnormalities).

In muscle, the cytopathic effects of parathion arise from a combination of pre- and postsynaptic events, such as excessive release of acetylcholine plus repeated binding of unhydrolized acetylcholine to receptors, both leading to excessive depolarization of endplate receptors.

Organophosphorous insecticides commonly produce rapid poisoning and in large doses may be rapidly fatal. However, they are quickly metabolized and excreted so that chronic poisoning is not a major problem. Cessation of exposure results in complete recovery.

Organochlorine insecticides

These neuropoisons show a wide range of acute toxicities. Unlike the organophosphorous compounds, their mechanisms of action are not clearly defined; they are less acutely toxic and have a greater tendency to chronic toxicity. Organochlorine insecticides are now in disfavor because they persist in the environment and accumulate in animal tissue.

Intense use of dichlorodiphenyltrichloroethane (DDT) from the 1940s to 1960s led to chronic exposure of animals and man, with accumulation of DDT residues in adipose tissue. The significance of these residues is unknown. Despite its widespread use in human antilouse dusting in World War II, there is no record of fatal human toxicity. In contrast, the devastating effects of DDT on wild animals and birds has caused ecologic imbalances and governmental restrictions on DDT use.

In mammals, DDT has primary toxic action on the motor cortex of the brain and on peripheral nerve fibers (both motor and sensory). Manifestations of toxicity (hyperexcitability, tremor, and convulsions) result from prolonged and repetitive action potentials in individual nerves.

Fish are very sensitive to organochlorine pollutants, which inhibit osmoregulation in gill epithelium. Muscle may also be affected by interruption of muscular excitation related to deficient Ca^{++} uptake by sarcoplasmic reticulum; that is, the insecticide inactivates the Ca^{++}-dependent pump, causing loss of Ca^{++} from muscle.

Wild marine birds are commonly affected by organochlorine insecticides. Since DDT accumulates in adipose tissues, these carnivorous birds are at the end of the biologic accumulation line. Eggshell thinning results, and increased egg breakage contributes to bird population decline.

Herbicides
Chlorophenoxy compounds

Dichlorophenol (2,4-D) and trichlorophenol (2,4,5-T), used for control of broadleaf weeds, exert their action by suppressing plant growth hormones; 2,4,5-T is an important herbicide and an ingredient of Agent Orange, used as a military defoliant in the Vietnam war. The action of chlorophenoxy compounds on animals is poorly understood. In large doses they cause cardiac ventricular fibrillation and in small doses, muscle damage. Lesions at necropsy are those of general toxicity: gastric hyperemia and degenerative changes in hepatocytes and renal tubular epithelium. Chronic exposure in man has been associated with dermatitis, which probably results from effects of the contaminant dioxin. Dioxin is also a major factor in production of the teratogenic effects of these herbicides: in 1970 birth defects in animals were ascribed to 2,4,5-T, but the teratogenic compound was probably a dioxin.

Bipyridal compounds

Of the bipyridal compounds used as herbicides, paraquat most commonly causes toxicity, usually by accidental ingestion or, a recent development, by humans smoking marijuana that has been sprayed with paraquat to control illicit production. Acute poisoning in mammals by a single large dose leads to myocardiopathy, and

FOCUS

The hidden signs of DDT toxicity

A Swiss research chemist, Paul Muller, testing chemicals for insecticidal properties in 1939, discovered the extraordinary effectiveness of dichlorodiphenyltrichloroethane. It was highly toxic to insects, insoluble in water, and of low toxicity to mammals. By 1941, the Swiss were using the compound successfully to combat the Colorado potato beetle and it was widely used in World War II to control mosquitos and body lice. By 1948, when Muller received the Nobel prize for his discovery, "DDT" was used throughout the world.

Dangers had already been recorded in 1945 by biologists of the U.S. Fish and Wildlife Service who warned against use of DDT in marshes. By the 1960s clues began to appear around the world that DDT was accumulating in soils and tissues of wild animals. Furthermore, the "food chain effect" was proposed: plants accumulate toxin, herbivores get them from plants, carnivores from their food, and finally, man—if the rate of absorption is higher than the rate of loss. In one well-studied estuarine marsh, accumulation of DDT via the food chain was documented carefully. Marsh water had DDT residues of less than 0.001 ppm; plankton contained residues of 0.01–0.1 ppm; clams, up to 1.0 ppm; fish, a few ppm; and birds, especially carnivorous birds, contained 10–100 ppm. The long struggle to legislate against use of DDT began some time later when conspicuous effects were noted; peregrine falcons and osprey began to disappear from their North American ranges along the Atlantic Seaboard. DDT caused production of soft-shelled eggs, which were easily broken in the nest. Reproduction failed and bird populations declined.

transient neurologic signs. Subacute injury is more commonly fatal; the target organ is the lung, regardless of route of entry. Necrosis of pneumocytes and progressive fibrosis of the alveolar septa occur during exhalation of paraquat in the process of elimination of the toxin by the lung.

Carbamate herbicides

These compounds, which have low toxicity for animals, include a large number of aromatic and aliphatic esters. Experimental feeding of barban and propham to rats leads to some weight loss but little other evidence of toxicity. Substituted ureas such as diuron and monuron are likewise relatively nontoxic. The *triazines* simazine and atrazine, shown experimentally to be slightly toxic for cattle and sheep, will kill in large doses. Amitrol is similar to the trazines but is a potent antithyroid drug; it can produce significant depression of thyroid function and is prohibited for use near animals. Many herbicides that are nontoxic for adult animals can produce subtle teratogenic effects.

Rodenticides
Strychnine

Strychnine is in many rodenticides and several products for animal and human consumption including laxatives, sedatives, and tonics. Strychnine excites all of the central nervous system and clinically resembles tetanus. The important effects result from its anti-inhibition of spinal cord interneurons. Strychnine competitively antagonizes the inhibitory neurotransmitter *glycine* at the postsynaptic receptor sites of ventral horn motoneurons. In animals that survive even for a few hours there are profound lactic acidosis, hyperthermia, and rhabodomylosis.

ADDITIONAL READING

Collins, L. G., and Tyler, D. E. Experimentally induced phenylbutazone toxicosis in ponies. *Am. J. Vet. Res.* 46:1605, 1985.

Harrison, L. H., et al. Paralysis in swine due to focal symmetrical poliomalacia: Possible selenium toxicosis. *Vet. Pathol.* 20:265, 1983.

James, L. F., et al. Locoweed (*Oxytropis sericea*) poisoning and congestive heart failure. *J. Am. Vet. Med. Assoc.* 189:1549, 1986.

Middlebrook, J. L., and Dorland, R. B. Bacterial toxins. *Microbiol. Rev.* 48:199, 1984.

O'Brien, T. D., et al. Hepatic necrosis following halothane anesthesia in goats. *J. Am. Vet. Med. Assoc.* 189:1591, 1986.

Payne, B. T., ed. The toxicity of three gold-containing compounds in laboratory animals. *Vet. Pathol.* 15 (Suppl. 5):1, 1978.

Schwartz, W. L., et al. Toxicity of *Nerium oleander* in the monkey (*Cebus appella*). *Vet. Pathol.* 11:259, 1974.

Spangler, W. L., et al. Gentamicin nephrotoxicity in the dog. *Vet. Pathol.* 17:206, 1980.

Szczech, G. M., et al. Ochrotoxicosis in beagle dogs. *Vet. Pathol.* 11:385, 1974.

Tschirley, F. H. Dioxin. *Sci. Am.* 254 (2):29, 1986.

Wells, R. E., and Slocombe, R. F. Acute toxicosis of budgerigars (*Melopsittacus undulatus*) caused by pyrolysis products from heated polytetrafluoroethylene. *Am. J. Vet. Res.* 43:1243, 1982.

Wilson, T. M., and Drake, T. R. Porcine focal symmetrical poliomyelomalacia. *Can. J. Comp. Med.* 46:218, 1981.

Biologic Causes of Disease

VIRUSES

Introduction

Viruses produce disease by replicating inside cells to cause degeneration. The intact infectious particles, which are called *virions,* do not have ribosomes to synthesize protein and must use cellular organelles to reproduce. As they replicate, organelles in the host cell disappear and are replaced by viral proteins and other structures that are used to form new virions.

Viruses must bind to cell surfaces to infect.

To be pathogenic, viruses must be capable of specifically attaching to the surfaces of target cells. Attachment must alter the cell membrane so that a specific signal for uptake of virions occurs. After entering the cell, viruses must contain enzymes (or genomic codes to produce enzymes) that alter cell metabolism in favor of viral replication. Viruses shut down host cell synthesis and subvert it toward replication of new virus-induced nucleic acids and proteins. This causes an *acute lytic infection* of cells that, if uncontrolled, leads directly to tissue destruction and systemic signs of illness.

Viruses kill cells by shutting off protein synthesis.

In the process of viral replication, normal cell metabolism is disrupted as protein synthesis is shut down. Viruses contain either DNA or RNA as their genetic material. These nucleic acid templates are liberated into the host cell cytoplasm and are used as codes to create new viral genetic material, viral enzymes, and structural proteins that will become part of the external coat of the virion. Although some of the viral peptides are directly toxic to the cell, *most cellular injury arises from failure of the infected cell to produce critical enzymes and energy for its own metabolism.*

As viral replication proceeds, production of the various proteins used to assemble new virions becomes unbalanced. Masses of virus-induced proteins and other excess components of virions accumulate as *inclusion bodies* that distort the cell (see Fig. 4.6). Energy sources are depleted, electrolyte pumps on the cell surface decline, and intracellular pH drops. The result may be a shrunken necrotic cell or a lysed cell that has liberated its cytoplasmic debris into tissue spaces.

Viruses are released by cell lysis or budding from cell surfaces.

Viruses vary considerably in size and complexity (Fig. 28.1) and thus in how they replicate within cells. Most virions are released from cells when the cell dies and disintegrates. In herpesviral infections, cells are quickly killed and virions are released into tissue. Some of the RNA viruses allow the cell to survive to shed new virions over a longer period. For example, influenza virus is shed into the lumen of the airways to be coughed up in respiratory exudates. In influenza-infected cells, the surface membrane is altered at sites where virions are to emerge. Immature viral particles migrate to the cell surface, are stitched into the plasma membrane by special viral proteins, and are drawn into the membrane and surrounded. After total envelopment, the virion is pinched off from the cell and released into the respiratory tract.

DNA VIRUSES

RNA VIRUSES

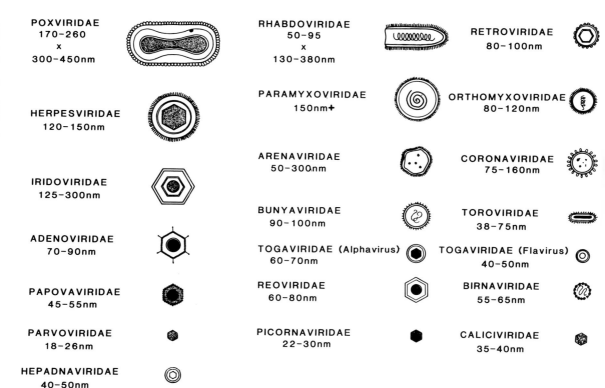

POXVIRIDAE
170-260
x
300-450nm

HERPESVIRIDAE
120-150nm

IRIDOVIRIDAE
125-300nm

ADENOVIRIDAE
70-90nm

PAPOVAVIRIDAE
45-55nm

PARVOVIRIDAE
18-26nm

HEPADNAVIRIDAE
40-50nm

RHABDOVIRIDAE
50-95
x
130-380nm

PARAMYXOVIRIDAE
150nm+

ARENAVIRIDAE
50-300nm

BUNYAVIRIDAE
90-100nm

TOGAVIRIDAE (Alphavirus)
60-70nm

REOVIRIDAE
60-80nm

PICORNAVIRIDAE
22-30nm

RETROVIRIDAE
80-100nm

ORTHOMYXOVIRIDAE
80-120nm

CORONAVIRIDAE
75-160nm

TOROVIRIDAE
38-75nm

TOGAVIRIDAE (Flavirus)
40-50nm

BIRNAVIRIDAE
55-65nm

CALICIVIRIDAE
35-40nm

Fig. 28.1. Diagram of virions in cross section.

Clinical signs of disease arise from death of infected cells.

Many signs of systemic disease are provoked when infected cells die. Clinical signs result from direct *tissue destruction* by viruses replicating inside cells, and from subsequent release of debris. Cell lysis releases different host and viral proteins into the lymphatic and blood-vascular systems. These include *biologically active peptides,* membrane fragments, and viral protein remnants that act on the vascular and nervous systems to produce inflammation. These substances act as pyrogens and chemoattractants for inflammatory cells and are responsible for many of the clinical signs of disease. For example, infection of monocytes by influenza virus causes this cell to release several peptides that act as cytokines to send signals to other tissue systems; for example, pyrogens act on the hypothalamus to produce fever, interleukins act on lymphocytes to induce immune reactions, and a

metabolism modulating factor induces gluconeogenesis in skeletal muscle (and the amino acid drain that explains some of the myalgia).

In addition to virus-induced cell injury, tissue may also be injured by severe inflammatory responses provoked by the virus. The disintegration of neutrophilic leukocytes and macrophages releases tissue destructive enzymes that enhance the primary viral injury.

Many viruses, especially those producing systemic disease, tend to replicate within leukocytes and endothelium; these cells release *cellular signal* molecules (e.g., cytokines, prostaglandins, and leukotrienes) that induce fever, anorexia, and myalgia (muscle pain).

Some viruses infect without producing disease.

Viral infection may occur without signs of disease. These infections are subclinical, or *asymptomatic.* Asymptomatic infection may occur because viral replication is very slow (without inducing cell degeneration) or because a virus does not replicate at all. Viral genetic material may hide at some location in the cell until later provoked to replicate and thus produce an acute lytic infection. Herpesviruses often act in this way. They remain latent until some stressful event occurs (often associated with adrenal corticosteroid release) that stimulates viral replication.

Tumor-producing viruses act in this way except that their association with the nucleus eventually leads to the uncontrolled cell replication of *neoplasia*. Neoplastic disease occurs long after infection and usually involves the integration of viral genetic material into the chromosomes of the host cell.

Diagnosis of viral infections at necropsy.

Analysis of the cellular changes and the character of the inflammatory response all lead to the proper diagnosis. The presence of *inclusion bodies* is a major factor in pinpointing the virus group involved. *Immunolabeling* of viral proteins present in tissue sections will establish a specific diagnosis. In the *fluorescent antibody* test, globulins are precipitated from serum of immunized animals, and the antibody molecules are conjugated with fluorescein isothiocyanate. Smears or frozen sections of tissue are fixed,

---

FOCUS

Viruses spread in characteristic pathways.

Viruses require living cells to replicate but persist in nonliving material. Some viruses are "cell-associated"; that is, they survive very short periods outside living cells. Retroviruses such as the feline leukemia virus and human immunosuppressive viruses pass from host to host chiefly within living cells in exudates. At the other extreme, some of the slow viruses live for years, even inside paraffin blocks after formalin fixation. The differences in how microbes pass within animal flocks or herds is determined by the hardiness of the virus and in what body fluid it is excreted.

Viruses that cause diarrhea usually spread by the *fecal-oral route;* for example, enteroviruses and rotaviruses that cause diarrhea in neonates replicate in the intestine, are shed in the feces, and infect new host animals when feces-contaminated food is ingested. Viruses that infect the respiratory tract are spread by oral secretions or the *oral/salivary-respiratory* route. Some herpesviruses are spread by genital secretions during mating, the *venereal* route.

Certain viruses are known to produce severe systemic disease because they produce viremia and are disseminated throughout the body. Some of the more important of these agents are canine distemper, infectious canine hepatitis, hog cholera, Newcastle disease of birds, myxomatosis of rabbits, rinderpest, and African swine fever. These viruses generally follow a course involving (1) *invasion* via skin, conjunctiva, intestine, or respiratory tract; (2) *spread* to regional lymph nodes where viral multiplication occurs; (3) *primary viremia* with entry of virus into bloodstream and lymph; (4) *tissue localization,* often in liver, spleen, and kidney; (5) *secondary viremia* with release of massive amounts of virus in spleen and often with secretion of virus in milk, urine, and semen; and (6) *peripheral tissue localization* in areas such as skin (rash), brain, and eyes.

stained with the conjugate, and examined under ultraviolet light, inducing fluorescein to fluoresce, thus indicating sites of viral proteins to which the antibody-fluorescein molecule is attached. With special care, this technique can be used on paraffin sections. *Immunoperoxidase techniques* have been developed by Drs. Ducatelle and Hoorens, at the State University of Ghent, Belgium, against several important viral pathogens of animals.

Poxviruses

Poxviruses are complex, DNA-containing viruses that have an affinity for epidermis (Table 28.1). Most produce local epidermal proliferative lesions that form vesicles and then pustules, which erode to leave a scab-covered ulcer. Within infected keratinocytes, large aggregates of virions develop that appear histologically as irregular, acidophilic, cytoplasmic inclusion bodies.

Poxviruses are transmitted mechanically to the skin and hematogenously within the animal. When scarified into skin, poxviruses enter the epidermis and dermal mesenchyme. After a latent period of 3–6 days, a small, focal, non-elevated area of erythema (the *macule*) appears. Proliferation of keratinocytes and subepidermal edema produces an elevation of the lesion above the level of normal skin (the *papule*). Infected epidermal keratinocytes progressively enlarge and develop hydropic degeneration and huge cytoplasmic inclusions. In the more cytopathic pox diseases, infected keratinocytes undergo lysis and serous fluid accumulates in tiny cystic spaces (microvesicles), which expand and coalesce to form *vesicles*. As a vesicle fills with neutrophils and fibrin, it becomes a *pustule*. Pustules erode to circumscribed ulcers, but barring complications these lesions heal, leaving a small hyaline connective tissue scar.

Some poxviral infections are more proliferative than others (they do not form vesicles). For example, swinepox, sealpox, benign monkeypox, and molluscum contagiosum all cause marked keratinocyte proliferation and epidermal nodules but not pustules. Poxviruses contain genes for cytokines (e.g., *vaccinia virus growth factor*) that use cell receptors for epidermal growth factor to stimulate keratinocyte proliferation. Leporipoxviruses produce fibroblastic nodules rather then epidermal nodules, and cytokines are probably involved in genesis of the lesion.

Poxviruses commonly cause viremia and virus spread hematogenously to skin. *Systemic disease* is rare, except for those poxviruses that cause major plagues (e.g., myxomatosis of rabbits, sheeppox, and human smallpox). In these diseases, virus is transmitted via the respiratory tract; there is local replication in the pharyngeal lymphoid tissues followed by secondary viremia with virus localization in the skin.

Some poxviruses that typically replicate only in skin can, under exceptional circumstances, produce systemic disease. The fetus is especially susceptible to hematogenous transmission of poxviruses. For example, swinepox is almost always a local infection but in pregnancy can become viremic in the sow, pass the placenta, and produce lesions in the newborn piglet.

Herpesviruses

Viruses in this large group are often highly pathogenic for in their animal host (Table 28.2). Herpesviruses tend to be epitheliotropic and to produce acute disease with much tissue damage. Most herpesvirus infections begin in epithelial cells of the upper respiratory tract, oropharynx, or skin. The characteristic lesion consists of a progressively enlarging focus of cell necrosis that destroys the epithelial layer and ends in an ulcer (see Fig. 4.1).

In infected epithelium, cells of the germinal or basal layers become swollen, loose cytoplasmic organelles and form pale, indistinct nuclear inclusion bodies. Large numbers of virions are released into intercellular spaces (Fig. 28.2). Spread of virus to neighboring cells quickly involves the entire thickness of the epithelium. Fluid arising from dilated subepithelial capillaries exudes into the epithelium to cause *vesicles*. The center of the lesion then becomes necrotic, sloughs away, and leaves in its place an *ulcer* filled at the base with necrotic cell debris. Cells with inclusions are best sought at the margins of the epidermal lesions.

Lymph nodes that drain sites of necrosis and ulceration also become infected and will have lymphocte depletion, many inflammatory cells, and foci of necrosis (see Fig. 24.9).

Table 28.1. Pathogenic viruses of the family Poxviridae

			Genera			
Orthopoxvirus	Parapoxvirus	Avipoxvirus	Leporipoxvirus	Capripoxvirus	Suipoxvirus	Unclassified
Vaccinia	Orf (contagious ecthyma)	Fowlpox	Myxoma	Sheeppox	Swinepox	Anteaterpox
Cowpox	Pseudocowpox	Canarypox	Rabbit fibroma	Goatpox		Benign epidermal monkeypox
Variola	Bovine papular stomatitis	Pigeonpox	Squirrel fibroma	Lumpy skin		Molluscum contagiosum
Rabbitpox		Juncopox	Yabapox			Raccoonpox
Ectromelia		Flickerpox	Hare fibroma			Marsupialpox
Pseudoswinepox		Et al.				Donkeypox
Horsepox						Dolphinpox
Buffalopox						Elephantpox
Monkeypox						Gerbilpox
						Sealpox

Table 28.2.   Pathogenic viruses of the family Herpesviridae

Host	Virus	Disease
Horse	Equine herpes 1 (rhinopneumonitis)	Abortion; systemic disease of fetus; rhinopneumonitis in foals; encephalitis; genital exanthem[a]
	Equine herpes 2	Inapparent infection in horses, keratoconjunctivitis[a]
	Equine herpes 3 (coital exanthema)	Sporadic genital vesiculopapular lesions
Pig	Pseudorabies	Inapparent infection, nasopharyngeal necrosis with abortion and encephalitis in newborn; fatal encephalomyelitis in cattle
	Cytomegalovirus (porcine)	Inclusion body rhinitis
Ruminant	Infectious bovine rhinotracheitis	Rhinotracheitis; upper alimentary disease; encephalitis; abortion; vulvovaginitis, et al.; dermatitis, particularly of teats
	Bovine mammillitis (bovid herpes 2)	Pseudolumpy skin disease; enteric lesions
	Wildebeest herpes	Inapparent infection in wildebeest; malignant catarrhal fever in cattle (African form)
	Ovine cytomegalovirus	Inapparent infection
	Ovine herpes[a]	Pulmonary adenomatosis
	Goat herpes	Gastroenteritis
Carnivore	Canine herpes	Inapparent infection in adult; fatal systemic disease in newborn
	Feline herpes	Feline viral rhinotracheitis
	Kinkajou herpes	Inapparent infection
Rodent	Rabbit herpes	Latent infection
	Guinea pig herpes	Malignant lymphoma;[a] inapparent infection[b]
	Guinea pig cytomegalovirus	Latent infection
	Ground squirrel herpes	
Bird	Infectious laryngotracheitis	Laryngotracheitis in chickens
	Owl herpes	Hepatosplenitis
	Duck plague (enteritis)	System infection with enteritis; liver necrosis
	Pigeon herpes	Systemic infection
	Marek's disease	Malignant lymphoma in chickens
	Turkey herpes	Inapparent infection
	Falcon herpes	Systemic infection
	Cormorant herpes	
Amphibian and reptile	Frog renal	Renal adenocarcinoma in frogs
	Iguana herpes	Systemic disease
	Turtle herpes	Liver and skin necrosis (gray-patch disease)
Fish	Channel catfish	Systemic disease, nephritis with tubular necrosis
	Carppox[a]	Skin lesions
Primate	*Herpesvirus B* (simiae)	Stomatitis in monkeys; fatal encephalomyelitis in man
	H. T (M)	Inapparent infection in squirrel monkeys, et al.; fatal disease in owl, marmoset, and tamarin monkeys
	H. aotus (types 1 and 2)	Inapparent infection in owl monkeys
	H. saimiri	Inapparent infection in squirrel monkeys; reticulum cell tumor in marmoset, spider, owl monkeys
	H. ateles (type 1)	Inapparent infection, with rare generalized fatal disease, in spider monkeys; experimental fatal disease in marmosets
	H. ateles (type 2)	Inapparent infection (high %) in spider monkeys; malignant lymphoma in marmosets
	H. ateles (type 3)	Inapparent infection (no known disease), natural in spider monkeys
	Varicellalike viruses[b]	Fatal disease in vervet monkeys with vesicular dermatitis
	Cytomegalovirus (several isolates)	Inapparent infection; systemic disease (pneumonitis, etc.) in immunosuppressed monkeys
	Rhesus leukocyte-associated herpes	Inapparent infection, associated with genome of circulating white blood cells
	Baboon EB herpes	Inapparent infection
Man	Herpes simplex type 1 (oral)	Stomatitis (common); encephalitis of infants (rare); fatal generalized disease in owl monkeys
	Herpes simplex type 2 (genital)	Vulvovaginitis; virus also associated with cancer of uterine cervix[a]
	Varicella-zoster	Chickenpox; herpes zoster dermatitis
	Cytomegalovirus	Inapparent infection; fatal systemic infection in newborn
	EB herpesvirus	Lymphosarcoma in children;[a] infectious mononucleosis

[a]Causal relationship not established.

[b]Cell-associated herpesviruses: Liverpool vervet virus, delta virus, macaque virus, patas herpesvirus, et al. All are related to varicella-zoster of man.

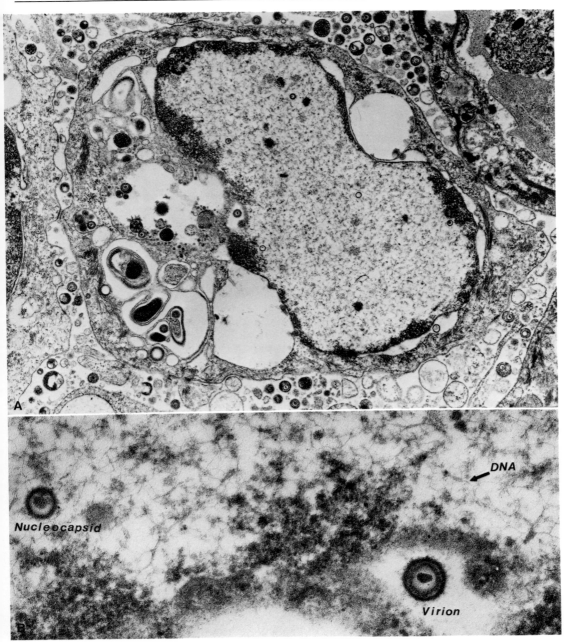

Fig. 28.2. Herpesvirus-infected esophageal epithelial cell, feedlot steer with infectious bovine rhinotracheitis virus. A. Viral DNA and viral structural proteins are combined in the nucleus to form immature viral particles called *nucleocapsids*. B. Nucleocapsids bud through the nuclear membrane to acquire an exterior coat and become complete viral particles called *virions*. Virions accumulate in vacuoles in the cytoplasm and are shed from the cell to the extracellular spaces.

Neonates are highly susceptible to herpesviruses.

There is a clear relationship between age and susceptibility to most herpesviruses. Neonatal animals may succumb during a disease to which they would be resistant a few weeks later. This marked change in susceptibility is related to immaturity in control of body temperature, immune systems, and capacity of macrophages to become activated. For example, canine herpesvirus rarely causes disease in adult dogs but produces widespread lesions in newborn pups. Duck plague rarely occurs except when large numbers of ducks or geese are stressed by a combination of lack of food, cold weather, and high population density. Infectious bovine rhinotracheitis and pseudorabies of pigs occur in adult animals without serious effects, whereas infection of the newborn leads to widespread viral dissemination, encephalitis, and death.

Disseminated herpesviral infection in neonates involves foci of necrosis in the liver, adrenals, and other organs. As parenchymal cells die they attract a few neutrophils, but lesions lack the purulent character of bacterial abscesses. Inclusion body–bearing cells are found only in degen-

---

FOCUS

Pseudorabies

Pseudorabies is an infection in the nasal cavity of swine that disseminates to cause encephalitis, especially in piglets. It is known as Aujeszky's disease, after the Hungarian veterinarian who first reported it. In adult pigs, the herpetic ulcers in the nasal mucosa often pass unnoticed. In other species, pseudorabies is often lethal (see Olander et al., *Vet. Pathol.* 3:64, 1966).

Infection of *pregnant sows* leads to typical necrotic and inflammatory foci in the nasal mucosa and infection in the fetus. Dr. John Kluge and colleagues, at Iowa State University, showed that pregnant gilts infected intranasally often died, and that those that survived often had mummified fetuses.

Pseudorabies in *cattle* of any age causes fatal encephalitis. Dr. R. M. McCracken and Charles Dow, at the Veterinary Research Laboratories at Stormont, near Belfast, Northern Ireland, examined nervous tissue from calves with pseudorabies by electron microscopy and found degenerate neurons and inflammatory infiltrates occur as early as 4 days after experimental infection; they concluded that viruses spread through the axoplasm of nerve fibers.

Pseudorabies can be fatal in cats and dogs. Dr. A. Sabo, at the Institute of Virology in Bratislava, Czechoslovakia, used a fluorescent antibody technique to show that viral antigens were in nasal and tonsillar mucosa by 24 hours after infection of *cats*. Virus spread from foci of epithelial necrosis to lymphatics and from peritonsillar nerves to the olfactory bulb and to the brain stem. Virus was present in the cats' saliva until they died. Pseudorabies virus in adult swine may persist as a latent infection but reappears after some episode of stress. Dr. M. Narita and colleagues, at the National Institute of Animal Health near Tokyo, treated infected but healthy pigs with corticosteroids and found that both pseudorabies virus and cytomegalovirus, a second latent herpesvirus that causes rhinitis, were reactivated.

erate cells at the periphery of the necrotic focus.

Acute herpetic encephalitis characteristically involves the cerebral cortex. Necrosis, perivascular lymphoid cuffing, and hemorrhage are typical. Gliosis and reactive astrocytosis surround areas of necrosis. Large, intranuclear eosinophilic inclusions occur in oligodendroglia and, less often, in nerve cells. Virions are best seen in biopsy specimens; inclusions present at the height of infection are often absent at necropsy.

Inapparent infection

A striking characteristic of some herpesviruses is their capacity to infect the host and remain clinically quiescent; that is, they can exist in their primary host in latent form yet cause serious disease during immunologic deficiencies or when transmitted to susceptible secondary hosts. Even some isolates considered highly pathogenic may persist as asymptomatic infections.

Recurrent herpesvirus disease is typical of many infections in adults. Despite the presence of circulating antibody and interferon, virus localizes, remains occult, and later, under a variety of stimuli, new virus is produced and vesicular lesions appear, often at the site of primary infection. Fever, malnutrition, immune deficiency, and any form of stress will cause *recrudescence* or exacerbation of herpes lesions. In herpes simplex fever blisters in man and herpes B virus blisters on lips of monkeys, viruses reside in nerve ganglia and after stress migrate down the nerve to replicate in epithelia of the lips. When present subclinically, these herpesviruses can be induced to cause disease by administering corticosteroids.

Oncogenic herpesviruses cause neoplasms.

Oncogenic herpesviruses include Marek's disease virus of chickens, the frog renal adenocarcinoma herpesvirus, a human virus associated with lymphoma and nasal carcinomas, and *Herpesvirus saimiri*, which induces a rapidly fatal lymphoma of the reticulum cell type in several nonhost species of marmosets and monkeys (see causes of neoplasms, Chapter 12).

Adenoviruses

Adenoviruses commonly infect the respiratory and enteric tracts (Table 28.3). Although infection is common, overt disease is rare. Immunosuppression and stress are often associated with outbreaks of disease in large animals. In horses, adenoviral pneumonia occurs chiefly in young foals with combined immunodeficiency disease. Adenoviruses isolated from different animals are similar in structure and are related (except for avian types) by a common protein antigen in the virion.

Large *nuclear inclusions* develop in adenovirus-infected tissues. They are composed of masses of virions. Unlike herpesviruses, which rapidly kill cells, adenoviruses have longer replication cycles. In general, infected cells survive longer and are more likely to develop large, dense nuclear inclusions. Marked *cytomegaly* with enormous eosinophilic nuclear inclusions are typical of avian adenoviruses and respiratory mucosa and placenta of sheep infected with ovine adenovirus.

Infectious canine hepatitis (ICH) is one of the few mammalian adenoviral diseases in which virulent virus (canine adenovirus-1, or CAV-1)

Table 28.3. Pathogenic adenoviruses

Host	Disease
Genus *Mastadenovirus* (mammalian)	
Dog	Infectious canine hepatitis (CAV-1)
	Respiratory disease; renal infection, with glomerulonephritis (CAV-2)
Horse	Pneumonia, especially in immunosuppressed neonates
Cow	Mild/inapparent respiratory and enteric infections
Sheep	"Contagious pneumoenteritis" of suckling lambs, diarrhea with respiratory signs; inclusions in nasal and bronchiolar epithelium
Goat	Mild/inapparent intestinal infection
Sea lions	Hepatitis
Genus *Aviadenovirus* (avian)	
Chicken	Inclusion body hepatitis
Turkey	Hemorrhagic enteritis with marked splenic hypertrophy
Goose	Inclusion body hepatitis
Pheasant	Marble spleen disease
Quail	Bronchitis

typically produces disease in susceptible hosts. Originally reported by Rubarth, at the Royal Veterinary College in Stockholm, ICH causes focal (or in severe cases, diffuse) necrosis of the liver with distinctive eosinophilic nuclear inclusions in hepatocytes. Virus enters the liver hematogenously and infects endothelium of the hepatic sinusoids (see Figs. 16.4 and 16.5). Endothelial cells are damaged, and platelets are trapped in the sinusoids. Virus rapidly spreads to and destroys hepatocytes. In late ICH, both platelets and coagulation factors are inhibited so that bleeding is common (see hemostasis, Chapter 16). Dr. N. G. Wright and colleagues, at the University of Glasgow, have shown that CAV-1 replicates in the kidney and is a significant cause of glomerulonephritis.

Canine adenovirus 2 (CAV-2) is a natural respiratory pathogen for dogs. Dr. William Castleman, now at the University of Wisconsin, has shown that viruses replicate in nonciliated epithelial cells to produce bronchitis and bronchiolitis within the lung. Eventually, many cell types are infected and the accumulation of debris produces obstruction in the lower airways.

A simian model of adenoviral pneumonia, first described by Drs. John Boyce, Ellis Giddens, and Marian Valerio, has been used to study viral lung disease. Dr. James Moe and colleagues, at the California Primate Research Center, infected rhesus monkey fetuses at various gestational ages and caused bronchiolar necrosis. Immunization of the pregnant mother largely prevented these lesions.

Papovaviruses

Introduced to group three small DNA viruses (derived from the first two letters of *pa*pilloma, *po*lyoma, and *va*cuolating agents), papovaviruses have slow growth cycles, replicate in the nucleus, and cause latent and chronic infection (Table 28.4). *Infectious papillomas* occur in skin, genital mucosa, and oral mucosa of many animals. Lesions consist of large, highly keratinized, warty growths that develop over a period of weeks and persist for some months before regressing. Histologically, lesions have *hyperkeratosis* (thickening of the stratum corneum), *parakeratosis* (extension of intact keratinocytes into the stratum corneum), and *acanthosis* (thickening of the stratum spinosum). In developing papillomas large "papilloma cells" occur in the granular layer of the skin, at the junction of the spinous and cornified layers (see Fig. 4.6). They are ballooned, with pale, structureless cytoplasm, marginated nuclear chromatin, and small clumps of basophilic material around degenerate nucleoli. The basophilic material, which is composed of virions, expands to form dense nuclear inclusion bodies.

Rarely, squamous cell carcinomas can arise within a viral papilloma (see causes of neoplasms, Chapter 12). Recent studies by Dr. John Sundberg, at the University of Illinois, suggest that papilloma viral agents are not present in cells of most viral papillomas.

Parvoviruses

Active DNA synthesis is required for parvovirus replication, and these viruses have affinity for dividing cells, especially in fetal and neonatal animals. Rapidly dividing cells of the bone marrow, intestine, and placenta are markedly susceptible to parvoviruses, and most parvoviruses are associated with enteritis, leukopenia, and fetal defects.

Parvoviruses cause disintegration of nucleoli, lysis of chromatin, and large nuclear inclusion

Table 28.4. Pathogenic viruses of the family Papoviridae

Virus	Host	Disease
Genus *Papillomavirus*[a]		
Bovine papilloma	Cow	Cutaneous papillomatosis; fibropapilloma of penis
	Horse	Equine sarcoid
	Hamster	Carcinomas or sarcomas at injection site (experimental), including osteosarcoma and meningioma
Papilloma viruses	Various mammals	Cutaneous or oral papillomatosis
Genus *Polyomavirus*		
Polyoma	Mouse	Inapparent infection; rarely, systemic disease with renal infection; sarcoma (experimental)
Viruses of progressive multifocal leukoencephalopathy	Human, monkey	Chronic CNS disease (BK, JC viruses)

[a]Most include viruses with several types based on viral DNA sequences.

bodies. The first inclusions are pale and lightly eosinophilic. Advanced inclusions are dense, basophilic, and stain intensely by immunofluorescence techniques. Inclusions usually are not present in late stages of disease; markedly enlarged nucleoli, which are evidence of repair of epithelial cells, may be mistaken for viral inclusions.

Feline panleukopenia and *mink enteritis* are caused by closely related parvoviruses that replicate in the intestine and spread systemically throughout the host. Lymphoid depletion is a serious effect of infection and the mortality is high. Infection by bacteria plays a role. In 1967, Drs. Michael Rohovsky and Richard Griesemer showed that specific pathogen–free cats infected with feline panleukopenia virus developed profound leukopenia, but did not die as field cats did.

In 1979, sudden death and myocarditis in pups was reported throughout the world caused by a previously unknown *canine parvovirus*. Pathologists reporting lesions included Dr. James Carpenter in Pennsylvania, Dr. Freddy Coignoul at the University of Liege in Belgium, and W. R. Robinson in Australia. The clearest report was by Dr. Michael Hayes, at the University of Saskatchewan, who clearly demonstrated parvoviruses in nuclei of myocytes and fluorescence in infected nuclei after staining with fluorescein-labeled anti–canine parvovirus antibodies (see *J. Am. Vet. Med. Assoc.* 174:1197, 1979).

Recent experiments by Dr. Paul Meunier, at Cornell University, showed that 5-day-old pups infected with canine parvovirus developed myocarditis even though the infection remained clinically inapparent. Myocardial lesions developed at the following times after inoculation: at 23 hours, myocyte degeneration and nuclear inclusions; at 51 hours, heavy lymphocytic infiltrates; and at 108 hours, fibrosis with regressed inflammatory lesions.

Iridoviruses

Iridoviruses are hexagonal, enveloped DNA viruses that develop in the cytoplasm. Pathogenic viruses include African swine fever, lymphocystis virus of fish, and tadpole edema virus. Associated with diverse disease, they have distinctive shapes as seen by electron microscopy. Lesions in the various iridoviral diseases do not resemble each other, and there is no common basis in their manner of cytopathology.

Hepadnaviruses

Hepadnaviruses are the hepatitis viruses of man, woodchucks, and ducks. The prototype virus is the small (42-nm) *hepatitis B virus* of man, which causes foci of hepatic necrosis and periportal infiltration of lymphoid cells. Virions are demonstrable in hepatocyte nuclei and in serum. Viral nucleocapsids fill the hepatocyte nucleus to cause clear, "ground glass" inclusion bodies. The presence of hepatic infection in most species correlates with the development of hepatic neoplasms (see neoplasia, Chapter 12).

Myxoviruses (influenza viruses)

Influenza viruses occur in birds and in four species of mammals: swine, horses, seals, and man. All produce disease by destroying epithelial cells of the respiratory tract. Soon after the initial foci of infection begin in epithelia of the nasal turbinates, virus spreads to involve the entire upper respiratory tract. An acute, intense, inflammatory response (rhinitis, tracheitis, and pneumonitis) is accompanied by coughing, fever, and myalgia. In the lung, epithelium of the terminal bronchioles is especially vulnerable to infection (see Focus: Influenza, Chapter 19). Affected epithelial cells swell and develop cytoplasmic basophilia, but definite inclusion bodies are not present (Fig. 28.3).

Paramyxovirus family

Paramyxoviruses contain surface spikes of hemagglutinins, fusion factors, and neuraminidase that are used to attach to and enter cells and for release of new viruses by budding from the cell surface (Table 28.5). Paramyxoviruses produce cytoplasmic inclusions and giant cells. The family Paramyxovirus includes the following genera: *Paramyxovirus* (Newcastle disease virus, parainfluenza viruses), *Pneumovirus* (respiratory syncytial viruses of several species), and *Morbillivirus,* (measles, canine distemper, and rinderpest viruses).

Virions of *Newcastle disease,* the prototype virus, attach to respiratory epithelial cells during infection by the complexing of viral hemagglutinin to cell membrane glycoproteins. Viral proteins develop as masses in the cytoplasm of infected epithelial cells, but inclusion bodies are not present in histologic sections.

Giant cells are characteristic of some myxovirus infections. In studies of measles, an im-

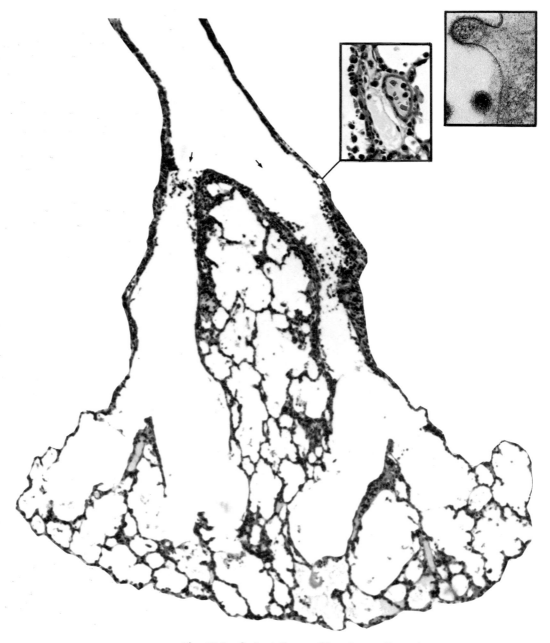

Fig. 28.3. Swine influenza. Virus first replicates in respiratory epithelium as it terminates in the ends of the bronchioles (*arrows*). As epithelial cells are destroyed (*left inset*), virions bud from cell surfaces (*right inset*) and are released into exudates in the airway.

Table 28.5. Pathogenic viruses of the family Paramyxoviridae

Virus	Host	Disease
Genus *Paramyxovirus*		
Newcastle disease	Chicken, turkey	Acute serous tracheobronchitis, systemic infection, encephalitis
Parainfluenza virus	Mouse	Pneumonitis (type 1 Sendai virus)
	Cattle	Pneumonitis, rhinitis (type 3)
	Horse	Nasal isolates (type 3)
	Man	Nasal isolates (types 1, 2, 3, 4); CNS isolates (type 1)
Mumps virus	Man	Parotitis, orchitis; oophoritis in adults, meningoencephalitis in children
Genus *Morbillivirus*		
Measles	Man	Acute systemic exanthem in children
		Postexanthematous encephalitis
		Giant cell pneumonia in immunosuppressed patients
		Congenital infection of newborn
		Subacute sclerosing panencephalitis
	Monkey	Giant cell pneumonia (common)
		Acute systemic exanthem (rare)
Canine distemper	Canidae: mink, raccoon, ferret	Acute systemic febrile disease with pneumonia and encephalitis
		Subacute demyelinating encephalitis
		Chronic encephalopathy
Rinderpest virus	Cattle	Acute systemic febrile disease with hemorrhage
Genus *Pneumovirus*		
Respiratory syncytial virus	Man	Bronchiolitis, pneumonitis (common cold syndrome)
	Chimpanzee	Bronchiolitis
	Cattle	Respiratory disease
Pneumonia virus of mice	Mice	Latent infection (widespread)
		Pneumonitis (rare)

portant disease of monkeys, Drs. W. C. Hall and Robert Kovatch found giant cells in the epidermis and hair follicular epithelium. Persistence of measles virus at these sites is related to poor immune reponses by the host, and in moderately immunosuppressed monkeys, *giant cell pneumonia* is the expected finding.

In chronic brain disease involving measles and canine distemper, *antigenic modulation* (the denuding of viral antigens from surfaces of infected cells) has been hypothesized to play a role. Viral antigens are removed by antibody, but virus continues to replicate inside the cell. While virus is prevented from budding from the cell surface, the viral genome can be slowly passed from cell to cell by fusion of infected cells to normal ones. These viruses produce a *fusion protein* that promotes this activity, bypassing the antibody response of the host. This may also promote mutant viruses formed with a defective outer coat that is not neutralized by antibody.

Rhabdoviruses

Rhabdoviruses (Table 28.6) are grouped together according to morphology of the virions and pathways of intracellular replication. Virions are bullet-shaped (i.e., planar at one end and hemispherical at the other). Several rhabdoviruses are important pathogens. Rabies and vesicular stomatitis viruses are the two important pathogens in this group.

Vesicular stomatitis occurs in horses, cattle, and swine as vesicular lesions in epithelium of the tongue, gingiva, snout, teats, and coronary bands and interdigital areas of the feet. Initial infection is followed by viremia, during which monocytes support the growth of virus. Papules appear initially but rapidly transform into large vesicles that coalesce into bullae. Microscopically, epithelial cells in the developing vesicle retract, become rounded, and are separated by intercellular fluids. Microvesicles form in the epidermis, in which keratinocytes and inflammatory cells float freely. Fluid disseminates through the epidermis and subepidermis to form larger, multilocular vesicles that erode, leaving shallow ulcers on the mucosa. In 1975, studies by Dr. James Proctor showed the virions formed on the surfaces of keratinocytes and budded into intercellular spaces.

Filoviridae (Marburg group)

This is a group of rare viruses (Marburg and Ebola isolates) that have been isolated from outbreaks of fatal hemorrhagic fevers of man in Africa (and subsequent fatal human laboratory

FOCUS

Canine distemper

Dogs with acute canine distemper enter the clinic with fever, anorexia, lethargy, and seropurulent discharges from the eyes and nose. Dyspnea, diarrhea, and dehydration are common, and there are often cutaneous vesicles and pustules that contain streptococci or staphylococci. Canine distemper virus (CDV) is disseminated throughout the animal, and viral antigens, as determined by fluorescent antibody techinques, can be found in nearly all tissues. Histologic examination reveals epithelial cells of the respiratory tract, urinary bladder, stomach (but rarely intestine), and other organs to contain multiple, round, eosinophilic *cytoplasmic inclusion bodies* (see Fig. 4.6). Dr. Anthony Confer, now at Oklahoma State University, has shown that inclusions are composed of masses of viral nucleocapids that aggregate in the cytoplasm.

Dogs usually die of *pneumonia* caused by the combined effects of CDV and pathogenic bacteria. Acute *encephalitis* may also cause death. Infection of the choroid plexus and dissemination of CDV via cerebrospinal fluid facilitates spread of virus in neural tissue. In neonates, viral replication in the heart produces foci necrosis and *myocarditis* that are lethal.

The pathogenesis of typical canine distemper involves (1) development of a local lesion in the upper respiratory tract, (2) transient, primary viremia, (3) an asymptomatic phase in which virus replicates in lymph nodes draining the respiratory tract, (4) secondary viremia with dissemination throughout the body of large amounts of virus, (5) viral replication throughout epithelial tissues and the reticuloendothelial system, (6) anergy, a phase of virus-suppressed immunologic function, and (7) either recovery or postinfectious syndromes. In animals with T lymphocyte depletion, distemper becomes chronic (see Chapter 24).

CDV causes widespread *lymphoid tissue destruction,* and immunosuppression results in secondary infections, especially toxoplasmosis. In 1965, John Gibson, then at Ohio State University, showed that germ-free dogs given virulent CDV developed only a mild, transient febrile disease with slight weight loss and lymphoid depletion. This suggested that the lesions in the lungs and intestine in natural canine distemper were probably associated with superinfecting bacteria.

Dogs that survive for 2–3 weeks develop *subacute encephalitis,* sometimes called "postinfectious encephalitis." Changes in the brain include *nuclear inclusions* in neurons, perivascular lymphocyte cuffs, and demyelination. Nuclear inclusions persist long after cytoplasmic inclusions in visceral organs have disappeared. Foci of necrosis develop in the neuropil, meningitis is constant, and chorioretinitis with proliferation of pigmented epithelium and degeneration of ganglion cells may cause visual disturbances. Giant cells (also called syncytia) are common in the anterior urea of the eye and in white matter of the brain; they probably arise from fusion of astrocytes.

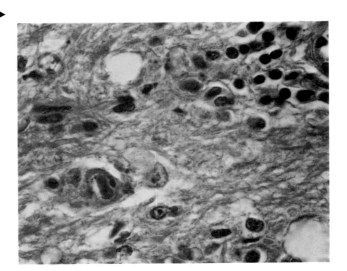

In 1942 Cordy reported a previously unknown progressive encephalopathy in dogs with ataxia, circulation, and episodes of convulsions. The cause was not determined, and the disease gradually became known as *old dog encephalitis*. In 1971, S. D. Lincoln and John Gorham, working at Washington State University, discovered fluorescent antigens of CDV in brains of dogs with old dog encephalitis. Recently, Dr. Steven Krakowka and Michael Axthelm, at Ohio State University, have shown that virus initially infects capillary and venular endothelium in the brain and then persists in neurons. Dr. Brian Summers, at Cornell University, proposes that CDV is also carried to the brain in lymphocytes. Virus is not present elsewhere in the animal with old dog encephalitis and is unusually difficult to isolate from brain. High titers of antibodies are in serum and cerebrospinal fluid of these dogs, but CDV is sequestered inside neurons untouched by the host's immune response.

Even though the dog produces an effective immune response and rids all other tissues of virus, CDV may persist silently in neurons of the brain for months. Chronic brain infection may follow not only acute distemper but may occur after inapparent infection or vaccination. The distinguishing features of old dog encephalitis are widespread foci viral antigens in both gray and white matter, demyelination, gliosis, and rare nuclear inclusions. Evidence from Krakowka, Summers, and Vandevelde and Zurbriggen in Switzerland indicate that demyelination is due to secondary, indirect damage to oligodendroglia. Although antibodies to myelin components appear in serum of dogs, an autoimmune mechanism of demyelination is probably not a mechanism. The brain lesions may be a response of a crippled immune system to persistent viral infection responsible for these lesions.

Table 28.6. Pathogenic rhabdoviruses

Virus	Host	Disease
Vesicular stomatitis	Horse, pig, cow	Necrosis with vesicles and ulcers on mucous membranes
Rabies	Warm-blooded animals	Encephalomyelitis, sialoadenitis
Ephemeral fever	Cow	Febrile systemic disease with lymphadenitis, arthritis, hemorrhages in myocardium and nasal cavity (arthropod borne); congenital deformities in utero
Viral hemorrhagic septicemia (Egtved disease)	Trout	Necrosis of lymphoreticular tissues
Infectious hematopoietic necrosis	Salmon	Necrosis of lymphoreticular tissues
Infectious aerocystitis	Carp	Swim bladder infection

Note: Other isolated rhabdoviruses not associated with known disease include Kern Canyon (bat) virus, Lagos bat virus, Flanders-Hart-Park (insect, bird) virus, and IbAn27377 (shrews).

FOCUS

Rabies

Rabies encephalitis has been a fearsome scourge of dogs, man, and other animals since the beginning of recorded history. Rabies persists in nature because of the unique duality of host infection. First, the encephalitis induces a change from the normal fearful attitude of the host to one of aggressive behavior in which, in carnivores at least, the host will attack other potential host animals. Second, virus replicates to high titer in the salivary glands of carnivores, and is excreted in the saliva.

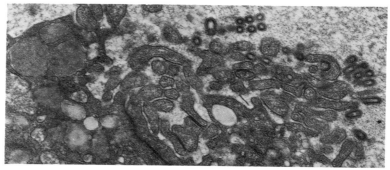

Virions at the surface of a ductal epithelial cell in the parotid gland of a fox. (Photograph: Richard Dierks, *Am. J. Pathol.*)

Rabies is nearly always transmitted by animal bites (in rare cases, aerosol infection has led to spread of virus via olfactory end organs in nares and tongue papillae). The location of the infecting bite wound determines different patterns of disease. In superficial bites, virus replicates in the stratum germinativum of skin and is transmitted to unmyelinated nerves. In deep bites, it first replicates in striated muscle cells with release of virus to neuromuscular spindles and motor endplates. Research by both Dr. Fred Murphy, at the Communicable Disease Center in Atlanta, and Dr. Ken Charlton, at the Animal Diseases Research Institute in Ottawa, have shown that rabies virus replicates locally in the myocyte, to provide a source of new virus for infection of the nervous system via peripheral nerves. Rabies virus ascends to the central nervous system by axonal flow through nerves and by transneuronal transfer. To enter nervous tissue it uses the normal *acetylcholine receptor* located at the synapse as the receptor for viral attachment.

▶

▶

Once signs of rabies develop, viral antigens (detected by fluorescent antibody stains) are found to be disseminated throughout the body, especially in skin, brain, salivary glands, nasal epithelium, pancreas, adrenals, and brown fat. Virus is usually absent from liver, spleen, kidney, and lung. Infected corneal epithelial cells provide the basis of a corneal smear immunofluorescent diagnostic test. Smears from snout epithelium are used to detect rabies infection in living dogs.

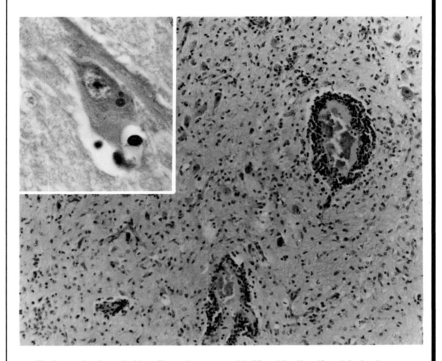

Perivascular lymphoid cuffs and neuron with Negri bodies (*inset*) in brain.

In the brain, virus has a predilection for the brain stem, where it produces an *acute, lymphocytic, leuko-* and *polioencephalomyelitis.* Neuronal degeneration is accompanied by perivascular lymphoid infiltrates and gliosis, often with glial nodules. The medulla, cerebellum, basal ganglia, spinal cord, and dorsal root ganglia may be severely affected, reflecting the clinical picture of ascending paralysis.

Neurons infected with virus undergo *cell swelling* and *chromatolysis.* Cell bodies may be well preserved despite the presence of large aggregates of dense granular viral proteins that develop in the cytoplasm. Called *Negri bodies,* these multiple, eosinophilic, cytoplasmic inclusion bodies are used histologically for the diagnosis of rabies.

infections). They are unusual, large, filamentous viruses that produce widespread tissue necrosis with large cytoplasmic inclusions in liver, lungs, and spleen. The hemorrhagic diatheses that occur in skin, mucous membranes, viscera, and gut lumen in terminal stages of disease reflect the generalized endothelial damage, thrombocytopenia, and depletion of coagulation factors. These, together with loss of plasma volume, dehydration, and hypoproteinemia, cause fatal shock and renal failure.

Coronaviruses

Coronaviruses are most often associated with diarrheal disease although several cause pneumonitis or encephalitis, especially in young animals (Table 28.7). There are three coronaviruses that are respiratory pathogens: avian infectious bronchitis, rat coronavirus, and human coronavirus. In the intestine, virus replicates in enterocytes. Villi become atrophic and fuse as virus is excreted.

Transmissible gastroenteritis (TGE) of swine involves vomiting, diarrhea, dehydration, and high mortality in neonates. The causal coronavirus replicates in and destroys absorptive cells on small intestinal villi. Degenerate cells are sloughed but are replaced by new cells migrating from the intestinal crypts that are not directly affected by TGE virus. Affected villi become shorter because the core of the villus contracts and because new cells are flattened as an

attempt to cover the naked villous surfaces. This lesion is called *villous atrophy*. The functional defect that results from atrophic villi is called *malabsorption*. The lesions of two coronaviruses other than TGE virus have recently been reported by Drs. Ducatelle and Hoorens, at the State University of Ghent, in Belgium.

Bovine coronavirus diarrhea was first reported by Dr. Charles Mebus, working at the University of Nebraska in the early 1970s with newborn calves with diarrhea. Using fluorescent antibody techniques, viral antigens were seen in epithelial cells of the small intestinal villi and surface of the colon. Infected calves produced large amounts of virus in their feces, which can be detected by electron microscopy.

In 1966, Dr. Lauren Wolfe, now at Auburn University, reported a new lethal disease of cats with ascites and diffuse fibrinous peritonitis. He reproduced the disease in germ-free cats and called it *feline infectious peritonitis.* Later shown to be a coronavirus, the infection is widespread among cats. Feline infectious peritonitis has an immunologic component. Kittens with antibody in their serum develop more serious disease than do kittens that have never been exposed to the virus.

Several important coronaviruses have been found in mice. *Mouse hepatitis virus,* with focal necrosis of the liver and encephalitis, has been extensively studied by Drs. Fujiwara and Goto, at the University of Tokyo. *Sialodacryoadenitis of rats,* which causes rhinitis and severe lesions in

Table 28.7. Coronaviruses pathogenic for animals

Virus	Host	Disease
Transmissible gastroenteritis virus (TGE)	Pig	Severe villous atrophy, especially jejunum; viral replication in cells of villi, crypt epithelium spared; mortality inversely related to age, with 100% death in newborn
Hemagglutinating encephalitis virus	Pig	Encephalitis in piglets
Bovine coronavirus	Cow	Enteritis and diarrhea
Infectious bronchitis virus (IBV)	Chicken	Acute serofibrinous tracheobronchitis and airsacculitis; chronic renal disease and oviduct hypoplasia
Transmissible enteritis (bluecomb)	Turkey	Enteritis, diarrhea with severe dehydration
Murine hepatitis virus[a]	Mouse	Various syndromes: acute liver necrosis, enteritis, acute demyelinating encephalomyelitis
Sialodacryoadenitis	Rat	Necrosis and inflammation of salivary glands
Canine enteritis	Dog	Acute enteritis and diarrhea (especially ileum), villous atrophy, and fusion of villi; nonlethal disease of pups
Feline infectious peritonitis (FIP)[b]	Cat	Acute or subacute systemic disease
Human enteric coronavirus (HECV)	Man	Mild enteritis
Human coronavirus (HCV)	Man	

[a]Serologically identical to "lethal intestinal virus of infant mice (LIVIM)."
[b]Closely related to TGE virus.

salivary glands, was first reported by Drs. Albert Jonas and Robert Jacoby.

Reoviruses

Reoviruses replicate in the cytoplasm, and many of them produce irregular, eosinophilic, cytoplasmic inclusion bodies. They are usually present in feces of healthy and sick mammals, and isolates are grouped serologically into three types. Natural infections are common in birds and many mammals (Table 28.8). Except for the avian and murine isolates, the relation of these viruses to natural disease is vague.

Rotaviruses

Rotaviruses are a major cause of diarrheal disease. They produce acute enteritis, atrophy of intestinal villi, and fluid loss into the gut lumen in neonates of most domestic mammals, birds, and man. Rotaviruses infect and destroy villous epithelial cells, especially of the middle and posterior parts of the small intestine. Evidence of viral infection occurs within 12 hours of infection and includes vacuolation and then loss of enterocytes. Aggregates of virions form in vacuoles in the cytoplasm of infected cells but are rarely large enough to be of diagnostic significance histologically. Enteric disease in most neonates is self-limiting, and epithelial regeneration begins within a few hours of injury.

Many other mammalian species have rotaviruses that cause diarrhea in neonates. Recently, Dr. Charles Johnson, Theron Snider, and colleagues have used scanning electron microscopy to study surfaces of intestinal epithelial cells in dogs infected with *canine rotavirus.* They found swollen epithelial cells on villi, denuded foci, and villous atrophy.

Three viruses have been recently grouped as *Birnaviruses:* infectious bursal disease of chickens, infectious pancreatic necrosis of fish, and eel skin tumor virus. Although these agents resemble reoviruses, they are smaller, have single capsid shells, and have a double-stranded RNA genome that is segmented into two pieces.

Arenaviruses

Arenaviruses (L. *arenosus,* sandy) are named through the fine granules in the virion seen by electron microscopy. Lymphocytic choriomeningitis (LCM), the prototype virus, has been extensively studied as a model because it produces lifelong inapparent but persistent infections in mice, with high death rates in adults due to an immunologically mediated encephalitis. LCM also infects pet rodents and primates and can cause fetal brain lesions. Disease-producing arenaviruses other than LCM virus are *Lassa*

Table 28.8. Pathogenic viruses of the family Reoviridae

Virus	Host	Disease
Genus *Reovirus*		
Mammalian reoviruses[a]	Man	Respiratory infection (types 1, 2, 3)
	Dog	Tracheobronchitis (type 1)
	Mouse	Hepatoencephalitis (types 1, 2, 3)
	Cat	Conjunctivitis
Avian reoviruses	Chicken	Arthritis, tendinosynovitis
	Turkey	Enteritis (?)
Genus *Orbivirus*		
Bluetongue	Sheep	Acute febrile disease with ulceration in oral cavity and coronary bands of feet (deer and cattle also susceptible)
Colorado tick fever	Man	Mild febrile disease with headache and muscle pain
Epidemic hemorrhagic disease	Deer	Highly fatal systemic disease with widespread vascular damage, edema, and hemorrhage
African horse sickness	Horse	Highly fatal systemic disease with widespread vascular damage, edema, and hemorrhage
Equine encephalosis	Horse	Encephalitis
Ibaraki	Cow	Febrile systemic disease; abortion
Rabbit syncytium	Rabbit	Inapparent infection
Genus *Rotavirus*		
Enteric rotaviruses[a]	Pig, calf horse, deer, etc.	Enteritis and diarrhea of neonates

[a]Inapparent infection in many species.

virus and the *Argentine hemorrhagic fever virus* of man.

Togaviruses

Most togaviruses were previously classified as *arboviruses* (for *ar*thropod-*bo*rne) because they are maintained in nature by cyclical transmission between susceptible vertebrate hosts and bloodsucking arthropods, with viral replication in both. Togaviruses are important causes of encephalitis and hemorrhagic fevers in animals and man.

Alphaviruses (subgroup A togaviruses)

These mosquito-borne viruses are serologically and structurally related. Important pathogens include agents associated with *equine encephalomyelitis* (Table 28.9). Inoculated subcutaneously as mosquitos bite, they replicate locally in macrophages. Viremia follows, which if of sufficient titer, results in infection of endothelial

cells and neurons in the brain.

Eastern and *Western equine encephalitis* (EEE and WEE) are transmitted to horses by mosquitos. The animal reservoir is chiefly wild birds, in whose circulating blood the virus reaches very high titers. In horses a highly transient viremia occurs, and the virus localizes in the brain. In animals dead of encephalitis, lesions are most common in the cerebral cortex, basal ganglia, hippocampus, and nuclei of the medulla oblongata. Neuronal degeneration and necrosis are accompanied by gliosis and infiltration of affected foci by plasmacytes, small lymphocytes, and a few neutrophils.

Flaviviruses (subgroup B togaviruses)

Flaviviruses fall into two groups, one requiring ticks, the other transmitted by mosquitos. There are enormous numbers of flaviviruses, but most are not known to cause overt disease in vertebrates; they are isolates obtained from serologic surveys of birds or mammals.

Table 28.9. Pathogenic viruses of the family Togaviridae

Virus	Host	Disease
Genus *Alphavirus* (arbovirus group A)		
Eastern, western, and Venezuelan equine encephalitis	Horse, man	Encephalitis
Semliki Forest		
Sindbis		
Genus *Flavivirus* (arbovirus group B)		
Mosquito borne		
Yellow fever	Man, monkey	Hepatic and lymphoid necrosis
Dengue	Man	Hemorrhagic fever; shock
Wesselsbron disease	Sheep	Hepatic necrosis; abortion
St. Louis encephalitis	Man	Encephalitis
Japanese B encephalitis	Man	Encephalitis
Tick borne		
Louping ill	Sheep, pig	Encephalitis
Nairobi sheep disease	Sheep	Febrile systemic disease
Kyasanur Forest disease	Monkey	Febrile systemic disease
Genus *Rubivirus*		
Rubella	Man	Acute systemic disease with rash; fetal anomalies; congenital syndrome
Genus *Pestivirus*		
Bovine viral diarrhea	Cow	Acute febrile systemic disease with lymphoid necrosis and enteritis; chronic multiorgan disease; congenital infection
Hog cholera (swine fever)	Pig	Acute systemic vascular disease
Border disease	Sheep	CNS disease
Unclassified		
Equine viral arteritis	Horse	Upper respiratory syndrome (mild); fatal systemic vascular disease; abortion
Simian hemorrhagic fever	Monkey	Fatal systemic vasculitis
Lactic dehydrogenase	Mouse	Inapparent infection
Akabane	Cow	Congenital encephalopathy

Bunyaviruses

The Bunyaviridae family includes the genera *Bunyavirus, Phlebovirus* (Rift Valley fever and sandfly fever); *Nairovirus* (Crimean hemorrhagic fever); and *Uukuvirus* (uukuniemi and related viruses). In their vertebrate host, most replicate locally, often in skeletal muscle, and then become viremic, pass the blood-brain barrier, and infect the brain to cause encephalitis.

Toroviruses

Toroviruses (Berne and Breda viruses) have recently been isolated from neonatal horses and cattle with diarrhea. Large numbers of bean-shaped virions are excreted into feces, but their role in disease is not clear. Dr. Joachim Pohlenz and colleagues, then at Iowa State University, inoculated newborn germ-free calves experimentally and found vacuolated enterocytes containing virions and viral antigens at 48–60 hours after infection.

Picornaviruses

Small, omnipresent picornaviruses are grouped into enteroviruses, rhinoviruses, cardioviruses, and others (Table 28.10). *Enteroviruses* are common infections of the gut and rare infections of the brain. While strains of enteroviruses show striking differences in virulence and invasiveness, tissue invasion depends on stresses or immaturity of immune mechanisms in the host. Pregnancy, immunosuppression, corticosteroid therapy, and surgical procedures markedly increase the risk of paralytic disease.

The nervous system is the target organ for enteroviruses of pigs, chickens, cattle, and man. Although virions replicate in many tissues, the resultant cytopathic effects are limited and not manifested as clinical disease. Within the brain, infection of neurons is preceded by involvement of vascular endothelium. Subsequent infection of neurons induce cell swelling, chromatolysis, and cell death. Cell loss is a direct cause of the paralysis observed clinically.

Caliciviruses

Caliciviruses develop in the cytoplasm. *Feline calicivirus,* a common cause of upper respiratory disease in cats, replicates in epithelium of conjunctiva, oral mucosa, and tongue. It produces vesicles, ulcers, and acute inflammation. The calicivirus of swine (vesicular exanthema) is closely related to, and probably originated from, the calicivirus of sea lions.

Table 28.10. Pathogenic viruses of the family Picornaviridae

Virus	Host	Disease
Genus *Enterovirus*		
Porcine polioencephalomyelitis	Pig	CNS inflammatory disease; abortion
Murine polio	Mouse	CNS disease
Avian encephalomyelitis	Chicken	CNS disease
Human enterovirus		
Polio	Man	Asymptomatic enteric infection with sporadic encephalomyelitis
Coxsackie	Man	Vesicular exanthem; aseptic meningitis; respiratory disease; myocarditis and renal infection
Echo	Man	Febrile systemic disease with diarrhea
Genus *Cardiovirus*		
Encephalomyocarditis	Pig	Systemic febrile disease
Murine encephalomyelitis	Mouse	Encephalitis
Genus *Rhinovirus*		
Human rhinovirus	Man	Upper respiratory infection (common cold)
Bovine rhinovirus	Cow	Upper respiratory infection
Genus *Aphthovirus*		
Foot-and-mouth disease	Cow, pig	Acute febrile disease with necrosis and ulceration of mucous membranes with epidermis
Unclassified picornaviruses		
Hepatitis A	Man, marmoset, chimpanzee	Hepatic necrosis and inflammation ("infectious hepatitis" via anal-oral route)
Duck hepatitis	Duck	Hepatic necrosis and inflammation

FOCUS

Porcine polioencephalomyelitis

In 1930, a new transmissible disease of suckling piglets dying with nervous signs was reported from Teschen, Czechoslovakia. Immediately the disease was recognized throughout central Europe, and pathologic lesions were reported in 1942 by the veterinary pathologist Dobberstein as a nondemyelinating, lymphoplasmacytic polioencephalomyelitis. Interest in the disease was given impetus by its similarity to human poliomyelitis, which killed or left crippled large numbers of young children, particularly in the more developed countries in the 1930s and 1940s.

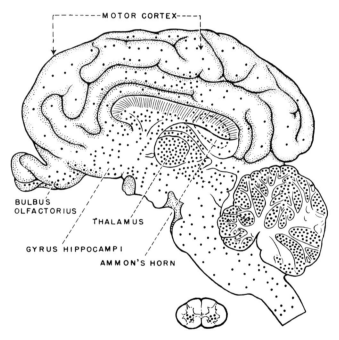

Distribution of lesions in porcine polioencephalomyelitis. (Drawing: Elias Manuelidis, *Am. J. Pathol.*)

▶

Astroviruses

Astroviruses, tiny viruses that resemble 5- or 6-pointed stars, have been identified in enterocytes of the intestine of lambs, calves, and human infants. The first animal astrovirus was found in feces of lambs with diarrhea, and the disease was reproduced by passing infected feces. In cattle, the ability to cause diarrhea has not been clearly shown.

Retroviruses

The family Retroviridae (Table 28.11) includes many oncogenic viruses, human immunodeficiency viruses, visna viruses associated with chronic infection of the central nervous system and lungs of sheep and goats, and the foamy viruses that are not associated with disease. Oncogenic (see causes of neoplasms, Chapter 12) and immunosuppressive (see immunodeficiency,

▶

   In 1957, reports from England by Harding and Done and from
Canada by W. P. C. Richards pointed to two important characteristics:
(1) in newborn pigs there was high mortality with loss of entire litters,
while the disease was less severe in older suckling pigs, and (2)
piglets farrowed late in individual outbreaks did not sicken. The
causal agent was identified as a small RNA-containing virus, which
was later classified as an enterovirus. The typical disease progressed
through (1) viral multiplication in intestinal epithelium and mesenteric lymph nodes; (2) viremia; (3) neural infection, with necrosis of
neurons, especially in ventral horns of the spinal cord; and (4) recovery.

   Porcine enteroviral polioencephalomyelitis was first reported in
the United States by Adalbert Koestner and colleagues in Ohio. Using silver impregnation techniques and germ-free piglets, he and Dr.
John Holman and John Long showed that necrosis of neurons in the
ventral horns of the spinal cord was followed by infiltration of microglia and then by proliferation of astrocytes. The end result was a paucity of neurons, aggregates of lymphoid cells, and astrocytic
meshworks.

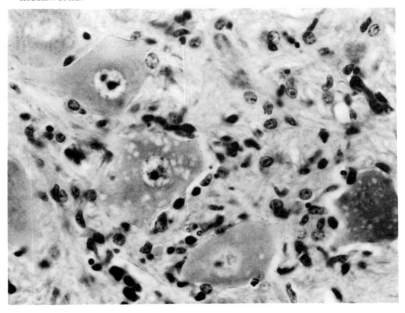

Chapter 24) characteristics are dealt with elsewhere. Many of these viruses are associated
with chronic demyelinating disease of the brain.
This was first reported in mice infected with
murine leukemia viruses. Recently a spongiform
polioencephalomyelopathy caused by a neurotropic murine leukemia virus has been reported

by Zachary and colleagues, at the University of
Illinois (see *Am. J. Pathol.* 124:457, 1986).

Subviral proteins

   The infectious agent that causes scrapie in
sheep, once considered to be a possible viroid,

Table 28.11.   Family Retroviridae

Subfamily Oncovirinae
  Genus (Type C oncovirus group)
    Subgenus mammalian
      Feline leukemia/sarcoma
      Murine leukemia/sarcoma
      Bovine leukemia
      Baboon oncovirus
      Gibbon ape leukemia
      Woolly monkey sarcoma
      Guinea pig, pig, and rat oncoviruses
    Subgenus avian
      Avian leukemia/sarcoma
      Avian reticuloendotheliosis
      Pheasant oncovirus
  Genus (Type B oncovirus group)
    Mouse mammary tumor
  Genus (Type D oncovirus group)
    Mason-Pfizer monkey
Subfamily Spumavirinae
  Bovine and feline syncytial
  Human and simian foamy
Subfamily Lentivirinae
  Visna-maedi
  Caprine arthritis-encephalitis
  Ovine progressive pneumonia
  Human immunosuppressive virus (AIDS)
  Equine infectious anemia

has recently been classified as a *prion* (for small, proteinaceous infectious particle). Prions contain a single major protein required for infectivity (they lack nucleic acids) and are highly resistant to most disinfectants. Three animal diseases are caused by prions: scrapie, transmissible mink encephalopathy, and chronic wasting disease of elk and mule deer. All are chronic, progressive diseases of the central nervous system and lead to reactive astrocytosis and (usually) vacuolation of neurons.

Viroids are small, naked, infectious RNA molecules that, despite their small amount of genetic material, replicate in plant cells and produce disease. They do not contain protein coats and do not form virions visible by electron microscopy. No animal viroids have been described.

PROKARYOTIC PATHOGENS

Prokaryotic pathogens range from simple cells that resemble viruses and require intracellular phases of development to highly complex cells that have some characteristics of eukaryocytes. The small rickettsiae and chlamydiae have evolved transport mechanisms that enable them to exploit host-generated ATP and other intermediates for their own use. In contrast, the large spirochetes move with highly complex fla-

gellae in a free-living manner similar to protozoa. The true bacteria lie between these extremes in size and metabolism.

Rickettsiae

These small, coccobacillary prokaryocytes cause febrile systemic disease in man, usually by infecting vascular endothelium. Once considered transitional between bacteria and viruses, rickettsiae are unable to grow in the absence of living host cells. In tissue sections or smears they stain by Giemsa or Macchiavello's methods. Most rickettsiae pass through arthropods as an obligate part of their life cycle; for example, classic epidemic typhus (*Rickettsia prowazekii*) is transmitted by lice, and Rocky Mountain spotted fever (*R. rickettsii*) by ticks.

Rocky Mountain spotted fever makes up 95% of human rickettsial infections in North America and has been reported in dogs. Lesions are characterized by widespread vasculitis of muscular arteries. *R. rickettsii* replicates in endothelial cells, causing vasculitis and liberation of pyrogens and kinin-generating enzymes that induce fever and increased capillary permeability. Dr. James Moe, studying experimental infections in monkeys, found vasculitis and thrombosis to be prominent in nares, pinna of the ear, scrotal skin, and testes.

Q fever

The way in which rickettsiae replicate in cells has been studied by Dr. W. C. Hall, at the U.S. Army Medical Research Institute at Fort Detrick. Using the agent of human Q fever (*Coxiella burnetii*), he infected nude mice, which are deficient in T lymphocytes. Organisms replicated in phagocytic vesicles of macrophages, especially in the liver and spleen, and the presence of a thymus and normal T lymphocytes proved to be important in the ability of the macrophage to clear organisms from the host.

Ehrlichiosis

Canine ehrlichiosis is endemic in semitropical areas of the world. In the United States its range coincides with that of the brown dog tick *Rhipicephalus sanguineus*. Clinical features are thrombocytopenia, anemia, decreased serum total protein, and increased γ-globulin. M. J. Reardon and Kenneth Pierce, at Texas A&M University, in experimental ehrlichiosis found interstitial pneumonia, subendothelial aggregates of mononuclear cells in lung blood vessels, and perivascular lymphocytes and plasmacytes in many organs.

Equine ehrlichiosis was first reported as Potomac fever in the 1970s. Fever, leukopenia, lethargy, and diarrhea were clinical signs. Disease was caused by *E. risticii,* which parasitized circulating monocytes. Dr. Donald Cordes reported the lesions of enterocolitis as patchy hyperemia, petechiae, and erosions throughout the intestine.

Mycoplasmas

The causal organism (*Mycoplasma mycoides*) of the great plague of cattle called *pleuropneumonia* was isolated at the turn of the century and became the prototype for this group. They are the smallest cellular form of life and have no membranous organelles and no cell wall. Pathogenic mycoplasmas infiltrate among, attach to, and destroy cilia of the respiratory tract. The names of the clinical syndromes they cause attest to their role in respiratory disease: swine enzootic pneumonia, chronic infectious catarrh of rodents, chronic respiratory disease of chickens, infectious sinusitis of turkeys, and primary atypical pneumonia of man.

Chlamydiae

Chlamydiae are small bacteria that have many properties of free-living bacteria but require enzymes present in living cells to multiply (Fig. 28.4). There are two species: *Chlamydia trachomatis,* a human pathogen, and *C. psittaci,* which produces various respiratory, genital, and intestinal infections in birds and mammals (Table 28.12). Inside cells, chlamydiae use some of the biochemical reactions that produce energy, especially of the glycolytic cycle. Most virulent chlamydial strains produce toxins. Uncharacterized isolates of *C. psittaci* are commonly isolated from animals with disease, but the precise role in causing disease is vague. For example, chlamydia are common inhabitants in the intestines of calves, and although incriminated as a cause of diarrhea, the pathogenesis of infection is often not clearly established.

Spirochetes

Once considered intermediate between bacteria and protozoa, spirochetes differ from protozoa in their lack of nuclear membrane and the presence of muramic acid in their cell walls. They are best detected live, swimming in darkfield preparations of exudates. Pathogenic genera are *Leptospira, Borrelia* (the cause of spirochetosis of horses, cattle, and birds), and *Treponema* (which contains the agents of human and rabbit syphilis). Treponemes are common inhabitants of the alimentary tract of mammals, particularly the oral cavity, stomach, and colon.

Treponema hyodysenteriae, the primary etiologic agent of swine dysentery (bloody scours), produces extensive but superficial necrosis of epithelium in the cecum and colon. Denudation of epithelium leaves villi composed only of lamina propria and a covering basement membrane. Grossly, the mucosa is rugose and covered by mucus, fibrin, neutrophils, and flecks of blood. In severe cases, this material combines with tissue debris and forms a pseudomembrane over the mucosal surface. In 1974, Dr. Robert Glock, then at Iowa State University, reported large spirochetes in the lumen of the colon. Clusters were attached to and inside epithelial cells, especially in the acute phases of the disease.

True bacteria

Pathogenic bacteria are classified according to characteristics they show in laboratory tests (Table 28.13): cell shape, growth in the presence or absence of oxygen, and the ability of the cell walls to retain or lose the Gram stain. In tissue sections bacteria are found in interstitial tissue, within cells (especially phagocytic cells), and on epithelial surfaces. Although especially common on lumina of intestine and respiratory tract, they are usually washed away during routine tissue processing.

Bacteria in tissue are characterized by the Gram stain (a dark blue crystal violet–iodine complex) that separates them into two major groups. Dye is trapped within *gram-positive* bacteria and cannot be removed by alcohol because of the thick cell walls composed of mucocomplexes containing muramic acid. *Gram-negative* bacteria have thin cell walls that permit removal of the dye by alcohol treatment; they stain pink with the Gram stain. Special stains are useful in diagnosis of some pathogenic bacteria (e.g., silver impregnation techniques for spirochetes, the Giemsa stain for rickettsiae, and the acid-fast stain, which uses basic fuchsin and phenol, for mycobacteria.

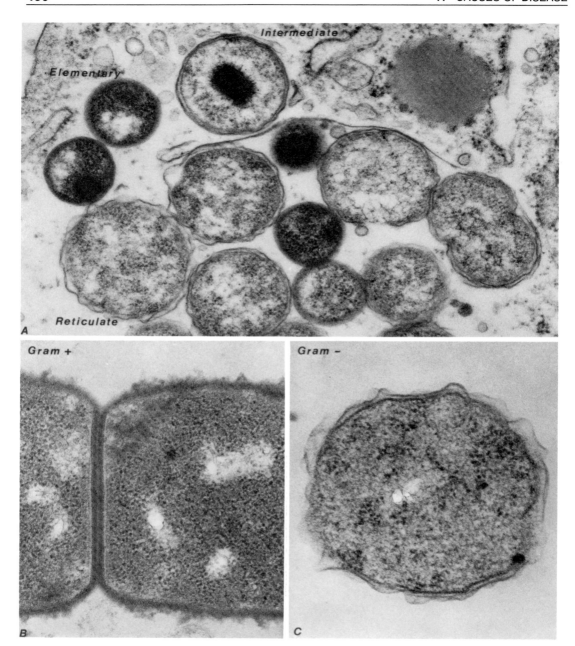

Fig. 28.4. Bacterial structure. A. Chlamydia, lamb polyarthritis. There are large, fragile reticulate bodies, intermediate bodies, and small hardy elementary bodies. (Photograph: Randall Cutlip) B. Gram-positive bacterium, two rods joined at attached peptidoglycan layers. C. Gram-negative bacterium, cytoplasm surrounded by plasma membrane and an outer undulant layer.

Table 28.12.   Diseases caused by _Chlamydia psittaci_

Disease	Animal	Lesions
Chlamydiosis	Turkey	Fibrinous pericarditis, peritonitis, airsacculitis (Beasley, _Am. J. Vet. Res._ 20:341, 1959)
	Man	Pneumonitis, patchy pneumonia
Feline pneumonitis	Cat	Acute upper respiratory infection with nasal and conjunctival fibrinopurulent exudates; foci of pneumonia (Hoover et al., _Am. J. Vet. Res._ 39:541, 1978)
Epizootic abortion	Cattle	Abortion (Kennedy et al., _Cornell Vet._ 50:417, 1960)
Sporadic bovine encephalomyelitis		Meningoencephalitis (McNutt et al., _Cornell Vet._ 30:437, 1940)
Chlamydial pneumonia	Sheep, cattle	Pneumonitis, patchy pneumonia (Dungworth and Cordy, _J. Comp. Pathol._ 72:71, 1962)
Enzootic abortion of ewes	Sheep	Abortion (Stamp, _Vet. Rec._ 62:251, 1950)
Polyarthritis	Sheep	Synovitis, arthritis (Cutlip, _Am. J. Vet. Res._ 34:71, 1973)

Colonies of bacteria may be present in tissues, especially if a terminal or comatose state existed prior to death. When they are found in the renal glomerulus, lung capillaries, and other vascular tissue, they may indicate an origin from septic emboli. Bacterial replication also continues after death, particularly the large saprophytic rods that are found in foci of postmortem degeneration in visceral organs.

Bacteria-host relationships determine the type of disease.

Pathogenic bacteria produce disease in several different ways. They may be _pyogenic_ (pus-producing), _toxigenic_ (releasing exotoxins that give rise to disease), or _intracellular._ The nature of the exudate in infected tissue provides clues to the identity of bacteria. Pyogenic streptococci and staphylococci release factors that strongly affect blood vessels and that release substances that are chemotactic for neutrophils and stimulate large amounts of pus. Toxigenic bacteria produce little pus but cause cell death, which varies from discrete killing of specific neurons to widespread destruction of muscle. Intracellular bacteria do neither of these but replicate inside macrophage or parenchyma cells to produce subacute or chronic disease.

Intracellular bacteria

Bacteria that grow in artificial media, yet, when in animal tissue, grow inside living cells are called _facultative intracellular bacteria._ Mycobacteria, brucellae, and salmonellae all replicate within cells of the host. Like other bacteria, they are taken up by macrophages as they enter tissue, but they are able to survive within the cytoplasm of macrophages and replicate to produce disease. Although macrophages kill most of these intracellular bacteria within a few hours, a small residual population survives and begins to multiply intracellularly to slowly produce a granulomatous or pyogranulomatous lesion.

Table 28.13.   Classification of pathogenic bacteria

Order	Family	Genera
Mycoplasmales	Mycoplasmataceae	_Mycoplasma_
Rickettsiales	Rickettsiaceae	_Rickettsia, Neorickettsia, Ehrlichia, Cowdria, Coxsiella_
	Chlamydiaceae	_Chlamydia_
	Anaplasmataceae	_Anaplasma, Paranaplasma_
	Bartonellaceae	_Bartonella, Eperythrozoon, Hemobartonella_
Eubacteriales	Streptococcaceae	_Streptococcus_
	Micrococcaceae	_Staphylococcus, Neisseria_
	Corynebacteriaceae	_Corynebacterium, Rhodococcus, Listeria, Erysipelothrix_
	Bacillaceae	_Bacillus, Clostridium_
	Brucellaceae	_Brucella, Pasteurella, Francisella, Bordetella, Actinobacillus, Bacteroides, Hemophilus, Moraxella, Fusobacterium_
	Enterobacteriaceae	_Escherichia, Aerobacter, Proteus, Klebsiella, Salmonella, Yersinia, Citrobacter_
	Pseudomonadaceae	_Pseudomonas, Bivrio, Legionella, Campylobacter_
Actinomycetales	Mycobacteriaceae	_Mycobacteria_
	Actinomycetaceae	_Actinomyces, Nocardia, Dermatophilus_
Spirochetales	Spirochaetaceae	_Leptospira, Treponema, Borrelia_

Pyogenic bacteria colonize skin and body orifices.

Streptococcus spp. cause inflammatory lesions in the skin, lymph nodes, heart valves, and meninges. These are important agents of mastitis in cattle, strangles and other respiratory diseases of horses, and many diseases of pigs, including septicemia, meningitis, arthritis, endocarditis, and lymphadenitis. Streptococci can colonize normal skin for long periods and then, after some minor trauma, cause *pyoderma.* The initial lesion is a microabscess or small pustule that expands into adjacent areas.

Staphylococcus spp. are residents of normal skin, nasal passages, and lower gut, depending on individual species. They are frequent causes of infection of skin and body orifices. Some strains of staphylococci produce toxins that cause vacuolar changes and microvesicles in epithelium (see Fig. 20.3). Dogs with diabetes mellitus commonly develop severe staphylococcal infections because their neutrophils are inhibited by persistent hypoglycemia (see Fig. 24.2). *Exudative epidermitis* (greasy pig disease), a subacute generalized neutrophilic dermatitis of pigs in the first month of life, is caused by infection with streptococci. Pathologic lesions were independently reported in 1968 by Anna-Lisa Obel, in Stockholm, and Charles Mebus, then at the University of Nebraska.

Granulomatous lesions of chronic infections of pyogenic bacteria, such as staphylococci and *Pseudomonas aeruginosa,* and by *Actinomyces* spp. and *Actinobacillus* spp. often contain peculiar but diagnostically useful granules formed from bacteria, debris, and proteins of plasma. Called *sulfur granules,* they stain bright red with eosin and have a central mass of amorphous debris from which club-shaped processes radiate outward. Reactions of antibodies with antigens in these masses produce aggregates of hyalin material.

FOCUS

Brucellosis

Bacteria of the genus *Brucella* cause acute and chronic febrile diseases in several species of animals, including man. *Brucella abortus,* the most important pathogen, causes relapsing disease characterized by fever, lymphadenopathy, and, in pregnant females, abortion. In chronic disease, bacteria are sequestered in phagocytic cells of the lymphoreticular organs and infected animals remain as carriers for long periods. Despite effective immunization programs using avirulent strains of *B. abortus,* brucellosis remains a leading cause of economic loss to the livestock industry and an important cause of chronic debilitating human disease. Like tuberculosis, it masquerades as a perplexing group of syndromes.

In typical bovine brucellosis, cattle are infected via the alimentary canal from infected uterine, placental, or fetal exudates. Acute regional lymphadenitis (at first neutrophilic, then plasmacytic) develops and is followed by bacteremia that leads to infection of the spleen, lymphoid tissues, mammary glands, and the pregnant uterus. Brucellosis involves long-lasting and intermittent bacteremia and results in persistence of the bacterium by virtue of its residence in macrophages. *B. abortus* produces substances in the cell wall that inhibit the bactericidal effect of macrophage lysosomes either by preventing phagosome-lysosome fusion or by depressing the effectiveness of lysosomal antibacterial substances.

▶

An unusual feature of *B. abortus* infection is an extraordinary replication to high titers in genital tissue, especially during pregnancy. Chorioallantoic fluid from infected cows may contain up to 1 × 10^{13} colony-forming units of bacteria. Abortion is common, and the infected placenta is inflamed and edematous. In the 1960s Drs. Joe Mollelo and Rue Jensen, then at Colorado State University, studied the infected ruminant placenta. The placental surface is covered with sticky brown exudate and contains yellow foci of necrosis. Chorionic epithelial cells are vacuolated and bear extraordinary numbers of bacilli. Cells of the interplacentome are more severely affected than those covering the placentome. Tips of maternal villi are necrotic, and the bases are infiltrated with leukocytes. The endometrium is not severely afflicted despite the severity of the placental inflammation. The tropism of *B. abortus* for the placenta is due, in part, to replication of bacteria within the trophoblast cytoplasm.

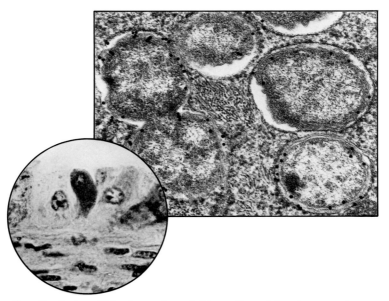

Brucella abortus within placental trophoblasts. Bacterial surface proteins are labeled with dense gold particles. Circle: Histology published in 1919 by Theobald Smith. (Tim Anderson, *Vet. Pathol.*)

In the circle above is a reproduction of a photograph of bacilli in placental trophoblasts published by Theobald Smith in a 1919 issue of the *Journal of Experimental Medicine*. In 1985, Dr. Tim Anderson, working at the National Animal Disease Center, demonstrated that *B. abortus* resides in the endoplasmic reticulum (within rectangle above) of the trophoblast and suggested that these bacteria require some unknown glycosylating enzyme found on the membranes of this organelle.

Bacteria normally colonize mucosal surfaces.

Surfaces of the upper respiratory tract, urogenital tract, oropharynx, stomach, and intestine have normal bacterial populations. The microflora of the tongue, orifices of salivary glands, and teeth are similar among different individuals. Tiny microbial plaques occur at the gingival margins of teeth when streptococci cling to tooth surfaces. They secrete enzymes that cleave sucrose (into glucose and fructose), and enzymes called glycosyltransferases in the bacteria polymerize the glucose into long chains called glucans. Glucans adhere to enamel and trap other bacterial species. Each animal species has its characteristic plaque population (see Fig. 21.2).

Some parts of the alimentary canal are important fermentation areas whose microflora is of great diversity (e.g., the rumen in many species and the colon in the pig and horse). These normal microflora are changed markedly in disease. The colon of healthy pigs contains streptococci (about 55% of the bacterial population), *Bacteroides* spp. (18%), and lactobacilli (12%), with over 15 other species present in small numbers. In pigs with dysentery this population shifts so that the dominant species are *Escherichia coli, Fusobacterium* spp., *Eubacterium* spp., *Acetovibrio* spp., and *Selenomonas* spp. This microbial shift probably plays an important secondary role in the diarrhea of dysentery. Staphylococci and streptococci are the most commonly isolated aerobic bacteria obtained from the vagina, prepuce, and urethral orifice of dogs; during genital disease of the female, *E. coli,* which is normally present in low numbers, replicates to much larger numbers.

Bacterial virulence factors

Surfaces of bacteria contain structures that are important *virulence factors* (e.g., pili, capsules, cell walls) (Fig. 28.5). Virulence factors function to enhance bacterial attachment and colonization in tissue, to inhibit phagocytosis, or to depress host immunity. When produced in sufficient concentrations, these substances cause the organism to resist the opsonic and lytic effects of antibody and complement. Although true virulence of bacteria is detectable only in living animals, microbiologists use those components that develop in cultures as markers of virulence (Table 28.14).

Bacterial secretions (exotoxins, coagulase, hyaluronidase) are also important virulence characteristics. They suppress the natural antimicrobial effects of glucosaminoglycans and enable bacteria to dissect through connective tissue.

Pili are small filamentous appendages that

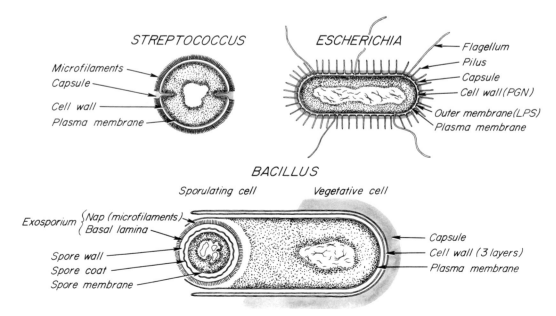

Fig. 28.5. Ultrastructure of *Streptococcus, Escherichia,* and *Bacillus.*

Table 28.14. Bacterial virulence factors

Factor	Mechanism
	STRUCTURAL COMPONENTS
Capsule	Inhibit phagocytosis (streptococci, anthrax bacilli)
Peptidoglycans	Degranulate platelets (streptococci, staphylococci)
Lipopolysaccharides (endotoxin)	Bind to and destroy cell surface membranes; pyrogen release; prostaglandin release
Lipoteichoic acid	Adhere to epithelium
Cytoplasmic lipids	Inhibit phagosome-lysosome fusion (tuberculosis)
Fimbrial proteins (pili)	Adhere to epithelium; promote colonization
	SOLUBLE FACTORS
Protein synthesis inhibitor	Split NAD to suppress elongation factors that catalyze translocation of peptide chains emerging from ribosomes
Phospholipase D	Membrane lysis (*Listeria* spp., *Corynebacterium ovis, Clostridia* spp.)
Sphingomyelinase	Sphingomyelin lysis (staph *β* toxin)
Cholesterol lysin	Cholesterol lysis (streptolysin O)
Hyaluronidase	Proteoglycan disintegration (staphylococci)
Coagulase	Activate fibrinogen, coat bacteria with fibrin, inhibit phagocytosis; promote intravascular coagulation (staphylococcal coagulase)
Streptokinase	Activate plasma; initiate fibrinolysis
IgA protease	Neutralize antibodies (streptococci, *Hemophilus* spp., *Neisseria* spp.)
Protease	Degrade fibronectin, inhibit phagocytosis (*Pseudomonas aeruginosa*)
Adenyl cyclase stimulator	Stimulate adenyl cyclase in membranes to produce cylic AMP and enhance electrolyte secretion (*Vibrio cholera, E. coli*)

project from the surface; they are important in adhesion of bacteria to the gut lumen and colonization of tissue surfaces. In several species of bacteria, virulent isolates are piliated while nonvirulent isolates lack pili. Pili may be composed of different proteins that function in adhesion. Pili on enteropathogenic *E. coli* of swine contain a protein called K88 that promotes attachment to intestinal epithelium. Vaccines made of purified K88-containing pili have been effective in colibacillosis of pigs and calves.

Several bacteria possess a slimy amorphous *capsule* of complex polysaccharides that inhibits phagocytosis (Fig. 28.6). The capsule of *Bacillus anthracis* effectively prevents phagocytosis by neutrophils and macrophages so that septicemia can develop. Other pathogenic bacteria elaborate soluble factors that suppress the host's cellular defense mechanisms. Tubercle bacilli contain complex lipids that in some way inhibit the fusion of phagocytes and lysosomes. Intracellular killing and digestion are suppressed, and bacteria can replicate to produce disease.

Gram-negative bacteria contain lipopolysaccharides in the cell walls, known as *endotoxin*, that greatly modify the host's inflammatory responses. Cell degeneration and death may be caused by *exotoxins* (toxic components of the bacterium) or by soluble toxins released during bacterial replication. The ultimate pathogenicity of a bacterium is largely determined by how effectively it produces these toxic factors (Table 28.14).

FUNGI

Fungi are single-celled, nucleated plant organisms that include not only a wide variety of pathogenic species but also yeasts, molds, mushrooms, and mildews. The simplest form is the single-celled budding yeast. In culture, most fungi consist of networks of hyphae called mycelia. Individual hyphae form by elongation of the fungal cells without separation into new cells. Fungi grow by producing new hyphae at the edge of the mycelium (vegetative growth). Many fungi form specialized reproductive bodies, or *spores*. Asexual spores arise by differentiation of cells of spore-bearing hyphae without fusion; sexual spores are produced by fusion of two cells.

With few exceptions, fungi pathogenic for vertebrates are classed as *Fungi Imperfecti;* the two important groups are the pathogenic yeasts and the dermatophytes (Table 28.15). Most of the important pathogens are *dimorphic;* that is, their typical growth forms are different in tissue and in saprophytic stages in culture. For example, in histoplasmosis, the causal organism, *Histoplasma capsulatum,* is found as small, budding yeast cells within macrophages. In culture, this organism grows as septate mycelia with microconidia and tuberculate chlamydospores.

Fungi cause three types of disease in animals: (1) *mycosis,* the direct invasion of tissue by fungal cells; (2) *allergic disease,* the development of hypersensitivity to fungal antigens; and (3)

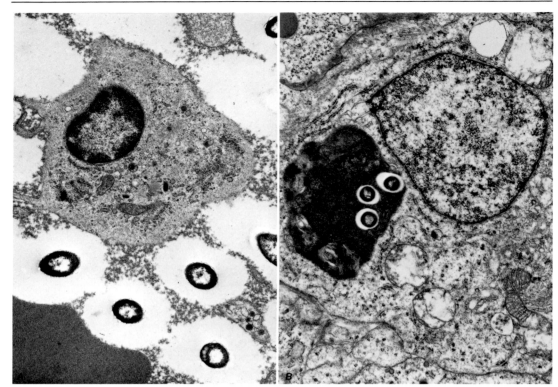

Fig. 28.6. Bacteria suppress macrophage function by different mechanisms. A. Anthrax. *Bacillus anthracis* produces a thick capsule that is antiphagocytic and prevents uptake by the monocyte or macrophage. B. Tuberculosis. *Mycobacterium* spp. are taken into macrophage phagosomes but produce cell wall lipids that prevent fusion of lysosomes with bacteria-containing phagosomes.

mycotoxicosis, the ingestion of toxic fungal metabolites. It is not unusual for mycosis and allergic disease to occur together, especially when infection of the lung is involved.

Imperfect immune responses lead to fungal infections.

Most fungi are omnipresent in the environment, so host resistance is a dominant factor in disease. Opportunistic fungal infections result when animals are immunosuppressed, when their mechanisms of inflammation are inhibited, and when stress is placed on their systems over long periods. Newborn and very old animals are most often affected by these factors. In immunosuppression produced by drugs, *Aspergillus* spp. and *Candida* spp. commonly produce complicating systemic infections. While aspergillosis usually occurs in the lungs, candidiasis commonly involves the kidneys. Localization in renal tissue involves attachment by specialized glycoproteins on the surface of the fungal spore, and tissue invasion occurs by specialized germ tubules that form and penetrate between and directly through surface epithelium of the renal cortex (Fig. 28.7).

Aerosol exposure is especially dangerous.

Inhalation is the most significant factor in enabling fungal infections to become established. The size of the fungal cell inhaled is important. In the mammalian lung, nothing over 10 μm that penetrates the nose reaches the lungs, while almost everything under 2 μm reaches the alveoli and is retained. The gastrointestinal tract, despite the ingestion of large numbers of spores, is seldom the site of primary fungal infection. One notable exception involves fungi associated with

FOCUS

Colibacillosis

Escherichia coli, a major pathogen in mammals and birds, causes *diarrhea* in young animals, *mastitis,* and *purulent infections* of the umbilicus and genitourinary tract. Because some strains of *E. coli* enter the bloodstream, they not only cause *septicemia* but lodge in organs and produce organ infections such as meningoencephalitis, osteomyelitis, and pyelitis. In the intestine, two distinct mechanisms of disease are caused by *E. coli*: *diarrhea* results from *enterotoxin* production, and *dysentery* from direct invasion of the gut wall.

Acute *enterotoxic colibacillosis* occurs in pigs, calves, lambs, and man as profuse water diarrhea that can lead to fatal dehydration and acidosis. Bacteria adhere tightly to the surface of intestine and are not washed out of the gut by peristalsis. Dr. Harley Moon, at the National Animal Disease Center, has shown that even though bacteria are confined to the gut they secrete *enterotoxins* that produce little or no structural damage. They do cause absorptive cells of the small intestine to secrete increased water and electrolytes, and when secretion exceeds the capacity of the colon to absorb water, diarrhea occurs.

Enteroinvasive colibacillosis is rare compared with enterotoxin disease. It occurs when *E. coli* attach to and actually invade absorptive cells of the gut to cause dysentery. The lesions involve severe inflammation of the mucosa, often with microulceration. J. E. Peeters and colleagues, at the National Institute of Veterinary Research in Brussels, studied enteropathogenic *E. coli* isolated from rabbits and showed that it was closely attached to apical surfaces of epithelial cells of dome epithelium of Peyer's patches in the ileum, and later to enterocytes of the distal small intestine, cecum, and colon.

Poorly characterized toxins of *E. coli* are associated with angiopathy and *edema disease* of baby pigs. Dr. Harry Kurtz and colleagues, at the University of Minnesota, have shown that degenerative angiopathy of arterioles and small arteries in several tissues develops as necrosis of smooth muscle cells of the media is followed by exudation and inspissation of albumen and other plasma proteins in the necrotic media. Common in arteries in the mesocolon and colic lymph node. Vascular degeneration in the brain causes ischemia, focal necrosis (malacia), and hemorrhage.

In birds, *E. coli* is a common cause of *septicemia.* It is an inhabitant of the intestinal tract of the normal bird. Most of these bacteria are nonpathogenic, and *E. coli* is rarely implicated in diarrhea in birds. Colisepticemia is especially devastating in turkeys. It involves three different but overlapping syndromes: *acute colisepticemia, subacute fibrinopurulent serositis* with lesions of airsacculitis and pericarditis, and *chronic granulomatous* pneumonitis/hepatitis/enteritis. Disease arises by extension of inhaled, feces-contaminated litter dust to the lower respiratory tract and then to the bloodstream. It is a respiratory tract disease that is maintained by carrier status of *E. coli* within the intestine. Dr. Larry Arp, at Iowa State University, has shown that bacteria are trapped in the liver and spleen and produce widespread lesions throughout the bird.

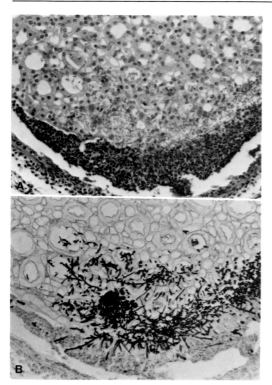

Fig. 28.7. Special stains identify fungi in tissue sections. A. Necrosis of renal papilla with neutrophil infiltration. B. Adjacent section stained for fungi, methenamine silver stain to show *Candida* sp.

bovine mycotic placentitis and abortion, in which the disease appears to follow ingestion of spores. The urogenital tract is rarely affected because fungi are swept away by mucous secretions. The bovine teat is an important orifice for infection, and mycotic mastitis results from several species of fungi.

PROTOZOA

The phylum Protozoa is composed of one-celled animals. Only a few of the thousands of protozoal species are pathogenic for animals, and most pathogenic species are associated with diseases of the blood, reticuloendothelial system, or intestinal tract. The major classes of pathogenic Protozoa are (1) flagellates, (2) amebas, (3) telosporea, (4) piroplasms (plasmodia, babesia, and other blood cell parasites), and (5) toxoplasmas.

Phylum Sarcomastigophora
Amebiasis

Amebae commonly infect the intestine of animals but are rarely implicated in disease. Parasites replicate in the gut lumen and live on digested food, erythrocytes, and other microorganisms. They are amorphous, large (15–50 μm) cells that move by the extension of pseudopodia. *Entamoeba histolytica,* a pathogen for primates, kills host cells on contact, allegedly by using its own lysosomes. Other free-living amebae can cause disease in immunosuppressed hosts or by gaining access to the brain.

Trypanosomiasis

All pathogenic hemoflagellates require a bloodsucking insect vector as an intermediate host. During their life cycle, these protozoa display a variety of structural manifestations typical for the growth phase in a particular host and tissue. Four forms are known, based on the type and position of the flagellum: crithidial, leptomonad, leishmanial, and trypanosomal (Table 28.15 and Fig. 28.8). In general, the flagellated stages inhabit body fluids in vertebrates and the alimentary canal in insects; leishmanial stages are found intracellularly.

Trypanosomiasis, a group of diseases important in tropical regions, involves a vertebrate host (which at some stage manifests a parasitemia) and a bloodsucking invertebrate. When taken into the gut of the latter, the parasite undergoes transformation through one or more

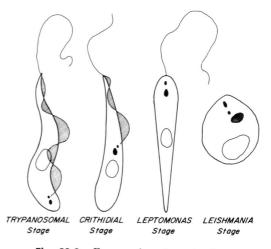

Fig. 28.8. Forms of pathogenic flagellates during phases of their life cycles.

Table 28.15. Classification of pathogenic protozoa

Subphylum	Subclassification		Genera
Sarcomastigophora	Amebas		*Entamoeba*
	Flagellates		
	Hemoflagellates		*Trypanosoma, Leishmania*
	Mucosoflagellates	Diplomonads	*Giardia*
		Trichomonads	*Trichomonas*
Apicomplexa	Hemosporidians	Piroplasmoses	*Babesia, Theileria, Cytauxzoon*
		Malarias	*Plasmodium, Leukocytozoon, Haemoproteus, Hepatocystis*
	Coccidia		*Eimeria, Isopora, Cryptosporidia, Toxoplasma, Sarcocystis, Frenkelia, Hammondia, Besnoitia*
Ciliophora			*Balantidium coli, Ichthyophthirius*
Microspora			*Encephalitozoon*

stages (the leishmanial, leptomonad, or crithidial forms) that are not infective to the vertebrate host. The final infective stage is the trypanosome stage. Trypanosomes localize in the brain, myocardium, subcutis, lymphoid organs, and mesenchymal tissues.

Flies inject trypanosomes into a cow's bloodstream. The cow makes antibody that destroys nearly 99% of the organisms, but a few survive by changing the proteins on their surfaces. Trypanosomes are able to switch surface coats at regular intervals so that every time the host develops antibodies to the trypanosomes' surface proteins, the antibodies have no effect. The trypanosomes remain one step ahead of the host's humoral immune defenses. By defying vaccination, these organisms prevent certain breeds of cattle from living in a large area of Africa.

Dr. V. Valli, at the Ontario Veterinary College, used *Trypanosoma congolense* in calves as a model to show that blood vessel damage was the primary lesion and that there was a generalized dilatation of the microvasculature, which was most prominent in the liver and mesentery. Anemia was common, and the number of circulating erythrocytes varied directly with the degree of parasitemia. The liver was the major site of erythrocyte destruction. Lymphoid hyperplasia was a prominent lesion in infected calves.

Leishmaniasis

Leishmaniasis is characterized by cutaneous, visceral, and ophthalmic lesions in mammals. The causal organisms of human cutaneous (*L. tropica*) and visceral (*L. donovani*) leishmaniasis also produce lesions in dogs. Lesions consist of aggregates of infected macrophages throughout the reticuloendothelial system. The large foamy macrophages contain protozoa and mimic the lesions of systemic fungal infections such as histoplasmosis.

The life cycle of *Leishmania* spp. involves two distinct stages. Flagellated promastigotes live extracellularly in the gut of insect phlebotomes. On transmission to a vertebrate host they are taken up by macrophages and transform into nonflagellated amastigotes. Amastigotes are obligatory parasites of macrophages and lodge in modified phagolysosomes called *parasitophorous vacuoles.*

Circulating erythrocytes and leukocytes are affected in visceral leishmaniasis. Dr. Roger Broderson, working at the Communicable Disease Center in Atlanta with owl monkeys infected with *L. donovani,* reported anemia, granulocytopenia, thrombocytopenia, and lymphocytosis. Parasitized macrophages were most prominent in the liver, spleen, bone marrow, and lymph nodes. The intense antigenic stimulus that persists in chronic leishmaniasis often leads to amyloidosis. Drs. Jeanne George and Svend Nielsen have reported widespread secondary amyloid in a Great Dane with chronic leishmaniasis.

Phylum Apicomplexa
Malaria

Plasmodium spp., the cause of malaria of reptiles, birds, and mammals, require two hosts for survival: an invertebrate, in which sexual reproduction occurs, and a vertebrate, in which they multiply asexually. A bite by an infected female mosquito introduces sporozoites into the vertebrate host.

An *extraerythrocytic phase* is initiated by infection of different tissues. In birds, the reticuloendothelial system is usually involved and in mammals, the liver. During this phase, the organism goes through several asexual reproductions: sporozoites transform to trophozoites, to multinucleate schizonts, and finally to mature schizonts. The end result is an immense host cell containing unicellular merozoites. On their release, the extracellular merozoites then either invade new cells and repeat the extraerythrocytic cycle or begin the *erythrocytic phase* by infecting red blood cells.

Fever, weakness, and anemia are signs of malaria. Characteristic periodic fever results from the synchronous release of merozoites and toxic peptides produced by plasmodia. In some infections, groups of parasites lodge in and block capillaries. When sequestered in the *brain,* they can cause death.

Coccidiosis

All members of the class Sporozoa are parasitic. They produce spores that contain one to several sporozoites. In coccidia, whose life cycle is completed in one host, the spore membrane is thick and resistant and protects the sporozoites while they are outside the host. The spore membrane is always thin and fragile in species that require two hosts. The organism is protected in an invertebrate host, where replication is required for it to infect the primary vertebrate host.

In general, the three stages in the sporozoan life cycle are (1) *schizogony* of sporozoites to produce many merozoites, (2) *gametogony,* or sexual reproduction, and (3) *sporogony,* in which the zygote divides to form multiple sporozoites. Sporogony may take place within delicate oocysts in the body of invertebrates or take place outside the body of the host in protective oocysts. In either case, the sporozoites are infective when swallowed by or injected into the appropriate host.

Coccida are a significant cause of diarrhea and death in suckling pigs. Lesions vary from atrophy of intestinal villi to foci of necrosis of the mucosa that are associated with bacterial invasion. Dr. Scott Eustis and colleagues inoculated *Isospora suis* in piglets and produced tenacious white fibrinonecrotic membranes covering the surface of the distal jejunum and ileum.

Toxoplasmosis

Toxoplasma gondii, a coccidian parasite, has an intestinal epithelial cycle for the production of oocysts only in cats and other Felidae. It under-

goes schizogony and microgametogony in the feline ileum. Oocysts are shed in the feces and are infectious after sporulation occurs. These asexual forms can propagate in macrophages and myocytes of different mammals.

On entering the secondary host, endozoites spread to muscle and other tissue after infecting circulating monocytes. Once inside the muscle cell, the organism is confined to a parasitophorous vacuole. Encysted cystozoites appear in muscle in about 2 weeks, as immunity becomes detectable. Crescent-shaped daughter parasites develop from the infecting ones. The thick cyst wall seen in inapparent chronic infection is a dense outer layer of host cell origin and an inner thin membrane of parasite origin. The host reaction consists of necrosis of infected cells and an attendant accumulation of macrophage and neutrophils (see Parker, *Vet. Pathol.* 18:786, 1981).

Sarcosporidiosis

Sarcocystis spp. parasitize cardiac and skeletal muscles of mammals, birds, and reptiles. Typically, there is no inflammatory reaction around encysted organisms in myocytes, and cysts are found incidentally at necropsy. Visible as white dots or streaks, these intracellular organisms are surrounded by a thick cyst wall of both host and parasite origin.

In the 1970s, studies by Drs. Anthony Johnson and Paul Hildebrandt, at the Walter Reed Army Institute of Research, and by Paul Frelier, at Cornell University, focused attention on *acute bovine sarcocystosis,* a febrile disease that occurs during schizogony of *S. cruzi* within vascular endothelium. Blood studies by Dr. Keith Prasse, at the University of Georgia, showed anemia, decreased serum proteins, and increased tissue enzymes during acute disease; platelets and coagulation factors were abnormal just prior to death. *Abortion* in pregnant cows occurs 30–40 days after sporocysts are ingested. Edema and foci of necrosis occur in placentomes. Experiments in pregnant cattle by Dr. Dean Barnett revealed that ovarian corpora lutea are infected and that luteal regression is correlated with diminished plasma progesterone and abortion.

Microsporidia

Encephalitozoon cuniculi infects the brain of rabbits, dogs, and wild carnivores. Although most infections are subclinical and have little inflammatory reaction around the parasites, *E.*

FOCUS

Cryptosporidiosis

Cryptosporidia have been described as parasites of mice since 1843. In 1971, Roger Panciera, Robert Thomassen, and Floris Garner reported these tiny organisms adhering to the surfaces of epithelial cells in the intestine of calves. Reports in other species followed in rapid succession: Robert Kovatch found them in intestine of monkeys, Oscar Fletcher discovered them in chicken tracheas in Georgia, and David Brownstein reported them in the stomach of snakes in zoos in Baltimore and Washington, D.C.

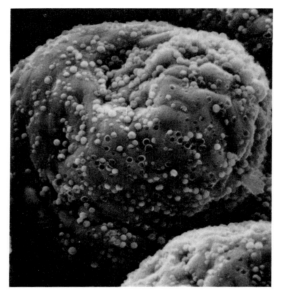

Scanning electron micrograph of atrophic villi to which cryptosporidia adhere. (Micrograph: Joachim Pohlenz, *Vet. Pathol.* 15:417, 1978)

Stanley Snyder, at Colorado State University, reported cryptosporidia in foals with combined immunodeficiency, suggesting that immunosuppression enhances infection. This was also reported in man, and in 1982, Dr. Harley Moon, collaborating with physicians, transmitted cryptosporidia from persistently infected humans to pigs via fecal material. The infected pigs had organisms in the ileum, cecum, and colon and were associated with atrophic ileal villi and flattened colonic surfaces.

Cryptosporidia appear to be attached to cell surfaces outside the cell. However, recent electron microscopic studies using the freeze fracture technique have shown that plasma membranes of the host cells fold upward and surround the protozoa. They are thus intracellular parasites.

cuniculi can cause encephalitis. Parasite cysts are surrounded by lymphoplasmacytic infiltrates and form tiny granulomas. Encephalitozoonosis is most serious in young pups, in which it causes weakness, circling, and convulsions. Drs. John Shadduck and Ray Bendele were the first to isolate *E. cuniculi* from pups and grow it in culture. The kidney is the target organ and chronic interstitial nephritis is typically present in fatal cases. Dr. Knut Nordstoga, at the Veterinary School in Oslo, Norway, has reported transplacental transmission of encephalitozoonosis in blue foxes. Dr. W. S. Botha has recently reproduced the disease in South Africa by feeding urine to young dogs.

ALGAE

Algae are aquatic, nonvascular plants. The most serious pathogenic group is *Prototheca* spp., colorless algae that replicate freely in stagnant water and decaying organic matter. They are associated with focal and disseminated granulomatous lesions of animals and man, generally as a rare, isolated disease in an immunosuppressed host. In tissue, algae occur as single endospores or as large sporangia containing multiple sporangiospores (daughter cells); both occur in macrophages. Protothecal cells have thick cell walls, large nuclei, and large numbers of starch granules.

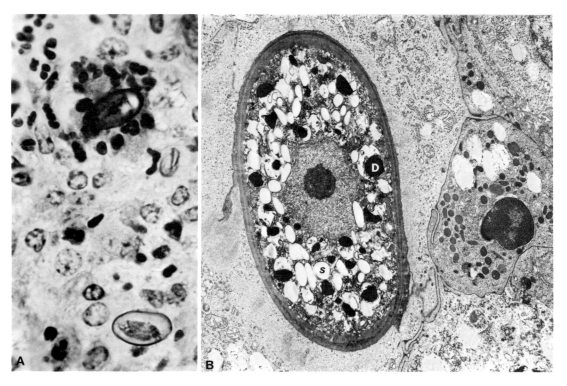

Fig. 28.9. *Prototheca zopfii,* cow with chronic granulomatous mastitis. A. Algae are killed by neutrophilic leukocytes when they are extracellular (*top*). When phagocytized by macrophages (*bottom*), the algae are protected from neutrophil activity. B. Within the macrophage the thick outer wall of glycoproteins prevents fusion with lysosomes and permits replication. Starch granules (*S*) and dense bodies (*D*) are in algae. Note vacuolated, granular neutrophil (*right*), which has cell membrane interdigitated with that of the macrophage.

Prototheca are an important cause of *mastitis* in cattle (Fig. 28.9) and occur incidentally in most other species. Dr. Herbert Van Kruiningen, at the University of Connecticut, reported severe enterocolitis in dogs, in which masses of organisms occupied the tunica propria. Dr. David Tyler and others, at the University of Georgia, described severe nervous system lesions associated with lodging and growth of prototheca.

Blue-green algae

In ruminants, ingestion of large amounts of blue-green algae can cause enteric infection, liver necrosis, and death. Dr. A. R. Jackson, at the Regional Veterinary Laboratory at Armidale, Australia, inoculated young sheep intraruminally with an algal bloom of *Microcystis aeruginosa*. The sheep developed elevations in serum enzymes and reduced blood glucose. They died 18–24 hours later with widespread hemorrhages and acute cell swelling and necrosis of hepatocytes.

INVERTEBRATE PARASITES

Metazoan parasites of vertebrate animals fall into five major groups: arthropods, penta-stomids, platyhelminths (flatworms), acanthocephalids, and nematodes (roundworms) (Table 28.16). The last group, which deserves special emphasis because it causes the most serious economic losses, is the largest and most diverse. Each group of parasites has gross characteristics and produces typical eggs or young that parasitologists use for identification.

In tissue sections, parasites are identified by comparing their integument, musculature, body cavities, digestive tracts, and reproductive systems. *Eggs* are commonly present in tissue sections and are an important aid in diagnosis; for example, eggs of *Trichuris* spp. have a double polar cap while those of *Oxyuris* spp. have a single polar cap. *Larvae,* which are also used for identification, may be present surrounding the parasite or in cross sections of the ovary or uterus of the female. In viviparous nematodes, ova embryonate and hatch in the uterus. Ovoviviparous nematodes produce ova that are embryonated but with larvae remaining within the eggshell as the eggs are deposited.

Invertebrate parasites produce disease by a wide variety of mechanisms (Table 28.17). Most parasites damage the host by mechanically obstructing ducts or vascular channels. Obstruction may result from masses of parasites or from the granulomas produced by the parasites' presence. Parasites nearly always are themselves in-

Table 28.16. Classification of pathogenic metazoan parasites

Phylum	Subclassification	Important Pathogens
Arthropoda	Class Arachnida	
	Metastigmata (ticks)	*Ixodes* spp.
	Mesostigmata (mites)	*Pneumonyssus* spp.
	Astigmata (mites)	*Sarcoptes* spp.
	Prostigmata (mites)	*Demodex* spp.
	Class Insecta	
	Siphonaptera	Fleas
	Anoplura	Sucking lice
	Mallophaga	Chewing lice
	Diptera	Flies
		Mosquitos, order Culicidae
		Bot flies, order Gasterophilidae
		Black flies, order Simuliidae
Nematoda	Order Ascarida	*Ascaris* spp.
	Order Ancyclostomida	*Ancyclostoma* spp.
	Order Rhabditida	*Strongyloides* spp.
	Order Spirurida	
	Superfamily Trichuroidea	*Trichinella spiralis*
	Superfamily Filarioidea	*Dirofilaria* spp.,
	Superfamily Trichostrongyloidea	*Ostertagia* spp., *Haemonchus* spp.
Platyhelminthes	Class Cestoda	*Taenia* spp., *Echinococcus* spp.
	Class Trematoda	*Fasciola* spp., *Schistosoma* spp.
Acanthocephala		*Macrocanthorynchus* spp., *Prosthenorchis* spp.
Annelida	Class Hirudinea	Leeches

Table 28.17.   Mechanisms of tissue injury by metazoan parasites

Mechanism	Parasite	Animal
Obstruction of lumina	*Dirofilaria immitis*	Dog (heart)
	Ascaris spp.	Pig (intestine)
	Metastrongylus spp.	Pig (lung)
	Liver fluke	Several (bile duct)
Irritation	Fleas	Many (skin)
Epithelial destruction	*Trichostronylus* spp.	Sheep (stomach)
	Hookworms	Dog (intestine)
	Strongylus spp.	Horse (large intestine)
Anemia	Hookworms	Dog (intestine)
	Strongyles	Horse (intestine)
	Stomach worms	
Carry pathogenic viruses	*Culicoides* spp.	Many (skin)
Bluetongue		
African horse sickness		
Bovine ephemeral fever		
Viral encephalitides		
Carry pathogenic protozoa	Several spp.	Mammals, birds, etc.
Haemoproteus		
Leukocytozoon		
Hepatocystis		
Carry pathogenic nematodes	*Culicoides* spp.	Dog
Dirofilaria immitis		Man
Wuchereria bancrofti		
Onchocerca cervicalis		

fected with bacteria. After creating wounds in epithelium they carry pathogenic bacteria into tissue (see Fig. 1.9).

Parasites that suck blood produce chronic anemia.

Chronic anemia caused by bloodsucking nematodes or insects may be lethal, especially in young animals. Some bloodsucking nematodes release an anticlotting substance that promotes blood flow. Adult hookworms, using a buccal cavity and hooklike teeth, attach to villi of the small intestine. The hookworm secretes a protease that inhibits fibrin clot formation and even promotes dissolution of clots as they form. Each worm can extract 0.2 ml blood per day, and in heavy infestations, this eventually leads to both hypoalbuminemia and chronic iron-deficiency anemia (see anemia, Chapter 17).

Parasites can alter the host's immune response.

Parasite surfaces are especially important in recovery stages because they contain substances that make the parasite refractory to an immune response. Large amounts of proteins shaved off the parasite surface may inhibit re-

sponses of inflammatory cells. On the other hand, some parasites release fragments of surface proteins or secrete toxins that act as potent antigens to induce *hypersensitivity reactions.* For example, ascaris surface antigens cause the host to become hypersensitive. Smashing ox warbles in the skin of cattle releases enough surface antigens to cause *anaphylaxis.*

Nematodes

Nematodes are unsegmented worms that are usually dioecious (male and female sex organs in different individuals). They have a body cavity (pseudocoelom) lined by a single layer of muscle attached to the body wall. The hypodermis is thinner than the somatic musculature. Internal hypodermal projections (chords) are present that usually separate somatic muscles into fields (Fig. 28.10).

Ascariasis

Adult ascarids (roundworms) parasitize the intestinal tract of mammals and birds. They feed on ingesta and cause growth retardation by depriving the host of nutrients. Adult worms are motile and may enter the biliary system and

FOCUS

Trichinosis

James Paget, a first-year medical student at St. Bartholomew's Hospital in London in 1835, discovered larvae of the roundworm *Trichinella spiralis*. Dissecting a human cadaver, he noted that small white specks in muscle were cysts with tiny worms inside. It was not until 1859 that clinical trichinosis was diagnosed. A German girl, preparing meat for Christmas, developed fever and myalgia. Brought to a Dresden hospital, she died after 15 days of excruciating muscle pain. When the pathologist Zenker removed a sliver of muscle from her arm, crushed it, and examined it microscopically, he saw dozens of tiny worms wriggling about. Once established as a disease, several severe outbreaks of trichinosis were recorded and the life cycle of the parasite was determined.

The adult life of *T. spiralis* is spent in the small intestine of many species of carnivores. Adult worms lie *within* the cytoplasm of absorptive and goblet cells. Threaded through rows of enterocytes, they often cannot be seen on the mucosal surface. The viviparous female burrows into the lamina propria of the intestinal villi and deposits her larvae directly into the intestinal lymphatics. Larvae exit in lymph, pass through the mesenteric lymphatics and thoracic duct, and enter the bloodstream. During circulation through the skeletal muscles, they enter myocytes and become *encysted*.

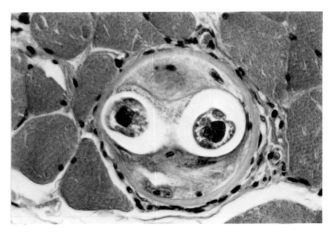

Early cyst of *Trichinella spiralis* in muscle.

The cyst both nourishes and protects the larvae from host defense mechanisms. Eosinophilic and neutrophilic leukocytes and plasmacytes (which contain antitrichina antibody) develop around the cysts, but their effect on encysted larvae is negligible. When the host is killed and its muscle eaten by a new potential carnivore host, intestinal enzymes digest the capsule, and the liberated larvae burrow into the intestine to begin their life cycle anew.

▶

▶

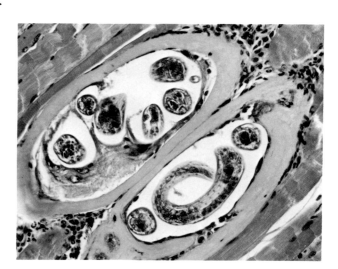

Late lesion with lymphoid cells surrounding the parasite.

Trichinosis is transmitted by eating raw or undercooked meat that contains larvae of *T. spiralis*. Every mammal is susceptible to the disease, but pigs are one of the few carnivores that people eat, so pork is the main source of human infection. Members of an arctic expedition around 1900 died when they ate raw *Trichinella*-infected polar bear meat. In North America, trichinosis causes several deaths each year. Sixty cases were reported to the Centers for Disease Control in 1984 (only about 1 in 3000 cases of human infection is diagnosed).

In the late 1800s, Europeans began using "trichinoscopes" to diagnose larvae in commercial meat, using pork diaphragm muscle. Another diagnostic method involved digestion of pork muscle with acidified pepsin, which releases the worms. In 1891, the United States began inspecting pork using the trichinoscope. Inspection was done on pork to be exported but not pork to be sold domestically (it added 64 cents to each pound of meat). Europe enacted other protective laws to keep American pork from flooding their markets, and in 1906, inspection in the United States ceased.

Infection stimulates specific immune responses at various stages of the life cycle, each of which can inhibit development of the parasite at several points in the life cycle. Recently, glycoproteins secreted by stichocytes (secretory cells that discharge products into the parasite esophagus during early intestinal infection) have been used to prepare vaccines. Mice immunized with these antigens expel adult worms from the intestine and inhibit fecundity of adult females.

pancreatic ducts to produce blockage.

Ascarid eggs are eaten by a new host and pass to the intestine where larvae emerge. Most ascarid species follow a unique *tracheal migration* route: larvae penetrate the intestine, pass to the liver, enter the lungs, break through pulmonary capillaries, enter alveoli, ascend via the airways to the trachea, are coughed up and swallowed, and pass to the intestine where they develop into adults.

Most of this pathway does not produce clinical disease, although hemorrhage and pneumonic areas occur during passage through the lung. Aberrant larvae also migrate through somatic tissues to produce granulomatous reactions. Prenatal infections can occur and infections of neonates can occur through passage of larvae into the mammary gland and out in the milk.

Adults of most ascarids are host-specific but larvae are not. Migrating larvae cause disease in other animal species. *Visceral larva migrans* is a disease of children infected with larvae of *Toxocara canis* that may produce serious disease in the eye.

Platyhelminths

Platyhelminths are tapeworms and flukes. They are the only tissue parasite with a body cavity filled with parenchyma. In tissue sections, they are flattened dorsoventrally; they have smooth muscles and are monoecious (both sex organs in one individual). Several criteria differentiate cestodes and trematodes (Table 28.18).

Cestodes

Cestodes parasitize nearly all vertebrate species. Adults exist as multiple flat segments called *proglottids,* joined at the ends in a long chain, and adhered to intestinal walls by the *scolex,* which is used in classifying different species. The scolex may have two or more elongate suctorial grooves, sucking discs and a proboscis,

often with hooklets. In tissue, the presence of a germinal tissue layer containing scoleces (or brood capsules with scoleces) is diagnostic for cestodes.

As the tapeworm grows, the most caudal proglottids are released into feces. Tapeworms produce little effect on the host, except in massive infestations. Lesions in affected intestine include erosions in the mucosa and atrophic villi. Larvae of some of the more important tapeworms produce *cysticercosis* ("beef measles"). The adult tapeworm (*Taenia saginata*) is a tapeworm of man; the intermediate stages are larvae (with a different speciation, *Cysticercus bovis*) that embed in cardiac and skeletal muscle of cattle, the intermediate host. *Cysticercus cellulosae,* found in pork muscle, is the intermediate stage of *Taenia solium,* another tapeworm of man. *Coenurus cerebralis* is the larval stage of the dog tapeworm, *Multiceps multiceps,* the etiologic agent of a brain infestation of sheep.

Echinococcus spp. are important tapeworms of cats, canidae, and other carnivores. Intermediate hosts are ruminants, horses, pigs, man, rodents, and others. Larvae form cysts in the liver, brain, and other viscera (see Fig. 3.5). Like neoplasms, the cysts grow slowly but expand to produce pressure injury on tissue.

Trematodes (flukes)

Distomiasis includes infestations of the genera *Fasciola* (common, large African, and large liver flukes) and *Dicrocoelium* (lancet liver fluke). Metacercaria of *F. hepatica* are ingested, pass the gut wall into the peritoneum, and migrate to the liver. Adult flukes are in the liver, bile ducts, and gall bladder, especially of cattle and sheep. Flukes reproduce by depositing ova in biliary canals. Free-living *miracidia* are formed, which penetrate snails. Metacercariae emerge from the snail, encyst on plants, and are ingested by cattle and sheep. They pass to the intestine, escape from the cyst, penetrate the gut wall, and migrate to the liver.

Table 28.18. Differentiating characteristics of platyhelminths

Character	Cestodes (tapeworms)	Trematodes (flukes)
Calcareous corpuscles	+	−
Segmented, ribbonlike	+	−
Digestive tract	−	+
Attachment mechanism	Scolex	Oral or ventral sucker
Cuticle	Thick	Thinner
Reproductive organs	Elaborate	Simple

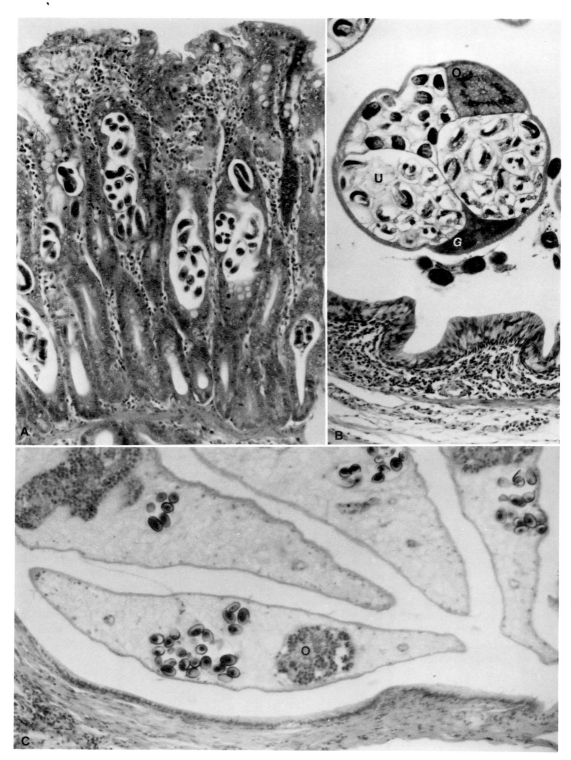

Fig. 28.10. Parasite structure. A. Nematode: *Strongyloides* sp., intestine, chimpanzee. Ova and developing larvae invade deeply into the mucosa. B. Nematode: *Metastrongylus* sp., lung, pig. Uterus (*U*), ovary (*O*) with rachis, and gut (*G*). Mucous hyperplasia of epithelium with underlying lymphoeosinophilic peribronchiolitis. C. Trematode, *Athesmia foxi,* liver, monkey. The dilated bile duct contains parasite; eggs are in the uterus. Ovary (*O*).

Arthropods

Two classes of the phylum Arthropoda are parasitic: Insecta and Arachnida. Insects include mites, fly larvae, and ticks (which usually do not penetrate tissue). *Myiasis* is invasion of living tissue by larvae of flies of the order Diptera; it occurs in skin (ox warbles), stomach (equine bots), nasal cavity (nose bot of sheep), and in wounds. *Acariasis,* infestation of ticks and mites, is most often cutaneous (see scabies in the fox, Fig. 20.5), although pulmonary acariasis of monkeys is caused by *Pneumonyssus simicola* (see Fig. 7.3).

Spiders secrete venoms that cause inflamma-tion in the bite area and in rare infestations, neurologic diseases (see arthropod toxins and venoms, Chapter 27).

The morphologic characteristics of arthropods that are used in identification in tissue section include (1) chitinous exoskeleton, (2) striated muscles, (3) small or vestigial body cavity (haemocoel), (4) jointed appendages, (5) metameric segmentation, and (6) malpighian tubules and tracheoles. Most arthropods have other distinguishing characteristics; for example, *Pneumonyssus* spp. have no external segmentation and a poorly chitinized exoskeleton; *Sarcoptes* spp. have spines on the dorsum (*Psoroptes* and *Chorioptes* do not).

FOCUS

Mechanical versus biological transmission of microbes by insects

Most insects carry bacteria and fungi and pass them, via *mechanical transmission,* from animal to animal. Their feet contain thousands of tiny hairs to which microbes attach. As flies flit from host to host, bacteria drop onto and infect new hosts. The likelihood of this occurring is enhanced by a preference to feed on fluids around wounds or body orifices.

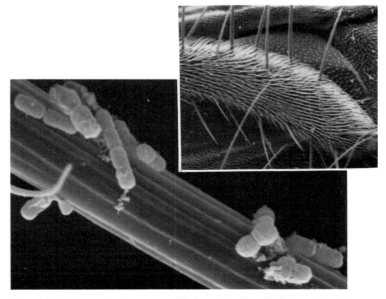

Moraxella bovis attached to external hairs of the face fly *Musca domestica.*

▶

The most common means of transmission of bacteria is through the gut of the insect. This is particularly important in the case of wounds, infected milk round teats, and aborted placentas. In brucella placentitis enormous numbers of *Brucella abortus* are swarming. Fluids from the placenta in bovine brucellosis can be milky because of the high content of bacteria. Flies of the genera *Musca* preferentially feed on placental exudates. Infected fluids sucked into the mouthparts pass rapidly into the midgut of the fly, where they are stored for several hours and the residue excreted by the fly. As fly feces contaminated with pathogenic bacteria are excreted on a new host, the disease is passed to mucosae of the conjunctivae or other body orifices.

Biological transmission, in which microorganisms replicate inside the insect, is a required part of the life cycle of certain viruses. Taken into the fly during a blood meal, the virus must first bind and fuse to cell surfaces of *midgut epithelium*; if glycoproteins on the virus do not match and bind with those on midgut cells, replication of virus will not occur. Once cells in the midgut are infected, new virus is disseminated into the hemocoel and then to the *salivary glands*. It replicates to high titer in gland cells and passes into a new host as the insect feeds again. Infection of the insect *ovary* is also important in those diseases that are transmitted through transovarian infection.

ADDITIONAL READING

Boothroyd, J. C. Antigenic variations in African trypanosomes. *Ann. Rev. Microbiol.* 39:475, 1985.

Chandler, F. W., et al. Differentiation between *Prototheca* and morphologically similar green algae in tissue. *Arch. Pathol. Lab. Med.* 102:353, 1978.

Chitwood, M., and Lichtenfels, J. R. Identification of parasitic metazoa in tissue sections. *Exp. Parasitol.* 32:407, 1972.

Keenan, C. M., et al. Visceral leishmaniasis in the German shepherd dog. *Vet. Pathol.* 21:74, 1984.

Middlebrook, J. L., and Dorland, R. B. Bacterial toxins. *Microbiol. Rev.* 48:199, 1984.

Pospischil, A., et al. Attaching and effacing bacteria in the intestines of calves and cats with diarrhea. *Vet. Pathol.* 24:330, 1987.

Prusiner, S. B. Prions. *Adv. Virus. Res.* 29:1, 1984.

Rogers, D. G., et al. Pathogenesis of corneal lesions caused by *Moraxella bovis* in gnotobiotic calves. *Vet. Pathol.* 24:287, 1987.

Smith, H., et al. The determinants of bacterial and viral pathogenicity. *Philos. Trans. R. Soc. Lond.* [Biol.] 303:63, 1983.

Southern, P., and Oldstone, M. B. A. Medical consequences of persistent viral infection. *New Engl. J. Med.* 314:359, 1986.

Walzer, P. D. Attachment of microbes to host cells. *Lab. Invest.* 54:589, 1986.

Nutritional Disease

THE clinical diagnosis of most nutritional deficiencies is difficult for three reasons: (1) it is not possible to find a precise etiologic agent, as it is in infectious diseases; (2) the functions of all nutrients are ultimately connected in cellular metabolism so that a deficiency of one nutrient will be compensated for by another; and (3) the precise lesions of an experimental nutritional deficiency are rarely identical to those in the naturally occurring disease. The great amount of nutritional research has furthered our understanding of the many and complex factors that lead to deficiency disease. However, much of the work has been done in laboratory rodents given purified diets, and the more complex situations that arise clinically have different signs and tissue lesions. This chapter deals with naturally occurring nutritional disease.

When the tissue concentration of a nutrient falls to a critical level, evidence of deranged metabolism appears. Abnormal metabolites first appear in tissue and then in blood, urine, and feces. As the deficiency progresses, microscopic tissue changes develop, especially in *rapidly metabolizing tissues* such as skeletal muscle, myocardium, and brain. *Immature animals are most susceptible* to nutritional disease, and rapidly growing tissues such as bone are also markedly affected. Cellular lesions slowly progress so that lesions can be seen grossly. In some nutritional disease, gross and microscopic changes are not present and the animal may sicken and die with only electrocardiographic abnormalities in the heart or brain.

The time required for a nutritional deficiency disease to develop influences the course and character of the tissue changes. Lesions of *acute* and *chronic deficiencies* are often markedly different. Swine with acute thiamine deficiency may die suddenly of cardiac failure with few lesions in cardiac muscle, while those with chronic deficiency have marked lesions in the myocardium.

Multiple deficiency is the usual case in animals; that is, a diet of poor quality is apt to be lacking in several important nutrients. When a deficiency of several essential factors occurs, syndromes develop that differ from the combined effects of individual deficiencies.

Nutritional imbalance is more common than a simple deficiency of one particular dietary factor. Some of the delicate interrelationships in nutrition are those of calcium and phosphorus, fat and calcium, and iron and phosphorus. Overlying all of this is the prospect of protein, fat, or carbohydrate excess, which ultimately influences the metabolism of other dietary constituents.

Protein/calorie malnutrition is the most common and serious nutritional disease in animals. It is a consequence of a dietary deficiency in total quantity or quality of food, and in primary form arises because there is no food available or animals are unable to feed. Protein/calorie malnutrition arises secondarily from disease. Nonnutritional diseases that are prone to be complicated by nutritional deficiency include intestinal *malabsorption diseases,* increased nutrient loss from *diarrhea, increases in demand for nutrients* due to excessive heat, cold, or work, and diseases that suppress tissue storage of nutrients (Table 29.1).

Loss of body fat and *muscle wasting* are the dominant signs of calorie deficiency. To determine the nutritional state of sheep, stockmen

Table 29.1. Factors that contribute to nutritional deficiency

Interference with intake	Anorexia
	Gastrointestinal disease
	Food allergy
	Tooth disease
Interference with absorption	Intestinal hypermotility
	Insoluble complexes forming in food (e.g., fat/Ca^{++})
Interference with storage	Hepatic disease (vitamin A)
	Thyroid disease (iodine)
Increased excretion	Polyuria
	Sweating
	Endocrine imbalances
	Lactation
Increased requirements	Fever
	Hyperthyroidism
	Pregnancy and lactation
Natural inhibitors	Thiaminases

palpate the longissimus dorsi because the spaces over the back and lateral to the vertebral spines should be filled with this muscle. Dr. Tom Hulland, at the Ontario Veterinary College, studied the longissimus dorsi in progressive atrophy of cachectic sheep and found that an early change was loss of type II muscle fibers; the reduced muscle volume resulted from alternate episodes of atrophy and hypertrophy that caused marked variation in fiber size.

CALORIE DEFICIENCY

Starvation

Food deprivation is characterized by emaciation, loss of musculature, serous atrophy of fat, subcutaneous edema, cardiac muscle degeneration, and atrophy of viscera. The liver and pancreas are markedly reduced in size, and individual hepatocytes are small. After a few days of food deprivation, hepatocyte volume decreases about 50% and the total volume of the energy-producing mitochondria may fall by 50%.

In *starvation,* the long-continued deprivation of food, fatty degeneration of the liver, anemia, and skin lesions develop but often involve mechanisms other than calorie deficiency. Fatty livers are especially common in animals on low-protein diets, in which total calorie intake is near normal but the diet is so deficient in protein that body tissues are broken down and the fats and

carbohydrates are transported to the liver to be used to synthesize protein.

There are great age and species differences in deaths during starvation. Very young and old animals are much less able to withstand food deprivation. Homeothermic animals can withstand starvation for about 2 weeks (unless hibernating), but poikilotherms can survive several months. Fish, for example, are able to survive long periods of fasting.

Food deprivation in pregnant animals may cause development to be retarded in the fetus. In starvation, abortions can occur. The neonatal period is also very important, and food deprivation may lead to failure of development of lungs and other viscera. Experimentally, intermittent starvation of rat pups leads to decreased lung size.

Intestinal involution occurs early.

Fasting has a rapid effect on renewal of epithelial cells of the intestine. Absorptive cells shrink, and their nuclei become pyknotic. Villi become shorter, and the basement membranes underlying the epithelium are markedly thickened. These changes may be due to lack of the hormonal stimulation of gut epithelium that is induced by food. Changes in the intestine closely resemble atrophic changes in other tissues (e.g., the involuting mammary gland at the cessation of lactation).

Atrophy of muscle and fat releases substitutes for food.

In early starvation, weight loss is due largely to decreases in muscle mass. Muscle protein breakdown is accompanied by loss of water (associated with loss of Ca^{++}, K^+, and Mg^{++}). As starvation progresses, the greater weight losses are accounted for by consumption of body fat, a much richer source of energy than is protein. Cortisol causes adipocytes to increase lipolysis and to liberate fatty acids. Circulating fatty acids are oxidized in the liver to acetoacetic acid and other ketones, and ketosis signals a response to depletion of body glucose. The brain of a starved animal uses ketones as a substitute source of energy.

Gluconeogenesis is an early event in food deprivation.

In early fasting, blood glucose drops (Fig. 29.1). *Insulin* levels are low, and *glucagon* levels high (relative to insulin). A consequence of the

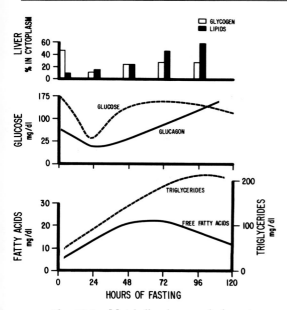

Fig. 29.1. Metabolic changes during starvation.

high glucagon:low insulin ratio is hepatic glycogen depletion. Insulin, a potent inhibitor of adipose tissue lipolysis, is the primary determinant that regulates liver changes in early starvation.

The glucocorticoid *cortisol* helps to maintain blood glucose by stimulating gluconeogenesis, chiefly in the liver. This anabolic effect on liver includes stimulation of enzymes required for gluconeogenesis and for shunting of glucose to glycogen. Cortisol has catabolic effects on skeletal muscle, adipose tissue, lymphoid tissue, and most other tissues.

In muscle, amino acids are produced to provide substrates for the liver. Of the amino acids appearing in plasma, alanine is the principal substrate for hepatic glucose production. Given by injection, alanine can increase synthesis of glucose in the liver. An alanine cycle (the conversion of alanine to glucose and reconversion to alanine) recycles a fixed supply of glucose and is an efficient means of transporting nitrogen to the liver from amino acids liberated by muscle breakdown.

Liver atrophy of food deprivation is followed by marked metabolic alterations as starvation occurs.

Within 24 hours of food deprivation, glycogen in hepatocytes and glucose in the bloodstream

are markedly decreased. Within the liver cells, there are simultaneous increases in glycogen phosphorylase (for glycogen degradation) and decreases of glycogen synthetase (for synthesis). As fasting continues, there are profound changes in other enzyme systems relating to utilization of glucose and fatty acids.

As excessive mobilization of fatty acids from adipose tissue continues in response to the negative energy balance, the liver begins to accumulate fat. Decreased protein synthesis by the atrophic hepatocytes contributes to fat accumulation by reducing the amounts of apoprotein available for secretion of triglycerides into the blood. After entering the hepatocyte, fatty acids are shunted to mitochondria where they are oxidized to acetyl CoA. Acetyl CoA formed during fatty acid oxidation enters the citric acid cycle, if fat and carbohydrate degradation are balanced. As fat breakdown predominates as the energy source, acetyl CoA accumulates and undergoes a different fate. If carbohydrate is not available, oxaloacetate is reduced and is unavailable for condensation with acetyl CoA. Thus acetyl CoA cannot enter the citric acid cycle and is diverted to acetoacetate and hydroxybutyrate (ketone bodies), which leave the cell and circulate in the bloodstream.

The prime factor leading to *ketosis* in starvation is the *insulinopenia* that develops with fasting. It leads not only to lipolysis but to changes in hepatic ketogenic enzymes and impairment of mechanisms for peripheral utilization of ketones. All three events act in concert to cause ketones to accumulate in the circulation.

As ketone production rises, ketones are increasingly utilized by the nervous system as alternative fuels to glucose. This permits reductions in gluconeogenesis and sparing of protein and is a crucial adaptive mechanism that prolongs survival in starvation.

Several factors spare energy in starvation.

The starving animal attempts to adapt to the low level of caloric intake. Diminished physical activity, loss of metabolically active tissue (with decreased caloric need), and lowering of the basal metabolic rate all play major roles. The metabolic rate is reduced in part by lowering of the serum thyroid hormone T_3 (with concomitant increase in noncalorigenic T_3 metabolites). The decrease in plasma insulin and increase in glucagon also attempt to conserve energy. In prolonged starvation, there is a shift of glucose from liver to kidney cortex; the kidney is able to synthesize glucose from amino acids.

Starvation is accelerated by trauma and infection.

Food deprivation that is associated with trauma or severe systemic infection develops more rapidly into a wasting disease. Some of this effect is mediated through the autonomic nervous system. Glucagon secretion is enhanced, insulin secretion is impaired, and the release of epinephrine is increased; free fatty acid release from fat tissue is stimulated and gluconeogenesis is accelerated. In addition to the marked hyperglycemia, there is an increase in vasopression and corticosteroid secretion during trauma, which causes decreased water excretion and sodium resorption by the kidneys.

In infections, monocytes release cytokines that selectively enhance muscle breakdown. The protein released from this process is transported to the liver where it is used both for gluconeogenesis and for synthesis of proteins released as "acute phase proteins" by the liver.

Brain respiratory centers are depressed in starvation ketosis.

Ketones dissociate to yield hydrogen ions, which use bicarbonate and depress plasma pH. At about pH 7.2, the respiratory center in the brain is stimulated. The resulting hyperventilation is an attempt to depress pH (increased loss of carbon dioxide reduces plasma carbonic acid). Further decline of pH is associated with depression of cerebral function, coma, and death.

VITAMIN DEFICIENCY

When protein/calorie nutrition is adequate, more specific nutritional deficiencies may appear. Vitamin deficiencies accompany most cases of starvation and add to the mortality of malnutrition. In specific vitamin deficiencies, animals may appear well nourished but exhibit specific signs of disease.

There are two groups of vitamins: the fat-soluble ones, A, D, E, and K, and the water-soluble ones, which include the vitamin B complex and vitamin C. The biochemical roles of the water-soluble vitamins are relatively well established, and most are components of coenzymes; for example, vitamin B_{12} (riboflavin) is a precursor of flavin adenine dinucleotide.

Vitamin A

Vitamin A alcohol (retinol) or its precursors, the carotenes, occurs in most normal diets. Both are present in plants containing yellow pigments and in animal fats and liver (e.g., cod liver oil). Beta carotene, the most important, is cleaved in the gut mucosa into two molecules of retinal (vitamin A aldehyde). After absorption, large amounts are stored in stellate, interstitial cells of the liver (liver disease impairs storage).

Squamous metaplasia of epithelium causes widespread lesions.

Squamous metaplasia of epithelial surfaces is the dominant lesion in vitamin A deficiency. Throughout the body there are widespread changes of simple types of epithelium to stratified squamous epithelium. This is most easily detected at body orifices but also occurs in viscera such as the pancreas, bladder, and other organs. It is especially important in ductal structures and has been incriminated as a cause of urolithiasis in cats, although this has not been confirmed.

From their studies on vitamin A deficiency in calves during the 1960s, Drs. Jungherr and Helmboldt, at the University of Connecticut, concluded that metaplasia of the parotid duct was pathognomonic. This was later confirmed by Dr. Svend Nielsen in calves only marginally deficient in A. In calves, clinically significant changes occur in arachnoid villi of the meninges; outflow of cerebrospinal fluid is inhibited, causing increased intracranial pressure.

Vitamin A exerts a controlling influence on development of epithelial cells. It has a steroidlike effect on nuclear transcription that causes dedifferentiation of cells followed by redifferentiation along a different pathway.

In *respiratory epithelium,* goblet cells are eliminated and replaced with keratin-synthesizing squamous cells. Foci of hyperplastic basal cells develop and expand, causing cells to desquamate. As basal cells enlarge, they gradually convert to keratin production.

Teeth are often abnormal in young animals with vitamin A deficiency. Ameloblasts show abnormal differentiation, which in turn adversely affects odontoblast development. Lesions induce hypoplasia of enamel, deficient mineralization of teeth, and retarded eruption.

Vitamin A deficiency in pregnant animals has been associated with stillbirth and abortions, particularly in swine.

Vitamin A deficiency causes night blindness.

Retinol (vitamin A) is the precursor of retinal, the light-absorbing group in visual pigments. Retinol deficiency leads to deterioration of the other segments of rods. Retinal is the prosthetic group of the photosensitive pigment in both rods and cones. The differences between the photosensitive pigments in rods (rhodopsin) and in cones (iodopsin) is in the protein bound to it. Sight involves isomerization in the dark of all-trans retinal to the 11-cis form, which in combination with opsin form rhodopsin. During light absorption, the 11-cis isomer is converted back to the all-trans form. During this cycle some retinal is reduced to retinol and lost to the reaction; thus vitamin A must be continually added to this visual reaction. In vitamin A deficiency the retinal used in rod vision is rapidly depleted and vision in low intensity light is lost—the explanation for human "night blindness."

Vitamin A toxicosis promotes the opposite effect.

Mucous metaplasia occurs in vitamin A excess. Normal squamous epithelium is converted to mucus-producing epithelium. This is not brought about by inducing mitosis, but by influencing postmitotic cells to abandon keratinization and to differentiate to mucous glandular epithelium. One striking change is formation of increased numbers of tight and gap junctions between cells. The normal tight junction-deficient squamous epithelium transforms by progressive emergence of large numbers of tight junctions between cells.

Vitamin D

Diet is the important source of vitamin D_3 (cholecalciferol) in most mammals and birds, although some is formed in skin by light-induced nonenzymatic photolysis of dehydrocholesterol. In the bloodstream, D_3 is bound to an α_2-globulin and transported to the liver. Vitamin D_3 is hydroxylated to $25(OH)D_3$ in hepatocytes and further hydroxylated to $1,25(OH)_2D_3$ (dihydroxycholecalciferol) in the kidney. Circulating $25(OH)D_3$ serves as a substrate for either 25(OH)-1-hydroxylase or 25(OH)-24-hydroxylase, both of which are in the renal cortex. The steroid hormone and active metabolite $1,25(OH)_2D_3$ is taken up by receptors within cells of target organs (intestine, bone, and kidney). The hormone-receptor complex passes into the nucleus, binds to specific portions of chromatin, and initiates gene expression and protein synthesis. The peptide that results produces the biologic action on calcium.

Vitamin D and its two chief metabolites, $1,25(OH)_2D_3$ and $24,25(OH)_2D_3$, interacting with calcitonin and parathyroid hormone, maintain calcium and phosphorus homeostasis (Fig. 29.2). Both of the biologically active metabolites of vitamin D are produced in the proximal convoluted tubules of the kidney.

The steroid hormone $1,25(OH)_2D_3$ induces Ca^{++}-binding proteins.

In kidney, synthesis of a calcium-binding protein is stimulated in cells of the distal tubule. In small intestine, $1,25(OH)_2D_3$ induces epithelial cells to produce another calcium-binding protein that passes into the microvillous glycocalyx, migrates to the cell surface, and causes Ca^{++} to pass from lumen into the bloodstream. Vitamin D metabolites produce two effects on *bone*: calcification of osteoid on trabecular surfaces and osteoclastic resorption for Ca^{++} mobilization. They also directly interact with *parathyroid* to suppress secretion of parathyroid hormone, which in turn inhibits formation of $1,25(OH)_2D_3$ in the kidney (Fig. 29.2).

The conversion $25(OH)D_3 -(1\text{-hydroxylase})\rightarrow 1,25(OH)_2D_3$ is the rate-limiting step in vitamin D metabolism and explains the delay between injections of vitamin D and a biologic response. Conversion is controlled by secretion of parathyroid hormone and calcium. Parathyroid hormone increases and calcitonin decreases the production of $1,25(OH)_2D_3$. Other steroid hormones, such as estrogens, increase renal hydroxylase action and play roles in special demands for calcium.

Vitamin D deficiency causes rickets in young and osteomalacia in adults.

These syndromes are no longer common but occur when errors are made in dietary formulations or as part of food deprivation during general debilitating disease. Rickets is commonly seen in birds, where it is characterized by retarded growth, hypocalcemia, parathyroid hyperplasia, and fibrous osteodystrophy (Fig. 29.3). There is marked expansion of growth plates, with failure of calcification of cartilage and osteoid. Although osteoclasts are increased, they may be less functional in late disease, a

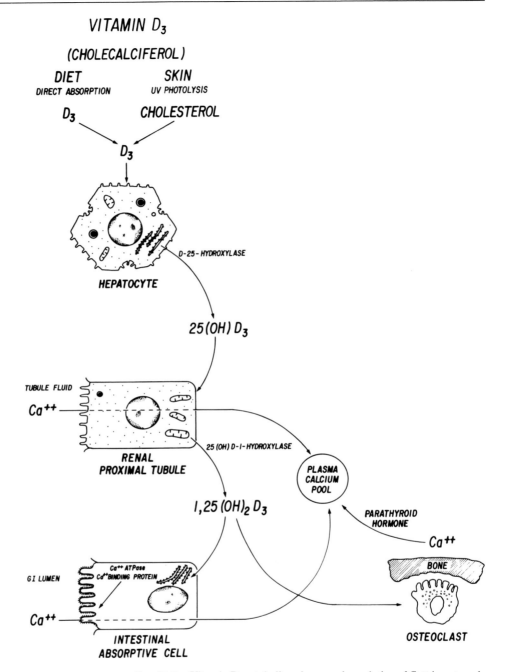

Fig. 29.2. Vitamin D metabolism: hormonal regulation of Ca^{++} in extracellular fluids.

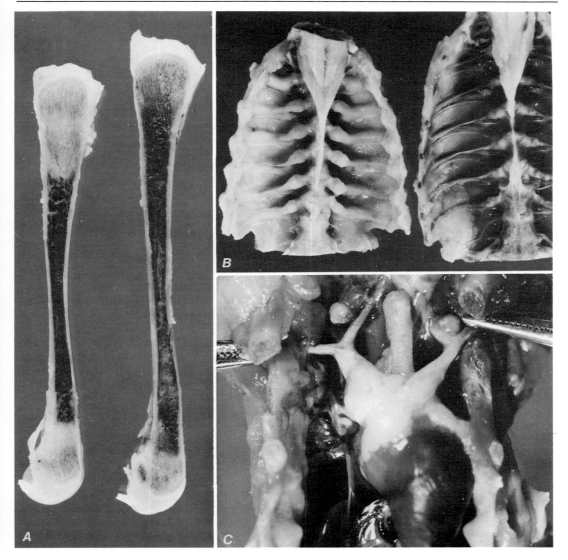

Fig. 29.3. Vitamin D deficiency, tibia, chicken. A. Expansion of metaphysis and shortened length (*top*). B. Distortion of vertebrae and ribs. C. Parathyroid hyperplasia in response to calcification defect and need to maintain plasma calcium.

defect probably related to parathyroid exhaustion.

Vitamin E

Vitamin E occurs in eight natural forms, four tocopherols and four tocotrienols. Alpha tocopherol is biologically the most active and is the important metabolite in vitamin E deficiency in animals. Early biochemical studies recognized the antioxidant property of tocopherols; for example, in vitamin E–deficient rodents, body fat was susceptible to oxidation and treatment with E prevented this oxidation.

Major lesions of vitamin E deficiency occur in muscle, brain, and skin. In addition, the reproductive system of some species (especially rodents and swine) require E for normal function, and reproductive failure has been ascribed to vitamin E deficiency in these species. Muscle dystrophy, the best-known disease syndrome associated with vitamin E deficiency, is common in ruminants, swine, and poultry and is rare in carnivores and nonhuman primates.

Myodystrophy

"White muscle disease" was first described as a disease in ruminants. In advanced disease, skeletal muscle becomes irregularly pale with blotches of white among areas of varying pallor (Fig. 29.4). Degeneration of skeletal muscle cells begins in the mitochondria, which in early phases of deficiency enlarge and then, as the myocyte fails, show disintegration. Lesions of necrosis are most prominent in the cerebellum.

In primates, the nervous system is also af-

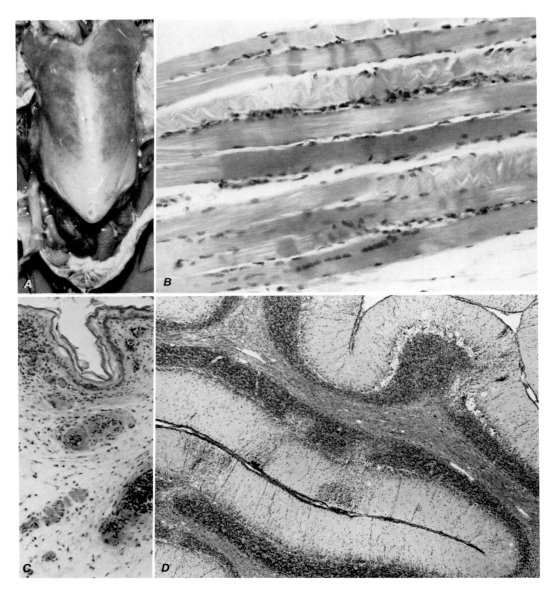

Fig. 29.4. Three syndromes associated with vitamin E deficiency, chicken. A and B. Myodystrophy, skeletal muscle degeneration. C. Exudative epidermitis, vascular degeneration, and edema in subcutis. D. Encephalomalacia, focal demyelination, and necrosis of the neuropil.

fected although clinical signs often arise from lesions outside the brain. Loss of sensory axons in posterior columns, sensory roots, and peripheral nerves leads to a syndrome of *sensory neuropathy.*

Vitamin E deficiency complex of birds

Vitamin E deficiency is associated with three different clinical syndromes: myopathy, encephalomalacia, and exudative dermatitis (Fig. 29.4). All are variants of the same injury, and all occur to some degree in each case, although the dominance of one usually determines the clinical diagnosis applied. Which form develops is largely controlled by the amount of fats in the diet (Fig. 29.5). Rations high in saturated fats predispose to encephalomalacia because of the increased oxidation stimulated by the fat.

Vitamin K

Vitamin K occurs in three forms: K_1, phylloquinone; K_2, menaquinone; and K_3, menadione. The first two are in green plants and animal tissues and are synthesized by gut microbes. K_3 is a synthetic compound. Since all are fat-soluble, uptake in the intestine requires normal fat absorption including bile salts and pancreatic enzymes.

Vitamin K deficiency leads to abnormal prothrombin.

Vitamin K is required by hepatocytes to synthesize prothrombin (factor II) and also factors

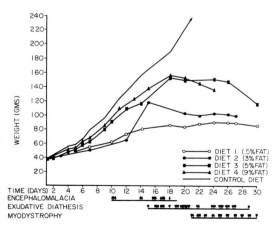

Fig. 29.5. Dietary fat determines the pathologic lesions and clinical syndrome that develops in chickens as a consequence of vitamin E deficiency.

VII, IX, and X. Vitamin K deficiency is referred to as hypoprothrombinemia. Abnormal prothrombin is synthesized in the absence of vitamin K. Although its amino acid sequence is normal, the carboxyglutamate amino terminus that binds Ca^{++} is defective because the vitamin K is an integral part of the enzymes that carboxylate the glutamate residues.

Vitamin B complex

The vitamins play roles in energy-releasing mechanisms in mitochondria that provide ATP, especially in cells involved in hematopoiesis. Deficiencies of B vitamins tend to produce changes in tissues with high rates of metabolism.

Thiamine

Thiamine is a component of *thiamine pyrophosphate* (TPP), the prosthetic group of three important enzymes (pyruvate dehydrogenase, α-ketoglutarate dehydrogenase, and transketolase) that transfer activated aldehyde units. Most importantly, TPP (as a component of the pyruvate dehydrogenase complex) serves as the initial catalytic cofactor in the oxidative decarboxylation of pyruvate: pyruvate + CoA + NAD $-(+$ TPP$)\rightarrow$ acetyl CoA + CO_2 + NADH. Blood levels of pyruvate and a-ketoglutarate are abnormally high in thiamine deficiency because of depressed activities of the pyruvate and α-ketoglutarate dehydrogenases. Transketolase activity of erythrocytes is also low; this is the basis for a useful diagnostic test.

Lesions of deficiency center on early mitochondrial hypertrophy and degeneration. Thiamine deficiency affects metabolically active cells of brain and myocardium, which is reflected in clinical signs of ataxis. Astrocytes and oligodendrogliocytes are the most susceptible; glial swelling is the initial change in experimental disease. Neural lesions, which progress from edema to hyperemia, hemorrhage, and necrosis, are the most prominent in the periventricular gray matter, cerebral cortex, and corpora quadrigemina.

Thiamine deficiency is a disease of ruminants and carnivores, especially foxes, cats, and mink. Deficiencies develop from (1) *dietary deficiencies* (e.g., beriberi of humans, caused by thiamine-deficient diets of polished rice, and Wernicke's encephalopathy accompanying alcoholism); (2) *thiaminases in the diet* (e.g., Chastek paralysis of mink, foxes, and cats, due to the thiaminase in fish muscle, and the central nervous system disease of horses associated with the thiaminase in bracken fern); and (3) toxicity of *thiamine-splitting drugs,* notably the thiamine analog amprolium, which is used as a coccidiostat and is causally associated with polioencephalomalacia in cattle and sheep.

Riboflavin

Riboflavin (vitamin B_2) is a component of several enzymes, all associated with oxidation-reduction reactions (e.g., cytochrome reductase and xanthene oxidase). Deficiency is associated with malfunction of the nervous system. "Curled toe paralysis" of chicks is one of the few documented syndromes. Swelling of sciatic and brachial nerves is associated with axonal swelling, Schwann cell proliferation, and demyelination.

Niacin

Niacin (nicotinic acid, nicotinamide) has an essential role in electron transport in the mitochondrion. Deficiency in man causes *pellagra* (L. *pelle,* skin, plus *agra,* rough) characterized by dermatitis, diarrhea, and dementia. Pigs fed purified diets deficient in niacin lose body weight, become anorexic, and develop diarrhea and anemia. At necropsy the gastrointestinal tract has mucous hyperplasia and in severe cases is congested with tiny hemorrhages.

Pyridoxine

Pyridoxine (vitamin B_6) deficiency has not been established as a clinical disease. Pyridoxine deficit occurs in uremia and is associated with amino acid imbalances in plasma.

Pyridoxine toxicity is generally considered a laboratory disease. No clinical disease has been reported but pyridoxine is widely used as a model to study human sensory neuropathies. Recently ataxia and neuropathy have been reported in humans consuming large daily doses of pyridoxine but the pathologic lesions remain unknown. Dr. D. M. Hoover, at Purdue University, produced ataxia in dogs given 150 mg/kg body weight/day for 100 days, a dose unlikely to occur naturally.

Vitamin C

A deficiency of *vitamin C* (ascorbic acid) markedly retards fibroplasia because this vitamin is required as a cofactor for proline hydroxylase. In animals, *scurvy* is seen only in guinea pigs fed on old stale feeds. Affected bones have excessive fibroblasts and ground substance but very few mature collagen fibers (Fig. 29.6). Fibroblasts do not form in parallel arrangement, and the resulting signs of disease are related to delayed wound healing and abnormal bone. In the classic medical literature, human scurvy patients were afflicted with breakdown of very old scars, a fact that emphasizes the active metabolism of collagen that occurs even in dense connective tissue.

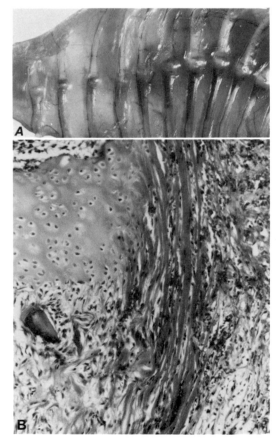

Fig. 29.6. Vitamin C deficiency (scurvy) in a guinea pig that had been given stale feed. A. Knobby bone growths are at costochondral junctions. B. Fibroblast proliferation and hemorrhage adjacent to cartilage of the growth plate.

MINERAL DEFICIENCY
Calcium

Dietary deficiency of calcium in animals with immature skeletons leads to skeletal deformities. Naturally occurring bone disease due to dietary deficiencies of calcium are relatively common because unsupplemented, all-meat diets are still used for some pet animals. The syndrome of hypocalcemia–parathyroid hyperplasia–bone disease can also be secondary to vitamin D deficiency or to excesses of phosphorus.

Nutritional secondary hyperparathyroidism

This end result of calcium deficiency occurs in cats, dogs, horses, primates, birds, and reptiles and is manifest as severe bone disease, often complicated by other deficiencies. Drs. Capen and Rowland, at Ohio State University, placed kittens on a diet of beef heart and distilled water (which provides large amounts of phosphorus but is severely deficient in calcium). The kittens developed hypocalcemia and hyperactive parathyroids in 1 week. Excess parathyroid hormones developed and led to generalized fibrous osteodystrophy.

FOCUS

Parturient paresis of dairy cattle

The dairy cow secretes about 1 g/kg calcium in milk. At parturition, the sudden needs of lactation (colostrum is rich in calcium ions) must adapt the plasma Ca^{++} balance to this drain. Plasma levels of Ca^{++} drop from preparturient amounts of 10–12 to 7–9 mg/100 ml; these cows develop the characteristic syndrome of paresis, collapse, and unconsciousness known as *parturient paresis,* or "milk fever." (*Tetany,* the spasm of skeletal muscle, is a sign of puerperal hypocalcemia in dogs but not in cattle.)

The mechanism by which hypocalcemia induces parathyroid hormone secretion (which stimulates bone resorption for calcium release) is too sluggish to meet the explosive demands for calcium brought on by lactation. Animals may die if they are not treated by giving intravenous solutions of calcium.

Parathyroid glands of affected cows are hyperactive, and elevated PTH levels occur in plasma. Parathyroids of cows fed high-calcium diets (especially if the diet is alkaline) have inactive or atrophic chief cells; they are prone to develop milk fever near parturition. Their ability to secrete PTH in response to a hypocalcemia challenge is reduced, compared with cows fed prepartum diets with the required amounts of calcium and phosphorus. Conversely, prepartum diets low in calcium reduce the incidence of milk fever near parturition, and chief cells in the parathyroids are predominantly in the actively synthesizing stage of the secretory cycle.

In milk fever, severe hypocalcemia develops in spite of hyperparathyroidsm and elevated levels of PTH. Treatment with large doses of exogenous PTH does not elevate plasma Ca^{++}. Thus PTH fails to stimulate bone resorption sufficiently to replenish blood calcium lost in milk. This is due not only to the sluggish response of chief cells in cows on high-calcium diets but also to suppression of osteoclastic and osteocytic activity in bone by other humeral factors. When bone resorption is inhibited pharmacologically, cows become hypocalcemic and hypophosphatemic shortly after parturition.

Phosphorus

Excess phosphorus in the diet (in proportion to calcium) leads to *hyperphosphatemia,* and this in turn causes a decrease in blood calcium. Hypocalcemia causes secondary hyperparathyroidism indirectly; that is, the decrease in plasma calcium directly stimulates parathyroid hyperplasia, which eventually leads to generalized fibrous osteodystrophy.

Equine nutritional secondary hyperparathyroidism, variously called "osteodystrophy fibrosa," "bran disease," or "bighead," is caused by excessive dietary phosphorus and secondary hypocalcemia. The parathyroids are hyperplastic in direct relation to the hypocalcemia, and the gland is dominated by hypertrophic chief cells. Osteoclastic resorption is prominent in the skull bones but also occurs in ribs and metaphyses of long bones. The leading feature is transformation of bone into a fibrous tissue of high collagen content, with rebuilding of bone in a more primitive pattern rather than into highly organized haversian systems.

High dietary phosphorus is associated with tissue mineralization. Ectopic mineralization occurs in pigs on high dietary phosphorus. Calcified lesions occur in the left atrial endocardium and in diaphragmatic and pulmonary pleura.

Iron

The amount of iron in most plants and grains plus the capacity of the animal to conserve iron is usually adequate to maintain iron concentrations within normal ranges. Most iron deficiencies occur in neonates and are related to dietary disorders. Blood loss may deplete tissue iron, but the loss must be severe or prolonged because dietary iron will compensate for iron lost in hemoglobin.

Several factors affect iron: (1) *dietary content,* that is, whether iron is present in sufficient amounts and in the form for absorption; (2) *intestinal absorption,* which requires the presence of normal gastric HCl and pancreatic juice for action; (3) *sufficient percent absorption* by intestinal absorptive epithelial cells; (4) adequate *transport proteins* in plasma; and (5) amount of *iron excreted* or *lost* in blood and sloughed epithelial cells.

Dietary iron deficiency is common in baby pigs.

Piglets are born with low iron in tissue. Their extraordinarily rapid rate of growth coupled with low iron levels in sow's milk require that they obtain large amounts of dietary iron. Plasma iron, which is normally 100–300 $\mu g/100$ ml may drop to 50 μg in anemic piglets. The iron-binding capacity of plasma is increased (when iron is given therapeutically, it is rapidly complexed to transferrin and accepted by erythroblasts). *Anemia* is the major sign of dietary iron deficiency in piglets. Mucous membranes are pale, and systemic signs such as dyspnea and cardiac abnormalities occur. At necropsy, there are cardiac pallor, dilatation, and hypertrophy of vetricular walls (see anemia, Chapter 17).

Other mechanisms of iron deficiency

Reduced iron absorption occurs in mink kits fed raw marine fish. Insoluble crystalline ferric oxide-hydroxides are formed by trimethylamine oxide in the fish.

Plasma iron versus ferritin

In plasma, iron is complexed to the protein *transferrin,* which has the electrophoretic mobilization of a B_1-globulin and serves as an iron carrier. Plasma iron represents the balance between iron of hemoglobin breakdown and iron absorbed from the intestine minus iron removed by heme synthesis, cell metabolism, and storage.

Determination of serum iron may be misleading. *Pseudo–iron deficiency* is diagnosed when tests for serum iron give low values, but tests for serum ferritin show normal or high values. This has been documented in horses; it is due to inflammatory processes that deplete serum iron but do not cause iron deficiency.

Selenium

Selenium is a component of the important antioxidant *glutathione peroxidase,* which is a scavenger of toxic oxygen radicals in the cytosol. When glutathione peroxidase is deficient, the cell becomes overly susceptible to almost all toxins. In fact, the toxicity of many poisons can be correlated with the degree to which glutathione peroxidase is depleted in tissue.

Selenium and vitamin E have overlapping

functions and the deficiency of one leads to or is accompanied by depletion of the other. As a result, the lesions of selenium toxicity are remarkably similar to that of vitamin E deficiency.

Selenium deficiency

Myopathy, particularly of the skeletal muscles, follows the same species distribution and lesion pattern of avitaminosis E. In chicks, atrophy and fibrosis of the pancreas is also an important lesion. Activity of glutathione peroxidase in the pancreas declines in selenium deficiency coincident with mitochondrial degeneration in the pancreatic acinar cells.

In cattle, selenium deficiency has been associated with anemia. Cattle grazing St. Augustine grass growing on peaty soils of the Florida Everglades developed Heinz body anemia associated with low serum Se values. Se supplementation corrected the anemia and returned growth to normal.

ADDITIONAL READING

Capen, C. C., et al. The pathology of hypervitaminosis D in cattle. *Vet. Pathol.* 3:350, 1966.

Das, R. M. The effects of intermittent starvation on lung development in suckling rats. *Am. J. Pathol.* 117:326, 1984.

Divers, T. J., et al. Blindness and convulsions associated with vitamin A deficiency in feedlot steers. *J. Am. Vet. Med. Assoc.* 189:1579, 1986.

Enwonwu, C. O., et al. Protein-energy malnutrition in infant nonhuman primates (*Macaca nemastrina*). *Br. J. Exp. Pathol.* 58:78, 1977.

Goedegebuure, S. A., et al. Morphological findings in young dogs chronically fed a diet containing excess calcium. *Vet. Pathol.* 23:594, 1986.

Goodman, D. S. Vitamin A and retinoids in health and disease. *N. Engl. J. Med.* 310:1023, 1986.

Grey, R. M., et al. Pathology of skull, radius and rib in hypervitaminosis A of young calves. *Vet. Pathol.* 2:446, 1965.

Gries, C. L., and Scott, M. L. The pathology of thiamine, riboflavin, pantothenic acid, and niacin deficiencies in the chick. *J. Nutr.* 102:1269, 1972.

Haschek, W. M., et al. Vitamin D toxicity. *Cornell Vet.* 68:324, 1978.

Hunt, R. D., et al. A comparison of the toxicity of ergocalciferol and cholecalciferol in rhesus monkeys (*Macaca mulatta*). *J. Nutr.* 1102:975, 1972.

McKenna, M. C., et al. Cellular localization of liver vitamin A in rats given total parenteral nutrition (TPU) solutions intravenously or orally. *J. Nutr.* 113:1176, 1983.

Maltin, C. A., et al. Mitochondrial abnormalities in muscle from vitamin-B_{12}-deficient sheep. *J. Comp. Pathol.* 93:429, 1983.

Michel, R. L., et al. Dietary hepatic necrosis associated with selenium–vitamin E deficiency in swine. *J. Am. Vet. Med. Assoc.* 155:50, 1969.

Nafstad, I. The vitamin-E-deficiency syndrome in pigs. *Vet. Pathol.* 8:239, 1971.

Okada, H. M., et al. Thiamine deficiency encephalopathy in foxes and mink. *Vet. Pathol.* 24:321, 1987.

O'Sullivan, B. M., and Blakemore, W. F. Acute nicotinamide deficiency in the pig induced by 6-aminonicotinamide. *Vet. Pathol.* 17:748, 1980.

Pion, P. D., et al. Myocardial failure in cats associated with low plasma taurine. *Science* 237:764, 1987.

Read, D. H., and Harrington, D. D. Experimentally induced thiamine deficiency in beagle dogs. *Am. J. Vet. Res.* 47:2281, 1986.

Smith, J. E., et al. Serum ferritin and total iron-binding capacity to estimate iron storage in pigs. *Vet. Pathol.* 21:597, 1984.

Woodard, J. C., et al. Effect of diet on longitudinal bone growth and osteochondrosis in swine. *Vet. Pathol.* 24:371, 1987.

Gene Defects and Diseases of Growth and Development

GENETIC DISEASE

Genetic disease develops from abnormalities in DNA, the cell's genetic material. The total genetic information, or genome, is partitioned into specific numbers of chromosomes, which are transmitted by gametes through generations according to the laws of Mendel. In this section we are concerned with *germ-line defects,* hereditary disorders that, by definition, are transmitted in the gametes from one generation to another. They arise from mutations that are considered familial when passed through several generations.

Stable alterations of genes within mitotically active *somatic cells* also occur. These changes, the subject of somatic cell genetics, are not transmitted to future generations and will not be discussed.

From the clinical point of view, genetic diseases may be placed in three major categories. (1) Diseases due to *abnormalities of chromosomal structure of function* are detected by the analysis of cellular chromosomes, that is, cytogenetic analysis. Change in chromosomal structure implies breakage followed by rearrangement. Abnormal numbers of chromosomes are due to nondysjunction, either during meiotic division (which results in an aneuploid gamete) or during postzygotic, mitotic division (anaphase lag). Many of these changes are incompatible with life and result in death of the fetus. (2) Diseases related to *mutant genes of large effect,* the so-called Mendelian disorders, include the rare storage diseases and inborn errors of metabolism that result from a single gene mutation. They are really diseases of abnormal chromosomal structure, but the defects are so small that they cannot be detected by chromosomal

analysis. (3) The final category is diseases of *multifactorial or polygenic inheritance. Polygenic inheritance* involves traits that are solely due to two or more genetic loci (e.g., neural tube defects, cleft palate, and some congenital heart defects). *Multifactorial inheritance* involves traits governed by the additive effect of many genes of small impact and usually involve nongenetic environmental factors that influence the phenotypic expression of disease. Diabetes mellitus and congenital hip dysplasia of dogs are diseases in which polygenic inheritance, coupled with predisposing environmental influences, underlie development of disease.

Gene function

A *gene* is simply a specific sequence of base pairs in DNA. The subunits of DNA are four nucleotides, each of which contains one of four bases: adenine, guanine, thymine, or cytosine. The sequence of bases along the DNA strand (say CTG or AGC) defines the gene. These triplets or gene code words are called *codons.* Each codon specifies an amino acid, and the long series of codons on DNA supplies instruction for assembling an entire peptide chain.

Genetic information for synthesis of protein is not arranged in a continuous sequence of DNA codons. Genes are split, and patches of coding sequences are separated by noncoding DNA. After each gene is transcribed onto mRNA, the transcript mRNA molecule is spliced and the coding sequences are joined directly to form a coherent mRNA and to eliminate noncoding sequences. The many different proteins produced in cells require more information than can be provided by an unaltered linear gene. This diversity is provided by shuffling various combinations of gene segments and by selective RNA transcription.

In transcription, DNA codons are copied onto a newly forming mRNA molecule by action of an enzyme, RNA polymerase. When completed, the mRNA strand moves from nucleus to cytoplasm carrying its codon copies to the ribosome, where they direct assembly of amino acids into peptide chains.

From patterns present in mRNA, the cell is able to replicate thousands of different proteins, each with several hundred amino acids arranged in a highly specific sequence. Newly completed peptides are either released into the cytoplasm for local use (such as hemoglobin in erythrocytes) or, if produced on the rough endoplasmic reticulum, passed through the cytocavitary network for further refinement (usually for addition of carbohydrate moieties and for folding of the peptide chain).

The DNA in different cells of an individual contain the same genetic information, but only a limited amount is expressed. The cell's genetic program can be switched on and off (as in mitosis) but also can be selectively expressed. Thus the neuron and keratinocyte have the same genome, but very different expressions of it.

Selective expression is illustrated by classic nuclear transplantation experiments done in the 1960s. Nuclei extracted from tadpole gut epithelium were transplanted into frog ova from which the nuclei had been removed. Some ova developed into normal adults, showing that intestinal epithelial nuclei contained all the genes required for development. These studies provided the foundation for current experiments that control genetic expression by injecting ova with purified extracts containing mRNA, which can instruct the cell to make specific proteins.

Abnormal chromosomes

Subtle aberrations involving discrete changes within single genes (point mutations) cannot be detected by examining chromosomes structurally. However, when large numbers of genes are rearranged, abnormalities can be seen on cytogenetic analysis. These gross chromosomal abnormalities may then lead to several consequences. Fetal death with spontaneous abortion is common because most of these conditions are lethal. Only in rare instances is the animal born alive. In man, in which several specific changes are known, congenital malformation syndromes often involve mental retardation (Table 30.1).

Neoplastic cells, although usually aneuploid, sometimes are associated with specific chromosomal abnormalities (see neoplasia, Chapter 10).

Cytogenetic analysis

Cytogenetic evaluation is done by examining the chromosomes of circulating lymphocytes. Blood samples collected by venipuncture are centrifuged to separate the cells. Lymphocytes are then incubated in culture medium to which a mitotic stimulant (mitogen) has been added. After 3 days, colchicine is added to stop all dividing cells in metaphase. The cells are fixed,

Table 30.1.   Classification of chromosomal abnormalities

Abnormality	Description
	ABNORMAL NUMBER
Polyploidy	Abnormality in multiples of the haploid number
Triploidy	Three of each instead of normal pair
Tetraploidy	Four of each; occurs normally in some animal tissues
Aneuploidy	Increase or decrease in normal (euploid) number of chromosomes but not involving haploid sets; may involve autosomes or sex chromosomes
Monosomy	Only one chromosome in particular pair
Trisomy	One chromosome present 3 times instead of 2; congenital malformations associated with specific trisomies (Down's syndrome in man has 21); trisomy in calves with brachygnathia; number 11 trisomy in fetal runted cats
Mosaicism	Presence of more than one karyotype variety of cell in same individual derived from single zygote; arises from postzygotic mitotic nondisjunction
Chimerism	Two genotypes present in one individual as a result of maternal-fetal cross circulation or postnatal transfusion (bovine freemartin)
	ABNORMAL STRUCTURE
Translocation	Separated chromosomal fragments attached to another chromosome
Deletion	Absence of piece of chromosome
Isochromosome	Chromosome separated in wrong plane at centromere: short arms attached to short arms and long to long
Inversion	Segments within a chromosomal arm not arranged in proper order

dried, and flattened to spread out the chromosomes, which are then stained to emphasize the shape and banding patterns. The number of chromosomes of about 20 well-spread cells is counted, and the presence of the sex chromosomes noted. Chromosomes in metaphase appear in various structural patterns, according to the position of the centromere (kinetochore), which determines the length of the chromosomal arms. *Acrocentric* chromosomes have centromeres at one end and thus have two long arms. In *telocentric* chromosomes, centromeres are near the end. *Metacentric* chromosomes have centromeres approximately in the middle, and *submetacentric* chromosomes have two short and two long arms (Fig. 30.1).

Special stains are used in banding techniques that help to differentiate specialized portions of the chromosome for proper identification. Q banding utilizes quinicrine fluorochromes that bind specifically to adenine-thymine bases in DNA. Differences in base compositions of DNA

segments provide variations in shades of brightness on ultraviolet fluorescence microscopy. Giemsa (G) banding gives patterns similar to Q banding. Other banding techniques are used to augment these common procedures (Fig. 30.2).

Sex chromatin is detected in stained smears of oral epithelium.

A useful technique for screening the number of X and Y chromosomes is the staining and evaluation of buccal smears. The female sex chromatin (Barr or X body) is a condensed chromatin mass about 1 μm in diameter along the nuclear membrane in nuclei of female cells. The X body is seen in about 20% of female nuclei; its presence indicates two X chromosomes, one of which is inactivated and condensed. The male Y chromosome in buccal smears can be detected only with special fluorescence microscopy. Only one X chromosome of the female is active during interphase; the second is inactive and pushed aside in the nucleus. This explains the equality of gene products in male and female. In

Banding Patterns in Chromosomes of Neoplastic Lymphocytes

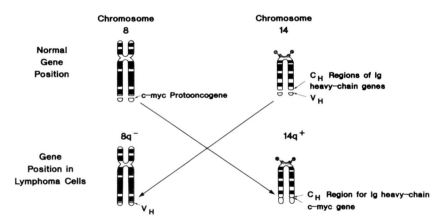

Fig. 30.1. Staining of bands aids in studies of abnormal chromosomes. Lymphocytes of the human Burkitt's lymphoma have translocations of chromosomes 8 and 14. The oncogene c-*myc* on chromosome 8 is transferred to a position adjacent to a gene for heavy chains of immunoglobulin molecules (C_H and C_V) on chromosome 14. The breakpoint in chromosome 8 is at the terminal part of the long arm (band q24). Transfer next to the active immunoglobulin gene allows the oncogene c-*myc* to come under the influence of enhancer genes of the immunoglobulin loci. Loss of control of c-*myc* (which encodes a protein involved in growth regulation of lymphocytes) is called deregulation. Deregulation of c-*myc* is related to the abnormal growth of neoplastic lymphocytes.

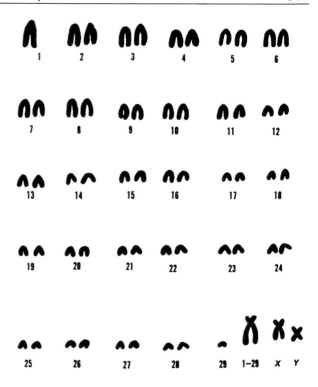

Fig. 30.2. Chromosome spread of leukocytes from a cow with a chromosomal translocation.

theory, if both female X chromosomes were active, females would have twice the amount of gene product as do males.

The karyotype is a code for chromosome numbers.

The karyotype is designated by writing the total chromosome number and the sex chromosomes; for example, the normal male cat is 38,XY. In defining structural abnormalities, the short arm of a chromosome is designated "p" and the long arm "q." Thus 38,XY,5p − indicates a male with 38 chromosomes and number 5 has a deletion of the short arm. A female cat with trisomy of chromosome 18 would be designated 38,XX, + 18. Chromosomal *mosaics* (the presence of more than one karyotype in one individual) are identified by separating the cell types by a slash: 38,XX/39,XXY is a mosaic with cells of normal female chromosomes and cells with an extra chromosome.

Species differ markedly in chromosome types.

Cattle have 60 chromosomes per cell (2n = 60). All autosomes are telocentric (although sex chromosomes are metacentric), making it difficult to identify individual chromosomes (Fig. 30.1).

Avian chromosomes fall into two distinct classes, macro- and microchromosomes. The microchromosomes are very small and easily lost in metaphase chromosomal spreads. In birds, the growing pinfeather has a very high mitotic index and provides material for the "feather pulp technique." Avian embryos at 16–72 hours of development can also be used for chromosome preparations.

Populations of lower vertebrates may naturally be polyploid.

Triploidy is a rare but naturally occurring phenomenon in fish, amphibians, and reptiles. This development of diploid-triploid mosaic individuals has benefits that enhance reproductive output. Triploid populations are unisexual (all females) and reproduce by *parthogenesis* (reproduction by development of an unfertilized gamete) or *gynogenesis* (in which the embryo contains only maternal chromosome due to activation of the egg by a sperm that degenerates without fusing with the egg nucleus).

Spermiogenesis is abnormal in mules and hybrid horses.

Hybrids between horses and donkeys are called mules or hinnies depending on the species of the dam. If a jack (male donkey) is mated to a mare, the resulting offspring is a mule. If a stallion is bred to a jenny (female donkey) the offspring is a hinny. Spermatogenesis is arrested in male mules and hinnies. At meiosis there are markedly abnormal pairings of chromosomes at the pachytene stage of meiotic prophase due to dissimilarity of the parental karyotypes; that is, the horse (*Equus caballus,* 2n = 64) has 26 metacentric and 36 acrocentric autosomal chromosomes while in the donkey (*E. asinus,* 2n = 62), 38 are metacentric and 22 acrocentric.

The Przewalski horse of Siberia has 66 chromosomes. F_1 hybrids between *E. caballus* and *E. przewalskii* (2n = 66) are fertile and have a diploid chromosome number of 2n = 65. A single Robertsonian translocation occurs, transforming 4 acrocentric chromosomes of *E. przewalskii* into 2 metacentric chromosomes in *E. caballus.* A trivalent chromosome is formed at meiosis by pairing of the three elements involved in centrix fusion rearrangement.

Diseases related to chromosomal aberrations

Few diseases of animals are associated with identifiable abnormalities in karyotype. This may be largely due to the lethality of such large genetic errors and loss of the embryo without detection. Most embryos with abnormal karyotypes are lost at the time of implantation. In some breeds this may be a major cause of embryonic death. Chickens have up to 9% abnormal karyotypes (breeds vary from 0.5 to 9%), and pigs may have up to 12% abnormal karyotypes with coincident loss of embryos.

Most chromosomal aberrations are related to the reproductive system.

In *X monosomy* one homologous X chromosome is missing, giving XO instead of XX. It has been seen most commonly in horses. Affected mares are infertile and have small reproductive organs: ovaries lack follicles, the uterus is small and flaccid, and there are irregular periods of estrus, often with no cyclic ovarian activity. Although the Arabian breed is chiefly affected, monosomy has been seen in Belgian mares and

several other equine breeds. Known as Turner's syndrome in man, XO monosomy has been reported in pigs, cats, sheep, monkeys, wallabies, and rodents.

In *trisomy* there is an additional (third) chromosome of one type in an otherwise diploid cell (2n + 1). *Trisomy-17* in cattle is associated with brachygnathia (short jaw) and is called the "lethal brachygnathia trisomy syndrome." Other trisomies have been suggested as being related to individual cases of cardiac anomaly, intersex, and arthrogryposis. In many instances 100% of the cells are not trisomic, and most reports are too incomplete to provide a clinical understanding of these diseases.

The 1/29 translocation of cattle is associated with reduced fertility.

This chromosomal abnormality was first found by Gustavsson, at the Royal Veterinary College in Stockholm, during studies of lymphocytes and bovine leukemia. It has been reported in nearly 40 breeds. Its frequency is near 0 in major North American breeds but is 30% in some breeds and as high as 66% in some herds of British white cattle. The 1/29 translocation, which is transmitted from heterozygous parents in a standard Mendelian pattern as a dominant, is associated with a subtle reduction of breeding ability. Affected females return to estrus early. The nondysjunction may occur during meiosis, and the resulting germ cells have a deficiency or duplication; zygotes resulting from such germ cells die early as embryos. No live monosomic or trisomic animals have been found in progeny of 1/29 parents.

In Sweden, screening all males to eliminate 1/29 heterozygotes and homozygotes from artificial insemination programs has reversed a trend to lowered fertility in Swedish red and white cattle. Approximately 25 other translocations in bovine chromosomes has been reported. None has been associated with defined clinical disease or altered reproductive function.

Chimerism

Chimeras (or "allophenic animals") have cells of more than one genotype. The bovine freemartin is a genetic female with genital hypoplasia, born co-twin with a male. Anastomosing placental circulations allow exchange of bloodborne cells during fetal life. The newborn freemartin is normal except that chimerism results in an intersex phenotype. Tubular genitalia of the Mullerian duct system fail to develop because of the influence of androgens produced by the male twin, which arrived in the female due to fused placental circulation. The testicle develops earlier than the ovary and suppresses female genitalia. Ovaries are rudimentary and contain vestigial seminiferous tubules.

Evidence of mingling of blood supplies is found in circulating blood cells of freemartins. The hematopoietic chimerism can be demonstrated by karyotyping bone marrow cells. If 100 cell spreads are counted, over half may contain XXY sex chromosomes, while the remainder will be normal female karyotypes with XX. The XX/XY karyotype is not found in solid tissues. The bull twin will also have XX leukocytes in its circulation; chimeric bulls are often sterile or produce only abnormal sperm. Freemartins also occur in swine, sheep, and goats.

Tortoiseshell cats have extra X chromosomes and primary hypogonadism.

Male tortoiseshell cats are infertile because of hypoplastic testicular tubules and aspermatogenesis. Their chromosome anomaly is an additional X chromosome, 39,XXY. Karyotypes of these cats actually reveal several mosaic varieties, including 38,XX/38,XY and 38,XY/39,XXY. Male tortoiseshells may also be 38,XY/38,XY, presumed to be somatic chimerics, that is, to have arisen from early embryonic fusion of what should have been two separate individuals.

"Tortoiseshell" signifies a mix of orange and black, usually blended together. Two sex-linked alleles determine color in the cat's hair coat, orange (O) and black (O+). These alleles are codominant, for each is expressed in the heterozygote, the tortoiseshell. The homozygous female may be black (O+O+) or orange (OO), but the hemizygous male must be orange (O) or black (O+). The normal heterozygous female (OO+) is tortoiseshell, but for the male to be tortoiseshell, there must be an additional sex chromosome and at least two sex chromosomes of differing color genes.

Modifying genes affect the pattern and intensity of black and orange; identification of the phenotypes must be done carefully. Calico (tricolor—orange and black, plus white) cats are similar except for the white patches, which are inherited and do not influence orange-black color inheritance.

Dr. T. C. Jones, a veterinary pathologist at Harvard Medical School, has studied male tortoiseshell cats as a model for Klinefelter's syndrome of human males, which includes testicular degeneration, infertility, enlarged breasts, and a karyotype of XXY. Similar syndromes of extra sex chromosomes and testicular abnormalities have been reported in mice, pigs, sheep, dogs, and cattle. The Y chromosome is male determining, promoting testicular development from the medullary part of the primitive gonad. With two X chromosomes, the cortex of the gonad develops into an ovary. The importance of the Y chromosome is seen in these XXY males, which are male despite the presence of two X chromosomes.

Mutant genes of large effect
Pedigree analysis

Pedigree analysis using Mendelian laws is used in the establishment of probable genetic cause, to predict the degree of risk of individuals, and to indicate possible abnormal genetic mechanisms even when biochemical mechanisms are unknown. Mendel's concepts of dominance and recessivity were derived from phenotypes and not from molecular mechanisms of inheritance.

Rediscovered in 1900, Mendel's laws of 1860 stated that (1) a unit of genetic information is transmitted unchanged from one generation to another and (2) alternate forms of this gene (later called an *allele*) must segregate during gamete formation and recombine independently in the offspring to provide a 1:2:1 ratio. Mendel's observations were made on the self-fertilizing pea plant, of which he had many true-breeding varieties. He crossed hybrids derived from true breeders and made quantitative calculations of disparate characters that appeared in succeeding generations. When plants containing wrinkled seeds were crossed with plants containing smooth seeds, he found that only smooth-coated seeds were present in the F_1 generation. When he self-fertilized smooth-seeded F_1 plants, he found one-fourth true-breeding smooth plants, one-fourth true-breeding wrinkled plants, and two-fourths smooth, impure breeders, which, when self-fertilized, produced the same 1:2:1 ratio. The wrinkled coat, although phenotypically not present in the F_1 hybrid, was transmitted unchanged from parent seed to the F_2 hybrids. He thus proposed that the physical expression (*phenotype*) differed from the genetic constitution (*genotype*) and that the genotype must be determined by two transmissible characters or genes.

Dominance and recessivity

By plotting incidence of animal disease in a related population, the pattern of inheritance can be determined as autosomal dominant, autosomal recessive, or sex-linked. *Autosomal dominant* diseases are those in which heterozygotes express the mutant allele. Both males and females are affected, and both transmit the disease. When an affected animal is mated to an unaffected animal, one-half the offspring will be affected. Some dominant conditions do not invariably manifest themselves in the heterozygote, a phenomenon called "incomplete penetrance."

Only homozygotes express autosomal recessive traits.

In transmission of *autosomal recessive* traits, disease typically occurs in offspring of unaffected parent animals (with a 1:4 risk). The great majority of inborn errors of metabolism are autosomal recessive, and the heterozygote in many of these show a partial deficiency of the enzyme that is lacking in the homozygote.

Chondrodysplasia of Alaskan malamute dwarfs is transmitted as a simple *autosomal recessive trait with complete penetrance and variable phenotypic expression.* It is a generalized symmetrical defect in endochondral ossification of cuboidal bones (which have wide, flat, irregular physes). Hypertrophic and degenerative zones in affected bones are irregular and widened proximally to microfractures in the primary spongiosa. Histologically, dwarf proliferative chondrocytes occur in clumps separated by wide areas of extracellular matrix. Ultrastructurally, the proliferating chondrocytes are vesiculated and surrounded by a matrix that is deficient in matrix granules. Proteoglycans extracted from growth plate cartilage have abnormal glycosaminoglycan rations; that is, there is increased chondroitin-6-sulfate and galactosamine, an indication of immature cartilage matrix.

Sex-linked diseases are transmitted from mother to son.

Sex-linked (or X-linked) diseases are transmitted by heterozygous carrier females only to sons who are hemizygous for the X chromosome. Very rarely, a female is affected if the male transmits a mutant dominant gene or if both parents transmit mutant recessive genes. No Y-linked diseases are known.

The relationship between sex determination and the presence of abnormal genetic traits was founded in the early 1900s on the hemophilia model based on the lineage of Queen Victoria of England, in which females were unaffected carriers of classic hemophilia A. In 1950 Brinkhous showed that hemophilia of dogs was also sex-linked and, through crossbreeding, hemophilic but viable homozygous females could be produced (negating the assertion the females bearing two hemophilic genes on their X chromosomes were probably inviable).

Sex-linked traits are known for many animal species. *Glucose-6-phosphate dehydrogenase* production is sex-linked in primates (man, gorilla, chimpanzee), horse, donkey, kangaroo, and several rodent species. The X-linked disease glucose-6-phosphate dehydrogenase deficiency is found in these animals. In general, a gene found to be X-linked in one mammal can be expected to be X chromosome–linked in other mammals. Many other X-linked traits of animals are known (Table 30.2).

Proteins as mutant gene products

Mutation of genes controlling protein synthesis, particularly of enzymes, can have widespread pathologic effects. The consequences of amino acid substitution vary from trivial to lethal. Some variants in protein do not produce functional impairment. Many normal, functioning variants have been reported for hemoglobin. The defects that arise from abnormal protein synthesis may be expressed in several different ways (Table 30.3).

The first molecular genetic disease to be described was human *sickle cell anemia,* in which an abnormal gene causes valine to be substituted for glutamic acid. This amino acid substitution results in the abnormal hemoglobin S. When deoxygenated, hemoglobin S polymerizes into aligned fibers, which form a gel and distort the erythrocyte into abnormal sickle shapes. Sickled erythrocytes have short life spans, and their lysis is manifest as hemolytic anemia.

Disorders of *amino acid metabolism* are among the most common (but less serious) of the inborn errors of human metabolism; very few have

Table 30.2.   **Sex-linked traits and disease in animals**

Gene Product or Disease	Animal Species Affected[a]
Glucose-6-phosphate dehydrogenase deficiency	Primate (man, gorilla, chimpanzee), horse, donkey, sheep, cattle, pig, hare, mouse, hamster, kangaroo
α-galactosidase deficiency	Sheep, cow, pig, rabbit, hamster, mouse
Coagulation factor VIII deficiency	Dog
Coagulation factor IX deficiency	Dog
Phosphoglycerate kinase deficiency	Horse, hamster, mouse, kangaroo, chimpanzee
Hypoxanthine-guanine phosphoribosyl transferase deficiency	Horse, hamster, mouse, chimpanzee
Anhidrotic ectodermal dysplasia	Cow
Copper transport deficiency	Mouse (Menkes kinky-hair syndrome)
Testicular feminization syndrome	Cow, dog, rat, mouse
Vitamin D–resistant rickets	Mouse
Ornithine transcarbamoylase deficiency	Mouse
Muscular dystrophy (Duchenne's)	Mouse

    [a]All syndromes have been identified in man.

been reported in animals (Table 30.4). They are caused by a single enzyme deficiency based on a single genetic mutation. Most aminoacidopathies are subclinical disorders discovered during amino acid analyses of urine.

Multifactorial disorders

Many genetic diseases are *polygenic,* or multifactorial, disorders; that is, the trait is determined by more than one gene and results from the blending of several genes. In Mendel's experiments the color trait was manifest in the following way. When purple-petaled and white-petaled plants were crossed, an intermediate mauve color resulted in the hybrid. When this F_1 hybrid was self-fertilized, a range in color was determined by more than one gene.

Many of the herditary malformations have this kind of inconsistent mode of inheritance.

Polydactyly (excess digits) of Simmental cattle develops as a polygenic disorder. *Porcine encephalocoele* follows a similar pattern (Fig. 30.3). Cleft palate, spina bifida, and pyloric stenosis occur in human populations with frequencies suggesting a multifactorial genetic disease.

Multiple defects transmitted together

Several independent abnormal traits may be transmitted together, presumably because of their close relationship on the chromosome. In the gray collie syndrome, a condition called cyclic hematopoiesis is transmitted as an autosomal recessive disease. Blood cells, chiefly neutrophils, disappear from the bloodstream in 11-day cycles, and the affected animal eventually succumbs to bacterial infection. Affected dogs also have traits for abnormal gray-silver coat color and microophthalmia, which are transmitted together with the blood disorder.

Table 30.3.   **Defective proteins as mutant gene products**

Defect	Example
Missing enzymes fail to catalyze metabolic pathways	
Accumulation of precursors due to enzyme block	Lipid storage disease
Deficiency of end products	Albinism
Accumulation of toxic by-products	Phenylketonuria[a]
Abnormal enzymes fail to catalyze membrane transport	
Sodium not absorbed in erythrocytes	Hereditary spherocytosis
Phosphate not absorbed in kidney	Hypophosphatemic rickets
Glucose not absorbed in kidney	Renal glycosuria
Cystine not absorbed in kidney	Cystinuria/renal lithiasis
Missing components of coagulation	
Factor VIII and IX deficiency	Hemophilia
Fibrinogen deficiency	Congenital afibrinogenemia
Failure to maintain structural proteins	
Collagen enzymes missing	Dermatosparaxis

    [a]Reported only in man.

Table 30.4. Aminoacidopathies

Amino Acid Detected	Primary Disorder	Secondarily Increased in
Alanine	. . .	Lactic aciduria Hyperammonemia
Arginine	Arginase deficiency	Ornithinemia
Carnosine	Carnosine deficiency	. . .
Cystine	Cystinosis (transport defect)	Renal disease
Glycine	Hyperglycinemia (nonketotic)	Ketosis
Ornithine	Ornithine-oxoacid aminotransferase deficiency	. . .
Phenylalanine	Phenylalanine hydroxlase deficiency (phenylketonu-ria) Dihydropteridine reductase deficiency (hyperphenyl-alaninemia)	High-protein diet in newborn
Phosphoethanolamine	Hypophosphatasia (alkaline phosphatase deficiency)	Bone disease
Proline	Hyperprolinemia	. . .

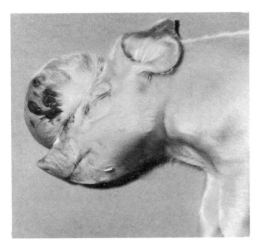

Fig. 30.3. Growth disturbance: encephalocoele in a newborn pig. A bony defect in the cranium allows the protrusion of the meninges and nervous tissue into a skin-covered sac. Dark areas in the skin are vascular malformations with stasis of blood.

Polygenic inheritance makes genetic analysis difficult.

Ocular dermoids are solid, skinlike masses in or on the eye. Typically, they occur as unilateral hairy growths adhered to the anterior surface of the globe, astride the ventrolateral limbus. They are especially common in some cattle breeds; it has been shown that in Hereford cattle, they are transmitted according to autosomal recessive and polygenic inheritance.

Genetic transmission is indicated by the following: (1) a high incidence in one geographic location without increased incidence in other breeds, (2) bilateral expression of the defect, (3) common ancestry of affected cattle, (4) occurrence in males more than females, (5) independence of season, and (6) inability to demonstrate teratogenic environmental patterns.

ADDITIONAL READING

Barkyoumb, S. D., and Leipold, H. W. Nature and cause of bilateral ocular dermoids in Hereford cattle. *Vet. Pathol.* 21:316, 1984.

Gustavsson, I. Banding techniques in chromosome analysis of domestic animals. *Adv. Vet. Sci.* 24:245, 1980.

Rousseaux, C. G. Developmental anomalies in farm animals. *Can. Vet. J.* 29:23, 1988.

Vonderfecht, S. L., et al. Congenital intestinal aganglionosis and white foals. *Vet. Pathol.* 20:65, 1983.

INDEX